THIRD EDITION

Undergraduate
Pharmacology

for Medical Students

THIRD EDITION

Undergraduate
Pharmacology

for Medical Students

K Mukhopadhyay MD FCGP PGCCHFWM

Professor and Head
Department of Pharmacology
College of Medicine and JNM Hospital
Kalyani, Nadia, West Bengal

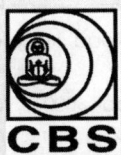

CBS

CBS Publishers & Distributors Pvt Ltd

New Delhi • Bengaluru • Chennai • Kochi • Kolkata • Mumbai

Bhopal •Bhubaneswar •Hyderabad •Jharkhand •Nagpur •Patna•Pune •Uttarakhand • Dhaka (Bangladesh)

Undergraduate
Pharmacology

ISBN: 978-93-87085-20-6

Copyright © Author and Publisher

Third Edition: 2018
 Reprint: 2019
First Edition: 2010
Second Edition: 2015

Published by Satish Kumar Jain and produced by Varun Jain for
CBS Publishers & Distributors Pvt Ltd
4819/XI Prahlad Street, 24 Ansari Road, Daryaganj, New Delhi–110 002, India.
Ph: 23289259, 23266861, 23266867   Website: www.cbspd.com
Fax: 011-23243014   e-mail: delhi@cbspd.com; cbspubs@airtelmail.in

Corporate Office: 204 FIE, Industrial Area, Patparganj, Delhi–110 092
Ph: 4934 4934   Fax: 4934 4935 e-mail: publishing@cbspd.com; publicity@cbspd.com

Branches

- **Bengaluru:** Seema House 2975, 17th Cross, K.R. Road, Banasankari 2nd Stage, Bengaluru-560 070, Karnataka, India
  Ph: +91-80-26771678/79   Fax: +91-80-26771680   e-mail: bangalore@cbspd.com
- **Chennai:** 7, Subbaraya Street, Shenoy Nagar, Chennai–600 030, Tamil Nadu, India
  Ph: +91-44-26680620, 26681266 Fax: +91-44-42032115   e-mail: chennai@cbspd.com
- **Kochi:** 42/1325, 1326, Power House Road, Opposite KSEB Power House, Ernakulam–682 018, Kochi, Kerala, India
  Ph: +91-484-4059061-65   Fax: +91-484-4059065   e-mail: kochi@cbspd.com
- **Kolkata:** 6/B, Ground Floor, Rameswar Shaw Road, Kolkata–700 014, West Bengal, India
  Ph: +91-33-22891126, 22891127, 22891128   e-mail: kolkata@cbspd.com
- **Mumbai:** 83-C, Dr E Moses Road, Worli, Mumbai–400018, Maharashtra, India.
  Ph: +91-22-24902340/41   Fax: +91-22-24902342   e-mail: mumbai@cbspd.com

Representatives

- **Bhopal**   0-8319310552   • **Bhubaneswar** 0-9911037372 • **Hyderabad** 0-9885175004   • **Jharkhand** 0-9811541605
- **Nagpur**   0-9021734563   • **Patna**   0-9334159340 • **Pune**   0-9623451994   • **Uttarakhand** 0-9716462459
- **Dhaka (Bangladesh)** 01912-003485

Printed at Glorious Printers, Delhi, India.

to

Late Satish Chandra Mukherjee

Late Dr Ram Nath Banerjee

Late Tulsi Das Mukherjee

Late Basudev Mukherjee

Preface to the Third Edition

Like any other branches of medical science, pharmacology is also developing tremendously in last couple of years. I have tried to incorporate all those I have heard in different seminars, and read in different books in this book so that it can be easily be grasped. Special emphasis has been given to must know area of the pharmacology for undergraduate medical students and for general practitioners.

My colleagues in my college Dr Chanchal Kumar Dalai, Dr Agnik Pal, Dr Abhishek Ghosh, Dr Kushal Banerjee and in other medical college Dr Abhijit Das, Professor Dipak Sarkar, Professor Dipankar Bhattacharjee. Professor RN Chatterjee (my teacher) all gave me important feedback to improve the book. I thank them all. My students too have given important feedback. My DNB student Dr Kishore Mazumdar also encouraged me and helped me proofreading.

I must thank Mr SK Jain, Mr YN Arjuna, Mr RN Mondal, Mr CD Bhattacharya, Mr Bandhu of CBS publishers for publishing the third edition of this book.

I thank Mrs Sabita Biswas for typing my manuscript.

K Mukhopadhyay

Preface to the First Edition

Like any other branch of medical sciences, pharmacology has also developed tremendously in the couple of years and therapeutic breakthrough in pharmacology is a frequent item nowadays. Knowledge of pharmacology is required for all clinical specialities or super-specialities for prevention, diagnosis and cure of disease. I bestow this book *Undergraduate Pharmacology* upon undergraduate medical students and general practitioners for quick review of the subject.

I am grateful to my undergraduate pharmacology teachers Professor MS Dey, Professor Robin Chatterjee, Professor BN Das, Professor RN Chowdhury, Professor S Banerjee; and my postgraduate teachers Professor (Late) AK Sanyal, Professor PK Das, Professor SS Gambhir, Professor SB Acharya, Professor SK Bhattacharya, Professor RK Goel and Professor BL Pandey; whose lectures were of immense help in preparing this book. My special thanks to Professor PK Mukherjee, MGM Medial College, Kishanganj; Professor AK Chakraborty; Professor SK Tripathy; Dr Anil Jaiswal; Dr NG Goswami and Dr D Bhattacharya for suggestions and encouragement. Professor JN Neogi, Professor KK Kundu, Professor KK Agarwal and Professor Ashim Dutta of CMS Nepal encouraged me to go about writing this book.

I am grateful to Dr (Mrs) Barnali Mukherjee and Dr (Mrs) Srabani Mukhopadhyay, my sisters-in-law; Dr (Mrs) Seba Mukhopadhyay, my wife; Dr Jhulan Mukhopadhyay; and Dr Angshuman Mukhopadhyay who were professional critics outside and loving family members in home.

I am thankful to Late Bina Mukherjee, Late Basudeb Mukherjee, Smt Kajoli Mukherjee, Smt Jayanti Sinha, Late GCP Sinha, Dr Tirthankar Deb, Dr BR Ghosh, Mr P Ghatak, Mr Baladeb Mukherjee, Mr S Chatterjee, Professor K Bhattacharya, Dr Mrityunjoy Halder, Dr Alok Kr Vishwakarma, Mr Alok Paul, Professor S Chattopadhyay, Professor A Ahmed and Dr Jyotirmay Biswas.

My cousins Smt Aditi Banerjee, Smt Lakshmi Chatterjee, Smt Arundhati Banerjee, Smt Nandini Pandit, Anuradha and Mrinal; all encouraged me with their unending enthusiasm.

My kisses and love to my son Sanak, nieces Esha, Adrija and Archisman, for their encouraging giggles and smiles.

I would acknowledge my mother Late Smt Baidbani Mukherjee who went through infinite patience and always stood by me.

I must thank Mr Satish Jain, Mr YN Arjuna and Late BR Sharma of CBS Publishers and Distributors who helped me to compile this book.

K Mukhopadhyay

Contents

Section 4:   Central Nervous System

Section 5:   Drugs Used in Anesthesia

Section 6:   Gastrointestinal System

Section 7:   Respiratory System

Section 8: Hemopoietic System

Section 9: Drugs Acting on Kidney, Water and Electrolyte Metabolism

Section 10: Cardiovascular System

Section 11: Drugs of Endocrinal Diseases

Section 12: Female Hormones and Drugs of Pregnancy and Lactation

Section 13: Antimicrobials and Chemotherapy

Section 14: Miscellaneous

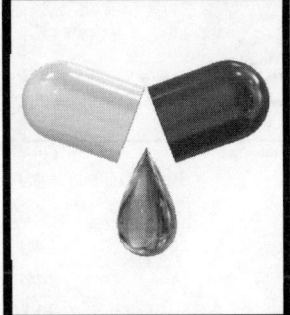 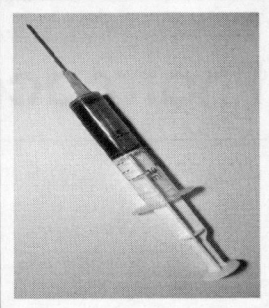 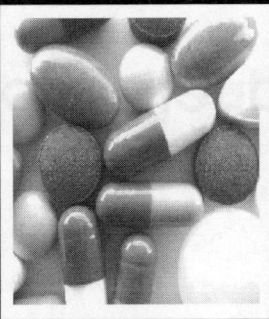 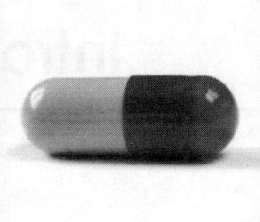

SECTION 1

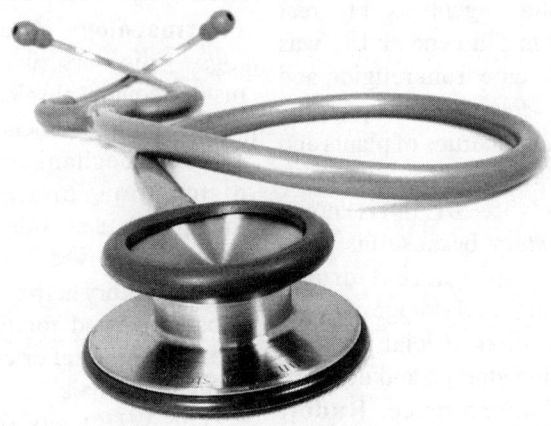

GENERAL PHARMACOLOGY

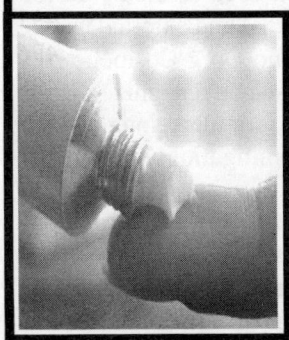 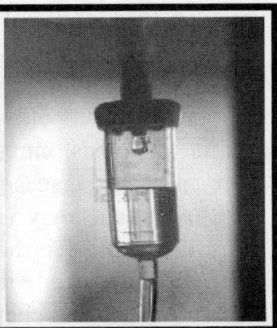 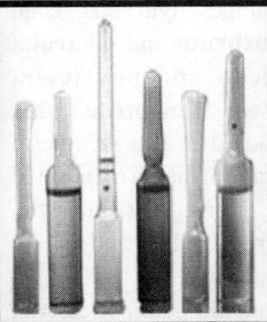 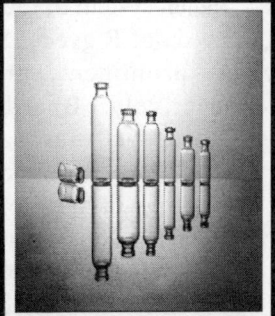

Introduction to Pharmacology

Man's endeavor to fight against diseases is as old as civilization. All civilizations had their own system of medicine. Primitive men used to believe that diseases were due to displeasure of supernatural agents and the priest was supposed to please those supernatural agents used to treat diseases. **Hippocrates** in 5th century BC was the first to separate medicine from religion and so he is called *Father of Medicine*. **Theophratus** (300 BC) identified different drugs of plants and animal origin so he is known as *Father of Pharmacognosy*. **Galen** (135–201 AD) is known as *Father of Polypharmacy* because his prescriptions contain multiple herbal drugs. Apotheray, *i.e.* procurement and storage of drugs was practised in Arab. First official pharmacopoeia, *i.e.* identification storage and doses of drugs was developed in Florence. **Rudolf Bucheim** (1846) first established experimental pharmacology. **Oswald Schmiedeberg** of Germany (1838–1921) was the first professor of pharmacology and is called *Father of modern Pharmacology*. **Paracelsus** (1493–1541) stated that wrong dose makes the poison.

Indian system of medicine "Ayurveda" is an Upaveda of Rigveda. **Sushruta** and **Charaka** were prominent surgeon and physician, respectively. Bhardwaj transmitted his knowledge to Atreya, and Atreya to Agnivesa. **Charaka** was contemporary of Galen mentioned 2000 drugs in his book. During Muslim rule, many ayurvedic literature was lost and Unani Tibb system came into limelight.

Britishers introduced an allopathic medicine in their period. First medical school in India was established in Kolkata and the first pharmacopoeia is Bengal Pharmacopoeia. Dr Ram Nath Chopra is the *Father of Indian Pharmacology*.

SOME DEFINITIONS

Pharmacology (Greek: *Pharmacon*—drugs; *logos*—discourse in) covers the knowledge of history, source, physical and chemical properties, compounding, biochemical and physiological effects, mechanism of action, absorption, distribution, biotransformation, exertion, therapeutic uses, side effects of a drug.

Drug (Derived from the French word *Drogue Vate* means dry herb): It is defined as the chemical substance used for the purpose of diagnosis, prevention, relief or cure of a disease in human being or animals.

The WHO has defined drug—"As any chemical substance or product that is used or intended to be used to modify or explore physiological system or pathological state for the benefit of the recipient".

According to Webster dictionary—"Drug is a substance or preparation used as medicine for treating diseases by internal and external use".

According to Food and Drug Cosmetic Act (1938)—"Drug is a substance recognized in an official pharmacopeia or formulary, intended for use in diagnosis, cure, mitigations, treatment, prevention of a disease".

Pharmacognosy (Pharma + Cognosy = Identification): It is the science dealing with the source, cultivation, identification, botanical characteristics and chemical constituents of the drug of vegetable and animal origin.

Pharmacy: It is the science and art of preparing and compounding drugs for the administration to patient. It also embraces the identification, selection, preservation, combination, analysis and standardization of drugs.

Pharmacist: Authorized and qualified person to practice pharmacy.

Pharmaceutics: Science and art of dealing with manufacture of drug.

Pharmaceutist: Skilled person in pharmaceutics.

Legal pharmacy: It covers legal laws controlling trade and profession of pharmacy.

Therapeutics: The branch of medicine concerned with cure of disease or relief symptoms including drug treatment.

Toxicology: It is the study of measurement, detection and treatment of poisons.

Materia Medica (Materials for medicine): It is an out of use terminology due to tremendous advancement of pharmacology, concerned with source, description and preparation of drugs.

Pharmacopoeia (Pharmacon—drug; poieen—to make): It is a book published by recognized authority of any country containing a list of accepted drugs and formulae for medical preparation with their average doses and description of their characteristic tests for their identity, purity and potency, viz. IP, BP, USP.

Social Pharmacology: It is the study of the use of drugs in relation to the social and cultural milieu. It is predominantly concerned with drug used for non-medical purposes illegally.

Pharmacodynamics: Effects of drugs on the body, i.e. complete action effect sequences, dose response curve and modification of drug action by other drugs.

Pharmacokinetics: Effects of body on drugs, i.e. absorption, distributions metabolism and excretion of a drug.

Prescription: It is written in order for one or more medical agents along with direction to their pharmacist for the preparation and to the patient for the use of the medicine at a particular time. (Parts of prescription are shown in Table 1.1.)

E-Prescription: It has started in some developed countries like USA which provides electronic flow of information from prescriber pharmacy, health plan (like medical history, formulary cost benefit, etc.) direction for uses etc. Pharmacist if thinks appropriate supplies prescription. Its benefits are prescribers gets information like drug interaction, cost of the drug, etc. It is clear, renewal of prescription if required can be done. Time to process prescription supply is less. Only registered medical practitioner with identification proof with unique PIN number biometrics of retinal scan and fingerprint can prescribe. It will prevent diversion of drug.

Pull down drug list can create errors.

Table 1.1: Parts of a Prescription		
1. Name of patient	: Mr/Mrs	
2. Superscription	: R_x (Take thou or Astronomical sign for Jove or Jupiter, God of healing)	
3. Inscription	: • **Base** (Ephedrine sulfate, 0.4 gm)	→ Chief active ingredient
	• **Adjuvant** (Potassium iodide, 15 gm)	→ Which assists the base
	• **Corrective** (Potassium bromide, 20 gm)	→ (Decreases undesirable effects of the base)
	• **Vehicle** (Syr. Glycyrrhiza 200 mL)	→ (Add to dilute the preparation to a reasonable dose)
4. **Subscription** (Mft. Mist.)	: Mix and make mixture.	Direction to pharmacist for compouding ingredient.
5. **Sigma** (Signature)	: (1 teaspoon with a glass of water, thrice daily)	Direction to patient including method of administration, dose and time of administration.
6. **Physician signature** and date, address, registration number. The prescriptions in this form are rarely written because of proprietary medicine.		

In USA Drug enforcement administration framing rules for it. There should be business association between pharmacy and insurance plan.

Source of Drugs

The different sources of drugs are:

1. Minerals   : Iron
2. Animals   : Insulin, thyroid extract
3. Synthetic   : Aspirin
4. Microbial   : Antibiotics
5. Plants   : Oil, glycosides, alkaloid, *etc.*
6. Within the   : Hormones, vitamin D
   body
7. Genetic   : By recombinant DNA
   engineering   technology, *viz.* human
                     insulin
8. Hybridoma   : *viz.* monoclonal antibodies.

The drugs which are not synthesized within the body are called **Xenobiotics** (Greek: *Xeno* = Stranger).

Poisons are drugs with harmful effects. According to Paracelsus, dose makes the poison,

Table 1.2: Liquid Dosage Forms

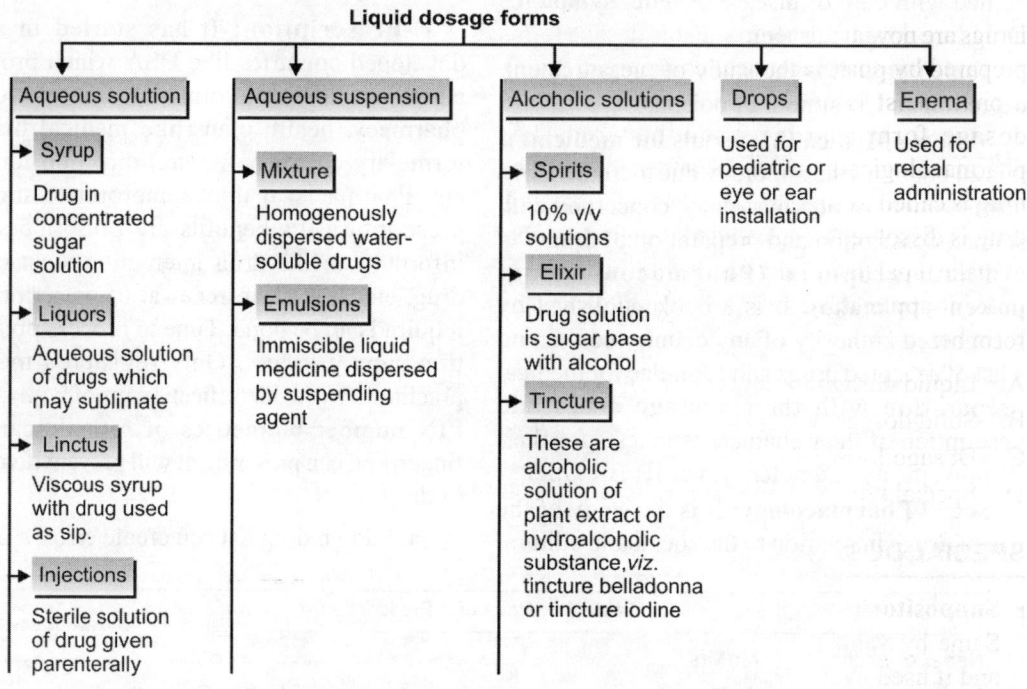

Table 1.3: Solid Dosage Forms

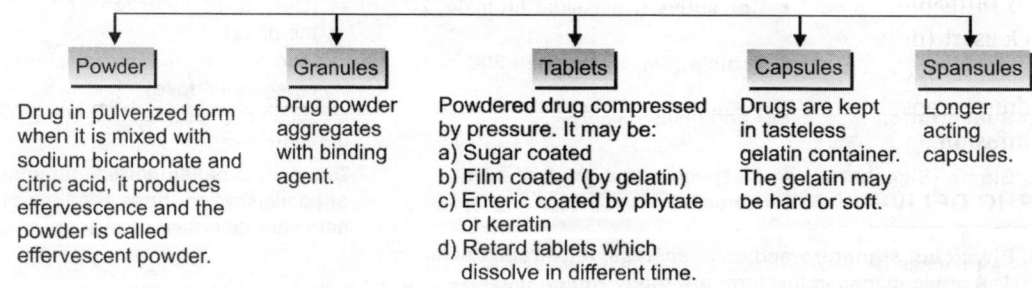

Table 1.4: Dosage foms for external use

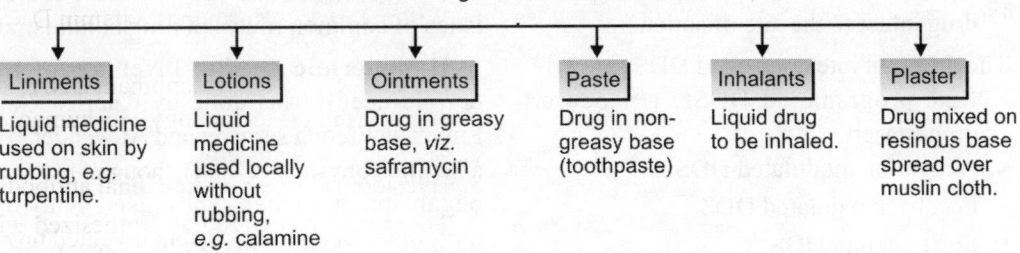

Liniments	Lotions	Ointments	Paste	Inhalants	Plaster
Liquid medicine used on skin by rubbing, *e.g.* turpentine.	Liquid medicine used locally without rubbing, *e.g.* calamine lotion.	Drug in greasy base, *viz.* saframycin	Drug in non-greasy base (toothpaste)	Liquid drug to be inhaled.	Drug mixed on resinous base spread over muslin cloth.

i.e. all drugs are poison on overdose. **Toxins** are poisons of biological origin.

DOSAGE FORMS

Drugs are now available in suitable dosage forms prepared by pharmaceutical companies. Rarely a pharmacist is called upon to prepare it. In dosage form a drug is administered. The pharmacologically inert substances added to the drug is called excipient. The substance in which drug is dissolved or suspended is called vehicle to make it palatable, *viz.* syrup, gum acacia or to make it applicable as in ointment. The dosage form be:

A. Liquid dosage form (Table 1.2)
B. Solid dosage form (Table 1.3)
C. Dosage form for external use (Table 1.4)
D. Special type of dosage form

SPECIAL DOSAGE FORMS

- **Suppositories** are dosage forms for rectal use. Same by vaginal applications are **pessaries,** and if used by urethra is called **Bougies**.
- In transdermal adhesive patch drug is incorporated in polymer and delivered into skin by diffusion.
- Ocusert (drug in a reservoir slowly released used in eye). Amphotericin B is available as drug encapsulated in liposomes for intravenous infusion.

DRUG DELIVERY SYSTEM (DDS)

It is a process of administering pharmaceutical compounds used to achieve therapeutic effects in human or animals by modifying in a drug release profile, absorption, distribution and finally to improve efficacy, safety and patient's compliance.

Problems with existing DDS are
- Reduce potency because of degradation.
- Toxic levels of administration which increases the cost because of excess dosing (Fig. 1.1).
- Compliance issues.

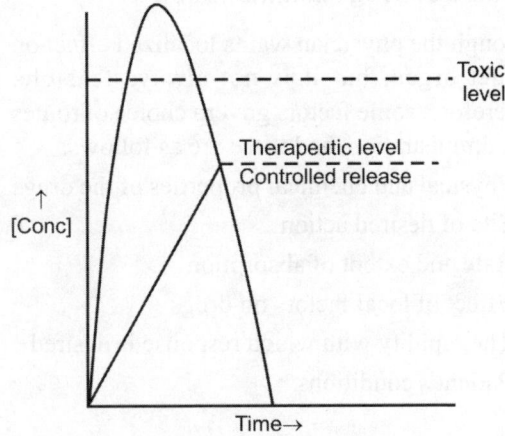

Fig. 1.1

Modern DDS's goals are:
- To deploy target site, and to limit side effects.
- Introduced in body through specific areas to avoid degradation.
- It should maintain therapeutic drug level for prolong period with predictable controlled release rate and decreases the dose frequency.
- It should be easy to administer.

- It should be stable and should transport the drug intact to the site of action.

The different rate controlled DDSs are:
- Rate programmed DDSs, *viz.* ocusert, progestasert.
- Activation modulated DDS
- Feedback regulated DDS
- Site targeting DDS

The vehicle which is used for DDS should be nontoxic, biocompatible, nonimmunogenic, and should not be cleared by reticuloendothelial cells.

The future trend of drug delivery system goes towards liposome encapsulation, antibody tagging and permeability enhancer to reduce systemic side effects and for its target action. With advancement of molecular biology, efforts are made to replace defective genes, receptors, enzymes and carrier responsible for the disease which will give more permanent solution.

Routes of Drug Administration

Though the physician wants localized effect on target organ, but it is not always feasible. Therefore, some factors govern choice of routes of administration, and these are as follows:
- Physical and chemical properties of the drugs
- Site of desired action
- Rate and extent of absorption
- Effect of local factors on drugs
- The rapidity with which response is desired
- Patient's conditions.

Flowcharts 1.1 and 1.2 give some characteristics of common routes of drug administration.

Hypodermic needle: Invention of hypodermic needle was done by Charles Gabriel Pravez, a French surgeon and Alexender Wood, a Scottish physician (1884), though the injection began much earlier. They used it to inject morphine. Benjamin A Rubin invented pronged vaccinating and testing needle. Arthr E Smith received patent for disposable syringe and needle made up of glass. Becton Dicknison and Co. first produced disposable syringe with needle for mass administration of salk polio vaccine.

Syringe and hypodermic needle (Fig. 1.2): These are used to introduce drugs into the body or to withdraw some fluids from the body. Syringe and needle both have three parts. The needle's one portion is bevelled, the next to bevelled portion is shaft followed by hub which is fitted to nozzle of the syringe. Fluid or drugs are drawn in barrel and pushed into the body or withdrawn from the body by plunger or piston. The barrel is graded. The hypodermic needle is hollow whereas suturing needles are solid.

Ampoules and vials: Ampoules are made up of glass generally contain liquid drugs. Vials are also glass made container with rubber cap containing multiple doses of drug or drug which has to be dissolved with solvent.

Different Routes of Drug Administrations
(Table 1.1) (Fig. 1.3 to 1.7)

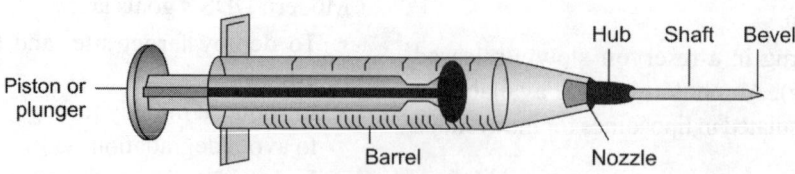

Fig. 1.2: Syringe with hypodermic needle

Flowchart 1.1: Routes of drug administration (Figs 1.2 to 1.7)

Routes

Local | Systemic | Special

Topical | Deeper tissues | Arterial supply

— Oral
— Rectal
— Sublingual
— Cutaneous (transdermal therapeutic system, TTS)
— Inhalation
— Nasal

(a) Iontophoresis — by galvanic current drug is penetrated into deeper tissues.
(b) Inunction — certain drugs are rubbed to penetrate into deeper tissues.

— Mouth and pharynx
— Eyes, ears, nose
— GIT
— Bronchi, lung
— Urethra
— Anal canal
— Vagina

Parenteral (Par — beyond, enteral — intestine)

— Subcutaneous
— Intradermal
— Intramuscular
— Intravenous
— Intramedullary
— Intraperitoneal
— Intrathecal
— Intracardiac

— Dermojet (for mass inoculation)
— Pellet implantation
— Sialistic implant (contraceptives)

Flowchart 1.2: Some characteristics of common routes of drug administration

Routes

	Intravenous	Subcutaneous	Intramuscular	Oral
Absorption	• 100% • Immediate effect	• Prompt • Slow for sustained form • Repository preparation	• Prompt for aqueous solution	• Variable
Special Utility	• Emergency • Permits titration of doses • Suitable for large volume and irritating substance	• Suitable for insoluble and for solid pellets	• Suitable for moderate volume, oily vehicles, irritating substances	• Most convenient • Economical • Safe
Limitations	• Increased risk of adverse effects • Not suitable for insoluble sub-stances	• Not suitable for large volume	• May interfere with interpretation of some diagnostic tests, *viz*. CPK may be increased.	• Requires patients cooperation • Availability variable; depends on hepatic metabolism.

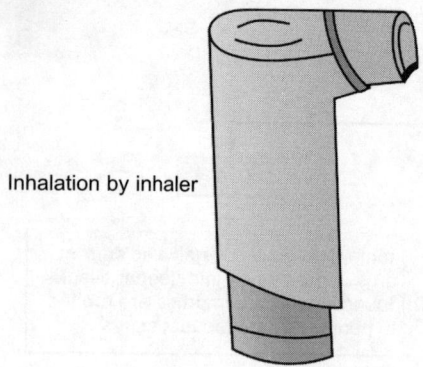

Inhalation by inhaler

Fig. 1.3

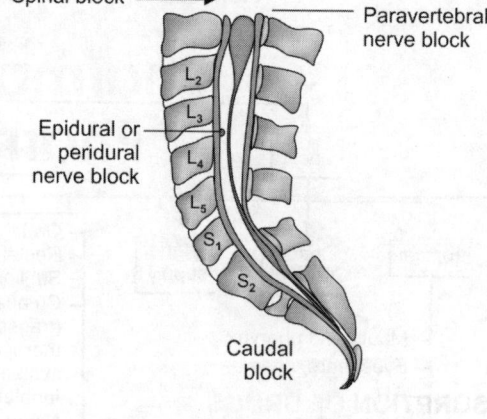

Spinal block

Paravertebral nerve block

Epidural or peridural nerve block

L_2
L_3
L_4
L_5
S_1
S_2

Caudal block

Fig. 1.6

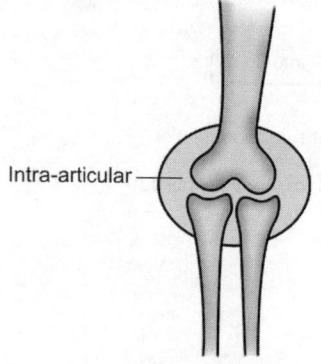

Intra-articular

Fig. 1.4

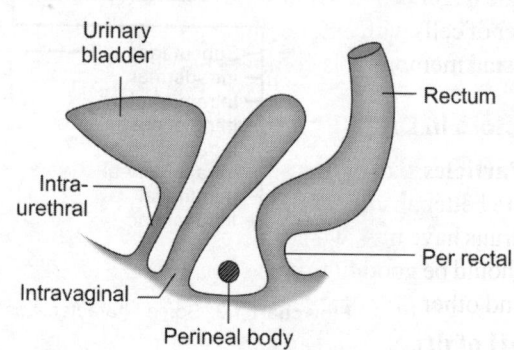

Urinary bladder

Rectum

Intra-urethral

Per rectal

Intravaginal

Perineal body

Fig. 1.7

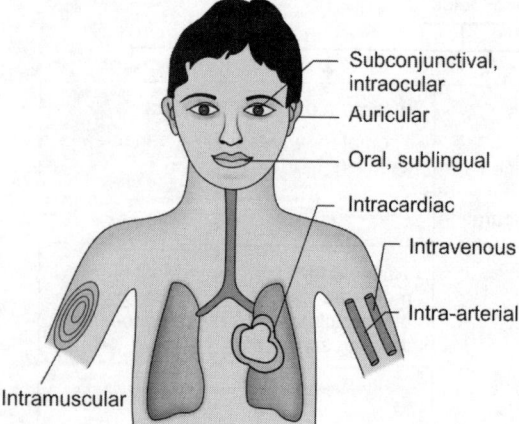

Subconjunctival, intraocular

Auricular

Oral, sublingual

Intracardiac

Intravenous

Intra-arterial

Intramuscular

Fig. 1.5

Figs 1.3 to 1.7: Different routes of drug administration

Pharmacokinetics and Pharmacodynamics

ABSORPTION OF DRUGS

The absorption of drugs are influenced by the following factors. The absorption may be through single larger cell as in intestine or through several layer of cells with extra-cellular protein like skin. Plasma membrane is common barriers.

Factors in Drug (Pharmaceutical factors)

- **Particles size of drug:** Smaller, fine particles are better absorbed, *e.g.* griseofulvin FP. Most drugs have mol. wt. between 100–1000. Drugs should be good fit for receptor in shape, charge and other proportions.
- **pH of drug:** Acidic drugs absorbed in acidic medium.
- **Disintegration and dissolution time**: Liquid drugs are better absorbed.
- **Adjuvant used in drugs influences the drug absorption.**
- **Concentration of the drugs:** Passive diffusion of the drug depends upon drug concentration.
- **Routes of drug absorption:** In case of IV drip drug is 100% absorbed.

Factors in Patients (Pharmacological factors)

- **pH of GI tracts:** Most of the drugs are weak electrolytes, so pH of the GI tract influences its ionization.
- **Ionization:** Ionized drug particles are less absorbed. Acidic drugs are less ionized in acidic medium and basic drugs are less ionized in basic medium. Electrostatic charge

of ionized molecule attracts water dipole to make it polar, water-soluble and lipid-insoluble. Since lipid diffusion depends on high lipid solubility, the drugs reduce their ability to permeate the membrane. Ionization of weak acid can be given by the formula

$$pH = pK_a + \log \frac{[H^-]}{[HA]}$$

$$\text{or } pH = pK_a + \log \frac{[\text{Protonated form}]}{[\text{Unprotonated}]}$$

where pK_a= Negative log of dissociation constant of weak electrolyte. [A] is an ionized drug and [HA] is non-ionized drug concentration. When $pH = pK_a$ then 50% of the drug is ionized. Acidic drug will accumulate on basic side of the membrane and basic drug will accumulate on acid side and the phenomenon is called **ion trapping**.

- **Motility of GI tracts:** GI hurry decreases absorption as in diarrhea.
- **Presence of other agents,** *e.g.* vitamin C enhances absorption of iron.
- **Enterohepatic circulation:** Increases bioavailability.
- **Area of absorbing surface:** Greater the area, more drugs are absorbed.
- **Metabolism of drug:** Drugs absorbed through gut wall may not be effective due to first pass metabolism.
- **Pharmacogenetic factors.**
- **Diseases states:** Like cirrhosis of liver, thyrotoxicosis, *etc.* may interfere with drug absorption.

Different Methods of Drug Absorption

1. **Simple diffusion or aqueous diffusion:** Rate of transfer across biological membrane is proportional to concentration gradient, *i.e.* according to Fick's law of diffusion and the process is not energy dependent.

   Fick's law

   Flux molecule per unit time =

   $$\frac{(C_1 - C_2) \times \text{Area} \times \text{Permeability coefficient}}{\text{Thickness}}$$

   Lipid aqueous partition coefficient determines how quickly drug moves between lipid and aqueous media; which is again dependent on pH.

2. **Lipid diffusion:** Aqueous partition coefficient determines how quickly drug moves between aqueous and lipid media.

3. **Active transport:** Energy dependent process of trans-biological membrane of transport, not proportional to concentration gradient. It may be carrier dependent, which acts as a ferry. It may be:

   (a) Primary active transport

   (b) Secondary active transport.

   (a) Primary active transport: Directly couples with ATP hydrolysis, *e.g.* Adenosine triphosphate **B**inding **C**assettes transporter (ABC transporter).

   (b) Secondary active transport: Here solute (S_1) is driven against concentration gradient energetically by transport of another solute (S_2) in accordance to its concentration gradient. If S_2 and S_1

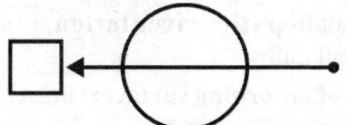

Fig. 2.1: Uniport

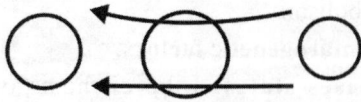

Fig. 2.2: Symport

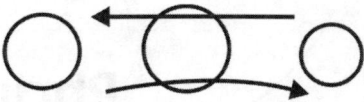

Fig. 2.3: Antiport

transporters are in the same direction it is *co-transporter or symporter* (Figs 2.1 to 2.3).

Antiport or exchanger moves their substrates in opposite directions.

4. **Pinocytosis or endocytosis:** Macromolecules are taken from surroundings into intracellular organism. They are engulfed by cell membranes forming vesicles. The reverse of endocytosis is **exocytosis** by which many neurotransmitters are released.

The knowledge of rate of absorption of drug is necessary to determine:

- Frequency of drug administration
- Duration of action of drug
- Predict onset of desired effect and side effects.

5. **Special carriers:** ABC, *i.e.* adenosine triphosphate binding cassette family contains multidrug resistance type 1 (MDR 1) transporter found in brain, testes and drug resistant neoplastic cells or MRP 1 (multidrug resistance associated protein). Transporters are important for excretion of some drugs or their metabolites into the urine.

Bioavailability of Drugs

The bioavailability of a drug (biologically active drug) is defined as the amount or percentage of drug that is absorbed from a given dosage form and reaches the systemic circulation following nonvascular administration. In case of intravenous administration, bioavailability is 100%. Bioavailability may be less than 100% in case of oral absorption due to:

 (i) Incomplete absorption or

 (ii) Rapid first pass absorption.

Thus drugs of different manufacturers or batch may be biologically inequivalent.

It can be calculated by comparing AUC (Area under plasma level time curve). It tells about extent of drug absorptions.

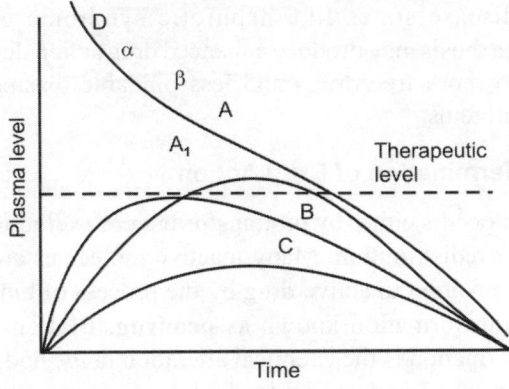

Fig. 2.4

Thus bioavailability (F) is determined by comparing AUC of oral and AUC of IV administration of the same drug.

$$\therefore F = \frac{\text{AUC after oral administration}}{\text{AUC after IV administration}} \times 100$$

In the graph (Fig. 2.4), drug A_1 is slowly absorbed, but reaches above therapeutic level than C. So drug A_1 is effective not B and C, though B is quickly absorbed.

In case of intravenous administration as depicted by D, there are two distributions of drug that determine the plasma concentration, first one is called α by its rapid dilution and second one is called β which is determined by different factors, viz. sequestration, elimination, etc.

Distribution of Drugs

After a drug is absorbed or injected into the bloodstream, it may be distributed into interstitial and cellular fluids, which is governed by affinities, it has various constituents of the tissues including aqueous solubility, lipid solubility, ionization at physiological pH, binding to extracellular substances and intracellular uptake.

A large molecular weight cannot move out of endothelial slits, so trapped in plasma which is 4 L in 70 kg individual; low molecular hydrophobic drug can move out of endothelial slits into interstitial space about 20%, i.e. 14 L of 70 kg individual. Low molecular weight hydrophobic can also move into cells distributed in 60% of body weight, i.e. 42 L in 70 kg individual.

Apparent Volume of Distribution (V_d)

Considering body as a single homogeneous compartment (V) in which drug gets uniformly and immediately distributed. Thus M is the total amount of drugs in the body, and C is the concentration in plasma, then the apparent volume of distribution is $V_d = M/C$. In some cases, the volume of distribution of a drug corresponds to an anatomy of physiological compartments. Drugs sequestered into other tissues may have apparent volume of distribution (V_d) much more than total body water and are not easily removed by hemodialysis.

The factors governing apparent volume of distribution are:
- Lipid water coefficient of the drug
- pK_a value of the drug
- Degree of plasma protein binding
- Affinity of drug for different tissues
- Diseases like CCF, uremia, cirrhosis, etc.

Sequestration of Drugs

Some drugs administrated may be sequestered by some tissues, viz.

(a) In blood cells:
  - Erythrocytes—chlorthalidone is sequestered by erythrocytes.
  - Platelets—srotonin is taken up by platelets
  - Leukocytes—mepacrine.

(b) Sequestration by tissue constituents:
  - Keratin : Arsenic, mercury, griseofulvin
  - Melanin : Chloroquine, chlorpromazine
  - Nucleic acid : Mepacrine
  - Collagen : Sulfasalazine

(c) Adipose tissues: Thiopentone, ether, DDT
(d) Bone: Tetracycline, lead, radium
(e) Hematopoietic tissue: Phosphate
(f) Pancreas: Selenium analogue of L-methionine is taken up by pancreas. Radioscans

after administration of 75Se-selenomethionine reveals morphological abnormalities and lesions of pancreas.

(g) Parathyroid: Selenomethionine, phenothiazine dye.

(h) Thyroid: Iodide.

Blood–brain Barrier

In 1885, Ehrlich showed that trypan blue injected into bloodstream of animals stained all tissues of body with the exception of most of CNS and CSF. The mechanism is generally referred as blood-brain barrier. The barrier is not absolute and represents quantitative rather than qualitative difference from other tissues in capillary permeability. The tight endothelial cells of the capillaries and astrocytes approximate of capillaries constitute the blood–brain barrier. The enzyme monoamine oxidase (MAO), cholinesterase and some other enzymes present in capillary walls do not allow catecholamine and acetyl choline to penetrate into the brain and act as enzymatic blood–brain barrier. The blood–brain barrier is deficient in CTZ, medulla oblongata and certain paraventricular sites. The CSF brain barrier is composed of epithetial cells lining the ventricles. There is no occluding zonulae.

Placental Barrier

Placenta is hemochorial, discoidal, fetoplacental membrane, allows lipophilic drug. Certain amount of nonlipid soluble drugs when present in high concentration for long periods in the material circulation gain access to the fetus. Therefore, it is an incomplete barrier.

Plasma Proteins

The acidic drugs generally bind to plasma albumins and basic drugs to glycoproteins. Binding of a drug to plasma proteins limits its concentration in tissues and its locus of action. It also limits its glomerular filtration. Thus plasma proteins act as nonspecific receptors for drugs. Any other drug replacing its attachments with plasma proteins may interfere with its action leading to drug interaction. In the same way, disease states like nephrotic syndrome or cirrhosis may produce enhanced drug action due to more free drugs and less bindable plasma proteins.

Termination of Drug Action

It occurs either by biotransformation, excretion or redistribution. Many inactive molecules are converted to active drug by the process of biotransformation known as **prodrug**. Biotransformation is the chemical alteration in the body where nonpolars (lipid-soluble) are converted to polars (lipid-insoluble) so that they are not absorbed. Liver is the main site for detoxification of drugs, other sites are kidney, intestine, lungs and plasma nasal mucosa. The biotransformation of xenobiotics detoxification may be: (1) Nonsynthetic (phase I reaction) or (2) synthetic conjugation (phase II reaction).

Nonsynthetic (Phase I) Reaction

Phase I reaction converts the main drug more polar by introducing or unmasking functional groups so that they are readily excreted and some phase I products undergo phase II reaction with endogenous substances (*viz.* glucuronic acid, sulfuric acid, *etc.*) before their excretion. Some examples of phase I nonsynthetic reactions are:

- Oxidation
  - Barbiturate
  - Phenothiazine
  - Steroids
- Reduction
  - Chloral hydrate
  - Halothane
  - Chloramphenicol
- Hydrolysis
  - Choline esters
  - Pethidine
- Cyclization
  - Proguanil
- Decyclization
  - Phenytoin
  - Barbiturates

DRUG METABOLISM

Foreign substances to the body called xenobiotics (*viz.* pollutants, food additives, cosmetics, chemicals used in agriculture, *etc.*) are metabolized by same enzymatic pathways as that utilized by dietary constituents.

Xenobiotic undergoes phase I reaction of oxidation, reduction, hydrolytic reaction and phase II reaction of conjugation in which product of phase I reaction conjugates with either sulfate, glucuronic acid, glutathione, methyl or acetyl group. The purpose of phase I reaction to decrease the biological activity of the drug or to make it biologically active (*viz.* prodrug) and phase II reactions facilitate easy elimination by improving water solubility. The xenobiotics metabolizing enzymes are present in GI tract (liver, small intestine, colon, *etc.*) other organs like nasal mucosa, lung, *etc.*

Phase I oxidation is catalyzed by CYP, flavin-containing monoxygenase (FMO); epoxide hydrolases (EH). CYP and FMO are super-families with multiple genes, CYPs are heme protein oxidizes the substrate and the electrons are supplied by NADPH-Cytochrome P450 oxidoreductase. CYPs carry the N-dealkylation, O-dealkylation, hydroxylation, oxidation, deamination and dehalogenation reaction aromatic hydroxylation.

There are 57 functional CYP genes and 58 pseudo-genes in humans. CYPs are inducible and it can be inhibited too. It engages itself to drug and food interaction.

There are six families of FMO.

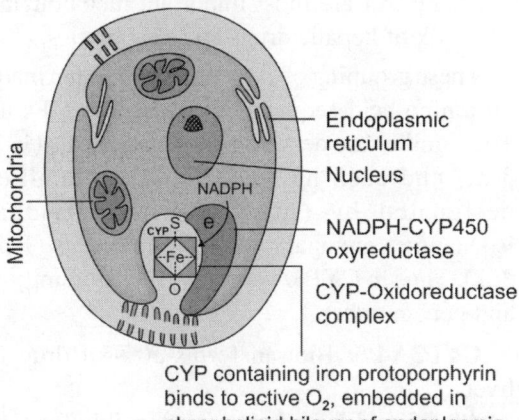

CYP containing iron protoporphyrin binds to active O_2, embedded in phospholipid bilayer of endoplasmic reticulum

Fig. 2.5: Location of CYP in the cell

FLAVIN-CONTAINING MONOOXYGENASE (FMO)

There are six families of FMO, involved in phase I reaction, with high levels in liver cell endoplasmic reticulum. It is neither inducable or inhibitable and not engaged in drug or food interaction. FMOs metabolises nicotine, cimetidine, clozapime Itopride etc. Since it is not inducible and inhibitible it is not involved in drug interaction.

HYDROLYTIC ENZYMES—EPOXIDE HYDROXYLASE (EH)

These are produced by CYP found in soluble form (sEH) and microsomal form (mEH) present in endoplasmic reticulum. It deactivates toxic derivatives of CYP metabolism, *e.g.* carbamazepine is metabolized to carbamazepine 10, 11 epoxide, is further metabolized to inactive form by mEH to dihydrodiol (inactive form). Carboxylesterase superfamily hydrolyzes ester and amide compounds. It is found in cytosol and endoplasmic reticulum. It is engaged in detoxification, activation of drugs, toxins and carcinogens.

PHASE II REACTION

Most of them are carried out in cytosol except glucuronidation which occurs in luminal side of endoplasmic reticulum. The characteristic features of glucuronidation is the participation of UDP-glucuronic.

A. GLUCURONIDATION

Nineteen genes encode UGT protein, out of which 9 are encoded by UGT_1 locus on chromosome 2 and 10 are encoded by UGT_2 gene in chromosome 4. UGT_2 acts more specifically on endogenous substance steroid. Some drugs are glucuronidated and excreted in bile and reenter circulation called **enterohepatic circulation**.

B. SULFATION

Sulfotransferase (SLUT) present in the cytosol- 13 isoforms SULTs are identified.

SULT1B1 present in skin and brain—carries sulfation of cholesterol and thyroid hormone. SULT1A3 is selective for catecholamine; oestrogen by SULT1E1; dihydroepiandrosterone is sulfated by SULT2A1. SULT1C2 and SULT1C4 are present in fetal tissue which declines with adulthood.

C. GLUTATHIONE CONJUGATION

Glutathione S. transferase catalyzes transfer of glutathione and protects cellular macromolecules to interact with electrophillic atoms O, N and S.

D. N-ACETYLATION

N-acetyltransferase (NAT) present in cytosol, metabolizes aromatic amine; environmental agents. NAT is polymorphic amongst all xenobiotic drug metabolizing enzymes, NAT_1 and NAT_2 are functional genes. Slow acetylator is attributed by NAT_2 polymorphism.

E. METHYLATION

Methyl transferases (MTs) are responsible for methylation. Catechol-orthomethyltransferase (COMT); phenylethanolamine N-methyl-transferase (PNMT) and thiopurine S-methyl-transferase (TPMT) are N-methyltransferases known in human.

Some Examples of Synthetic (Phase II) Reaction

Glucuronide conjugation: Aspirin, phenacetin and morphine undergo glucuronide conjugation, drug glucuronide is excreted by bile, may be hydrolyzed by intestinal bacteria. Liberated drug may be reabsorbed and may prolong drug action.

Acetylation: Sulfonamide and PAS. Multiple gene control the action of N-acetyl transferase, (NAT), slow and fast acetylator determine rate of acetylation.

Methylation: Adrenaline, histamine, nicotinamide. Methionine and cysteine act as methyl donor.

Glutathione conjugation: It inactivates highly reactive quinone formed during metabolism of certain drugs, viz. paracetamol poisoning.

Glycine conjugation: Drugs with carboxylic groups like salicylates, nicotinic acid conjugate with glycine is a minor pathway for metabolism.

Nucleotide synthesis: Important for activation of purine and pyrimidine antimetabolites used in cancer chemotherapy.

Enzymes

Drug metabolizing enzymes are located in the lipophilic endoplasmic reticulum of liver and other tissues. When they are fractionized and homogenized from cell they reform vesicles called microsomes. Some important enzymes present in microsome and non-microsome fractions are:

(a) **Microsomal:** Present in smooth endoplasmic reticulum, viz. monooxygenase, cytochromes P450.

(b) **Non-microsomal:** Present in cytoplasm, mitochondria of liver cells, viz. flavoprotein oxidase, esterase, etc.

In the oxidation–reduction process, two microsomal enzymes play a key role.

(a) NADPH—Cytochrome P450 reductase, and

(b) Cytochrome P450 which is a heme protein, serving as terminal oxidase. By immuno-blotting analysis several P450 isoforms are identified of which CYP1A2, CYP2A6, CYP2C19, CYP2D6, CYP2E1, and CYP3A4 are most important metabolizing bulk of hepatic drugs and xenobiotics.

These grouping of cytochrome P450 are made on amino acid sequence of cytochrome P450. The families are designated by numericals (1, 2, 3,...) and each having several subfamilies designated by (A, B, C,...). Individual isoenzymes are again allotted numericals (1, 2, 3,...). Thus in CYP3A4 family is 3; subfamily A and gene number 4.

CYP3A4/5: Biotransforms 50% of drug in liver.

Also found in intestine (responsible for first pass effect), kidney. Inhibited by erythromycin, ketoconazole, clarithromycin, etc. Induced by rifampicin, barbiturates, etc.

This inhibition and induction of CYP iso-enzymes responsible for many drug interactions.

CYP2D6: Metabolizes 20% of drug including neuroleptics, selective serotonin uptake inhibitors, beta blockers, opiates, *etc*. It is inhibited by quinidine so conversion of codeine to morphine is blocked.

CYP2C8/9: Metabolizes phenytoin; warfarin (low safety drugs) and ibuprofen; tolbutamide.

CYP2C19: Omeprazole; lansoprazole, *etc*. are metabolized by it. Induced by rifampicin; carbamazepine.

CYP1A1/2: Metabolizes theophylline; activates procarcinogens. Induced by rifampicin; cigarette smoke; polycyclic hydrocarbons.

CYP2E1: Metabolizes alcohol, paracetamol; chronic alcoholism induces it.

Hofmann Elimination

Inactivation of drug in the body fluids by spontaneous molecular rearrangement without any enzymes, *e.g.* atracurium.

Enzyme Induction and its Consequences

Many drugs, insecticides, carcinogens increase the synthesis of microsomal enzyme proteins, as a result rate of metabolism of drug is increased resulting in:

- Decrease intensity and duration of action
- Tolerance
- Interferes with dose adjustments
- Toxicity

Enzyme Induction

Xenobiotics can induce the expression of genes which encode drug metabolizing enzymes and may their own metabolism with losing their efficacy, *viz.* omeprazole, a proton pump inhibitor and a ligand for AHR induce **A**ryl **H**ydrocarbon **R**eceptor (AHR) and can induce and CYP1A1 and CYP1A2 activating toxins and carcinogens. In the same way phenobarbitone induces **C**onstitutive **A**ndrostane **R**eceptor (CAR) and Rifampicin and dexamethasone induces **P**regnane **X** **R**eceptor (PXR). Fibrates induce

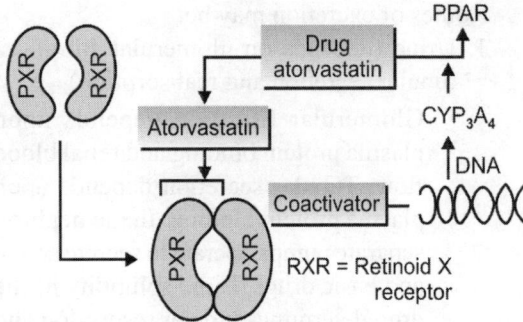

Fig. 2.6

Peroxisome **P**roliferator **A**ctivated **R**eceptor (PPAR).

Drug atorvastatin entering the cell to bind with nuclear pregnane X receptor (PXR). PXR forms complex with retinoid X receptor (RXR) which binds to DNA of target genes and recruits coactivator for transcription which targets CYP3A4 which metabolizes atorvastatin, therefore, its own metabolism is induced.

Members of PPAR family:

(i) PPAR α— targets gemfibrozil and feno-fibrate

(ii) PPAR γ — modulates genes involved in lipid and glucose metabolism

First Pass Presystemic Metabolism

The drug is metabolized during absorption in the GI tract wall by CYP3A4 enzyme system or liver, before reaching systemic circulation and is an important determinant factor for bioavailability. Liver may also excrete drugs into bile which may also alter bioavailability. Lower gut harboring microorganism may biotransform the drug, affecting their bioavailability. Gastric juice metabolizes penicillin; insulin is digested by digestive enzymes or catecholamine by gut wall enzymes. These drugs should be given alternative to oral routes, *viz.* sublingual, transdermal or suppositories in lower rectum which drains into inferior vena cava.

Excretion

It is defined as the passage out of systematically absorbed drugs and their metabolites.

Routes of excretion may be:

1. Urine (depends on glomerular filtration, tubular secretion and reabsorption)
   - Glomerular filtration depends upon plasma protein binding and renal blood flow. Tubular secretion depends upon plasma protein binding. In the nephron separate pumps operate to secrete acidic and basic drugs. Lipid solubility of the drug determines tubular resorption and lipid solubility depends on ionization. Ionized drug excretes *via* kidney.
2. Feces
3. Lungs
4. Saliva and sweat
5. Milk (may produce toxicity to infant fed on milk)

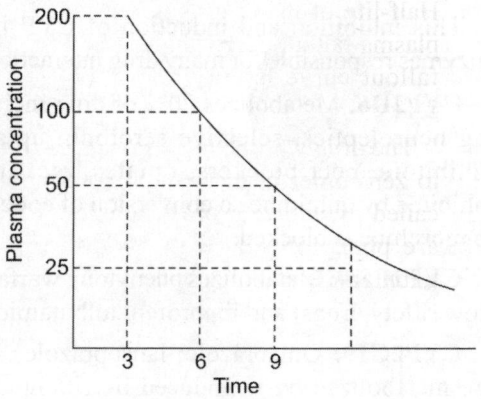

Fig. 2.7

KINETICS OF ELIMINATION

Clearance: It is the theoretical volume of plasma from which drug is completely removed in unit time. Clearance like volume of distribution may be in respect to blood (Clb); plasma (Clp) and unbound in water (Clu). Systemic clearance = (Cl renal) + (Cl liver) + (Cl other).

$$\text{Clearance} = \frac{\text{Rate of elimination}}{\text{Plasma concentration}}$$

Say plasma concentration is 8 mg/mL and rate of elimination 400 mg/min then rate of eliminaton is 50 mL/min.

- **First order kinetics:** A constant fraction of drug is eliminated in unit time. Hence full drug is dissolved in GI fluid and rate of absorption is proportional to GI fluid. It can be estimated by area under curve (AUC). At low doses drug metabolism is first order. t½ and clearance are constant in first order kinetics and rate of elimination is proportional to plasma concentration. Here plasma fallout curve is curvilinear and log plasma fallout curve is linear (Figs 2.7–2.9).
- **Zero order kinetics:** A constant amount is eliminated per unit time. Here rate of absorption is independent of amount of drug in the gut, but determined by rate of gastric

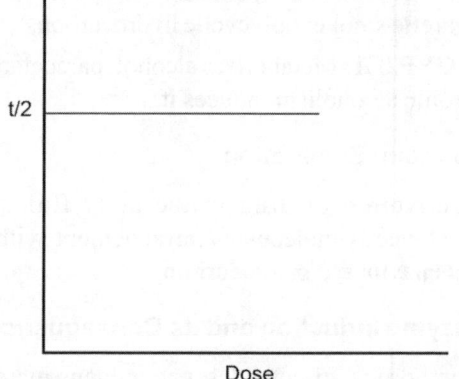

Fig. 2.8

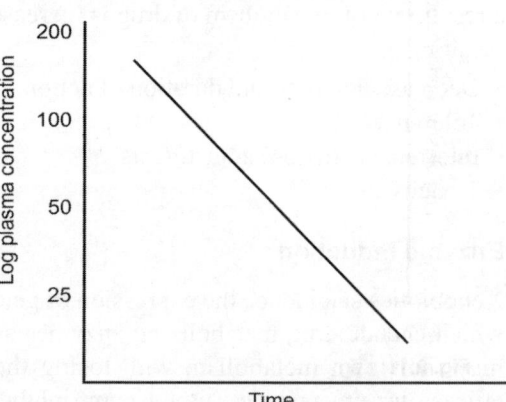

Fig. 2.9: Log plasma fallout curve in first order kinetics

emptying or controlled release formulation. Ethyl alcohol is eliminated by zero order kinetics. Elimination of some drugs approaches saturation over therapeutic range and their kinetics change from first order to zero order.

Half-life of the drug is never constant. Here plasma fallout curve is linear and log plasma fallout curve is curvilinear. Fig. 2.10 and 2.11

The drug whose kinetics changes from first to zero order in therapeutic concentration is called pseudo-zero order kinetics. The drugs are phenytoin, digoxin, warfarin, aspirin, tolbutamide and dicumarol.

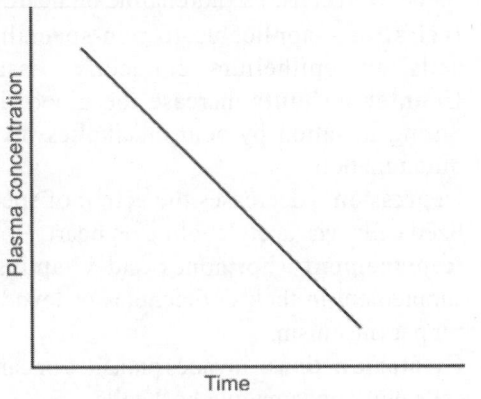

Fig. 2.10: Log lasma fallout curve in zero order kinetics

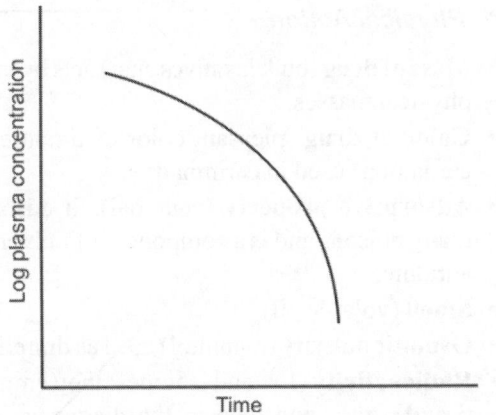

Fig. 2.11: Log plasma fallout curve in zero order kinetics

- **Plasma half-life (t½):** The time taken to reduce plasma concentration to half. Theoretically, four to five plasma half-lives are required for total removal of drug from body. When a drug is given through IV (considering body as single compartment and rate of elimination following 1st order kinetics), there will be two declines 1st α phase for rapid distribution and 2nd β phase for elimination. Elimination t½ is determined for β phase. Most of the drugs have multicomponent distribution and multiexponential decay. t½ is determined by the formula $(t½) = 0.693 \times \dfrac{V}{CL}$.

  (i) Plasma t½ is the time in which plasma concentration of the said drug is reduced to half.

  (ii) Biological effect t½ is the time where pharmacologic effect of the drug or its active metabolites are reduced to half. The effect of hit and run drug persists even long after drug is eliminated from plasma, *viz.* MAO-inhibitors, reserpine, *etc.*

  (iii) Elimination t½ is the time where the drug amount is reduced to half after equilibrium in plasma and other compartments (*viz.* muscles, fats, *etc.*) and can be measured by radioisotopes.

- **Repeated drug administration:** If a drug is administered in a short period before elimination then a steady state plasma concentration is achieved and drug will be accumulated in the body until dosing stops. Accumulation in practical terms occurs, if the dosing interval is shorter than four half-lives.

- **Loading dose:** Loading is single or in a few quick doses to attain target concentration. Durgs with high volume of distribution given with this strategy.

- **Maintenance dose:** It is a repeated dose at specified interval, after attaining target dose, keeping in mind the rate of elimination.

Therefore, loading dose = Target plasma concentration × a V_d and maintenance dose = Clearance (CL) × Target plasma concentration rate.

As a general principle drug with t½ 4–12 hours is given every t½ interval, with t½ of 12–24 hours given every 12 hourly, with t½ of 24 hours half the therapeutic doses are given 12 hourly and drugs wiht very short t½, *viz.* dopa-mine, oxytocin, etc. given by continuous IV infusion.

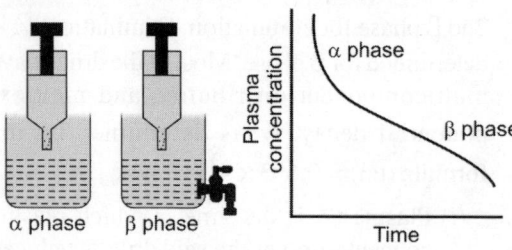

α phase   β phase   Time

Fig. 2.12

Importance of Monitoring Plasma Concentration of Drugs

- Low margin of safety drugs
- If the individual variation of drugs is large
- In case of renal failure for nephrotoxic drugs
- Poisoning cases
- Failure to response, *i.e.* resistance by anti-microbials
- To check patient compliance.

There is no justification in monitoring plasma concentration to antidiabetic, prodrug, hit and run drug or drug with irreversible action.

Prolongation of Drug Action

At times prolongation of drug action is required for patient's compliance and decreasing repeated drug administration. Prolongation of drug action can be achieved by:

1. Changing pharmacokinetics

- Retarding drug absorption
- Retarding metabolism
- Retarding excretion
- Making drug more protein-bound.

2. Changing drug delivery system

- Like ocusert
- Transdermal delivery system.

Structure-Action Relationship

The activity of a drug depends upon its chemical structure and its knowledge is important for:

- Synthesis of new compounds with more specific action
- Synthesis of competitive antagonist

- To know the mechanisms of action. Some examples of structure action relationships are mentioned in appropriate section.

PHARMACODYNAMICS

Effects of a drug on the body.

Principles of Drug Action

- **Stimulation**—enhancement of action of specialized cells, *viz.* adrenaline on heart.
- **Irritation**—applicable to non-specialized cells, *viz.* epithelium, connective tissues. **Counter irritants** increase the blood flow. Strong irritation by acid or alkalies invites inflammation.
- **Depression**—decreases the action of specialized cells, *viz.* acetylcholine on heart.
- **Replacement**—hormones and vitamins to supplement in their deficiencies or levodopa for parkinsonism.
- **Cytotoxic action**—invades parasites or cancer cells without damaging host cells.

MECHANISM OF DRUG ACTION

1. Physical Action

- **Mass of drug** (bulk laxatives agar) acts by their physical masses.
- **Color of drug** (pleasant color of tincture of cardamon) used in carminative.
- **Adsorptive property** (charcoal): It adsorbs many poisons and is a component of universal antidote.
- **Smell** (volatile oil)
- **Osmotic activity** (mannitol) used as diuretics.
- **Radioactivity** (I^{131} and isotopes; they emit α, β and γ rays and help in the diagnosis and treatment of many diseases.)
- **Radio-opacity** (barium sulfate used as swallow) to visualize stomach, duodenum and gastrointestinal tract.

2. Chemical Action

Chelators (BAL): Acid neutralizer antacids or iodine or potassium permanganate used as germicide.

3. Through Enzymes

A. Stimulation (adrenaline stimulating adenyl cyclase)

B. Inhibition (common mode of drugs action)

(a) Non-specific (heavy metals): Strong acids or alkalies inhibit enzymes non-specifically.

(b) Specific: Here particular enzyme is inhibited either competitively or non-competitively.

  (i) Competitive (Non-equilibrium type): Here enzyme inhibition occurs by the drug reacting with catalytic site strongly by covalent bond, *viz.* methotrexate and dihydrofolate reductase. Here K_M is increased, but V_{max} is reduced.

Equilibrium type (Fig. 2.13)

- Here the drug being structurally similar, competes with the normal substrate for the enzyme. Here KM is increased but V_{max} is unchanged.

- Allopurinol competing with hypoxanthine for xanthine oxidase.

- Carbidopa inhibiting dopa decarboxylase competitively with levodopa.

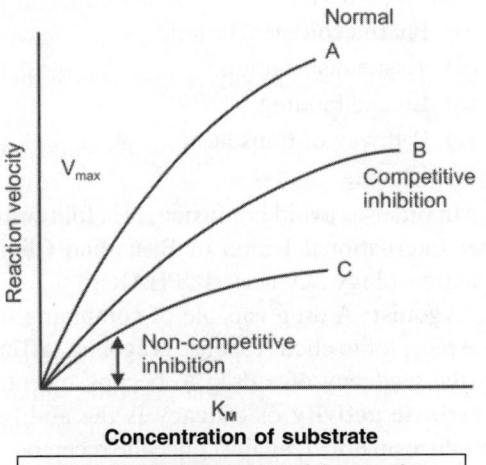

Fig. 2.13

where K_M = Rate constant of the reaction;
V_{max} = Maximum velocity of the reaction

  (ii) Non-competitive: Here the drug reacts with adjacent to catalytic site to loose its catalytic properties. Here K_M is unchanged, but V_{max} is reduced.

- Acetozolamide inhibiting carbonic anhydrase and aspirin inhibiting cyclo-oxygenase.
- Digoxin inhibiting Na^+/K^+-ATPase.

4. Through Receptor

(Discussed later)

 A drug does not impart new function to any system, organ or cells. It only alters the ongoing activity.

Factors Modifying Drug Action

1. Body size:

$$\frac{Individual}{dose} = \frac{Body\ weight\ (kg)}{70} \times \frac{Average}{adult\ dose}$$

$$or \quad \frac{BSA\ (m^2)}{1.7} \times Average\ adult\ dose$$

BSA = Body surface area can be calculated by DuBois formula.

Body weight $(kg)^{0.425}$ × Height $(cm)^{0.725}$ × 0.007184

Dose recommendation by BSA of some drugs (anticancer drugs) is available for rest of the drugs body weight is taken as index.

2. Age: *Child dose =*

A. $\dfrac{Age}{Age + 12} \times Adult\ dose$ (Young's formula)

B. $\dfrac{Age}{20} \times Adult\ dose$ (Dilling's formula)

C. $\dfrac{Wt.\ in\ pound}{150} \times Adult\ dose$ (Clark's formula rarely used)

In common practice for 20 years adult dose is given, for 15 years ¾; for 10 years, ½; for 5 years, ¼; for 2 years, ⅛ and for 1 year, ¹⁄₁₆ of adult dose are given, if the drug is indicated.

Child or infant shall not be considered as mini-adults because their mechanism of liver metabolism and renal excretion is less.

3. Sex: Ketoconazole decreases libido in man, pregnancy decreases GI motility leading to decrease absorption. Female requires smaller dose because of body size.

4. **Species and race:** Rabbit is resistant to atropine. Subacute myelo-optico-neuropathy (SMON) is reported with quiniodochlor in Japan, but inspite of its extensive use, it is less common in India.

5. **Genetics:** The slow acetylators are prone to INH and sulfonamide toxicity.

6. **Routes of administration:** $MgSO_4$ acts as purgatives when taken orally, decreases intracranial tension by rectal route and decreases swelling of inflammation, if applied to inflamed area. It inhibits convulsion if given by iv route in pre eclampsia patient.

7. **Psychological factors: Placebo** (I will please) inert substance produces effect equivalent to active drug. Placebo drugs are used by physician, if he thinks patient does not require treatment or in clinical trials. **Nocebo** is converse to placebo, opposes therapeutic effect.

8. **Pathological state:** Like liver disease, thyroid disease, kidney disease; heart failure may alter drug action.

9. **Concomitant use with other drugs:** If insulin and β blockers are used together, the features of hypoglycemia of insulin may be masked.

10. **Cumulation:** Prolong use of chloroquine may damage retina.

11. **Tolerance:** Here higher doses of the drug are required to produce effects. It may be cross tolerance, may be pharmacokinetics or pharmacodynamics.
    - Cross-tolerance (tolerance to related drugs, *e.g.* alcoholics require higher doses of general anesthetics).
    - Tachyphylaxis (Tachy—fast, phylaxis—protection). Repeated drug uses decrease drug action (*e.g.* ephedrine, tyramine).
    - Drug resistance: Applicable to tolerance of microorganism to antimicrobial to its inhibitory effect.

5. Receptors

Ehrlich and Langely introduced the concept of receptors. These are part of macromolecular complexes on effecter cells with which drug molecules interact to produce effect. A receptor may have a number of agonists in common, though their potency may vary. A neurotransmitter may have multiple receptor subtypes to interact, *i.e.* neurotransmitter is the master key capable to unlock multiple receptor subtypes. Drugs can be made to mimic neurotransmitter. The concept of receptor is important for development of drug to understand its action and for therapeutic decision. It may be briefed as follows:

(i) It mediates action of both agonist and antagonist.

(ii) It determines quantitative relation of dose and its pharmacological effect.

(iii) They are selective for drug action.

Ligands

Any molecule (whether agonist or antagonist) which attaches selectively to particular receptor or site. The receptors are classified using the following criteria:

(i) Pharmacological criteria

(ii) Tissue distribution

(iii) Ligand binding

(iv) Pathway of transducer

(v) Cloning

In order to avoid confusion, it is followed as per International Union of Basic and Clinical Pharmacology Sciences (IUPHAR).

Agonist: A drug capable of combining with the receptor to elicit response is agonist. **Affinity** is the tendency of a drug to occupy receptors. **Intrinsic activity** or **efficacy** is the ability to produce an effect, against once the receptors are occupied by agonist. Partial and antagonist may be compared with a table lamp with a rheostat (Figs 2.14A, B and C).

Pure agonists: It has intrinsic activity equals to one and affinity equals to one, *i.e.* it binds to receptor and activates the receptor in a fashion which directly and indirectly produces the effect. (Fig. 2.15)

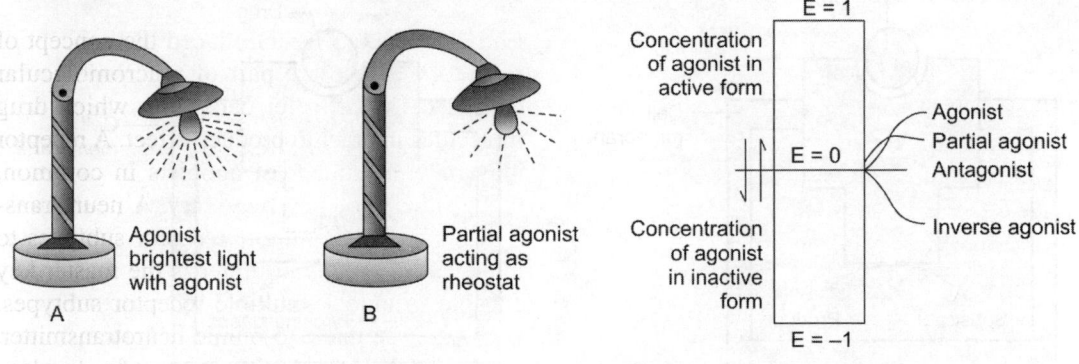

Figs 2.14(A to C): Light as an analogy of agonist spectrum

Partial agonist: It has intermediate intrinsic activity producing submaximal effect at full receptor occupancy. (Fig. 2.15)

Antagonist: It combines with receptor, but without intrinsic activity or zero, *i.e.* binds to receptor and prevents its binding to other molecule, *viz.* atropine antagonizes the action of acetylcholine binding with muscarinic receptor. (Fig. 2.15)

Inverse agonist: These drugs have affinity for the receptor, but intrinsic activity, a minus sign, *e.g.* DMCM on benzodiazepine receptor, *i.e.* inverse agonist do the opposite of agonists.

Functions of Receptor

1. To propagate regulatory signals from outside to inside of effecter cells and to amplify it.
2. To integrate various extracellular to intra-cellular regulatory signals.
3. To adopt short-term and long-term changes in the regulatory milieu to maintain hemostasis.

Receptor Theories of Drug Action

i. Occupation theories of Clark

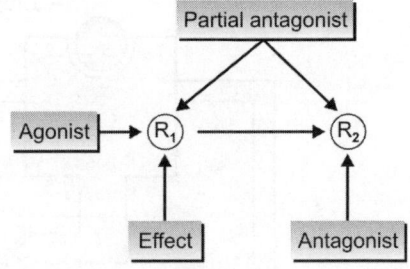

Fig. 2.15

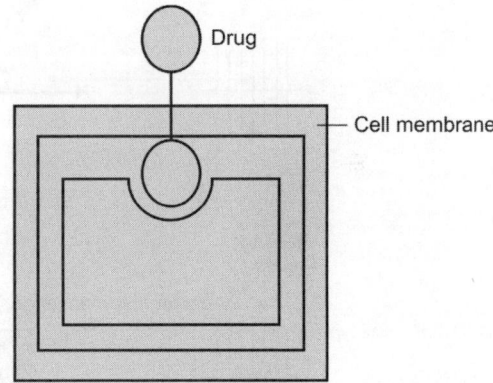

Fig. 2.16

$$\text{Drug} + [A] + \text{Receptor } [R] \underset{K_2}{\overset{K_1}{\rightleftharpoons}} AR \xrightarrow{K_3} \text{Response}$$

In affinity, the association : dissociation constant is one and determines potency, K_3 determines maximal effect of agonist.

ii. Rate theory of Paton: Response is the function of rate of association between drug molecule and receptors. Drug with high

dissociation constant K_2 is agonist, low K_2 is antagonist and which has intermediate K_2 is partial antagonist.

iii. Two state receptor model: Receptor exists in two interchangeable states R_1 and R_2. Agonist binds to R_1 to produce effect. Antagonist binds to R_2. Partial antagonist binds to both R_1 and R_2 (Fig. 2.15).

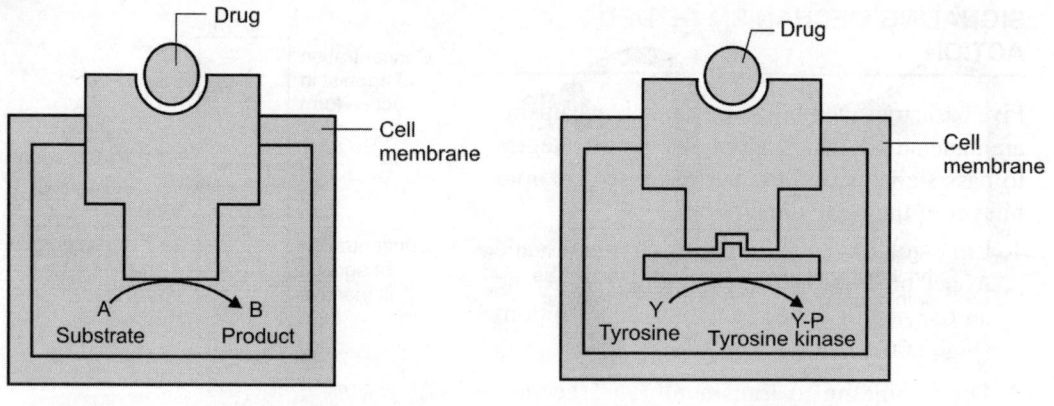

Fig. 2.17   Fig. 2.18

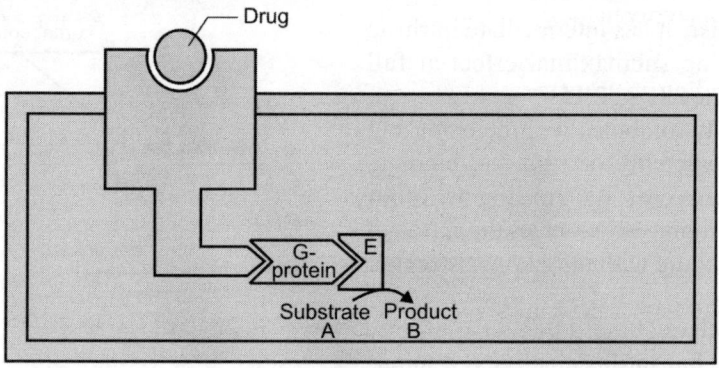

Fig. 2.19

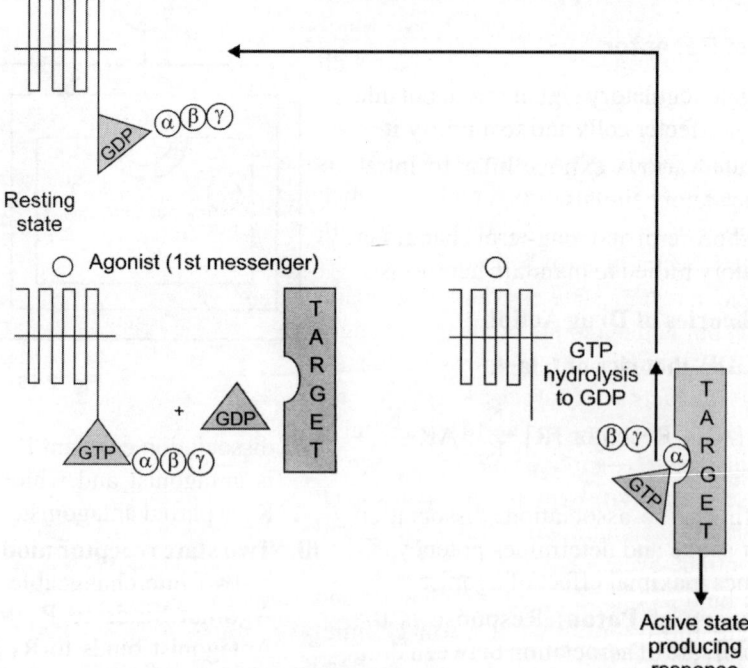

Fig. 2.20

SIGNALING MECHANISM OF DRUG ACTION

Five basic transmembrane signaling mechanisms are understood, which adopt different strategies to pass signal across the barrier posed by lipid bilayer of the plasma membrane.

1. Lipid-soluble ligand crossing the membrane to act on intracellular membrane (may be an enzyme or gene regulating transcription) (Fig. 2.16).

2. Drugs binding to transmembrane receptor protein allosterically regulating intracellular enzymatic activity in the cytoplasmic domain (Fig. 2.17).

3. Drugs binding to transmembrane receptor which binds to a protein tyrosine kinase and activates it (Fig. 2.18).

4. Drugs bind to transmembrane receptor linked to an effector enzyme by G-protein (Figs 2.19 and 2.20).

   G-protein coupled receptors (GPCRs) or metabotropic receptors are membrane-bound receptors coupled with enzyme or channel, i.e. effector system via GTP binding proteins GPCR, have seven transmembrane helices with extracellular domain to which drug binds and intracellular domain which couples with G-protein. G-proteins have three subunits α, β and γ, i.e. they are heterotrimeric. There are three main subunits of Gα proteins. Gs is stimulatory. Gi is inhibitory and Gq which controls Phospholipase-c (described with lithium's mecha-nism of action).

   While in resting state α, β and γ are bound to GTP, but while agonist binds it exchanges with GDP on α-subunits, β and γ dissociates. α-GTP interacts with target proteins to produce second messenger. The first messenger is agonist itself. α-subunits have got intrinsic GTPase, an activity which hydrolyzes GTP to GDP and α subunit which reunits to β and γ to continue cycle.

5. Drugs bind to ligand-gated ion channel and regulate the opening of the ion channel (Fig. 2.21).

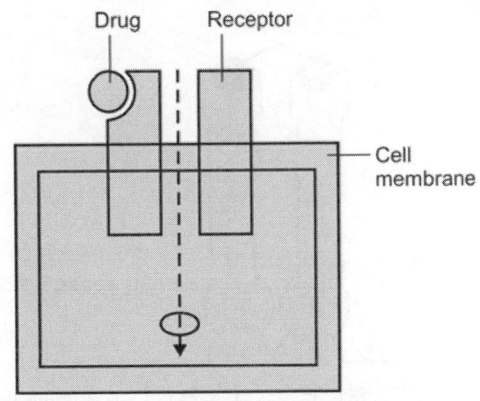

Fig. 2.21

INTRACELLULAR RECEPTORS FOR LIPID-SOLUBLE AGENTS

Many biologic ligands (corticosteroid, mineralocorticoids, sex steroids, vitamin D, thyroid hormone) are lipid-soluble, so easily cross the plasma membrane to act on intracellular receptor and stimulate the specific DNA sequence called response elements. For example, in absence of glucocorticoid hormone, the receptor binds to hsp90, a protein (heat shock protein) preventing active conformation of receptor. When glucocorticoid binds to receptor causing dissociation of hsp90 to make it active and ultimately alters transcription of specific genes.

DRUG OR LIGAND REGULATED TRANSMEMBRANE ENZYMES AND RECEPTOR TYROSINE KINASES

Signaling of insulin, platelet derived growth factor, epidermal growth factor, atrial natriuretic peptide (ANP) and transforming growth factor β (TGF-β) are mediated by this class of receptors. These receptors are polypeptides with extracellular domains binding hormones and intracellular domain (may be tyrosine kinase, serine kinase or guanylate kinase). The two domains are connected by polypeptide across the lipid bilayer of plasma membrane. When ligand binds to the receptor, changes its conformation and brings together the tyrosine kinase to make it enzymatically active by phosphorylation and additional downstream signaling

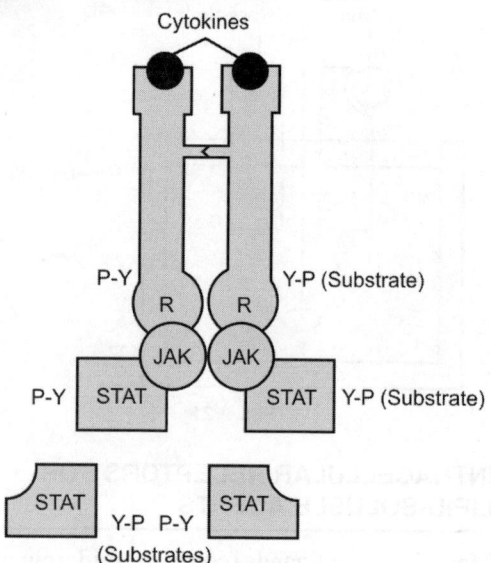

Fig. 2.22

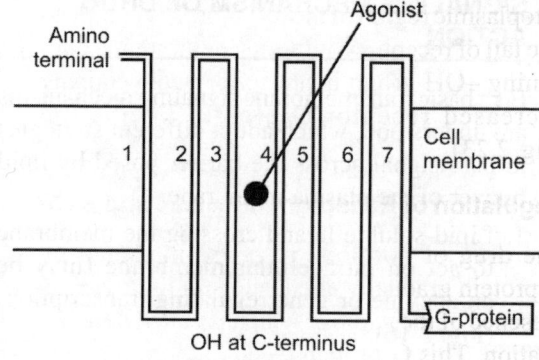

Fig. 2.23

protein to modulate several biochemical processes.

The intensity and duration of drugs acting *via* tyrosine kinase is limited by a process called downregulation. Ligand binding may induce endocytosis of receptor from cell surface followed by degradation. If the process of endocytosis and degradation is faster than *de novo* synthesis of receptor then surface receptors are reduced (downregulated).

Cytokine receptors (Fig. 2.22): Growth hormone, erythropoietin, interferon, regulators of growth and differentiation act through cytokine receptor. Here separate protein, tyrosine kinase from Janus kinase family binds to the receptor which on activation phosphorylates tyrosine kinase which signals it to another set of proteins called STATs (signal transducers and activator of transcriptions). Bound STATs are phosphorylated by JAK. Two STAT molecules dimerize dissociated from receptor, go to cell nucleus and regulate transcription of specific genes (Fig. 2.22).

Ligand-gated channels: Synaptic transmitter acetyl choline, 5HT; GABA and glutamate increase transmembrane conductance of relevant ion to alter electrical potential across the membrane. As for example, acetyl choline receptor is a pentamer made up of 4 polypeptides (two α chains and one β, γ and δ chains). Acetyl choline binds to α chain to open central aqueous channel.

Second messengers: Extracellular ligands may act by increasing intracellular concentrations of second messenger like cAMP, Ca^{2+}, phosphoinositide. Extracellular ligand combines to cell surface receptor which triggers activation of G-protein on cytoplasmic face of plasma membrane to change activity of the effector cell (either enzyme or ion channel).

The receptor coupled G-protein consisting of seven transmembrane polypeptide serpentine receptors (like snake). Agonist reaches receptor from extracellular fluid. G-protein interacts with

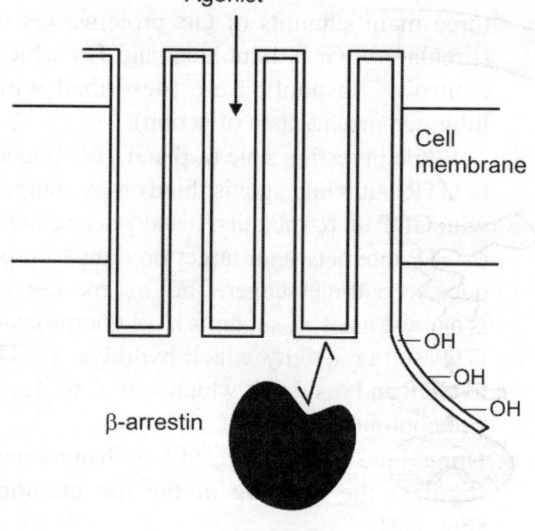

Fig. 2.24

cytoplasmic region of the receptor. The cytoplasmic tail of receptor with serine or threonine containing –OH group is phosphorylated causing decreased receptor G-protein interaction (Fig. 2.23).

Regulation of Receptors (Fig. 2.24 and 2.25)

The drug or hormone response mediated by G-protein gradually attenuate with time even in presence of the agonist, which is called desensitization. This G-protein receptor in presence of agonist causes conformation change in the receptor to make it active which acts as a substrate for G-protein coupled receptor kinases (GRKs). The activated GRK in turn phosphorylates serine residue of carboxy terminal of the receptor. The phosphoserine increases receptors affinity to another protein β-arrestin in cytoplasmic loop and decreases receptor ability to bind to G-protein (Fig. 2.24).

β-adrenoreceptors and some other serpentine receptors binding to β-arrestin, accelerate endocytosis of receptors from plasma membrane, and this endocytosis of the receptors promotes their phosphorylation by receptor phosphatase present in endosomal membrane and returns to plasma membrane and the receptor recovers from desensitization (Fig. 2.25).

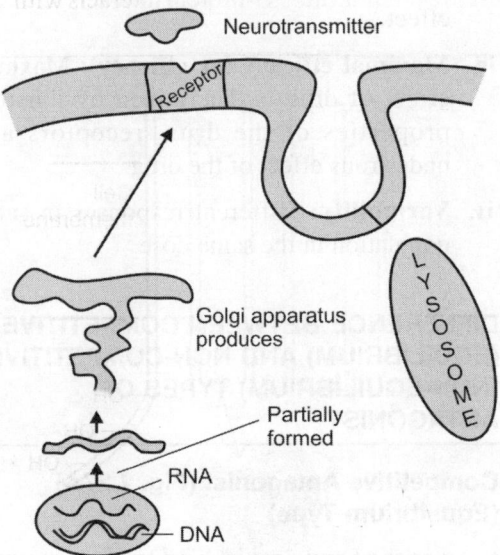

Fig. 2.25

Some serpentine receptors go to lysosomes after endocytosis and degraded.

DNA of cell nucleus is the command center for receptor protein production. The mRNA is transcribed which travels to endoplasmic reticulum to produce partially formed receptor which travels to cell membrane to be acted upon by neurotransmitter to produce second messenger. The bound neurotransmitter may cause pit in the cell membrane and it can be reversed or go to lysosomes and destroyed (Fig. 2.25).

Some Established Second Messengers

1. **Cyclic adenosine monophosphate: Involved in**
   - Mobilization of stored energy by β-adreno-receptor
   - Ca^{2+} hemostasis by parathyroid
   - Water conservation by vasopressin
   - Increases cardiac contractility
   - Regulates production of adrenal and sex hormones.

2. **Calcium and phosphoinositide: Inolved in**
   - Mediation of actions of some hormones and neurotransmitters
   - Growth factors by stimulating membrane enzyme phospholipase C (PLC) splitting phospholipid component of plasma membrane phosphatidylinositol 4, 5-biphosphate (P_1IP_2) into second messenger diacylglycerol (DAG) and inositol 1, 4, 5-triphosphate IP_3.
   - The DAG remains confined to membrane, but IP3 being water-soluble moves to cytoplasm and triggers Ca^{2+} release and regulates activites of enzymes.

3. **Cyclic guanosine monophosphate:** It is second messenger in some cells like intestinal mucosa, vascular smooth muscle. Here the ligand directed to cells surface stimulates membrane-bound guanylyl cyclase to produce cGMP.

Almost all second messengers undergo reversible phosphorylation for amplification or flexible regulation. There is interplay among different signaling mechanisms.

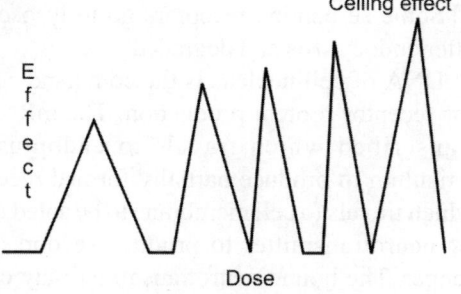

Fig. 2.26A

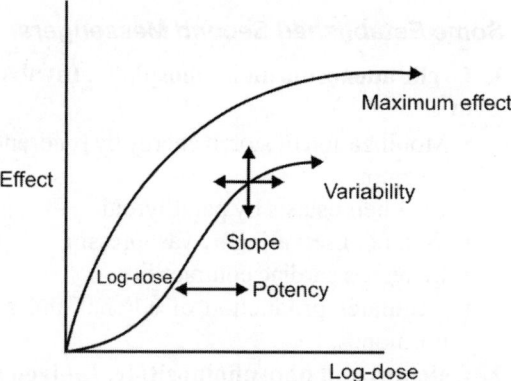

Fig. 2.26B

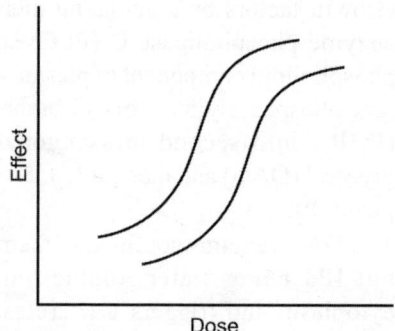

Fig. 2.27A

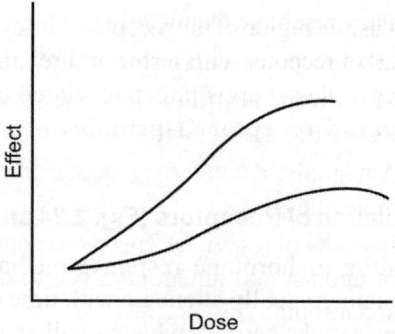

Fig. 2.27B

response is also increased till ceiling effect is observed (Fig. 2.26A). The log of dose and response curve, is a sigmoid curve, and has four characteristics: (i) Potency, (ii) slope, (iii) maximal efficacy and (iv) variability (see, Fig. 2.26A and B). In case of competitive antagonist, there is parallel shift of this curve to the right, but in case of non-competitive antagonist there will be flattening of dose response curve (Fig. 2.28).

i. **Potency:** Location of drug effect on dose axis. It is influenced by absorption, biotransformation, distribution and excretion of a drug.

ii. **Slope:** Reflects drug binding to receptor and mechanism of action. Steep dose-response curve means quick achievement of toxic effect.

iii. **Maximal efficacy (or efficacy):** Maximal effect of drug is determined by inherent properties of the drug, receptors and undesirous effect of the drug.

iv. **Variability:** Different responses in same population in the same dose.

DOSE–RESPONSE RELATIONSHIP

Generally, response of a drug increases with increase in dose, and the dose response curve is a rectangular hyperbola, because drug receptor inter-actions follow the Henry's law of mass action. The dose curve has two components, (i) dose-plasma concentration curve and (ii) plasma concentration-response curves. As drug concentration increases

DIFFERENCE BETWEEN COMPETITIVE (EQUILIBRIUM) AND NON-COMPETITIVE (NON-EQUILIBRIUM) TYPES OF ANTAGONIST

Competitive Antagonist (Fig. 2.27A) (Equilibrium Type)

• Antagonist and agonist bind to same receptor site.

- They resemble chemically.
- Dose-response curve shift to right.
- Maximum response can be attained by increasing dose of agonist (sur mountable).
- Antagonist apparently reduces some agonist molecules.
- Intensity of response depends on concentration of agonist and antagonist, *viz.* acetylcholine and atropine (Fig. 2.27A).

Non-competitive Antagonist (Non-equilibrium Type) (Fig. 2.27B)

- Binds to another site of receptor
- There is no chemical resemblance.
- Dose response curve flattens (Fig. 2.28).
- Maximal response is suppressed (Unsurmountable).
- Antagonist apparently reduces some receptors.
- Response depends on concentration of antagonists, *viz.* diazepam and bicucullin.

Therapeutic window phenomenon: Unusual feature seen with certain drugs where optimal therapeutic effect is exerted only over a narrow range of plasma drug concentration. Antihypertensive clonidine may rise BP at concentration above 0.2–2 ng/mL (Fig. 2.28).

Median lethal dose: It is (mg/kg) the dose which is expected to kill half of an unlimited population of same species or strain (LD50).

Median effective dose: This is the dose (mg/kg) which produces a desired response in 50% of test population (ED50).

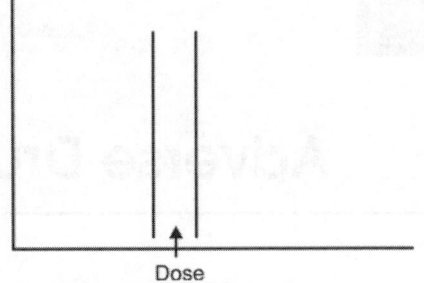

Dose

Fig. 2.28: Therapeutic window

Therapeutic index: This terminology is used for assessing safety of drug and it is expressed as ratio of median lethal dose to median effective dose.

$$\text{Therapeutic index} = \frac{LD_{50}}{ED_{50}}$$

For a drug to be safe, its therapeutic index should be more than one. The fallacy of therapeutic index is that it is applicable to experimental animals. For human studies it is calculated as

$$= \frac{\text{Dose which produces defined unwanted effect, } viz. \text{ tachycardia by beta agonist salbutamol, in 50\% of subject}}{\text{Dose producing airway reduction in 50\% of subject by salbutamol}}$$

Certain safety factor (CSF): It is assessed by ratio of extreme quantal response, *i.e.* effective dose of 99% by lethal dose of 1%,

$$i.e. \; CSF = \frac{LD_1}{ED_{99}}.$$

Adverse Drug Reactions (ADRs)

Undesirable clinical manifestation which arises as a consequence of drug administration. It may be abnormal sign, symptoms or laboratory test or cluster of all. In the USA, 2–5% patient admitted in hospital are for ADR. There are two main types of ADR: Type I or dose dependent and type II or dose independent.

ADVERSE DRUG REACTIONS (ADRs)

a. Dose dependent (Type I)

Chances of ADR increase with dose. Drugs with steep slope are more prone to ADR.

b. Dose independent (Type II)

- **Side effects** (unavoidable, but unwanted): Antihistaminics producing sedation, *i.e.* effects and adverse effects side by side.
- **Secondary effects** (corticosteroids flaring TB): These are indirect effects of a drug.
- **Toxic effects:** Excessive pharmacological action due to excessive dose (homicidal, suicidal, or accidental).
- **Intolerance** (toxic effect at therapeutic level): They fall in the left side of Gaussian frequency distribution curve, *viz.* single dose trifluoperazine producing extrapyramidal effects.
- **Idiosyncrasy** (abnormal reactivity to chemicals, phenobarbitone producing excitement instead of sleep): It is individuals genotypes.
- **Allergy** (immunological mediated reaction): Prior sensitization with the drug required.

- **Photosensitivity** (cutaneous reaction with UV radiation): It may be:
  - **i. Phototoxic** causing local tissue damage (*viz.* sunburn) or
  - **ii. Photoallergic** drug inducing cell-mediated immune response which on exposure to light wavelength of 320–400 mm UV light producing dermatitis like response.
- **Drug dependence:** Alters mood on withdrawal. Reinforcement is the ability of the drug to take it repeatedly.
- **Drug abuse:** Self-medication of drug. Deviating social and medical norms as in drug addiction or habituation.
- **Withdrawal response:** Sudden withdrawal producing symptoms. Clonidine producing severe hypertension, if withdrawn suddenly.
- **Teratogenicity:** Producing foetal abnormalities. Drugs may affect fertilization, implantation, organogenesis, growth and development.
- **Iatrogenic:** Doctor produced disease, *e.g.* Jaundice by INH.
- **Carcinogenic:** Drugs producing cancer.
- **Biotropism:** Combined effect of drugs and toxins produced by pathological process, *viz.* streptococcal tonsillitis treated with sulfonamide producing erythema nodosum.
- **Mutagenicities:** Drugs producing genetic changes.

Factors Influencing ADR

- **Formulation:** The other substances present in constituents of drug along with active ingredient called excipient may influence ADR, *viz.* water-soluble lactose used as an excipient, increases phenytoin toxicity compared to insoluble excipient calcium sulfate.

  Study of influence of formulation on therapeutic activity of drug is called **Biopharmaceutics.**

  The rate of break up of tablets or capsule is called **disintegration** time and the rate at which it goes into solution is **dissolution rate**.

- **Routes of administration:** Parenteral drug administration produces more ADR compared to oral drug use because of higher peak level.

- **Age:** Neonates or premature neonates are deficient of some enzymes cannot metabolize some drugs produce toxicity, *viz.* gray baby syndrome with chloramphenicol.

- **Difference in enzyme activity: Inherited** or acquired may influence ADR example.

  Inherited: Porphyria with barbiturate.

  Acquired: MAO-inhibitors producing hypertension crisis with tyrosine.

- **Kinetic of metabolism:** ADR is likely to occur when hepatoxic compounds accumulate, exhausting hepatic conjugating mechanism.

- **Protein binding:** Hypoproteinemic condition may increase toxicity of protein-bound drugs.

- **Excretion:** Alkalinization of urine decreases urinary excretion of acidic drug (aspirin) increasing their toxicity.

- **Local factors:** Hypocalemia increases toxicity of digitalis on heart.

- **Patient compliance:** Alters ADR which is influenced by formulation, number of drugs prescribed, age of patient and ability to comprehend instructions.

- **Drug interaction:** Drug interactions increase the chance of ADR.

  Other way to classify ADR by the cause and safety. **Type A: Augmented pharmacologic** (hypotension by β blocker), **Type B: Bizzare** effect (hepatitis by halothane), **Type C: Chronic effect** (tardive dyskinesia by antipsychotic), **Type D: Delayed effects** (ophthalmopathy by chloroquine), **Type E: End of treatment effect** (opioid withdrawal symptoms), **Type F: Failure of therapy** (increased hypertension because of treatment failure).

Monitoring ADR

Before labeling any sign or symptoms as ADR, doctor should confirm:

- Is clinical manifestation widely known, universally accepted ADR?
- Has enough experience accumulated with the drug?
- Is clinical manifestation a change, recurrence, complication, new manifestation in pre-existing condition present before?
- Is the disease followed by clinical manifestation?
- Is it a new alternative to etiology?
- Time since drug administration.
- Is there any evidence of overdose?

DOCTORS' RESPONSIBILITY TO REDUCE ADR

- Whether they should interface with patient?
- What alteration in patient condition they hope to achieve?
- Is the drug they intent to use, best capable of doing it?
- Can they administer the drug in such a way that right concentration can be attained a right place at right time for right duration?
- What other effect a drug can produce and whether they may be harmful?
- How they will decide to stop drug?
- Consider benefits versus risk.

Drugs' Combinations

When two or more drugs are given simultaneously or one after the other, the combined drug response may be either equal or more (synergism) or less (antagonism) than the sum of their individual response or they may interact.

a. **Synergism:** Here one drug effect is facilitated by others. It may be:
- **Additive:** The sum of two drugs response is equal to the algebraic sum of them, *viz.* Aspirin + Paracetamol.
- **Potentiation:** When response is more than sum of their individual response.

b. **Antagonism:** Here one drug inhibits the action of another. The antagonism may be:
- **Physical:** Charcoal adsorbs alkaloids due to its physical properties.
- **Chemical:** Acid + Alkali.
- **Competitive:** Atropine in muscarinic poisoning.
- **Non-competitive:** DFP + Acetylcholine.
- **Therapeutical:** Physiological histamine induced bronchospasm antagonized by adrenaline.

Drug Interactions

When two drugs are given simultaneously or one after another they may interact. The drug interaction is generally harmful to the patient so proper precaution has to be taken to reduce it.

Some examples of therapeutically desirable drug interactions

- **Addition:** Dopaminergic + Anticholinergic in the treatment of parkinsonism.
- **Synergistic:** Cotrimoxazole as antimicrobials.
- **Augmentative:** Penicillin + Probenecid or Carbidopa + Levodopa.
- **Facilitative:** Penicillin + Aminoglycosides
- **Reparative:** Aluminum + Mg salt for acid neutralization for smooth regular bowel as antacids.

Drug Screening

Regardless the source of drug molecule, the sequence of repeatative experimentation and characterization is called drug screening to define its pharmacological profile at molecular to origin level. Result of desired screening produces "lead compound", a successful new drug.

Expiry Date of a Drug

It is a legal requirement that all pharmaceutical products carry date of manufacturing and date of expiry, the period in between is called **life period.** The Drug and Cosmetic Act specifies the life period between 1–5 years. Self-life is dependent on drug itself and its storage condition. Drugs are not allowed beyond expiry date legally though they are not always toxic.

Pharmacovigilance

WHO has defined pharmacovigilance "as science and activities related to detection, assessment, understanding and preventing ADR or any drug related problem". Its activities include post-marketing surveillance, spreading of ADR data through drug alerts, labeling of medicine with warning and drug withdrawal. Pharmacovigilance center is present in almost all the countries. The Uppsala Monitoring Center in Sweden is an international collaborating center. In India, national collaborating center is present in the All India Institute of Medical Sciences (AIIMS). These centers are expected to provide standard algorithm and rating scales.

Counterfeit Medicine

A medicine is counterfeit, if produced with intention to cheat, *viz.* mislabeling, fudging expiry date, wrong ingredient or no ingredient or correct ingredient in insufficient quantity.

Central drug standard control organization is responsible for safety, efficacy, quality of drugs, their import, manufacture, distribution sale and standard of drugs.

Over the Counter (OTC) Drugs

In some advanced countries the drugs are divided by laws into those restricted to sale by prescription only and those which may be sold without prescription also are called OTC drugs. The knowledge of OTC drugs by general practitioner or by specialist is important because:
i. Some of the OTC products are cheaper.
ii. Some OTC drugs may worsen the clinical situation.

iii. They may interact with other drugs so while selecting following should be kept in mind:

- Select a product which contains effective dose.
- Simplest formulation
- Read the product and prescribe that which suits clinical condition.

Overuse or misuse of OTC drugs may produce severe medical problems.

In India, OTC drugs are very common.

Me-too drugs: These are the drugs with same chemical structure with mild variation, *viz.* omeprazole and esomeprazole which is enantiomer of omeprazole. Some of these drugs are pharmacokinetically superior, but in majority of cases it is produced by companies to get a market share.

Pharmacogenetics

PHARMACOGENETICS

It is the study of the basis of variation of drug response based on genetic variation.

PHARMACOGENOMICS

Surveying the entire genome to assess multigenic determinant of drug response is called pharmacogenomics.

Different genetic and environmental factors influencing drug response are:

- Age
- Infection
- Smoking habbit
- Other drugs
- Fever
- Gender
- CVS, GI, hepatic, kidney function
- Disease
- Circadian circle

POLYMORPHISM

This is a variation in DNA present at an allele. Variation in human phenotype may be:

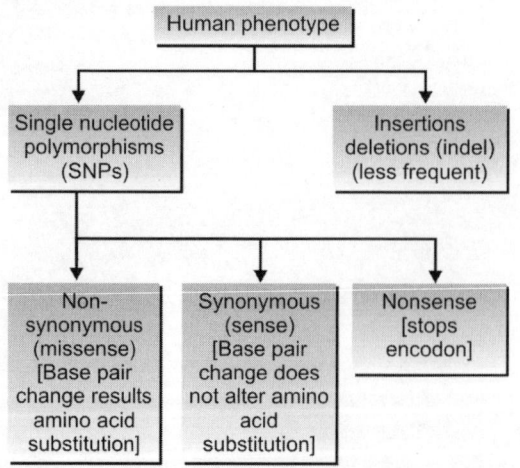

Ethnic Diversity

Polymorphisms may differ in the human population. Africans are believed to be the oldest population with highest population specific polymorphisms.

Applied Importance

i. If dextromethorphan is given orally and urinary ratio of parent drug is measured it will reflect CYP2D6 genes.

ii. The gene for therapeutic and adverse response can be devided into three groups.

   a. **Pharmacokinetic:** Effecting enzyme transporters to determine therapeutic and adverse drug reactions, *viz.* slow and fast acetylators.

   b. **Drug target:** Beta adrenergic receptor polymorphisms have been linked to responsiveness to asthma.

   c. **Disease modifying:** Polymorphism in ion channel may affect risk of cardiac dysrhythmia.

iii. Pharmacogenetics may help in the development of new drug.

iv. Clinical trial and pharmacogenetics: Drug dosing can be based on genetic testing directly rather than indirectly one measuring liver and kidney function.

Clinical Pharmacology

DEFINITION

It is an independent academic discipline and is concerned with effectiveness of drugs in man. The concerns include three principles:

- Pharmacology of drugs in man, *i.e.* deposition of drugs (absorption, distribution, metabolism, and elimination)
- The second involves the study of drug action to investigate the pathophysiology of the disease.
- The third and unifying approach deals with the documentation of the safety and efficacy of the drug in man.

DRUGS SCREENING BEFORE CLINICAL TRIALS

In earlier days, drugs are used in human being based on observations of its effects, but it should be done after.

Following types of tests are performed:

- Screening test: Rapidly performed test to see pharmacodynamics effect.
- Test on isolated organs, bacterial cultures.
- Test on animal models of the disease.
- Systemic pharmacology testing to see effects on different organs.
- Test to see dose response and pharmacokinetics.
- Toxicity studies (acute, subacute toxicity giving repeated doses and chronic toxicity, *etc.*)

Animal experimentation should be done as per good laboratory practice (GLP).

The potential candidate which is identified on screening is called **hit**. A few of the drugs come out as initial hit, turn out to be marketable because they have modest affinity for the target, may not have specific pharmacological properties or may not be pharmaceutically successful.

Potential drug, *i.e.* "hit" is tested on animals before its administration to people for potential toxicity by monitoring its activity on various systems in two species of animals (one rodent and one non-rodent) for extended period. The hit compound is also evaluated for its carcinogenicity, effects on genotoxicity and effects on reproductive system.

The test hit drug is now called a **"lead drug"**. In the USA, the sponsor now applies for its application in Investigational New Drug (IND) for its permission for clinical trial. The IND judges the efficacy of experimental system, pharmacology, chemistry, toxic effects, manufacturing process, *etc.* before permitting the clinical trial. IND may ask for more data otherwise, if they don't ask for more information on lead compound within stipulated periods from application, the clinical trial may be started by the sponsors.

It has been observed that from basic research and screening, if 10,000–25,000 molecules are searched after preclinical and different phases of clinical studies only one could get registered in market in 10–12 years of time. Some drugs are also **withdrawn from the market after post-marketing surveillance (phase IV clinical trials) because of its adverse effects.**

The clinical studies: It should be done according to ethics (which means first do not harm for greater overall happiness). It is designed to investigate or compare the two or more therapeutic measures or drugs. It is conducted after conducting all ethical considerations as per "Good Clinical Practice (GCP) guidelines", with informed consent of the patient or trial subject. The trial subject is always at liberty whether he or she will continue with it. The motive of the trial is to do good to the subject and not to harm or put the subject in undue risk. The inclusion and exclusion criteria at the end point should be properly settled before the experiment starts.

Experimental Design

Controlled trials: A comparative similar group should receive a placebo drug or comparable drug for comparison called control group. The control may be parallel control going simultaneously or cross over control where each group of subject gets chance to become control group when the drug administered group is totally free of the drug which is administered to them. The groups are randomized before the experiment starts to avoid the biasness.

The clinical trial may simultaneously go on several centers in different countries called multicentric trial.

The data on several similarly conducted data may be pooled for meta analysis.

Errors in interpretations: The type I (α-errors) is the difference between two groups when there is no such difference existing whereas in type II (β-error) there is no difference between two groups when there is actual difference.

Cohort study: Cohort is a group of people with some common features who have taken a particular drug and occurrence of event (either harmful and beneficial) is compared between users and non-users of drug.

Case control study: It is generally a retrospective study proceeds from effect to cause involving a few number of patients with quick results and is suitable to study rare diseases. It is relatively inexpensive. As for example, in a hospital patient admitted with a disease of agranulocytosis, and if we try to analyze how much of them are exposed to a particular drug (*viz.* phenylbutazone) then we can get a correlation between them.

DRUG TRIALS (FOUR PHASES)

First phase (1st human administration) 24–30 months (it is open trial)

Who   : Normal volunteers (if drug is very toxic, its first application may be on patients, *viz.* cancer drug on rare patient)

Why   : Determine biological activity and metabolism in man.

By whom : Clinical pharmacologist.

Second phase (12–24 months)
(It is single blind study)

Early

Who   : Selected patient

Why   : To determine potential, usefulness and dosage range

By whom : Clinical pharmacologist

Late

Who   : Large number of selected patients for long duration

Why   : For final dosage form, more data on metabolism

By whom : Clinical pharmacologist

Third phase (broad clinical trials) (It is difficult to design and execute because it is expensive and needs many patients)

Who   : Large sample of specified patient

Why   : To determine safety and efficacy

By whom : Clinical investigators.

If the above three phases' results are as per expectation, then application is made for new drug application (NDA). Generally, it takes five years or more for approval of making patent application to approve new drugs. In the USA, the lifetime of patent is 20 years. After five years, any company can manufacture the drugs with the approval of authority without paying license fees; that being paid by the original patent owner and called *generic products*.

Fourth phase: Conditional approval of new drug application (NDA) 12–36 months

Monitored release

Who : Patient under specified supervision

Why : Monitoring of drug impact under limited marketing

By whom : Selected medical centers by qualified persons.

Post-marketing surveillance (3 to infinity years)

Who : Patient under condition of actual drug use.

Why : To determine pattern of drug utilization and additional efficacy and toxicity after general marketing.

By whom : All physicians agreed to participate in organizing reporting.

Drug dosage

It is the appropriate amount of a drug required to produce certain degree of response. Different strategies are adopted for individual dosage.

- **Standard dose:** Same dose is appropriate for most patients, *viz.* chloroquine, mebendazole, oral contraceptive pills, amantadine.
- **Regulated dose:** Dosage is adjusted with measurement of physiological parameters, *e.g.* hypoglycemic, anticoagulant, antihypertensive.
- **Target level dose:** Response is demonstrated by certain range of drug concentration in plasma, *e.g.* digoxin, lithium.
- **Titrated dose:** Maximum level of drug cannot be given because of intolerable side effects. Dosages are adjusted either by step up or step down titration, *e.g.* anticancer, corticosteroids, levodopa, *etc.*

Fixed dose combination

A large number of pharmaceutical preparations are available in fixed dose ratio combination.

Advantages

- Better patient compliance.
- Certain drug combinations are synergistic.
- Side effects of one may be counteracted by other.

Disadvantages

- Patient may not require all the ingredients.
- Dose of each drug has to be adjusted.
- Time course of action of different drugs may vary.
- Adverse effect cannot be explained by a particular drug.
- Altered liver and renal function affect pharmacokinetics differently to the individual drug.
- Contraindication of one component contraindicates the whole preparation.
- Confusion of therapeutic aim.

Essential Drugs

The existing healthcare system fails to provide healthcare to all, so methods to provide it were discussed in the 1978 in Alma-Ata of USSR in a joint conference of the WHO and the UNICEF. According to Alma-Ata declaration, the object of primary healthcare includes:

- Education about prevailing health problems and methods to prevent and control them.
- Promotion of food supply and proper nutrition
- Adequate supply of safe water and basic sanitation.
- Mother and child care including family planning.
- Immunization against diseases.
- Appropriate treatment of common diseases and injuries.
- Promotion of essential drugs.

The WHO has defined essential drugs those satisfy the healthcare needs of majority of population and they should be available at all time in adequate amounts and appropriate dosage forms. The WHO has laid down certain criteria for selection of essential drugs.

- Adequate data on its efficacy and safety should be available.
- It should be available in a form which quality including bioavailability, stability on storage can be assured.
- The choice should depend upon pattern of prevalent disease, availability of facilities, trained person, financial resources, genetic, demographic and environmental factors.
- Choice should be influenced by local facility of manufacturing and storage.
- It should be single compound; fixed drug combination should be avoided.
- Selection of essential drug should be a continuous process. India has produced National Essential Drugs list in 1996 contianing 279 drugs adequate to meet the general health needs of the population.

The medicine in essential list are classified as 'core list' which are minimum list for basic health care system and 'complementary list' present essential medicine for priority diseases for which specialized diagnostic, monitoring, specialist training are required. Monitoring of safety of essential medicine is done by pharmacovigilance.

The essential medicine list for primary, secondary and tertiary are different categorized as P, S, T respectively.

Orphan Drug

These are drugs or biological products for diagnosis, treatment or prevention of a rare disease or condition. The costs of this are recovered from sales of those drugs, though these drugs may be life-saving for some patients, e.g. digoxin immune fab (antibody), desmo-pressin. These drugs are difficult to research, development and marketing. Since 1983, the USA has approved 268 orphan drugs to treat 82 rare diseases.

Hit and Run Drugs

The drugs whose effect lasts longer than drug itself, viz. reserpine, guanethidine, omeprazole, MAO-inhibitors, etc.

Nomenclature of a Drug

A drug may have a formal chemical name, new drug has generally a code name by pharmaceutical producer. And after launching in market, non-proprietary name is called generic name and when it is admitted in pharmacopeia it is called official name. A drug gets a name by manufacturer called trade name or proprietary name. International agreement of drug names are given by the WHO and pertinent health agencies. Only a few drugs (viz. levodopa, dextroamphetamine) give clue for stereochemistry. One should try to adopt non-proprietary or official drug name as far as possible.

PERSONAL DRUGS (P-Drugs)

A physician requires only 50–60 drugs in their day-to-day practice to treat common ailments. Personal drugs (P-drugs) are those chosen by physician to treat their regular patient and with which he/she becomes familiar.

P-treatment: It means personal treatment, which may vary from physician to physician.

6

Drug-Drug and Drug-Food Interactions

The response of a drug may be altered due to concurrent use of other drug or food known as drug-drug and drug-food interactions. Most of the time drug-drug interaction is not beneficial to the patient. Several mechanisms are known by which a drug can react with another drug, which are as follows:

A. It may occur *in vitro, viz.* succinyl choline and thiopental Na react in the syringe so should not be mixed.

B. *In vivo* drug interactions may be grouped into two heads.

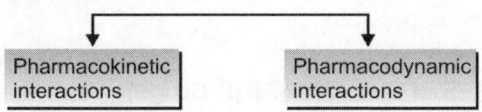

I. Pharmacokinetic interactions

It may occur in any label, *viz.* absorption, distribution, metabolism and excretion. Examples: At the label of absorption many drugs interfere with absorption, *viz.* calcium chelates tetracycline. In the same way pH of stomach, gut motility, transport proteins all determine absorption of a drug and any drug altering those may interfere with other drugs.

Drug distribution may be interfered by plasma protein binding or a drug may be displaced from target tissues which can transiently increase the blood concentration of the drug.

In the same way enzymes responsible for drug metabolism may be either induced or inhibited by the drug producing decrease or increase in their concentration.

Renal excretion may be a determining factor for drug label. Decrease in excretion of a drug increase the plasma concentration of the drug.

II. Pharmacodynamic interactions

Two drugs with same pharmacological effect will produce either additive effect or synergistic effect or with two drugs with opposite effect may produce antagonism.

Food similarly may produce drug-food interaction, *viz.* cheese and MAO-inhibitor or tyramine containing food and MAO-inhibitors may produce hypertensive crisis.

Some known enzyme inducers are phenytoin, phenobarbitone, griseofulvin, smokings, carbamazepine and **some known enzyme inhibitors** are INH, ketoconazole cimetidine, ciprofloxacin, erythromycin, *etc.* A drug prescriber should be well conversant with the drug-durg interaction. Then only he/she will be able to write safe prescription and can minimize adverse drug reaction and the best way to avoid it is writing minimal possible drug.

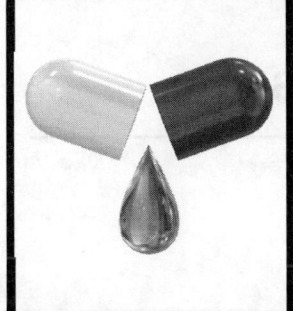
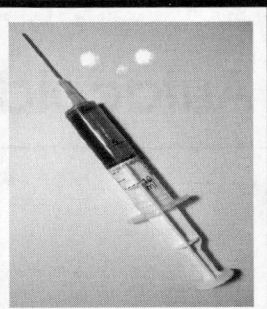
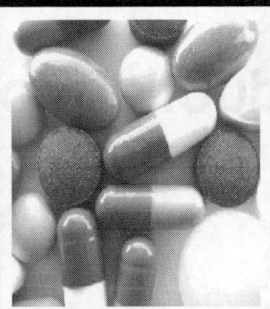
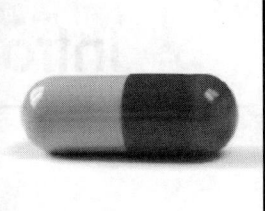

SECTION 2

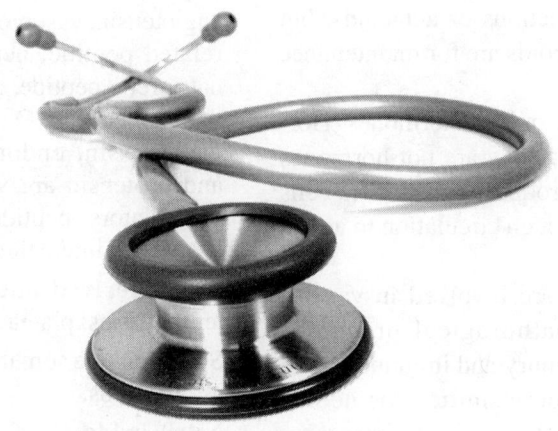

AUTACOIDS AND RELATED DRUGS

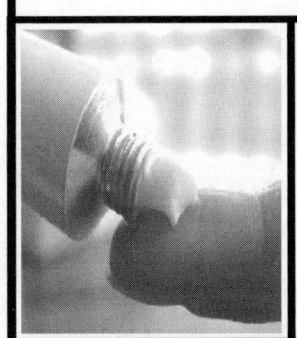
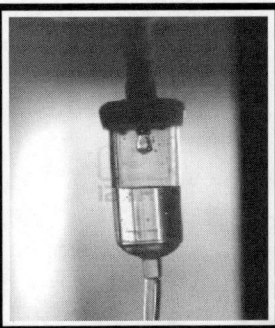
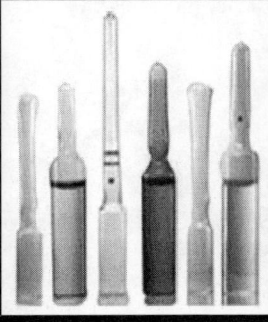
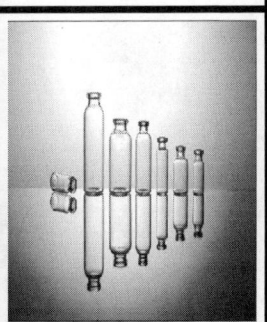

Introduction to Autacoids

The word autacoid is derived from the Greek words *autos* = self and *akos* = healing substance or remedy, which plays wide range of pharmacological activities in a vanishingly small amount. The pharmacologist disputes the rival claims of different functions of autacoids, but all will agree that autacoids are for maintenance of body economy.

Some gave the name of local hormones (Hormaein "to stir up"), but they are not hormones because they are not produced by specific cells and are transported through circulation to act on distant target tissues.

In brief, autacoids are involved in various physiological and pathological processes (specially reaction to injury and immunological insult or act as neurotransmitters or neuromodulator).

The classical autacoids can be classified as follows:

- **Amine autacoids:** Histamine, serotonin (5-hydroxytryptamine)
- **Peptide autacoids:** Bradykinin, kallidin, angiotensin, vasopressin, VIP; calcitonin gene related peptide, neuropeptide Y, urotensin, natriuretic peptide, substance-P; neurotensin, adrenomedullin. Out of which angiotensin II, vasopressin, endothelins, neuropeptide Y and urotensin are vasoconstrictors, rest are vasodilators, peptides are generally used by tissues for intercell communication.
- **Lipid derived autacoids:** Prostaglandins, leukotrienes, platelets activating factors.
- Some include somatostatin, gastrin, cytokines as autacoids.
- **Nitric oxide**.

Histamine

Histamine (Histos = tissue), the tissue amine are imidazole compound, which is widely present and its close relationship with certain allergic reactions are quite common. Present in mast cells in storage granules, abundantly present in skin, lungs, gastric and intestinal mucosa, liver, placenta. Non-mast cells histamine are present in brain, epidermis, gastric mucosa, blood, body secretions and pathological fluids.

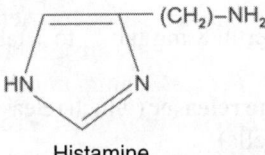

Histamine

It is synthesized from amino acid histidine by decarboxylation, degraded rapidly by oxidation to imidazole acetic acid and methylation to N-methyl histamine which is oxidized to imidazole acetic acid. Histamine (positively charged) held with negatively charged heparin within intracellular granules released by exocytosis. Intracellular cAMP inhibits histamine release. It is degraded in liver, if given orally.

Histamine acts through two types of receptors, H_1 and H_2. A third variety of receptor H_3 served as autoreceptor to control its release. H_4 receptors are found in leukocyte, bone marrow and circulating blood (Table 8.1). H_1 and H_2 receptors are postsynaptic in the brain but H_3 is presynaptic predominatly. H_4 receptors are also present in g.i. tract and CNS. Eosinophils change thier shape, chemotaxis and inflammatory response occurs when H_4 receptors are stimulated. H_1 and

H_2 are postsynaptic gererally but H_3 is presynaptic. All four receptor act through GPCR.

Table 8.1: Types of histamine receptor and their agonists and antagonists

Receptor subtype	Agonist (partially selective)	Antagonist (partially selective)
H_1	Histaprodifen	All antihistaminics
H_2	Amthamine	Ranitidine
H_3	(R)-α-methylhista-mine, Imetit	Clobenpropit
H_4	Clozapine	Thioperamide

Role of Histamine in Pathology

- Peptic ulcer by increasing HCl and gastric secretion. May cause diarrhoea.
- Allergic phenomenon responsible for urticaria, angioedema, bronchoconstriction and anaphylactic shock.
- Inflammation—promotes adhesion of leukocyte to vascular endothelium by expressing molecules P selection.
- As transmitter involved in awakefulness. maintaining body temperature, thirst, hormone release from anterior pituitary, *etc.*
- Tissue growth and repair
- Responsible for some vascular headaches.
- Implicated for inflammation
- May be having role for growth and repair.
- H_1 and H_3 receptor have important role in appetite. H_3 agonist **pitolisant** or **tiprolisant** reduces drowsiness in patient of narcolepsy. They are inverse against/

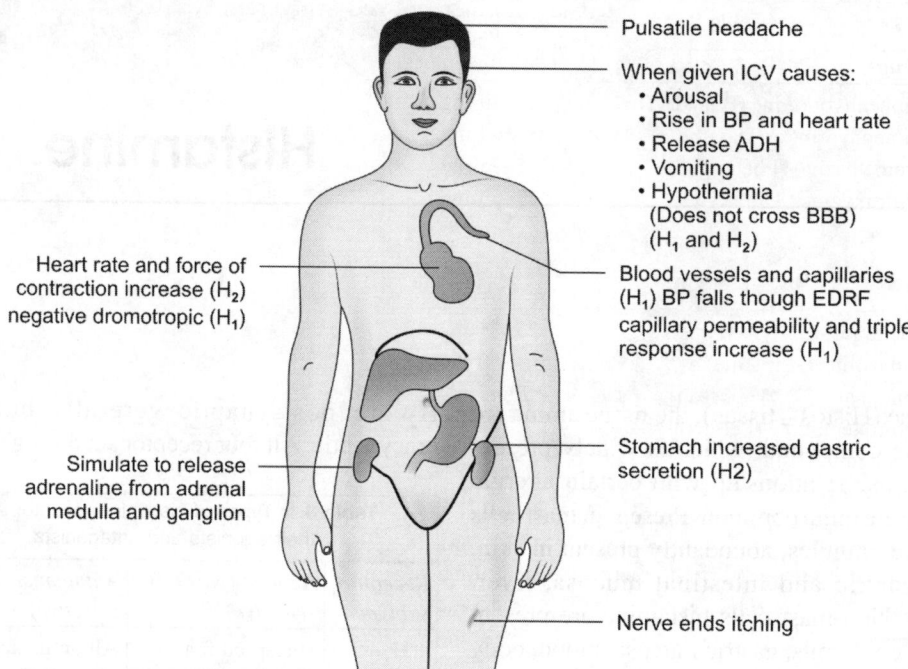

Fig. 8.1: Pharmacological actions of histamine

antagonist of selective H_3 receptor subtype, decreases releases of Ach, amine and peptides.

Pharmacological Actions of Histamine
(Fig. 8.1)

Histamine: Therapeutically rarely used, but some uses are:
- To test acid secreting capacity of stomach. Pentagastrin now preferred.
- In diagnosis of pheochromocytoma.
- Provocative test for bronchial asthma by aerosol.

Triple response: Histamine injected intra-dermally produces red spot, oedema and flare called triple response. Flare is said to be due to antidromically induced axon reflex. Histamine liberator 48/80, morphine also produces same effect. Reddening occurs due to dilatation of small vessels which is surrounded by edematous wheal.

- Betahistine an H_1 selective analogue of hista-mine used to control Ménière's disease and

vertigo (vertin 8 mg tab ½ to 1 tab QID given orally).

Histamine releaser (which releases histamine from mast cells)
- Antigen *vs* antibody reaction
- Tissue damage, *e.g.* venoms, stings, trauma
- Proteolytic enzymes, phospholipase A
- Polymers (dextran)
- Polyvinylpyrrolidone (PVP)
- d-tubocurarine
- Morphine
- Atropine
- Polymyxin B
- Vancomycin
- Surface acting agent Tween 80; compound 48/80.

ANTIHISTAMINICS

Conventionally, antihistaminics means which blocks H_1 receptors competitively. A big list of drugs name are there and used for a variety of purposes. Adrenaline is a physiological anta-gonist of histamine in anaphylactic shock.

Table 8.2: Some important antihistaminics (classified clinically)

	Drugs	Dose (orally)	Remarks and uses
Highly sedative	Diphenhydramine (Benadryl)	25–50 mg	• Moderate antispasmodic
	Dimenhydrinate (Daramine)	25–100 mg	• Marked sedation used for motion sickness
	Promethazine (Phenergan)	12.5–25 mg	• Long acting
	Hydroxyzine (Atarax)	25–50 mg	• Used for colic, vomiting, prurities, pre-anesthetic medication, post-operatively, general anxiety disorder
Moderate sedative	Pheniramine (Avil)	25–75 mg	• Allergic reaction
	Antazoline (Antistine)	50–100 mg	• Antiarrhythmic
	Trimeparazine (Vellergan)	2.5–5 mg	• Antipruritic
	Cyproheptadine (Periactin)	2–4 mg BD	• Antipruritic, apetizer (off label use)
	Meclizine (Diligan)	25–50 mg	• Motion sickness
	Buclizine (Buclifen)	25–75 mg	• Sedation, appetite stimulant
Mild sedative	Chlorphenramine (Pirition/Zeet)	5–20 mg	• Highly potent and sedative
	Methdilazine (Dilosyn)	8–16 mg	• Slight sedative, antipruritic
	Mepyramine (Pyrilamine)	25–50 mg	• Antipruritic
	Dimethindene (Foristal)	2–5 mg	• Antipruritic
	Triprolidine (Actidil)	2.5–7.5 mg	• Slight sedative
	Mebhydroline (Incidal)	100–300 mg	• Anti-allergic
	Cyclizine (Marezine)	50 mg	• Motion sickness
	Clemastine (Tavist)	1–2 mg	• Anti-allergic

2nd Generation

	Drugs	Dose (orally)	Remarks and uses
Non-sedative	Terfendadine (Trexyl)	10 mg	• Good for maintenance therapy, not for acute. Torsades de pointes may occur.
	Loratidine	10 mg	• Does not produce torsades de pointes desloratadine is active metabolite of loratatidine.
	Cetrizine (Incid-L Cetirizine)	10 mg	• Also inhibits release of histamine R (–) enantimer is levocetrizine.
	Rupatidine (Rupalist)	10 mg	• Also got PAF antagonist property.
	Mizolastine (Elina)	10 mg	• Non-sedating
	Ebastine (Ebast)	10 mg	• Rapidly converted to active metabolite carbastine. Has arrhythmogenic property and drug interaction with CYP3A4 substrates.
	Azelastine (Azep)	4 mg oral, 0.28 mg intra nasal	• Nasal spray produces symptomatic intra-nasal relief to perennial rhinitis
Anti-vertigo	Cinnarazine (Vertigon, Cintigo)	25–75 mg	• With anticholinergic, anti-5HT, vasodilator properties.

Pharmacological Actions of Antihistaminics

Some common antihistamines (Table 8.2)
- Antagonism of histamine
- Antiallergic actions—role doubtful. Adrenaline acts as physiological antagonist.
- CNS—depress CNS. Promethazine and a few other antihistaminics by virtue of anticholinergic and sedative property benefit rigidity and sialorrhoea of parkinsonism.
- Local anesthetic action: Mepyramine. Antazoline has strong membrane stabilizing property, but they are rarely used as local anesthetics because of irritation. Antazoline is used to relieve nasal congestion.
- BP may fall. If injected through IV.
- Some of them inhibit neuronal uptake of NAD and potentiate their action like cocaine.
- Anticholinergic action: Some antihistaminics have anticholinergic properties.
- Promethazine has alpha receptor blocking action.

Pharmacokinetics

- All classical H_1 blockers absorbed from oral and parenteral routes.
- They are metabolized in liver and exerted in urine.
- The newer compounds penetrate into brain poorly, so they are less sedative.

Side effects: Side effects of H_1 antagonists are frequent, but mild. Some tolerances develop to frequent administration. Common side effects are sleepiness, diminished alertness, light headedness, motor inco-ordination, fatigue, impaired psychomotor performance, therefore, they should be alerted not to drive vehicle and machine which require constant attention. They should be used with caution in pregnancy as documented for their teratogenic effects in animal studies. The antihistaminics with anticholinergic properties may produce dry month, blurred vision and urinary hesitancy. Overdoses may produce excitation, tremor, convulsion and flushing. Terfenadine is a second generation H_1 blocker may produce polymorphic ventricular tachycardia (torsades de pointes) because they block cardiac K^+ channels, which may be increased in liver disease or by cytochrome P450 inhibitors which increase its plasma concentration. Terfenadine is banned in some countries because

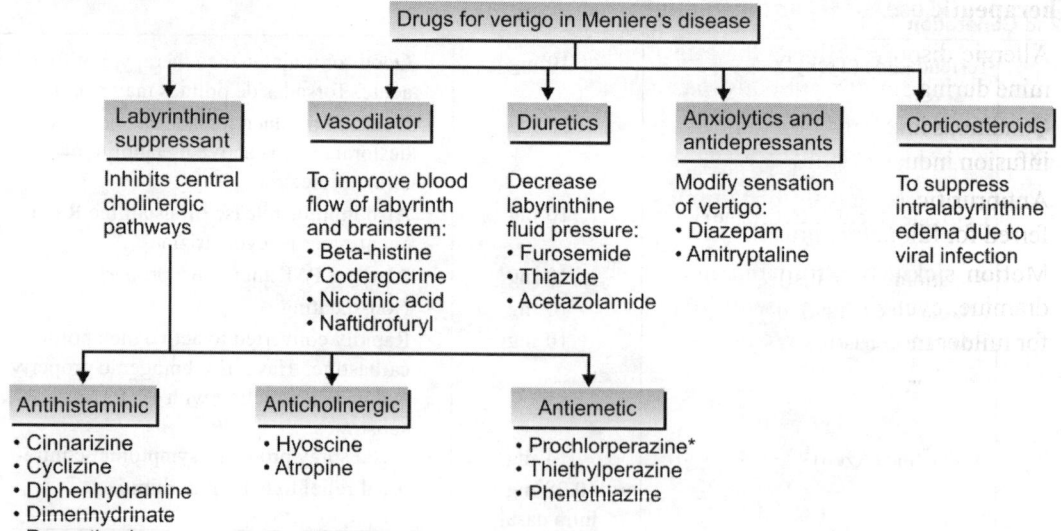

Prochlorperazine is most effective in controlling violent vertigo and vomiting, used parenterally.

Note: Combined preparations of antihistaminics and bronchodilators or with more than one antihistaminics is banned in India.

of its cardiac side effects and extensive interaction with erythromycin, clarithromycin, ketoconazole, itraconazole which precipitate cardiotoxicity.

Newer Introduction

- Fexofenadine (allegra 180/altiva 120 mg) used for rhinitis, itchy nose and red eyes.
- Desloratidine (loraday 5 mg): Chronic idiopathic urticaria, allergic rhinitis, non-sedative, fast acting, sustained action, OD dose.
- Luvistin (calciluvin 20 mg): All types of allergies, BD doses, rhinitis, chronic idiopathic urticaria, OD dose.
- Mizolastine (elina 10 mg): Seasonal allergic, rhinitis, chronic idiopathic urticaria, OD dose.
- Ketotifen (ketasma 1 mg): Mast cell stabilizer used for allergic rhinitis, dermatitis for allergies, urticaria, BD doses.
- Sodium cromoglycate (Fintal eyedrops, inhalation, nasal spray): Prophylaxis of asthma, exercise and cold induced asthma and allergic conjunctivitis as drops. It is a mast cell stabilizer.

Therapeutic uses of H$_1$ antihistaminics

- Allergic disorder: Blocks the effect of histamine during antigen-antibody reaction.
- Conditions involving histamine like insect bite, infusion induced rigor
- Antipruritic (older antihistaminics are preferred for idiopathic prurities)
- Motion sickness: Promethazine, diphenhydramine, cyclizine are used prophylactically for milder motion sickness.

- Common cold given for symptomatic relief to rhinorrhea
- Vertigo: Cinnarizine is used.
- Pre-anesthetics (Promethazine is preferred for its anticholinergic properties)
- Cough
- Release inhibitors of histamine are cromolyl and Nedocromil.
- Parkinsonism: Discussed with parkinsonian drugs.
- Sedative, hypnotic, anxiolytic
- Acute muscle dystonia. Hydroxyzine and promethazine reverse muscle dystonia of antidopaminergic and antipsychotic drugs.
- Appetite stimulator: Cyproheptadine is used. It is off label use.

Emedastine 0.05%, **Levocabastine** 0.05% are local H$_1$ receptors antagonist, used for conjunctivitis. Other drugs are cromolyl sodium 4%, Nedocromil sodium 2%. Ketotifen has both action used 0.025%, locally too.

For hereditary angioedema Ecallantide is used which is reversable kallikrein inhibitor.

H$_2$ Receptor Blockers

In human being, H$_2$ receptor antagonists are used for decreasing gastric acid secretion discussed with antipeptic ulcer drug.

H$_3$ Receptor

It is involved in autoregulation of histamine release. Its ligand may be of value for obesity, cognitive and psychiatric disorders, sleep disorder.

Release inhibitors of histamine are cromolin and Nidocromil.

5-Hydroxytryptamine (Serotonin)

5-hydroxytryptamine or serotonin, earlier known as enteramine, is widely distributed in plants and animals intestine, platelets and brain, higher concentration in pineal gland serving as precursor for synthesis of melatonin. Chemically, it is β-aminoethyl-5-hydroxyindole, synthesized from tryptophan.

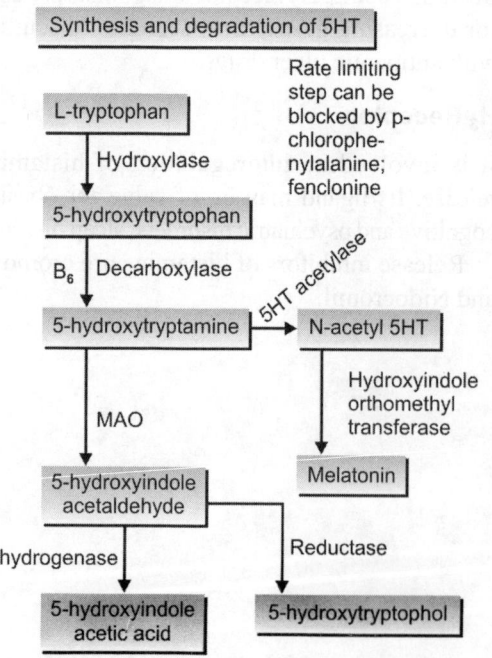

Serotonin

Synthesis and degradation of 5HT

L-tryptophan	Rate limiting step can be blocked by p-chlorophenylalanine; fenclonine

Hydroxylase

5-hydroxytryptophan

B_6 | Decarboxylase

5-hydroxytryptamine → N-acetyl 5HT (5HT acetylase)

Hydroxyindole orthomethyl transferase

MAO

Melatonin

5-hydroxyindole acetaldehyde

Dehydrogenase | Reductase

5-hydroxyindole acetic acid | 5-hydroxytryptophol

After synthesis, it is stored or degraded by MAO, reductase and by dehydrogenase. In the pineal gland, it serves as precursor of melatonin, a melanocyte stimulating hormone. 90% of it found in enterochromaffin cells of gastrointestinal tract. It is concentrated within vesicles of nerve ending and platelet by vesicle associated transporter (VAT) which can be blocked by reserpine.

5HT'S SIMILARITY WITH CATECHOLAMINE (CA)

The 5HT and CA both are decarboxylated before their synthesis and actively reuptaken by amine pump which can be inhibited by tricyclic antidepressants. Both are degraded by MAO.

5HT receptors: Gaddum and Picarelli classified 5HT receptors into D type (musculotropic) blocked by methysergide and cyproheptadine and M type (neurotropic). Seven families of 5HT receptors are known with given numeric subscripts from 1–7. Out of which 6 involving G-protein coupled of transmembrane serpentine receptor and one is ligand gated ion channel.

Some of 5HT receptor types

$5HT_{1A}$: Present in raphae nuclei and hippocampus. Buspirone (anti-anxiety drug) acts as partial agonist of this receptor.

$5HT_{1D}$: Maintains dopaminergic tone in substantia nigra, basal ganglia and cause constriction of cranial vessels. Sumatriptan (antimigraine) is a selective agonist of $5HT_{1D}$.

Types of 5HT receptors

These are of seven types $5HT_1$ to $5HT_7$ whereas $5HT_1$ and $5HT_2$ are classified further.

Important varieties of 5HT receptors.

cc	Location	Function	Mechanism	Agonist	Antagonist
$5HT_1$	Blood vessels of CNS	Pre-synaptic auto-receptor controls mood and vaso-constriction	GPCR $\downarrow$ CAMP	Buspirone is partial agonist of $5HT_{1A}$ sumatriptan agonist	Ergotamine $5HT_{1A/1D}$ (partial agonist)
$5HT_2$	Smooth muscles, platelets, CNS	Platelet aggregation, smooth muscle contraction	GPCR $\uparrow$ IP3, DAG	LSD	Ketanserin $5HT_{2A}$ Methysergide $5HT_{2A/2C}$ Clozapine Cyproheptadine 2A
$5HT_3$	CNS ENS PNS	Anxiety Excitation Emesis	Ion channels	2-methyl 5HT	Setrons like ondensetrons
$5HT_4$	CNS ENS	$\uparrow$ GI motility Excitation	GPRS	Metoclopramide, Cisapride, etc.	–

$5HT_2$: Functions are vasoconstrictions, contraction of intestine, uterine and bronchial smooth muscles, platelet aggregation. Ketanserin is a $5HT_2$ antagonist.

$5HT_3$: Corresponds to classical M type receptor of 5HT. Ondansetron (anti-emetics) blocks $5HT_3$.

$5HT_4$: Augments intestinal secretion and peristalsis. Cisapride and renzapride are $5HT_4$ agonists.

Physiological Roles of 5HT (Fig. 9.1)

1. Neurotransmitters involved in sleep, thought, cognitive functions, behavior and mood, vomiting, pain perception.

2. Precursor of melatonin in pineal gland which regulates biological clock.

3. Neuroendocrine functions to regulate release of anterior pituitary hormones.

4. Vomiting and intestinal motility.

5. Migraine: Produces vasoconstriction and precipitate inflammation.

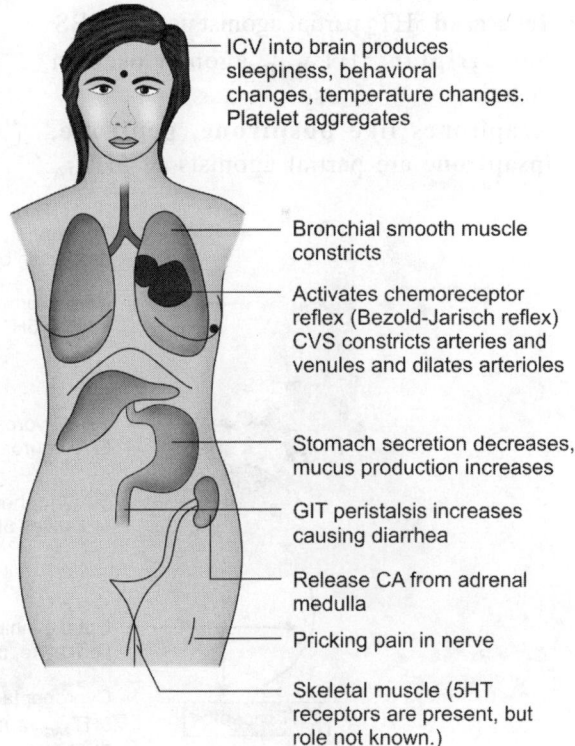

ICV into brain produces sleepiness, behavioral changes, temperature changes. Platelet aggregates

Bronchial smooth muscle constricts

Activates chemoreceptor reflex (Bezold-Jarisch reflex) CVS constricts arteries and venules and dilates arterioles

Stomach secretion decreases, mucus production increases

GIT peristalsis increases causing diarrhea

Release CA from adrenal medulla

Pricking pain in nerve

Skeletal muscle (5HT receptors are present, but role not known.)

Fig. 9.1: Actions of serotonin

6. Platelet aggregation and clot formation are accelerated.
7. Raynaud's phenomenon. Ketanserin may be used prophylactically.
8. Hypertension in pre-eclamptic
9. Variant angina: 5HT and thromboxane A2 are said to be responsible for coronary spasm of variant angina.
10. Carcinoid syndrome where there is massive release of 5HT.
11. Pellagra: Diversion of tryptophan to 5HT formation.
12. **Serotonin syndrome:** When 5HT agonist is given to a patient receiving MAO inhibitors causes severe muscle contraction and hyperthermia.

Some 5HT Agonists Used Clinically

- Agonist **LSD** abused as hallocinogens.
- **Buspirone** (antianxiety) $5HT_{1A}$ agonist
- **Cisapride** (prokinetic) $5HT_{1D}$ agonist
- **Renzapride** (prokinetic) $5HT_4$ agonist
- **Tegaserod** $5HT_4$ partial agonist used for IBS
- **Sumatriptan** $5HT_{1B/1D}$ agonist used in migraine
- Azapirones like **buspirone, gepirone, ipsapirone** are partial agonists of $5HT_{1A}$

receptor used as anxiety drugs.
- **Dexfenfluramine** is a 5HT agonist and 5HT uptake inhibitor and blocks 5HT transporter used to suppress appetite. Lorcaserin $5HT_{2c}$ agonist is also approved for weight losing.
- **Sibutramine** also inhibits 5HT transporter and inhibits reuptake also suppresses appetite.
- **Fluoxetine** used for depression

Some 5HT Antagonists Used Clinically (Fig. 9.2)

- **Cyproheptadine:** $5HT_{2A}$ blockers with anti-histaminic and anticholinergic properties. Used for antiallergic, appetite stimulant, dumping syndrome, carcinoid syndrome, priapism and orgasmic delay produced by fluoxetine and trazodone (the 5HT uptake inhibitor blockers). Confusion, weight gain, dry mouth, ataxia are the side effects.
- **Methysergide:** $5HT_{2A/2C}$ antagonist used to treat carcinoid and post-dumping syndrome and prophylaxis to migraine. Dose 2 mg BD. Side effects are abdominal pain, diarrhea, nervousness, pulmonary abdominal and endocardial fibrosis.
- **Pizotifen:** Inferior to propranolol as prophylactic to migraine $5HT_{2A/2C}$ antagonist.

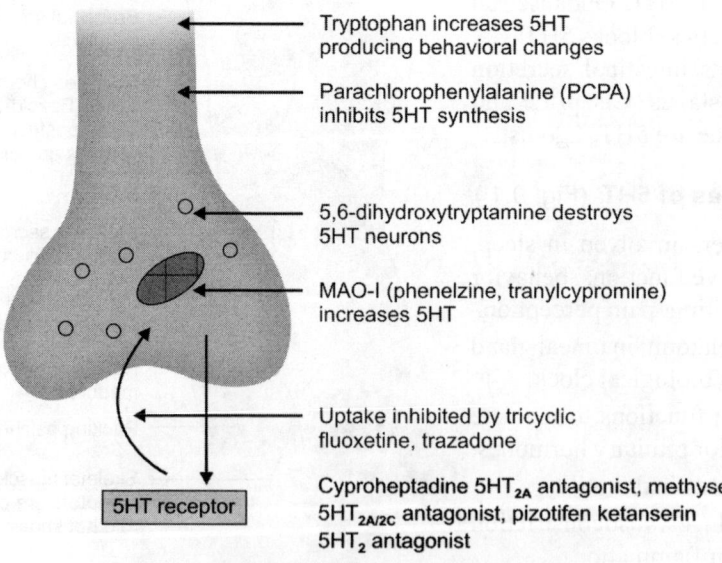

Tryptophan increases 5HT producing behavioral changes

Parachlorophenylalanine (PCPA) inhibits 5HT synthesis

5,6-dihydroxytryptamine destroys 5HT neurons

MAO-I (phenelzine, tranylcypromine) increases 5HT

Uptake inhibited by tricyclic fluoxetine, trazadone

Cyproheptadine $5HT_{2A}$ antagonist, methysergide $5HT_{2A/2C}$ antagonist, pizotifen ketanserin $5HT_2$ antagonist

5HT receptor

Fig. 9.2: Drugs affecting 5HT system

- **Ketanserin:** $5HT_2$ receptor blocker used as antihypertensive, may be due to α_1 blocking effects.
- **Ritanserin:** $5HT_{2A}$ antagonist selective, congener of ketanserin. Ritanserin $5HT_2$ antagonist reported to alter bleeding time.
- **Clozapine:** $5HT_{2A/2C}$ blockers used in schizophrenia. It has dopaminergic antagonist property.
- **Risperidone:** Used to treat schizophrenia ($5HT_{2A}$ and dopamine D2 blocker).
- **Ondansetron:** $5HT_3$ antagonist, used to treat chemotherapy and radiotherapy induced vomiting.

ERGOT ALKALOIDS

Obtained from fungus grown in rye or other grains known as *Claviceps purpurea*. It is a store house of pharmacologically active substances like alkaloids, LSD, histamine, ACh, tyramine and sterols.

Natural Ergot Alkaloids

- Amine alkaloids: Ergometrine (oxytocic)
- Amino acid alkaloids: Ergotamine, ergotoxine (mixture of ergocristine + ergocornine + ergocryptine) vasoconstriction + α-blockers.

Semisynthetic Ergots

- Dihydroergotamine (DHE): Dihydroergotoxine (codergocrine) [antiadrenergic, cerebroactive]
- Bromocriptine (dopaminergic agonist)
- Methysergide: 5HT antagonist
- Synthetic non-lysergic acid derivative resembling ergots are lisuride, pergolide, lergotrile and metergoline.

Actions

Ergotamine: Partial agonist and antagonist to an adrenergic, $5HT_1$ and $5HT_2$, but not with $5HT_3$ and DA receptors. Produces vasoconstriction, visceral smooth muscle contraction.

Dihydroergotamine (DHE): α-receptor blockers.

Dihydroergotoxine (codergocrine): α-blocker, partial agonist and antagonistic actions on 5HT receptor. Produces metabolic effects and enhancement of ACh release, so used for dementia.

Bromocriptine: D2 agonist on pituitary lactotropes and striatum, is used to suppress lactation and to treat parkinsonism.

Ergometrine: Used as oxytocic.

Pharmakokinetics: Slow and incompletely absorbed orally and have high first pass metabolism, crosses blood-brain barrier, metabolized in liver.

Doses and Preparations

Ergotamine 1-3 mg oral/sublingual or 0.25 to 0.5 mg IM or s/c. (Gynergen 1 mg tab, 0.5 mg/ml).

Dihydroergotamine (DHE, 1 mg tab; migranil, 1 mg/mL) for migraine 2–6 mg oral or 0.5–1 mg IM or SC.

Dihydroergotoxine 1–1.5 mg oral or sublingual for dementia or 0.15–0.6 mg IM.

MIGRAINE AND ITS TREATMENT

Definition: Migraine is a mysterious disease with pulsating headache of one side, comes in attack, may be associated with nausea, vomiting, sensitivity to light or sound, vertigo, loose motion, *etc.*

Types of Migraine

- **Classical** (headache preceded by visual and other neurological symptoms, *i.e.* with aura)
- **Common migraine:** Without aura

The pathogenic mechanisms are not well-understood, can be explained by:

(a) **Vascular theory:** Causing vasoconstriction and shunting of blood through carotid arteriovenous anastomosis.

(b) **Neurogenic theory:** Depression of cortical electrical activity followed by vascular phenomenon. 5HT plays an important role in its genesis. Other mediators responsible for inflammation are neurokinin, substance P, calcitonin gene-related peptide (CGRP) and nitric oxide.

Drugs of Migraine

1. **NSAID or analgesics:** Like aspirin, paracetamol, ibuprofen, naproxen.
2. **Antihistaminics:** Diphenhydramine
3. **Antiemetics:** Metoclopramide, domperidone or diphenhydramine or promethazine which serves dual purpose of sedation and antiemetic agents.

Ergot (Some Combination Preparations)

Ergotamine (Migranil; cafergot; ergotamine + caffeine) migril (ergotamine 2 mg; caffeine 100 mg; cyclizine 50 mg) (vasograin 1 gm, caffeine 100 mg, paracetamol 250 mg, prochlorperazine 2.5 mg tab)

Ergophen (ergotamine 0.3 mg; belladonna dry ext. 10 mg, phenobarbitone 20 mg tab)

Ergotamine given early in attack quickly relieves migraine by oral or sublingual route may be given, per rectal to patient who vomits. It constricts dilated cranial vessels, reducing shunting of blood from carotid artery. It acts as partial agonist of $5HT_{1B/1D}$ receptor and reduce neurogenic inflammation and leakage of plasma in dura mater due to retrograde stimulation of perivascular afferent nerves. Inhalation preparations are availale in some countries. Continuous use may be hazardous. Dihydroergotamine is preferred for parenteral administration, may be given orally. The ergot does not have any prophylactic role in migraine.

Sumatriptan (Migratan 50, 100 mg tab; Suminate 60 mg/5 mL): $5HT_{1B/1D}$ receptor agonist, better tolerated. It is rapidly absorbed by SC injection and 15% by oral route, metabolized by MAO-A iso-enzyme.

May produce tightness of head and chest, paresthesia, feeling of heat, weakness, rise of BP, bradycardia and coronary vasospasm. Should not be given in IHD; epilepsy, hepatic and renal impaired patient. Dose 50–100 mg at the onset. Do not give second doses, if not responding. Parenteral dose is 6 mg SC.

Sumatriptan, ergotamine, 5HT uptake inhibitor and lithium should not be given simultaneously.

Rizatriptan (Rizact 5 and 10 mg tab) is more potent, more bioavailable by oral route. Fast acting than sumatriptan. Other triptans available in different countries are **naratriptan** (dose 2.5 mg); **zolmitriptan** (dose 2.5 mg); **frovatriptan** (dose 2.5 mg); **almotriptan**; (6.25 mg); **eletriptans** (20–40 mg); **naratriptan** (1–2.5 mg).

Prophylactics for Migraine

- **β-blockers:** Propanolol, nadolol, timolol may be given. Pindolol is ineffective.
- **Tricyclic antidepressant:** Amitriptyline in patient suffering with depression.
- **Calcium channel blockers:** Flunarizine blocks Ca and Na channel (cerebroselective). Side effects are sedation, constipation, dry mouth, hypotension, weight gain and extrapyramidal symptoms. Nomigrain 5 and 10 mg cap. Dose 10–20 mg OD, children 5 mg OD.
- **5 HT antagonists:**
  (a) Methysergide: $5HT_{2A/2C}$ antagonist. May produce retroperitoneal fibrosis. Rarely used.
  (b) Cyproheptadine: $5HT_2$, histamine and cholinergic antagonist used to prevent migranious attack.
- **Anticonvulsants: Valproic** acid (400–1200 mg/day) **gabapentin** (300–1200 mg/day), **topiramate** have proprophylactic effect to migraine and are the new approach to treat migraine.
- Antagonist to calcium gene-related peptide antagonist BIB-4096BS has potential to treat migraine.

PHARMACOLOGY OF MELATONIN

Melatonin is methoxylated and acetylated product of serotonin, chemically N-acetyl-5-methoxytryptamine found in pineal gland responsible for diurnal cycles and sleep work behavior of humans. Melatonin acts on MT_1; MT_2 and MT_3 receptors.

Functions of different melatonin receptors are as follows:

MT_1 = Activation causes sleepiness

MT_2 = Light-dark synchronization and biological clocks.

MT_3 = Poorly defined function, probably related to intraocular pressure.

Ramelteon (agonist of MT_1 and MT_2) approved for the treatment of insomnia. It raises prolactin level. Another MT_1 and MT_2 agonists and $5HT_{2C}$ agonist agomelatine is approved for depression. **Tasimelteon** the newer MT_1 and MT_2 agonist may be used for sleep wake disorder.

Serotonin Syndrome

Clinical feature: Skeletal muscle contraction hyperthermia, hypertension, hyper reflexia, diarrhea, mydriasis, agitation, coma due to excess serotonin in the synapse. Drugs which may produce serotonin syndrome are as follows:

i. Inhibiting 5HT metabolism like MAO-I.

ii. Increasing 5HT release like amphetamine, fenfluramine.

iii. Inhibiting 5HT uptake like SSRI; TCA

iv. Serotonin agonist like buspirone, LSD; sumatriptan

v. Non-specific; Lithium therapy; Tramadol; ECT; Carbamazepine; Nefazodone. St. John's wort, Linezolid, ginseng

Treatments of serotonin syndrome

- Benzodiazepines
- Intubation
- Ventilation
- Serotonin $5HT_2$ blockers like cyproheptadine, or chlorpromazine.

Other hyperthermic syndromes are:

- **Malignant neuroleptic syndrome:** Occurs with D_2 blocking antipsychotics. Treated with diphenhydramine, sedation by benzodiazepines and cooling.

- **Malignant hyperthermia:** Occurs with succinylcholine, treated with dantrolene and cooling.

Prostaglandins

Kurzork and Leib, two American gynecologists in 1930, observed that human uterus contracts or relaxes when they are exposed to semen. Thinking that active is principal derived from prostrate, they called it prostaglandins. Bergstorm, Samuelson and Vane got Nobel Prize in 1982 for their work on prostaglandins and leukotrienes which are biologically active derivatives of 20 carbon atom polyunsaturated essential fatty acids, that are released from cell membrane phospholipids. The prostaglandins (PGs) are the derivatives of prostanoic acid. *Leukotrienes* with three double bonds (trienes) and were first isolated from leukocytes. The PGs, LTs and TXs are derived from eicosa (20 atom) called *eicosanoids* which are universally distributed autacoids in the body. The substrate for synthesis of eicosanoid (Greek eikosi = twenty) and platelet activating factor are supplied by membrane lipid. Eicosanoids are metabolites of arachidonic acid. These are not stored, but produced by cell to different stimuli, *viz.* physical, chemical and humoral which activate acyl hydrolases to make available arachidonate. Prostaglandins, prostacyclines and thromboxanes are called prostanoids. Its synthesis is shown in the Fig. 10.1.

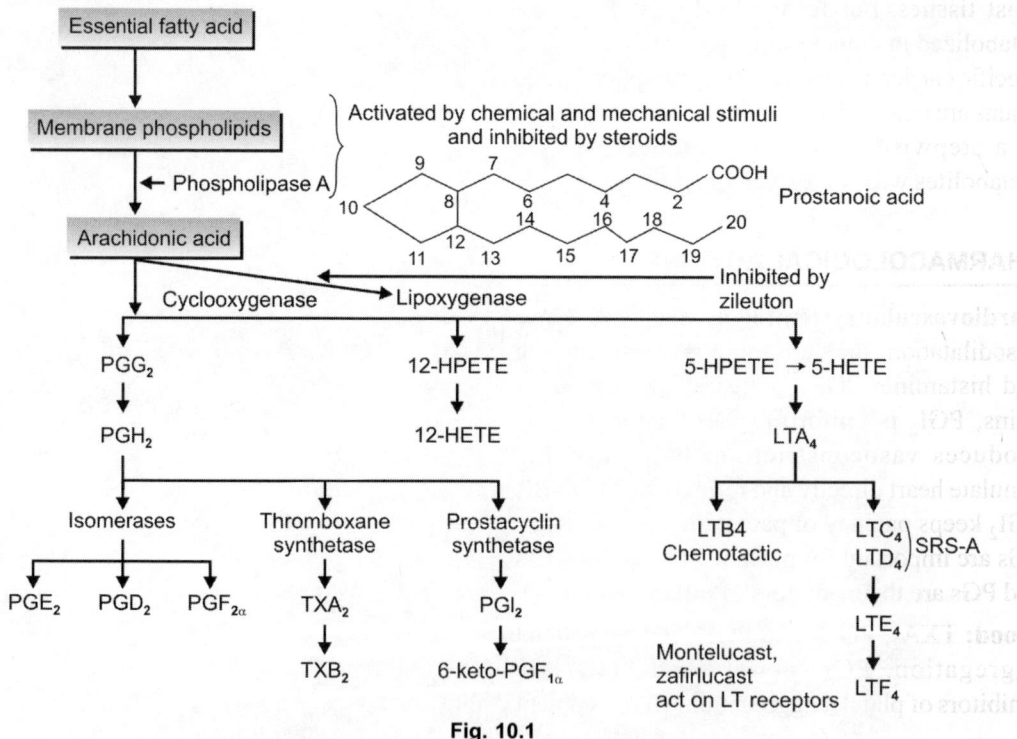

Fig. 10.1

The PGE is partitioned into ether, while PGF partitioned into phosphate (Fosfat) buffer, α-refers to position of –OH group.

Cyclooxygenase exists in two isoforms COX-1 and COX-2 which are **constitutive** housekeeping; and **inducible** respectively. COX-2 is responsible for inflammatory and pathological process. COX-2 has larger flexible substrate channel and large space where inhibitors bind. COX-2 gene transcription is induced by stress injury, ischemia and its expression is inhibited by glucocorticoid.

Some COX-2 inhibitors are celecoxib = diclofenac = meloxicam = etodolac < valdecoxib << rofecoxib < lumiracoxib

NSAIDs produce competitive, reversible inhibition of COX enzymes, while aspirin acetylates COX at a serine residue causing irreversible inhibition of COX.

Glucocorticoid stimulates lipocortin or annexin (peptide) which inhibits phospholipase A2 and production of all eicosanoids (PGs, TXs, LTs).

The arachidonates are rapidly destroyed in most tissues, but fastest by lungs. PGI_2 are catabolized in kidney, some uptake by cells in a specific carrier mechanism. After reuptaken, side chains are oxidized and double bonds are reduced in a stepwise manner to produce inactive metabolites which are excreted through urine.

PHARMACOLOGICAL ACTIONS

Cardiovascular system: PGE_2 and PGA_2 cause vasodilatation, they are more potent than ACh and histamine. $PGF_{2\alpha}$ constricts many larger veins, PGI_2 is uniformly vasodilatory. TXA_2 produces vasoconstriction. PGE_2 and $F_{2\alpha}$ simulate heart directly and reflexly by fall in BP, PGI_2 keeps patency of patent ductus arteriosus. PGs are important for placental blood flow. LTs and PGs are the mediators of inflammation.

Blood: TXA_2, PGG_2 and PGH_2 induce platelet aggregation. PGI_2 mainly and PGD_2 are inhibitors of platelet aggregation, LTB_4 is potent chemotactic agent for polymorphonuclear leukocytes. PGA_2, PGF_2 and $PGF_{2\alpha}$ induce erythropoiesis by stimulating release of erythropoietin. PGD_2, 5-HPETE and 5-HETE release histamines from human basophils, while PGI_2 inhibits histamine release.

SMOOTH MUSCLES

Uterus: PGE_2 and $F_{2\alpha}$ contract pregnant and non-pregnant uterus. Fetal tissues produce $PGF_{2\alpha}$ and initiates progression of labor. The semen contains high concentration of PGs, coordinate its migration from vagina during coitus. High level of PGs causing incoordinate uterine contraction, compress blood vessels and uterine ischemia causing dysmenorrhea.

Bronchial smooth muscle: $PGF_{2\alpha}$, PGD_2, and TXA_2 are bronchoconstrictors; PGE_2 and PGI_2 are bronchodilators.

GI tract: Longitudinal muscle contract, propulsive activity is enhanced resulting in colics and watery diarrhea (increases water, electrolyte and mucus secretion). PGE_2 reduces acid secretion, juice volume and pepsin content of gastric juice (histamine, gastrin induced secretion). Secretion of mucus and its blood flow is also increased.

Kidney: PGE_2 and PGI_2 increase water, Na^+ and K^+ excretion with diuretic effect, renal vasodilatation, inhibit tubular reabsorption and antagonizes ADH action. TXA_2 causes renal vasoconstriction. PGI_2, PGE_2, and PGD_2 release renin. The diuretic effect of frusemide is blunted by NSAID.

Bartter syndrome: Characterized by hypokalemia, hyperreninemia, hyperaldosteronism, juxtaglomerular hyperplasia, normotensin and resistance to the pressure effect of angiotensin II due to excessive production of renal prostaglandin, can be effectively treated by aspirin and indomethacin group of drugs.

CNS: Does not cross blood-brain barrier, causes sedation and produces fever. It acts as neuromodulator.

Peripheral nerves: It (PGE_2 and I_2) sensitizes nerve ending to chemical and mechanical stimuli and on applicatoin to mucous membrane produces dull long lasting pain.

Endocrine system: Growth, prolactin, ACTH, FSH and LH, insulin, adrenal steroid secretions are facilitated by PGE_2, $PGF_{2\alpha}$ causes leutolysis and terminates early pregnancy.

Metabolism: PGEs mobilize Ca^{2+} from bone, antilipolytic and exerting an insulin like effect on carbohydrate metabolism.

Eye: $PGF_{2\alpha}$ induces ocular inflammation and enhances uveoscleral outflow to lower intraocular tension. Non-irritating congeners like latanoprost is used for glaucoma. New drugs of this group are bimatoprost, travoprost, unoprostone.

Some prostaglandin analogues of clinical importance

Prostaglandin	Drug	Used for
PGE_1	Alprostadil	To maintain ductus arteriosus, Errectile disorder antiplatelet
PGE_2	Misoprostol, rioprostil	Peptic ulcer
PGE_2	Misoprostol & Mifepristine (Antiprogestin)	MTP
PGF_2	Latanoprost Travoprost. Bimatoprost Unoprostone	Glaucoma
PGI_2	Epoprostenol, iloprost, Treprostinil	Used for pulmonary hypertension
$PGF_{2\alpha}$	Carboprost, dinoprost	Second trimester abortion, to control PPH.
PGI_2	Beraporst	For peripheral vascular disease
PGE_1	Lubiprostone	Constipation

11

Leukotrienes

These are staight chain lipoxygenase products of arachidonic acid produced by neutrophils, LTB$_4$, LTC$_4$ and LTD$_4$ by macrophages. Lipoxygenases are non-heme iron-containing enzymes that catalyze oxygenation of polyenic fatty acids to lipid hydroperoxides.

Lipoxygenase operates mainly in lungs, WBC and platelets to produce leukotrienes (generated by 5-LOX). Membrane associated transfer protein called five lipoxygenase activating protein (FLAP) carries arachidonic acid to 5 LOX-LT$_4$, a product of 5-LOX can be converted to LXA$_4$ via 12 LOX in platelets. 15 LOX-1 prefers linoleic acid as a substrate forming 15-hydroxyoctadecanoic acid. HPETE produced by LOX can be converted to hepoxilin, trioxillin and lipoxin. Cytochrome P450 can metabolize arachidonic acid into 19- and 20-HETE and epoxyeicosatrienoic acid. Isoprostane is produced non-enzymatically from arachidonic acid by free radicals. In the brain cells, arachidonic acid couples to ethonalamine to produce anandamide possessing cannabinoid like action. Epidermal accumulation of 12(R)-HETE is a feature of psoriasis and ichthyosis.

Leukotriene receptors: Seperate receptors for LTB$_4$; LTC$_4$ and LTD$_4$ are identified all of which function through IP$_3$/DAG transducer mechanism. Montelukast and zafirlucast are leukotriene receptor antagonists used for bronchial asthma.

Functions of leukotrienes

When injected IV: Brief rise of BP followed by prolong fall. The fall is due to coronary constriction, causing reduction of cardiac output and circulatory volume due to increased capillary permeability by LTC$_4$ and LTD$_4$. Migration of neutrophils through capillaries and their clumping at inflammation site is promoted by LTB$_4$. Most of the smooth muscles contract (bronchial; GIT).

Increases mucus secretion of airways. Afferent nerves are sensitized to carry pain of inflammation.

Prostanoid receptors: PG and TX act on specific receptor on cell membrane which are G-protein coupled receptors.

DP has affinity of PGD$_2$, but with some actions on PGE$_2$ when stimulated increases cAMP which inhibits platelet aggregation.

EP has affinity for PGE$_2$. Enprostil is a selective agonist. EP are of two types.
- EP$_1$—smooth muscle contraction through IP$_3$/DAG pathway.
- EP$_2$—smooth muscle relaxation by increasing cAMP.
- EP$_3$ and EP$_4$ are identified by cloning.

FP has affinity for PGF$_{2\alpha}$. Fluprostenol is an agonist, causes smooth muscle contraction mediated through IP$_3$/DAG.

IP has affinity for PGI$_2$. Cicaprost is an agonist, increases cAMP. Inhibits platelet aggregation and causes smooth muscle contraction.

TP has affinity for TXA$_2$. PGH$_2$ also acts on it. Two types are known TP platelets, aggregate platelets and TP non-platelet, causing smooth muscle contraction.

Separate receptors LTB$_4$, LTC$_4$, LTD$_4$ are **differentiated and all function through transduction of IP$_3$/DAG.**

Therapeutic uses of PG analogue

- Abortion, molar gestation by PGE_2, vaginal pessary reduces trauma of abortion.
- Induction of labor in place of oxytocin in toxemia and renal failure patients because they do not retain fluid. Intravaginal routes are preferred to oral, IV, intra- and extra-amniotic routes.
- Cerical priming by applying intravaginally.
- Postpartum hemorrhage (carboprost, 15-methyl $PGF_{2\alpha}$, IM).
- Peptic ulcer PGE_1 (misoprostol, rioprostil) (PGE_2) (enprostil).
- To maintain potency of ductus arteriosus (PGE_1) (alprostadil).
- To avoid platelet damage (PGI_2) (epoprostenol) during hemodialysis and cardiopulmonary bypass; to harvest platelet for transfusion.
- Peripheral vascular diseases (PGI_2), IV (PGI_2) for Raynaud's disease.
- To reduce infarct size (PGI_2)
- Pulmonary hypertension PGI_2 (epoprostenol, treprostinil by continuous SC infusion.
- Impotence (PGE_1) under investigational level (alprostadil injected into penis).
- Glaucoma: Latanoprost, travoprost, unoprostone, bimatoprost. May causes brown pigment of iris, conjunctivitis, drying of eyes may occur.
- Inducing contraception
- Bronchial asthma (aerosolized PGE_2).

Side effects of prostaglandins

- Nausea
- Vomiting
- Watery diarrhea
- Uterine cramps
- Vaginal bleeding
- Flushing, shivering
- Fever
- Malaise
- Hypotension
- Chest pain
- Forceful uterine contraction.

Some preparations of PG used for induction of labor and abortion

- Vaginal gel 1 mg or 2 mg/2–5 ml, 1 mg inserted in posterior fornix, repeat after 6 hours, if required.
- Vaginal tab 3 mg inserted in posterior fornix to be repeated after 6 hours, if required.
- Extra-amniotic solution 10 mg/ml in 0.5 mL ampoule rarely used.
- Intravenous solution 1 mg/ml in 0.75 ampoule: 10 mg/ml in 0.5 ml ampoule used rarely.
- Oral tablet (primiprost 0.5 mg tab) 1 tab hourly till induction rarely used.
- Cervical gel (cerviprime 0.5 mg in 2.5 ml prefilled syringes) used for preinduction, inserted in cervical canal in patient with poor Bishop's score.
- Gemeprost (cervagem 1 mg vaginal pessary) for dilating OS or attempting dilatation.
- $PGF_{2\alpha}$ (dinoprost 5 mg/mL in 4 mL ampoule) for abortion or induction of labor.
- 15-methyl $PGF_{2\alpha}$ (Prostodin 0.25 mg/mL) every ½ to 2 hours for abortion or PPH.
- T-pill + MISO mifeprostone 200 mg (3 tabs + misoprostol 200 µg (2 tablets) for termination of pregnancy up to 49 days.

Recent Advances in PG; TX and Leukotrienes

Zileuton (Lox inhibitors) trialed for allergic rhinitis and inflammatory bowel disease and asthma.

Dazoxiben and Primagrel: TX synthetase inhibitors trialed for vasospastic, thrombotic, respiratory disorders; pre-eclampsia but without any encouraging results.

PG receptor antagonists: Sulotroban, vapiprost are TP receptor antagonists, inhibit platelet aggregation and have potential use of cardiovascular, renal and allergic diseases.

Search for PAF antagonist is going on.

12

Platelet Activating Factors

Platelet activating factor (PAF) is a cell membrane derived polar lipid with intense biological action. Membrane glycerophosphocholine derivative can modify enzymatically to produce PAF in some cells like endothelial cells, leukocytes and platelets.

Actions of PAF

- Platelet aggregation and TXA2 are released.
- Chemotactic to neutrophils, eosinophils and monocytes (LTs are involved)
- Blood vessels dilate due to EDRF leading to fall BP.
- Smooth muscle contracts directly and by LT release.
- Stomach—ulcerogenic and contracts gastric smooth muscle.

PAF acts through G-protein coupled receptor which acts through IP3/DAG and releases Ca^{2+}.

Many actions of PAF are mediated by LT and TXA, which are considered as their extracellular messengers.

SYNTHESIS AND DEGRADATION OF PAF (Fig. 12.1)

It is derived from cell membrane acyl glycerophosphocholine in WBC; platelet, vascular endothelium; kidney cells on demand, there is no preformed PAF.

It is degraded to lyso-PAF and then to acyl glycerophosphocholine which gets incorporated to the cell membrane by PAF acetyl hydrolase and acyl transferase enzyme respectively.

PAF antagonist: Ginkgolide-B, a Chinese plant, used for strokes, intermittent claudication, vertigo or Meniere's diseases, myocardial infarction, shock, gastrointestinal ulcer, asthma and contraceptive. Alprazolam and triazolam

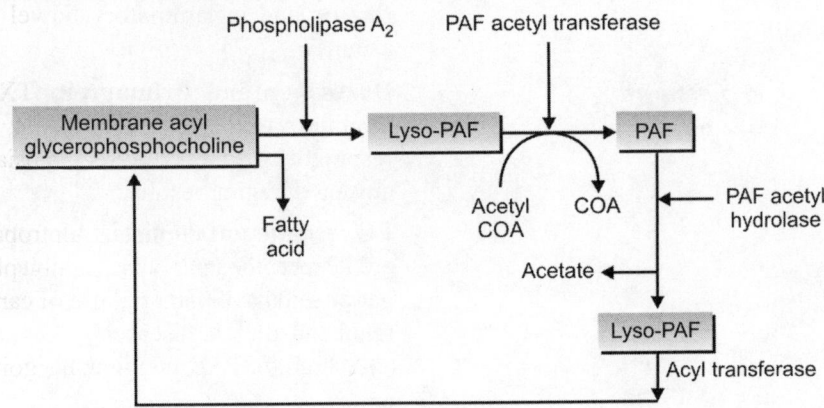

Fig. 12.1: Synthesis and degradation of PAF

antagonize some of the actions of PAF. Rupatadine has some PAF antagonist properties.

PAF has role in following pathological conditions

- Inflammation PAF causes vasodilatation, exudation, hyperalgesia and cellular infiltration.
- Bronchial asthma causes bronchospasm + edema.

- Anaphylactic shock (shock is associated high PAF).
- Stomach—ulcerogenic erosion and mucosal bleeding occurs with IV PAF injection. Stomach smooth muscle contracts.
- Hemostasis by promoting platelet aggregation.
- Rupture of mature Graafian follicle and implantation.
- Labor is delayed by PAF antagonists.
- Ischemic state of brain and heart.

13

Plasma Kinins

Plasma kinins are polypeptides derived from kininogen by the action of enzyme kallikreins. Kininogens are α_2 globulins present in plasma which also contains inactive prekallikrein activated by factor XII (Hageman factor) which itself is activated by tissue injury, collagen basement membrane, bacterial liposaccharides and urate crystals. Plasmin activates Hageman factor. Trypsin, snake venom also generate kinin present in kidney, pancreas, bradykinin (nonapeptide) generated from high molecular weight kininogen, while kallidin is produced by both low and high molecular weight kininogens. Removal of lysine residue by aminopeptidase also produces bradykinins from kallidin. Kinins are rapidly degraded in lungs by enzyme kininase II or angiotensin II converting enzyme (ACE) which spits off 2 amino acids from carboxy-terminal of peptide chain. Carboxypeptidase kinase I removes only one amino acid (arginine) producing des-Arg bardykinin and des-Arg kallidin which are degraded by peptidases.

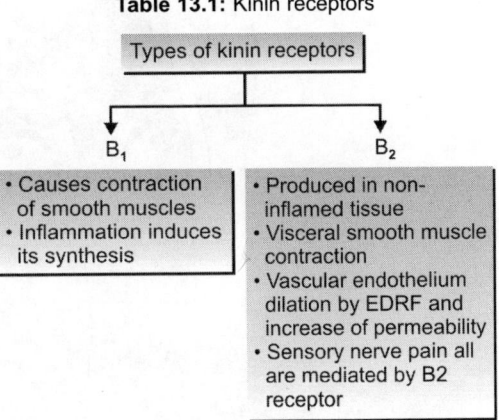

Table 13.1: Kinin receptors

Types of kinin receptors	
B₁	**B₂**
• Causes contraction of smooth muscles • Inflammation induces its synthesis	• Produced in non-inflamed tissue • Visceral smooth muscle contraction • Vascular endothelium dilation by EDRF and increase of permeability • Sensory nerve pain all are mediated by B2 receptor

Bradykinin has higher affinity for B_2, kallidin for both B_1 and B_2. des-Arg metabolites of bradykinin and killidin have affinity for B1 receptor. Both are GPCR

Kinins have no potential pharmacological actions, but they are involved in following pathological conditions:

• Mediators of inflammation, pain and hyperemia, production of inflammatory mediators like ILI and TNFα.

• Closely related to clotting, fibrinolysin and completement systems.

• Closes PDA and constriction of umbilical vessels and adjusts fetal to neonatal circulation.

• Shock, angioedema, asthma, ACE inhibitor induced cough, dumping syndrome, carcinoid syndrome, diarrheas, pancreatitis, immune reaction are also due to kinins.

Kinins have no therapeutic use.

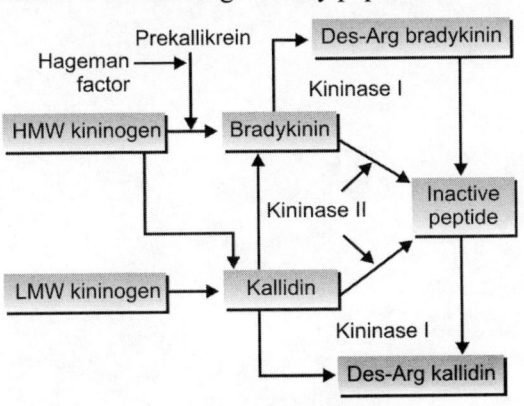

Fig. 13.1: Generation of kinin and its degradation

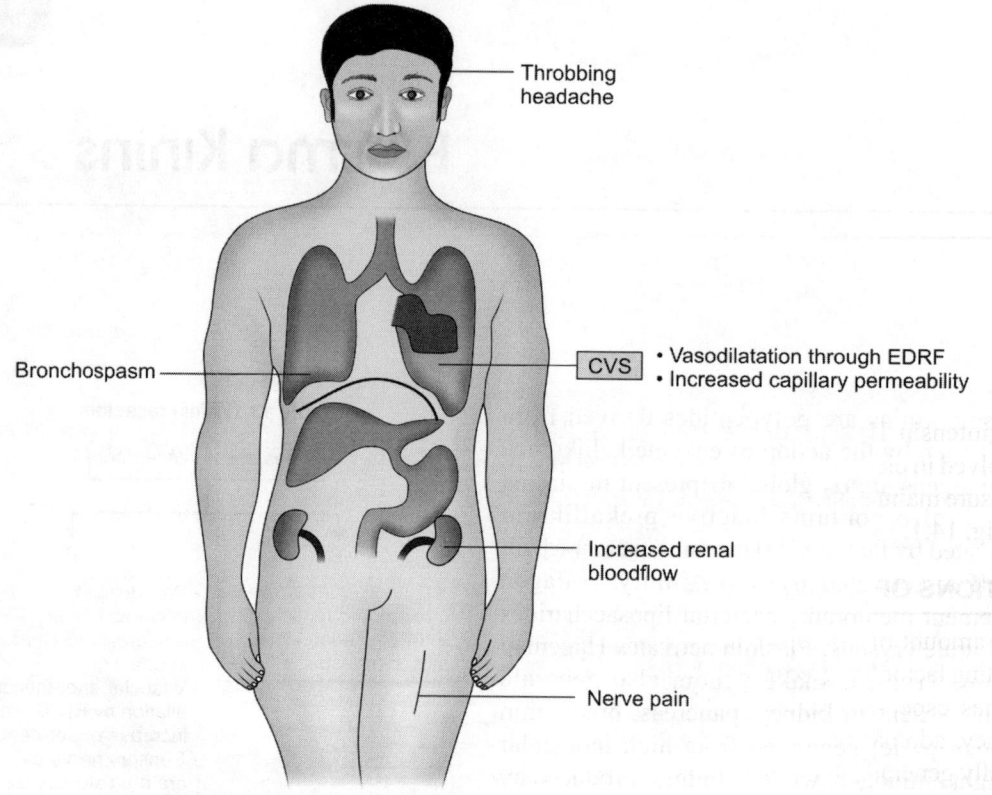

Fig. 13.1: Actions of kinins

Bradykinin antagonists : Several B_1 and B_2 receptor antagonists are produced. Icatibant is B_2 antagonist with long t/2. Icatibant; FR 173657 are orally active B_2 antagonist have undergone limited trial as analgesic, antiinflammatory in pancreatitis and head injury. **Icabitant** is approved for hereditary angioedama in Europe. Synthesis of kinins can be inhibited by **aprotinin, cinryze, berinert.** Which are used for prophylaxis or treatment of angioedema. ACE inhibitors enhances kinins action. **Ecallantide** is recombinant plasma kallikrein inhibitor.

Angiotensin

Angiotensin II is produced from α_2 globulin involved in electrolyte, blood volume and blood pressure maintenance, is produced as mentioned in Fig. 14.1.

ACTIONS OF ANGIOTENSIN

The amount of renin in plasma acts as the rate limiting factor for angiotensin II formation. Many tissues especially heart, blood vessels, brain, kidney, adrenals have all enzyme systems and locally generate angiotensin II.

Two types of angiotensin receptors are known and cloned.

Types of angiotensin receptors

AT1	AT2
• G-protein coupled receptor • Losartan selective antagonist	• PD 123177 selective antagonist, function not clear, found in adrenal medulla, CNS

Pathophysiological Role of Angiotensin

i. Mineralocorticoid secretion by angiotensin II and III.
ii. Increase BP by vasoconstriction—Na and H_2O retention.
iii. Development of hypertension.
iv. Secondary hyperaldosteronism.
v. Angiotensin II in brain regulates thirst.

REGULATION OF RENIN RELEASED BY DRUGS

• Vasodilator and diuretic stimulate PRA by lowering BP so does ACE inhibitors and AT1.
• Loop diuretics increase renin production by reducing entry of Na^+ into macula densa cells.
• Central sympatholytic and β blockers decrease renin by depressing β-adrenoceptor pathway.
• NSAID decreases PRA release by inhibiting PG production.

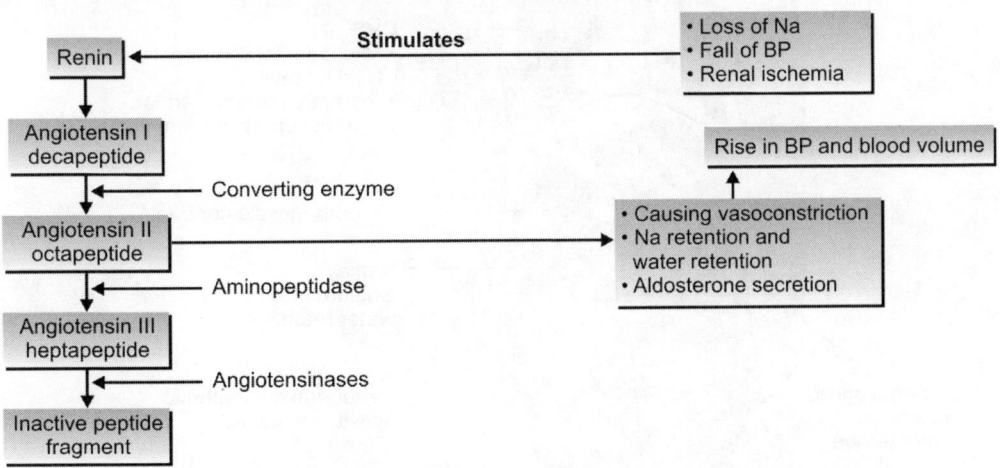

Fig. 14.1: Regulation of renin-angiotensin system

Therapeutic use: Angiotensin II is to counteract anesthesia-induced hypotension because it does not produce secondary hypotension, tissue necrosis on extravasation, however, it may precipitate myocardial ischemia. It is not commercially marketed.

Pharmacological actions of Angiotensin II shown in Fig. 14.1.

Inhibition of Renin-Angiotensin System

- Sympathetic blocker decreases renin release.
- ACE inhibitors prevent conversion of angiotensin II.
- Angiotensin receptor (ATI) antagonist blocks action of angiotensin II.
- Aldosterone antagonist blocks mineralocorticoid receptors.
- Direct renin inhibitors block renin action.

ANGIOTENSIN-CONVERTING ENZYME INHIBITORS (ACE-I)

Captopril was first orally active ACE inhibitor introduced in 1977. Since then a large number of ACE inhibitors has been produced and grouped into three classes.

Class I (Captopril): Lipid-soluble

Class II (Prodrug): Benazepril, cilazapril, enalapril are converted in body into active form to produce their action, *i.e.* prodrug.

Class III (Lisinopril): Water-soluble

All of them block conversion of angiotensin I to angiotensin II. They also inhibit degradation of bradykinin enkephalins, substance-p.

Pharmacokinetics (captopril as prototype): Up to 70% of the drug is absorbed orally, food interferes with absorption, brain penetration poor, partly metabolized and partly excreted unchanged.

Adverse effects: Hypotension, hyperkalemia, cough, rashes, angioedema, reversible loss of taste (dysgeusia), fetal damage, headache, bowel upset, proteinuria, granulocytopenia, acute renal failure in bilateral renal artery stenosis patient.

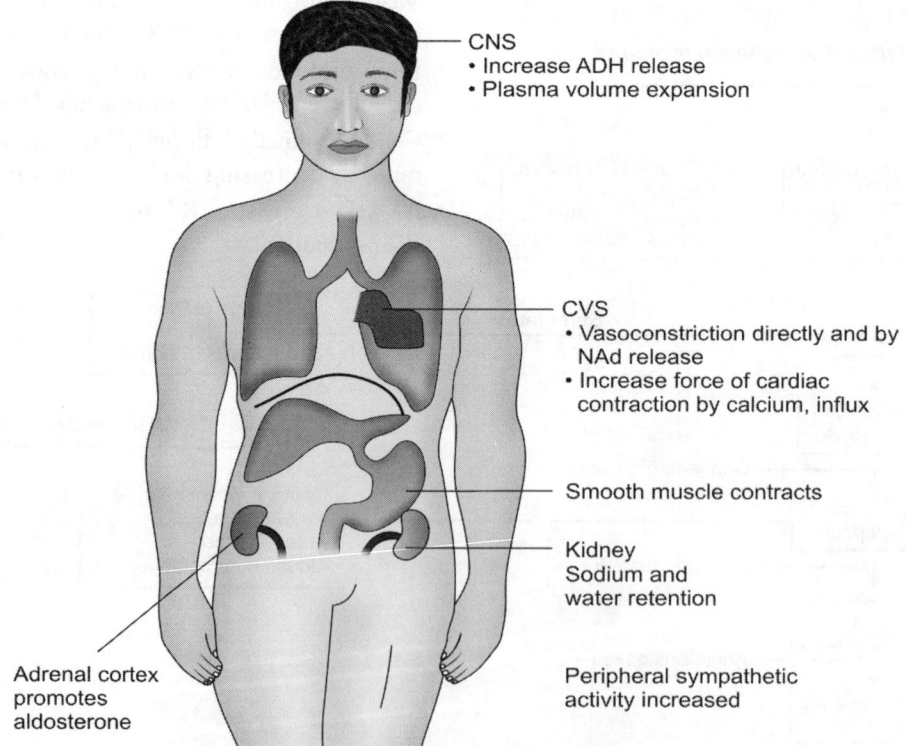

CNS
- Increase ADH release
- Plasma volume expansion

CVS
- Vasoconstriction directly and by NAd release
- Increase force of cardiac contraction by calcium, influx

Smooth muscle contracts

Kidney
Sodium and water retention

Adrenal cortex promotes aldosterone

Peripheral sympathetic activity increased

Fig. 14.1: Pharmacological actions of angiotensin

Therapeutic uses of ACE inhibitors

i. Hypertension with following advantages:
  - No postural hypotension, feeling of weakness and CNS effect.
  - Safe in diabetic, asthmatic, peripheral vascular disease, gouty arthritis, hyperlipidemic patient.
  - Renal blood flow maintained.
  - Reverse LVH
  - No rebound hypertension on withdrawal
  - No disturbances with sleep, sexual function, better quality of life.

ii. CHF and myocardial infarction

iii. Diabetic nephropathy

iv. Scleroderma crisis causing rise of BP and deterioration of renal function caused by angiotensin II can be treated with ACE inhibitors with dramatic improvement and life-saving.

v. Captopril test to diagnose renovascular hypertension .25 mg of captopril administered in sitting and PRA measured 1 hour before and after the drug. A post-drug PRA more than 12 ng/mL/hour or rise in 10 ng/mL/hour over baseline is positive test.

vi. Nondiabetic nephropathy.

ANGIOTENSIN ANTAGONIST

Saralasin is a first angiotensin II antagonist not suitable for clinical use because of partial agonist action. Recently, losartan, valsartan, zolasartin, candesartan are in market. All are AT1 receptor antagonists. Losartin is marked in India. Losartin has almost all side effects of ACE inhibitors.

Recently, many renin inhibitors like aliskiren, enalkiren, remikiren have undergone clinical trials.

ACE-I + β-blockers is BWA 575 C.

ACE-I + atrial natriuretic peptide potentiating glycopril, alatriopril are at research level with good potentialities for hypertension patient not adequately responding to ACE inhibitors.

Newer AT1 blockers

Valsartan (Valent 80 mg caps): AT1 receptor blocker, regresses left ventricular hypertrophy used for essential hypertension and heart failure.

Candesartan (Candelong 4, 8, 16 mg tab): Used once daily AT1 receptor blocker with good patient compliance.

Irbesartan (Irovel 150–300 mg): Oral bioavailability is high.

Telmisartan (Telvas 20; 40; 80 mg): It does not produce active metabolite. Action starts in 2 hours and last 24 hours.

Uses of Angiotensin (AT1) Receptor Blockers

- Hypertension
- CCF
- Myocardial infarction
- Diabetic nephropathy.
- Theoretically ACE inhibitor can be used with ARB.

Endothelins (ETs)

It was first isolated from aortic endothelial cells. Three isoforms are known ET1, ET2 and ET3 which are the products of different genes and synthesized as preproform and ultimately processed to peptide. Endothelin consists of 21 amino acids with two sulfide bridges.

It is rapidly cleared from circulation by enzymatic degradation and by ETB receptor.

ET1 gene expression increased by growth factors, cytokines, angiotensin II, vasopressin and mechanical stress and inhibited by nitric oxide, PGI2 and natriuretic peptide.

Action: Dose dependent vasoconstriction, positive ino- and chronotropic effects on heart, coronary vasoconstriction, renal vasoconstriction to decrease glomerular filtration, broncho-constriction, increased secretion of renin, vasopressin, aldosterone, atrial natriuretic peptide. ET1 is a mitogen for vascular smooth muscle cells, cardiac muscles and glomerular mesengial cells.

ENDOTHELIN RECEPTORS

There are two types of endothelin receptors ETA and ETB

ET_A = High affinity for ET1 and low for ET3. Present in smooth muscle cells.

ET_B = Has equal affinity for ET1 and ET3.

Bosentan is a non-selective antagonist of endothelin receptor. **Sitaxsentan** and **ambri-sentan** are two ET_A selective antagonists. Phosphoramidon inhibits endothelin formation by blocking endothelin coverting enzyme.

Therapeutic potentialities: Endothelin is involved in hypertension, heart hypertrophy, cardiac failure, atherosclerosis. CAD, bronchial asthma, pulmonary hypertension and many kidney diseases may be treated by endothelin antagonist.

Adverse effects of endothelin antagonist (Bosentan): Hypotension, tachycardia, edema, facial flush, headache, nausea, vomiting, constipation, teratogenicity. Bosentan is hepatotoxic. It should not be given to pregnant woman.

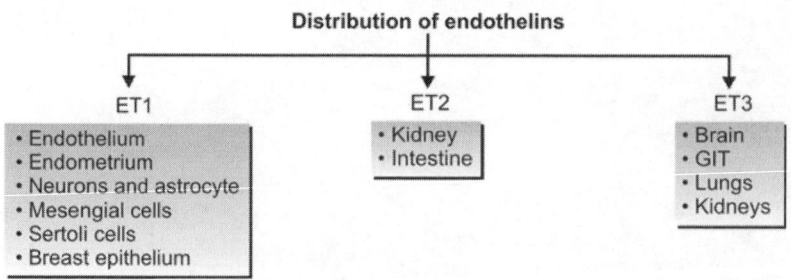

Distribution of endothelins

ET1
- Endothelium
- Endometrium
- Neurons and astrocyte
- Mesengial cells
- Sertoli cells
- Breast epithelium

ET2
- Kidney
- Intestine

ET3
- Brain
- GIT
- Lungs
- Kidneys

Vasoactive Intestinal Peptides (VIPs)

VIP is a 28AA peptide belongs to glucagon secretin family present in central and peripheral nervous systems and also in GI tract, heart, lung, kidney, thyroid gland and blood vessels. In the CVS, it produces vasodilation, coronary dilatation, positive ion and chronotrophic effects.

It acts on VPAC1 and VPAC2 receptors to produce cAMP, activating adenylyl cyclase causing vasodilation. Other actions are probably inositol triphosphate and Ca^{2+} mobilization mediated.

Specific VIP receptor agonist and antagonist are available for research purposes.

Aviptadil is a VIP analogue causes smooth muscle relaxation can be used with phentolamine for erectile dysfunction.

17

Substance P and Neurokinin

Substance P, neurokinin A and B all belong to tachykinin family with common carboxy-terminal. Substance P is undecapeptide and others are decapeptide. Substance P is a neurotransmitter in CNS and ENS.

It is implicated for anxiety, depression, nausea and vomiting. It causes vasodilation.

Actions of substance P and neurokinin are mediated by NK_1, NK_2, NK_3 receptors where NK_1 is present in brain and substance P is its preferred ligand.

NK_1 receptor antagonist, **aprepitant** is highly selective, orally active, penetrates brain, used for chemotherapy induced nausea and vomiting. **Fosaprepitant** prodrug converted to aprepitant given IV for same purpose.

These drugs have potentialities to treat depression.

Neurotensin (NT)

Neurotensin is a tridecapeptide, found in CNS, GIT and circulation, synthesized from larger precursor which also contains **Neuromedin N**. It acts as local hormone in periphery, but acts as neurotransmitter and neuromodulator. In CNS, it is in close association with dopamine so may be involved in schizophrenia, parkinsonism and drug abuse. It acts through neurotensin receptors NTR_1, NTR_2 and NTR_3.

Neurotensin agonist crosses BBB and has potential to treat **schizophrenia** and parkinsonism.

The neurotensin receptor may be blocked by antagonists SR 142948A and SR 48692, which block hypothermia and analgesia produced by centrally administered neurotensin and also block cardiovascular effects of neurotensin.

Calcitonin Gene-Related Peptide (CGRP)

CGRP (37AA), calcitonin, adrenomedullin and amylin belong to calcitonin family peptide. CGRP is present in C cells of thyroid, central and peripheral nervous systems, CVS and GIT and urogenital system. It decreases appetite and raises BP if injected into CNS, but in circulation it produces hypotension and tachycardia. It is most potent vasodilator. It is involved in migraine via Trigeminal Nerve. In human αCGRP and β CGRP forms exists which differ in amino acids and produced by different genes.It mediates its action via calcitonin receptor which is GPCR with receptor activity modifying protein ($RAMP_1$). It has got role in migraine. Selective serotonin agonist used in migraine normalizes CGRP level in cranium, **Olcegepant** and **Telcagepant** is effective in migraine. The later is given orally but it is hepatotoxic. These two are CGRP receptor antagonist.

Adrenomedullin (AM)

Calcitonin family of 52-amino acid peptides are widely distributed, highest concentration in adrenal medulla, anterior pituitary and hypothalamus. Also present in kidney, lung, CVS and GIT.

It dilates vessels, increases Na excretion in kidney, inhibits insulin and aldosterone secretion. It acts as a physiologic antagonist of angiotensin II and endothelin I to protect cardiovascular overload.

It acts through CGRP receptors and also via adrenomedullin receptors AM1 and AM2. Circulating AM levels increase during exercise, essential hypertension, septic shock, heart and kidney failures. It may be beneficial in the treatment of some cardiovascular diseases treatment.

Neuropeptide Y

Consisting of 36-aa, abundantly present in CNS and PNS, near noradrenergic neurons acting as cotransmitter.

It increases feeding, hypotension, hypothemia, respiratory depression, cerebral vasoconstriction, rise in BP, positive chrono- and inotropic actions of heart, renal vasoconstriction.

It acts through receptors Y_1, Y_2, Y_3, Y_4, Y_5 and Y_6.

Y_1 and Y_2 responsible for CVS and peripheral action.

Y_4 has affinity for pancreatic polypeptide.

Y_5 found in brain and controls food intake.

Y_6 has no significant role in human BIBP3226, which is a Y_1 receptor antagonist.

Y_1 and Y_5 are receptor antagonists have potential use in obesity. Others may have role in regulation of hemodynamics of hypertension and cardiac failure.

MECHANISM OF ACTION OF ANTIOBESITY DRUGS (Flowchart 21.1)

Orexin is a peptide with 33-aa acting on orexin receptor stimulates food intake. Ghrelin is an acetylated peptide from stomach mucosa stimulate GH to stimulates food intake. **M**elanocyte-**s**timulating **h**ormone (MSH) and **C**ocaine- and **a**mphetamine-**r**egulated **t**ranscript (CART) stimulate 5HT2 receptor to reduce food intake. Neuropeptide Y (NPY) and **A**gouti-**r**elated **p**eptide (AgRP) stimulate food intake and reduce energy expenditure and increase obesity. Cannabinoid through cannabinoid receptor stimulates NPY and AgRP.

Flowchart 21.1: Regulation of food intake (Physiological and Pharmacological basis)

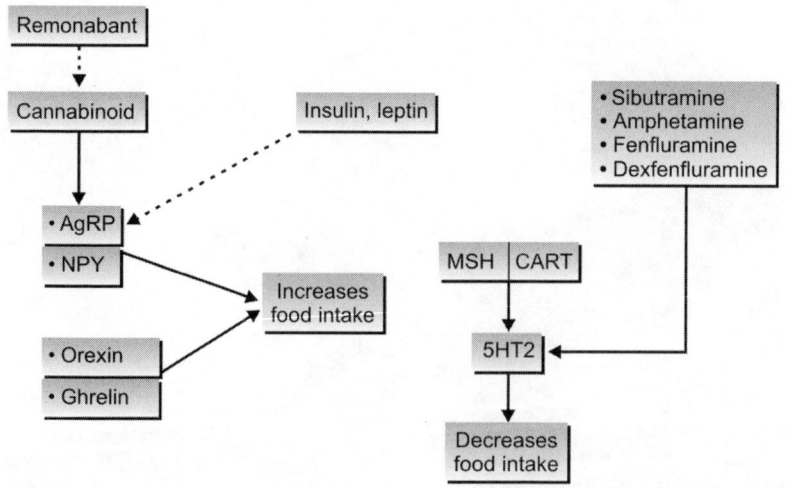

Urotensin (UT)

Urotensin II is 11AA peptide, expresses in brain, spinal cord, kidneys, plasma. It is potent vasoconstrictor. Its receptors are distributed in brain, spinal cord, heart, smooth and skeletal muscles and pancreas.

Palosuran is UT receptor antagonist. Urotensin II level is increased in hypertension; heart failure, diabetes mellitus and kidney failure atherosclerosis.Urantide a nonpeptide urotensin antagonist is penicillamine sustitute.

Nitric Oxide (NO)

Observations made that acetylcholine is not able to relax isolated strips of rabbit aorta when endothelium of it was removed, but can still relax it when nitroglycerine is applied. They call it endothelium-derived relaxation factor or (EDRF). Later, it was proved to be nitric oxide (NO).

Synthesis, Signaling and Inactivation of NO

Nitric oxide is a highly reactive signaling molecule present in neurons, skeletal muscle, endothelial cells and immune system cells. It is produced by NO synthetase (NOS, EC 1.14.13.49) with isoenzymes encoded with separate genes which generate NO from amino acid L-arginine in O_2 and NADPH dependent reaction involving heme, tetrahydrobiopterin and flavin adenine dinucleotide.

The enzyme synthetase has three isoforms, endothelial NOS (eNOS), inducible NOS (iNOS) and neuronal NOS (nNOS). iNOS is inducible in many inflammatory conditions whereas eNOS and nNOS are expressed constitutively.

Signaling mechanism: NO covalently modifies protein. Its targets are: (i) Metalloprotein (ii) thiols and (iii) tyrosine nitration.

Metalloproteins: NO binds to heme to stimulate guanylyl cyclase and increases level of intracellular cGMP which activates protein kinase G to phosphorylation of specific proteins for vasodilatation. NO inhibits cytochrome oxidase responsible for mitochondrial respiration. Heme containing cytochrome P450 is also inhibited by NO responsible for liver disease.

Thiols: NO produces nitrosothiol reacting with thiols (found in amino acid cysteine which can activate or inhibit the activity of these proteins). H-ras which regulates cell division is activated by S-nitrosylation while glyceraldehyde 3-phosphate dehydrogenase is inhibited by S-nitrosylation. Intracellular glutathione interacts with NO to generate S-nitrosoglutathione. Vascular glutathione is decreased in diabetes mellitus, responsible for vascular complications of diabetes.

Tyrosine nitration: Peroxynitrate is a powerful oxidant which can damage DNA and is produced when NO reacts to superoxide.

NO inactivation: NO is also inactivated by superoxide. Scavengers of superoxide anion like superoxide dismutase protects NO and enhances its potency and duration of action. NO reacts with heme and hemeproteins, including oxyhemoglobin which catalyzes NO oxidation to nitrate.

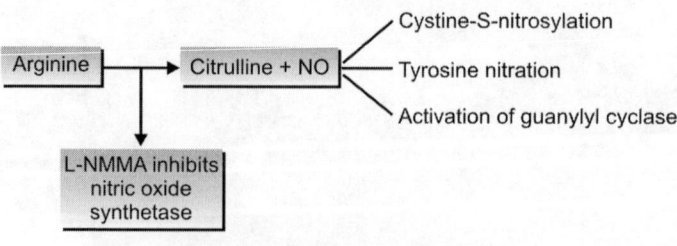

Pharmacological Manipulation of Nitric Oxide

Done by Inhibiting NO Synthesis

- In sepsis, inhibition of iNOS isoform is required, but in neurodegenerative condition eNOS inhibition is required.

NO Donors

- Organic nitrates may produce tolerance.
- Organic nitrites
- Na nitroprusside
- Hybrid NO donor (NOS cap incorporates captopril with nitrosothiol)
- NO gas inhalation in acute respiratory distress syndrome
- Alternate methods: Sildenafil inhibits 5-phosphodiesterase causing NO induce cGMP elevation in several tissues.
- Hydralazine: Acts by partly releasing NO and partly opening K^+ channel.
- Nebivilol: This β-blocker releases NO.

Nitric oxide in Diseases

Vascular effects: NO is a vasodilator. It inhibits thrombosis and atherogenesis, vascular smooth muscle proliferation and increases fibrinolysis.

Septic shock: Lipopolysaccharides of bacterial wall induce iNOS which causes hypotension and shock and can be reversed by NG-monomethyl-L-arginine (L-NMMA).

Inflammation: Numerous cytokines like TNF and interleukin-1 induce iNOS in leukocyte to produce NO which is responsible for vasodilatation, vascular permeability and edema. It stimulates synthesis of PGs in inflammatory site. Inhibitor of iNOS has dose dependent protection in arthritis, psoriasis, inflammatory bowel disease and asthma.

CNS: NO has role as neurotransmitters and neuromodulators or both in process in memory and behavior.

Peripheral nervous system: It acts as neuromediators in non-adrenergic, non-cholinergic neurons (NANC) and neurons of gastrointestinal and reproductive tracts.

Respiratory diseases: NO decreases pulmonary artery pressure to improve oxygenation of blood. In newborn, it is used when extracorporeal membrane oxygenation (ECMO) fails. It has role in adult respiratory distress syndrome also. **Sildenafil** reduces pulmonary hypertension.

Preparation available: Nitric oxide (INOmax) by inhalation of 100 and 800 ppm gas.

24

Natriuretic Peptides

The mammalian atria and other tissue contain some peptides with natriuretic and diuretic. Vasorelaxant properties are like atrial natriuretic peptide (ANP), brain natriuretic peptide (BNP) and C type natriuretic peptide (CNP) and urodilatin.

ANP is synthesized in cardiac atrial cells, ventricular myocardium, lungs, central and peripheral nervous systems from common precursor termed as prepro-ANP and is released by atrial stretch, volume expansion, exercises changing from standing to supine position, sympathetic stimulation *via* $\alpha 1$ adrenoceptor, endothelin *via* ETA receptor, glucocorticoids and vasopressin. Its concentration rises in heart failure, chronic renal failure, inappropriate ADH secretion syndrome and primary aldosteronism.

It produces sodium excretion and urinary flow, GFR with little change in renal blood flow, inhibits renin aldosterone and vasopressin secretion, causes vasodilatation and decreases atrial BP.

BNP also shows natriuretic, diuretic and hypotensive effects. CNP generally present in brain, vascular endoth\elium. It is potent vasodilator.

Urodilantin synthesized in distal tubules and posses diuretic, natriuretic and relaxes vascular smooth muscle.

ANP acts via ANP_A, ANP_B, ANP_C receptors. Primary ligands for ANP_A are ANP and BNP; for ANP_B primary ligand is CNP.

Nesiritide is a recombinant BNP when given to heart failure patient increases natriuresis and improves hemodynamics, but it causes renal damage. Synthetic urodilatin has beneficial effect on heart failure and cirrhosis patients when given IV.

Vasopeptidase inhibitors inhibit metallo-protease enzymes NEP 24.11 and ACE and thereby increase level of natriuretic peptide and decrease the level of angiotensin II and so decrease vasoconstriction and enhance vasodilatation and sodium excretion. Some vasopeptidase inhibitors are **omapatrilat**, **sampatrilat** and **fasidotrilat**.

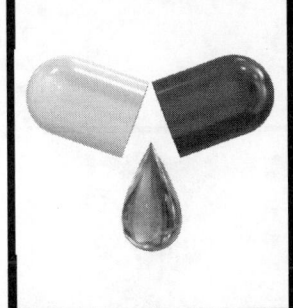
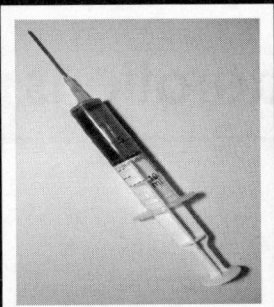
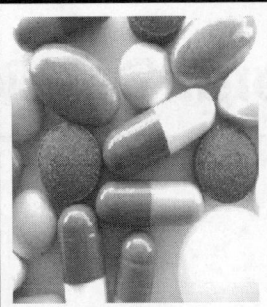
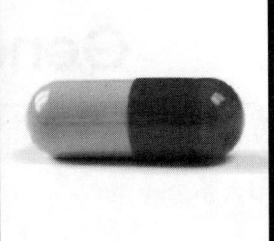

SECTION 3

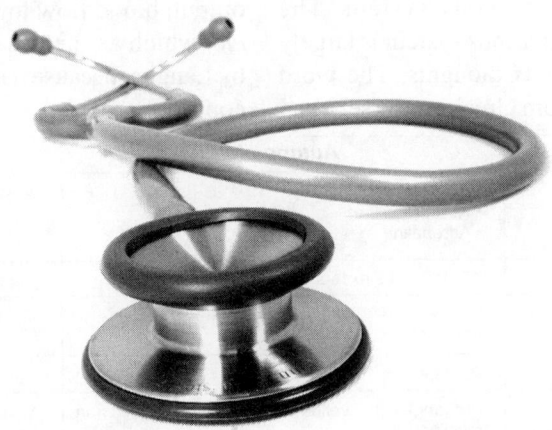

AUTONOMIC NERVOUS SYSTEM

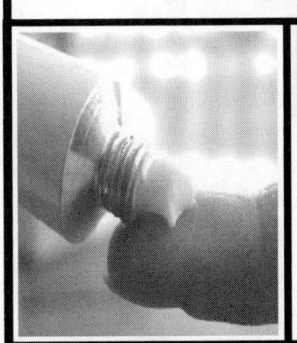
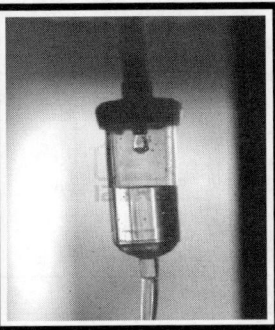
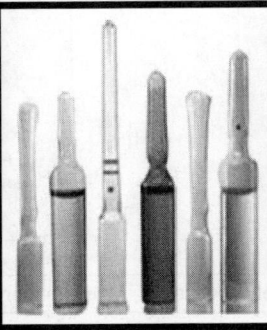
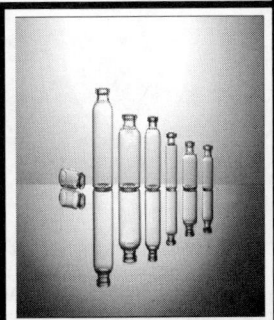

25

General Considerations

The nervous system as convention divided in (CNS) central nervous system (brain and spinal cord) and other outside CNS called peripheral nervous system (PNS). Two divisions (i) somatic and (ii) autonomic which belong to motor (efferent) portion of nervous system. The function of autonomic nervous system is largely independent of conscious thoughts. The word autonomic is derived from Greek *autos* (self) and *nomos* (law of governing). It regulates the activity of smooth muscle mass largely present in hollow viscera, exocrine glands, smooth muscles containing structures of eye pupil, ciliary muscles, pilomotor muscles of skin, cardiac output, blood flow to various organs, digestion, *etc.* which are necessary for life. It is so named by Langley because it is independent of volitional control.

	Autonomic	Somatic
1. Humoral transmitter	• Acetylcholine • Noradrenaline • Adrenaline	Acetylcholine
2. Organ	All structures except skeletal muscles	Skeletal muscle
3. Distal most synaptic junction	Outside cerebrospinal axis, *i.e.* autonomic ganglion	Inside cerebrospinal axis
4. Peripheral plexus formation	Present	Absent
5. Myelin sheath	Preganglionic myelinated and postganglionic non-myelinated	Myelinated
6. Results of nerve damage	Smooth muscle and glands maintain automatic activity	Skeletal muscles are paralyzed and atrophied.

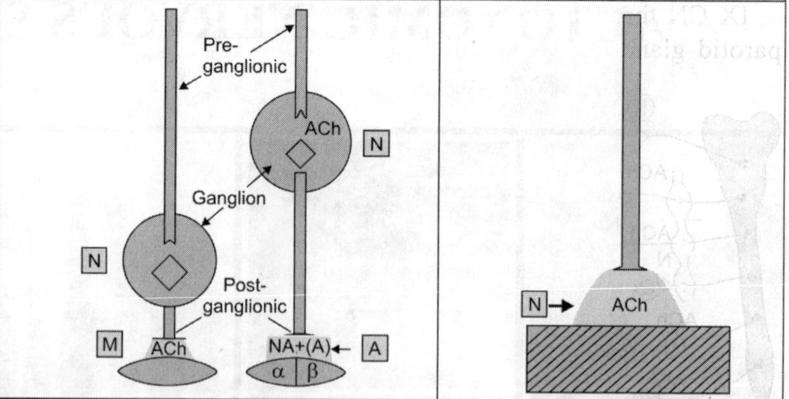

NB: N = Nicotinic, ACh = Acetylcholine, M = Muscarinic, NA = Noradrenaline

Fig. 25.1: Difference between autonomic and somatic nervous systems

Whereas somatic division consciously controls movement, posture and respiration. Both the divisions have afferent (sensory) inputs which modify efferent (motor output) *via* reflex arc.

The autonomic nervous system comprises two broad divisions:

i. Parasympathetic   ii. Sympathetic.

Similarities between nervous system and endocrine system

i. High level of integration in brain and influence distance organs.

ii. Both the systems use chemical transmitters which either stimulate or inhibit the target.

DISTRIBUTION OF PARASYMPATHETIC NERVOUS SYSTEM

Afferent impulses from the viscera, which reflexly modify the autonomic functions and efferent supplies to glands, smooth muscles, heart and viscera through craniosacral outflow. Midbrain through Edingar Westphal nucleus supplies to 3rd cranial oculomotor nerve terminates in ciliary ganglion. Postganglionic fibers from ciliary ganglion supply to ciliary muscle and circular muscles of sphincter pupilla.

From medulla through facial (VII CN); glossopharyngeal (IX CN) and vagus (X CN). VII CN supplies to submaxillary and sublingual, and lacrimal glands through submaxillary ganglion.

IX CN through otic ganglion supplies to parotid gland. X CN supplies secretomotor and vasodilator fibers to visceras of thorax and abdomen with exception of lower third of GI tract.

The sacral outflow supplies to lower third of GI tract, urinary bladder and sex organs. The terminal ganglion in parasympathetic system located near innervated tissues.

DISTRIBUTION OF SYMPATHETIC NERVOUS SYSTEM

The preganglionic fibers of sympathetic system originate from lateral column of 8th cervical to 2nd and 3rd lumbar segments (thoracolumbar outflow) to supply the sympathetic ganglia which are of five types:

i. **Paravertebral:** Twenty-two pairs on either side of vertebral column. The first three pairs of paravertebral ganglion, known as superior, middle and inferior cervical ganglia supply to sphincter pupilla, sublingual and submaxillary salivary glands.

ii. **Prevertebral:** Present in abdomen and pelvis are coeliac, superior, inferior mesenteric and aorticorenal ganglia. The postganglionic fiber from them supply to abdominal visceras, external genitalia and urinary bladder.

iii. **Terminal ganglia:** Postganglionic fibers from them supply to rectum and urinary bladder.

iv. **Intermediate ganglion:** Postganglionic fiber from them (1st to 4th thoracic) form cardiac, esophageal and pulmonary plexuses to supply those organs.

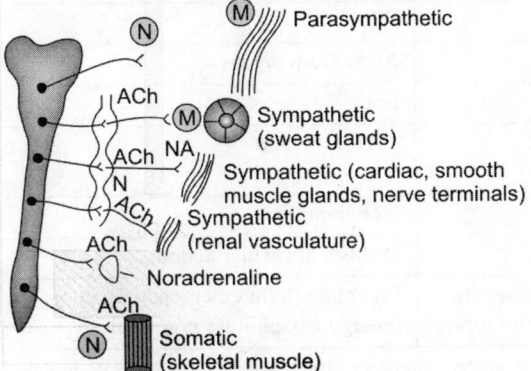

Fig. 25.2: Distribution of sympathetic nervous system

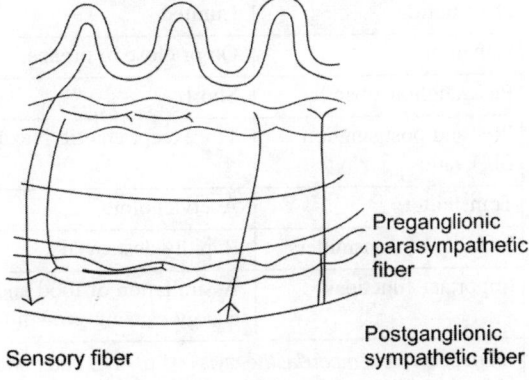

Fig. 25.3: Enteric nervous system

v. Adrenal medulla: Embryologically it belongs to sympathetic ganglion without any postganglionic fiber.

Enteric Nervous System (ENS) (Fig. 25.3)

It is highly a collection of organized neurons of gastrointestinal system and is said to be the third division of autonomic nervous system, includes submucous plexus and myoenteric plexus. They receive preganglionic parasympathetic, postganglionic sympathetic and sensory inputs from the gut wall and control motility and secretory cells. Parasympathetic and sympathetic fibers on enteric plexus play modulatory role. It acts as semiautonomous manner.

NEUROTRANSMITTER

Langley postulated there is excitatory and inhibitory substance in the effector organ.

Dubois Raymond (1877) first suggested about junctional transmission as either electrical or chemical. **Kunhe** (1888) showed skeletal muscle excitation by the current of nerve impulse. **Elliot** (1904) showed sympathetic nerve impulses are acted by liberation of adrenaline and **Dixon** (1906) proposed that parasympathetic activity by liberation of muscarinic like substance.

Otto Loewi (1921) and **Navratil** showed vagus stimulation inhibited the heart and allowed the perfusion fluid (donor) to second recipient frog heart and that heart arrested by stimulation of vagus of first frog. Since there was no connection between two frog hearts, they concluded it was due to chemical substance. They called it as vagusstoff which was later established as acetylcholine. **Barger** and **Dale** (1910) used the term sympathomimetic. Cardio accelerator neurohumoral transmitter nor adrenaline was established by **von-Euler** (1946).

The neurotransmitters are substances which transmit message across nerve synapses must satisfy the following criteria:

- The transmitter and the enzyme capable for their synthesis must be present at the nerve.
- The transmitter must be released when the nerves are stimulated.
- The transmitter given extrinsically, must mimic the effect of nerve stimulation.
- The enzyme or enzyme systems capable of inactivating the proposed transmitter must be present in the nearby tissues.
- The drug which alters the response to nerve stimulation, should alter the response of the proposed transmitter in the same way.

The neurotransmitters established for autonomic nervous systems are:

- **Acetylcholine:** A large number of peripheral ANS fibers synthesizes and releases

Table 25.1: Difference between parasympathetic and sympathetic nervous systems

	Parasympathetic	*Sympathetic*
Origin	Craniosacral	Thoracolumbar
Distribution	Limited	Wide
Ganglion	On or close to organs	Away from organs
Postganglion fiber	Short	Long
Pre- and postganglion fiber ratio	1:1 except enteric plexus	1:20 to 1:100
Transmitter	Acetylcholine	Noradrenaline
Stability of transmitters	Rapidly destroyed	Diffuses for wider action
Important functions	Assimilation of food and conserve energy causing growth (trophotropic)	Fight and flight emergency functions. (energy expenditure ergotropic)

In midbrain and medulla, the divisions of ANS and endocrine system integrate with sensory inputs and information from higher centers of CNS.

acetylcholine called *cholinergic fibers, viz.* preganglionic autonomic and non-autonomic somatic fibers, *i.e.* all fibers leaving CNS are cholinergic. Most postganglionic parasympathetic and a few postganglionic sympathetic fibers release acetylcholine. Some postganglionic parasympathetic fibers utilize nitric oxide or peptide.

- **Noradrenaline:** Mostly released by postganglionic sympathetic fibers. Adrenal medulla releases adrenaline and noradrenaline.

- **Dopamine:** It is an important neurotransmitter of CNS, also released by some sympathetic fibers. The actions of autonomic nerves are also moderated by several cotransmitters.

Steps in Neurohumoral Transmission
(Fig. 25.4)

1. **Impulse conduction:** Normal resting transmembrane potential (−70 mv negative inside) is due to increased K^+ inside and Na^+ outside. Nerve on stimulation causes its depolarization and increases Na^+ conductance inside becomes +20 mv inside and increase inside Na^+ concentration and an action potential, thus produced initiates local circuits which activate next excitable part, *i.e.* node of Ranvier and action potential is propagated.

↓

2. **Transmitter release:** The neurotransmitter stored in presynaptic nerve ending within vesicles are released by fusion with axonal membrane through entry of Ca^{2+} ion. Its release may be modulated by neurotransmitter and neuromodulator.

↓

3. **Transmitter's action on postjunctional membrane:** The released transmitters act on specific receptors on post- and prejunctional membranes producing excitatory postsynaptic potential (EPSP) or inhibitory postsynaptic potential (IPSP) by altering permeability of different ions.

↓

4. **Postjunctional activity:** EPSP produces propagated action potential in nerves, muscle or glands and IPSP resists depolarization stimuli.

↓

5. **Termination of transmitter action:** Activity of transmitter is either degraded by enzymes present locally or by reuptaken mechanism.

The synapses and neuroeffector junction have following properties:

1. Transmission across junction in one direction only.

2. There is delay of transmission across the junction.

3. Fatigue occurs more readily at junctions.

4. Many drugs act selectively at junction.

Presynaptic and postsynaptic regulations: Autonomic functions can be regulated by presynaptic feedback inhibition (α_2 or presynaptic blocks and β receptor of presynaptic region facilitates) or release of noradrenaline called

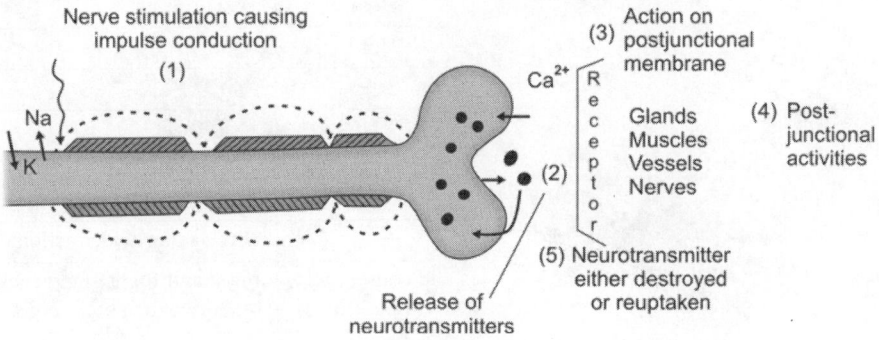

Fig. 25.4: Steps of Neurohumoral transmission

autoreceptors. Heteroreceptor at nerve terminals may be activated by transmitter, *viz.* vagus fiber of myocardium inhibits noradrenaline release.

In the same way, postsynaptic modulation of transmitter in the form of either down- or up-regulation of receptor may occur. It may be evoked by same or other transmitter acting on different postsynaptic receptors.

Surgical denervation of skeletal muscles causes proliferation of nicotine cholinoceptors causing denervation supersensitivity.

On depletion of noradrenaline by reserpine, increase in sensitivity of smooth muscles and cardiac muscles occurs.

The postsynaptic regulation can also occur through same or other neurotransmitter (*viz.* ganglion transmission discussed with drug acting on autonomic ganglion).

NEUROMODULATOR

One neuron releasing one transmitter is over simplification and it has been observed that many central and peripheral neurons have been shown to release more than one active substances when stimulated, *i.e.* neuron uses polypharmacy of its own. As for example, apart from acetylcholines,

noradrenalines, the autonomic fibers release ATP, vasoactive intestinal peptide, neuropeptide Y, substance P, prostaglandins, enkephalin as cotransmitters, acting as neuromodulators. Many abnormal findings after adrenergic or cholinergic blockade can be explained by cotransmission of neuromodulators. In some cases, they provide faster or slower response to supplement the effect of primary transmitter or may be responsible for feedback inhibition of adjacent nerves.

NONADRENERGIC, NONCHOLINERGIC (NANC) NEURONS

The gut, airway and bladder contain non-adrenergic and noncholinergic neurons in addition to cholinergic and adrenergic fibers. In the gut, neurons contain nitric oxide chole-cystokinin, neuropeptide, serotonin, gastrin releasing peptide, dyanorphin, enkephalin, somatostatin, calcitonin G related peptide (CGRP) and vasoactive intestinal peptide (VIP). Some neurons may contain as many as five transmitters acting as semi-autonomous manner, synchronizing impulses for forward propulsion of gut content and relaxation of sphincters when gut contracts.

26

Cholinergic/ Parasympathomimetic Drugs

The cholinergic neurons contain vesicles containing cotransmitters and acetylcholine. Acetylcholine is synthesized from acetyl-coenzyme A and choline, catalyzed by choline acetyl transferase enzyme. This enzyme is synthesized in ribosomes of nerve cells and transported to nerve terminals by axoplasmic flow. Acetyl coenzyme A is formed in mitochondria comes out of mitochondria by conversion into citrate where it is reconverted to acetyl coenzyme A by ATP citrate lyase. Choline is obtained from extracellular fluid by sodium dependent membrane choline cotransporter. In cholinergic axonal terminal, high affinity carrier facilitated transport mechanisms are present to supply sufficient choline. Glucose, oxygen and Na ions are necessary for optimal acetylcholine synthesis.

The vesicles are provided with vesicles-associated membrane protein (VAMP), which helps to align it to the release site on the inner side of the nerve membrane, the corresponding release site is called synaptosomal nerve-associated protein (SNAP).

Once acetylcholine is synthesized, it enters into vesicle by vesicle-associated transporter (VAT) which can be blocked by vesamicol.

Each vesicle contains 1000–50000 molecules of ACh. ACh released from vesicles depends upon extracellular calcium and occurs when action potential reaches the terminal to initiate influx of Ca^{2+} ions, which in turn interacts with VAMP to fuse with terminal membrane to release ACh.

Interfering Cholinergic System

A. Hemicholinium blocks reuptake of choline blocking choline symporter.

B. Vesamicol blocks VAT antiporter.

C. Botulinus toxin inhibits cholinergic transmission.

D. Black widow spider toxin induces massive release and depletion of ACh at cholinergic nerve terminals.

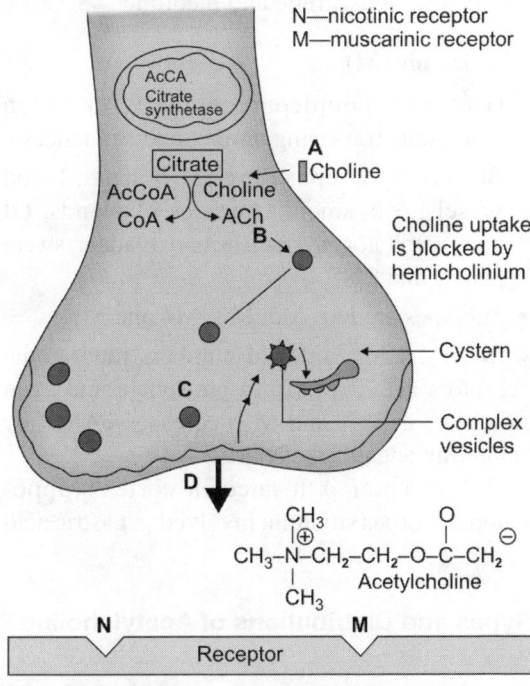

Fig. 26.1: Synthesis of acetylcholine

Acetylcholine immediately after release is hydrolyzed by cholinesterase and choline is recycled. Two types of cholinesterase are present.

A. True acetylcholinesterase

- Present in all cholinergic sites
- RBC

- Hydrolysis is fast to ACh and methacholine
- Inhibited by physostigmine
- Terminates ACh function.

B. Pesudo- or Butyrylcholinesterase

- Present in plasma, liver, white matter, intestines
- Hydrolysis process is slow.
- Hydrolyzes benzylcholine and butyryl choline
- Inhibited by organophosphorus
- It hydrolyzes ingested esters.

CHOLINOCEPTORS

Acetylcholine released from cholinergic nerve terminals acts on cholinoceptors, which are of two types—muscarinic and nicotinic.

Muscarinic (M)

- G-protein coupled receptor with seven membrane traversing amino acid sequences.
- Blocked by atropine. Present in heart, blood vessels, eye, smooth muscles of glands, GI tract, respiratory system, urinary bladder, sweat glands and CNS.
- Subtypes are M1, M2, M3, M4 and M5.

M1, M3, M5, i.e. odd numbers muscaranic receptors acts via inositol phosphate and even numbers, i.e. M_2 and M_4 decreases cAMP by inhibiting adenylate cyclase.

M1 receptor is located in cortex, hippocampus, corpus striatum; involved in gastric acid secretion, relaxes lower esophageal sphincter, learning and memory.

M2 receptor causes vagal bradycardia and auto-receptors are also M2 type in cholinergic nerve endings. It opens K^+ channel.

M3 receptor causes smooth muscles contraction and vasodilatation via EDRF. Present in eye, GIT, bladder, bronchus, glands and CNS.

Actions mediated by muscarinic receptors are:

Heart: Bradycardia and decreases force of contraction.

BP: Falls due to vasodilatation mediated by EDRF. Due lack of innervation of cholinergic nerves in blood vessels it is not a good drug for BP control.

Smooth muscles: Peristalsis increases, detrusor contracts and bronchial smooth muscle constricts.

Glands: Secretion increases, sweating increases, acid secretion, lacrymation and tracheobronchial secretion increase.

Eye: Miosis, reduces IOT; spasm of accommodation.

M1 agonist   : Oxotremorine

M1 antagonist : Pirenzepine, telenzepine

M2 agonist   : Methacholine

M2 antagonist : Methoctramine, tripitramine

M3 agonist   : Bethanechol

M3 antagonist : Hexahydro-sila-difenidol, darifenacin, solifenacin

Functionally; M1, M2 and M5 fall in one class and M2 and M4 in another class.

Types and Distributions of Acetylcholine Receptor

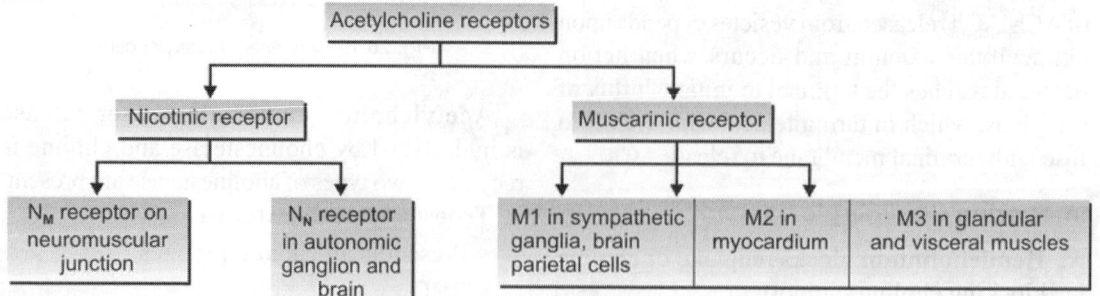

Nicotinic (N)

1. Ligand gated cation channels blocked by d-tubocurarine or hexamethonium.

2. **Subtypes N_M:** Present in skeletal muscles end plate, stimulated by phenyl trimethyl ammonium (PTMA) and blocked by tubocurarine. It mediates skeletal muscle contraction.

   - **N_N type:** Present in ganglionic cells, adrenal medulla, spinal cord, stimulated by dimethylphenylpiperazinium (DMPP) and blocked by trimethaphan hexamethonium. It mediates ganglionic transmission.

3. Actions are mediated by nicotinic receptors.

   - High dose of ACh after atropine causes tachycardia, rise of BP and contraction of skeletal muscles.

Classification of Parasympathomimetic Drugs

1. **Esters of choline:** Acetylcholine, methacholine, carbachol, bethanechol

2. **Alkaloids:** Pilocarpine, muscarine, arecholine.

3. **Cholinesterase inhibitors:** Neostigmine, organophosphorus compounds, *etc.*

Therapeutic Uses of Cholinergic Drugs

- **Methacholine:** Used to terminate paroxysmal supraventricular tachycardia. Hydrolised by AchE. Acts on muscarinic receptor.

- **Bethanechol:** Used to treat postoperative retention of urine (urotonin 10–40 mg oral) or 2.5–5 mg SC. Do not give IV. Not hydrolyzed by either cholinesterase.

- **Carbachol:** 0.75–3% drops to treat wide angle glaucoma. Contraindicated for bronchial asthma, hyperthyroid, myocardial infarction and peptic ulcer patients. Do not give intravenously.

- **Arecholine:** Obtained from *Areca catechu* or betel nut, tried for dementia. It possesses muscarinic and nicotinic actions.

- **Cevimeline:** Increases salivary and lacrimal secretion, used for dry mouth (Xerostomia) orally.

- **Demecarium:** User topically for glaucoma.

- **Pilocarpine:** Obtained from leaves of *Pilocarpus microphyllus* used as 0.5–4% eyedrops.

- **Oxotremorine:** Synthetic, stimulates muscarinic receptors used for experimental purposes.

- **Edrophonium:** Short acting, used for diagnosis of myasthenia gravis and to differentiate myasthenia and cholinergic crisis.

- **Physostigmine** used as eyedrops 0.25% with 2% pilocarpine nitrate (bimiotic). Apart from its use in eye, it is relatively safe in treatment of anticholinergic drug (atropine) poisoning

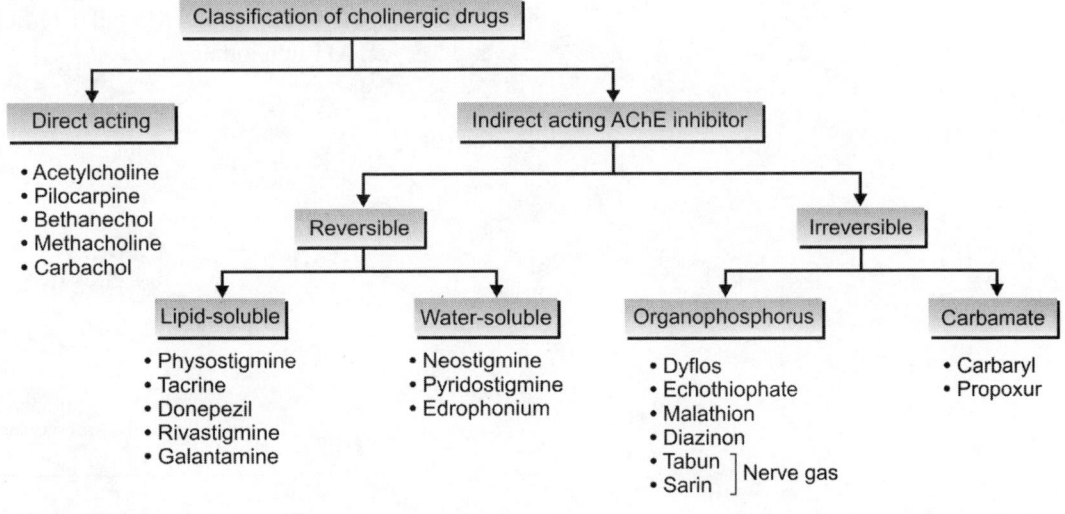

and poisoning of phenothiazines and anti-depressants specially with CNS symptoms of delirium.

- **Tacrine:** It increases brain ACh level and has been found to improve AD partially.

- **Pyridostigmine:** Oral bioavailability is more used for myasthenia gravis. Two moelcules of pyridostigmine joined together to form distigmine.

- **Donepezil:** Centrally acting Anti-AChE improves cognitive and behavioral improvements in Alzheimer's disease (AD).

- **Echothiophate:** Water-soluble 0.025–0.25% solution used in resistant glaucoma. It is potent and long-acting so used in 1–3 days.

- **Rivastigmine:** Lipophilic cerebroactive cholin- esterase inhibitor trialed for AD.

- **Galantamine:** Gives symptomatic improvement to AD. It is an alkaloid inhibits cerebral AChE.

- **Dyflos:** Potent and long-acting, used rarely as miotic. Its oily solution causes irritation.

MUSHROOM POISONING

Muscarine is found in poisonous mushroom *Amanita muscaria* and Inocybe species. Three types are known.

1. **Muscarinic type** due to Inocybe species (early mushroom poisoning). Treatment: Atropine.

2. **Hallucinogenic type** (due to isoxazole compounds). Manifestations are central.
   - They stimulate amino acid receptors and block muscarinic receptors of brain and have hallucinogenic property. No specific treatment. Atropine is not given.

3. **Phalloidin type** (or late mushroom poisoning due to peptide toxins inhibiting RNA and protein synthesis). Symptoms start late due to liver, kidney and GI damage.
   - Treatment: Supportive measures. Thioctic acid has antidotal effect.

Botulinum toxins A and B: Produced by *Clostridium botulinum* is a neurotoxin causes long-lasting loss of colinergic transmission localized injection of its A form (Botox) or its hemagglutinin complex (Dysport) is used for spastic conditions, belpharospasm, torticollis strabismus, hemifacial spasm, axillary hyper-hidrosis, age related facial wrinkles. May cause ptosis, diplopia, dry mouth, dysphagia, dysar-thria, even respiratory paralysis.

27

Anticholinesterase or Cholinesterase Inhibitor

These groups of drugs inhibit the enzymes true and pseudocholinesterase, thereby accumulate acetylcholine and mimic the action of stimulation of central, ganglionic and peripheral cholinergic components.

Classification of Anticholinesterase Drugs

I. *Reversible*

A. Carbamates:
- Physostigmine
- Pyridostigmine
- Edrophonium
- Rivastigmine
- Galantamine
- Neostigmine
- Ambenonium
- Demecarium
- Donepezil

B. Acridine:
- Tacrine

II. *Irreversible*

A. Organophosphorus:
- Dyflos
- Parathion
- Diazinon (Tik20)
- Sarin
- Metrifonate
- Echothiophate
- Malathion
- Tabun
- Soman

B. Carbamates:
- Carbaryl (Sevin)
- Propoxur (Baygon)

Active Center of Cholinesterase

Nachmanson and Wilson made extensive studies on acetylcholinesterase with different substances.

Anionic site makes bond with ionic positively charged cationic head of acetylcholine supplemented by van der Walls forces. The esteric site at 0.7 nm distance combines with ester groups containing glutamic acid, serine and alanine and probably by histidine groups.

The oxygen of serine donates electron to the electrophilic carbon of carboxyl group. Choline is then released. In the second stage, transient acetylated enzyme reacts with water to yield acetic acid and regenerates active enzymes. Histidine acts as proton acceptor.

The reversible anticholinesterase combines with anionic and esteric sites of cholinesterase. The complex they form with esteric site is readily hydrolyzed. The irreversible anticholinesterase combines with esteric site and consequently

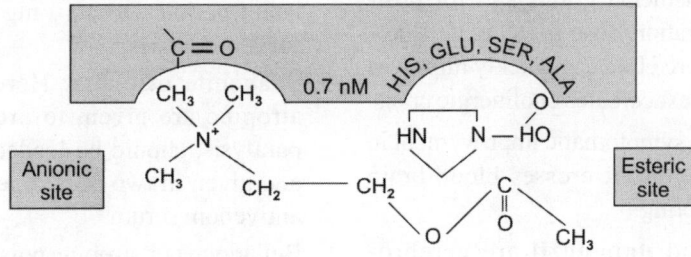

Fig. 27.1

phosphorylated. The hydrolysis of phosphoric acid is difficult or does not occur at all. Echothiophate forms complexes with esteric and anionic sites and is more potent. Lipid-soluble ACE-inhibitors (physostigmine and organosphosphates) have more marked muscarinic action and CNS effect than as lipid-insoluble ACE-inhibitors (neostigmine has marked effect on skeletal muscle and less prominent muscarinic effect).

Pharmacokinetics of Cholinesterase Inhibitors

- Physostigmine rapidly absorbed from GIT.
- Neostigmine poorly absorbed orally, does not cross blood-brain barrier or cornea.

Individual Anticholinesterase Compounds

Physostigmine (bimiotic eyedrop): 2% pilocarpine nitrate with 0.25% physostigmine.

Pyridostigmine: Less potent, but long acting, used for myasthenia gravis (60–180 mg orally or 1–1.5 mg IM or SC).

Neostigmine (Prostigmine 15 mg Tab) 0.5 mg/mL in 1 mL or 5 mL injection.

Pyridostigmine is structurally related to neostigmine, but shorter-acting lasting for 10 minutes and muscarinic side effects are countered easily by atropine. In myasthenia gravis patient, overdose may produce persistent depolarization called cholinergic crisis which has to be differentiated from myasthenic crisis where there is exacerbation of myasthenic weakness. **Distigmine** is longer acting neostigmine analog.

Edrophonium: Brief duration of action, used for diagnosis for myasthenia gravis and for postoperative decurarization, dose 1–10 mg IV. Edrophonium administered IV 2 mg quickly improves muscle power, but exacerbates cholinergic crisis.

Tacrine: Produces symptomatic improvement in Alzheimer's dementia. It crosses blood-brain barrier and long-acting.

Rivastigmine and **donepezil** are cerebroselective ACE-inhibitors used for Alzheimer's disease.

Galantamine: It has some agonistic actions on nicotine receptor used for symptomatic relief of Alzheimer's disease.

Demecarium: Two neostigmines linked by the chain of 10 methylene groups, potent and long-acting miotic (0.125–0.25% eyedrop).

Dyflos: 0.025% as miotic, rarely used because of irritation.

Echothiophate: 0.025–0.25% solution used in refractory cases of glaucoma. It is long-acting.

Metrifonate is an organophosphorus compound effective against schistosoma hematobium (bilharziasis). Cholinergic side effects of diarrheas, tremor, nausea, vomiting, bronchospasm may occur which can be tackled by atropine. Should not be used in pregnant mother or with succinyl choline.

Therapeutic Uses of Cholinesterase Inhibitors

1. Eye: • Glaucoma, miotics increases tone of ciliary muscle and sphincter pupilla to increase outflow of aqueous humor.
   • To counter effect of mydriatic after refraction.
   • To prevent adhesion between iris and lens or cornea. In case of iritis, corneal ulcer miotic and mydriatics are used alternatively.
2. Myasthenia gravis.
3. Postoperative paralytic ileus and retention of urine by neostigmine 0.5–2 mg subcutaneously.
4. Postoperative decurarization. Neostigmine 0.5–2 mg IV preceded by atropine to reverse neuromuscular blocking by curare group. Edrophonium is preferred because of short latent period. Dose 10 mg may be repeated for 2 or 3 doses.
5. Snakebite of cobra: Here neostigmine + atropine are given, to prevent respiratory paralysis, should be loaded in two syringes and given in two sites. Specific treatment is antivenom serum.
6. Belladonna or atropine poisoning (physostigmine is used). Because it penetrates BBB

and antagonises both central and peripheral effects.

7. To treat drug overdoses of antihistaminic, tricyclic antidepressant, phenothiazines. physostigmine are used.

8. Alzheimer's disease.

Drugs Used for Glaucoma (Wide Angle/Open Angle/Chronic Simple)

1. β-adrenergic blockers
- Timolol ($\beta_1 + \beta_2$) 0.25–0.5% eyedrops; BD eyedrops; BD (Glucomol)
- Betaxolol (β_1) 0.5% (Optipress) eyedrops; BD
- Levobunolol: Used once daily (Betagan 0.5% eyedrop) 1 drop OD.
- Carteolol (prevents optic nerve damage)
- Metipranolol (has corneal anesthetic property)

2. Miotics: These cholinomimetics cause ciliary muscle contraction, open trabecular network to increase aqueous humor outflow.
- Carbachol
- Physostigmine
- Pilocarpine
- Demecarium
- Ecothiophate

3. α-adrenergic agonist: Increases outflow.
- Adrenaline 0.5–1%
- Phenylephrine 10%
- Dipivefrine a prodrug for adrenaline better tolerated, longer-acting than adrenaline (propine 0.1%) 1 drop BD. Used as add-on drug.

4. α₂-selective agonist: Decreases aqueous secretion.
- Brimonidine used for post-laser or surgery patient topically.
- Apraclonidine 0.5–1% potent ocular hypotensive. Adrenergic drugs are used as adjuvant to miotics or β blockers.

5. Carbonic anhydrase inhibitors
- Dichlorphenamide 50–100 mg BD or TDS
- Methazolamide 50–100 mg BD or TDS
- Acetazolamide 0.25–0.5 gm orally BD
- Dorzolamide topically active carbonic anhydrase inhibitor. 2% eyedrops used TDS used as add-on drug with PG analogues, or β blockers.
- Brinzolamide: Topically used.

6. Prostaglandin analogues: Low concentration of $PGF_{2\alpha}$ lower intraocular tension by increasing outflow. Latanoprost, bimatoprost, travoprost, unoprostone are used.

Narrow Angle Glaucoma (Acute Congestive Glaucoma)

Occurs in individual of narrow irido corneal angle and shallow anterior chamber and should be lowered quickly.

Treated by

Drugs
- Topical β-blockers (Timolol)
- Miotics (Pilocarpine)
- Hypertonic mannitol 20% or glycerol 10% by IV infusion or 50% as retention enema.
- Acetazolamide orally 0.5 gm IV or orally BD
- Apraclonidine 1% installation topically.

Iridotomy

Definite treatment is iridotomy (surgery or laser).

Myasthenia gravis

Myasthenia gravis is an autoimmune disease due to deficiency of post-synaptic neuromuscular acetylcholine receptor complex, present with fatiguability and weakness of striated muscles with intermittent periods of exacerbations, due to postsynaptic neuromuscular acetylcholine receptor complex which are degraded and cleared faster. Diagnosed by 1–10 mg edrophonium administered IV improves symptoms.

Drugs which aggravate muscle weakness are aminoglycosides, phenytoin, phenothiazine, α-tubocurarine.

Treatment
- Neostigmine 15 gm 6 hourly or pyridostigmine, ambenonium (later two have longer duration of action)

- Corticosteroids (prednisolone 30–60 mg/day)
- Immunosuppressants (cycloslpoorine; azathio-prine) 25–50 mg TDS.
- Ephedrine and potassium chloride 1–2 gm TDS as adjuvants
- Thymectomy
- Plasmapheresis.

Lambert-Eaton syndrome is also of auto-immune nature occurs with small cell carcinoma of lung where calcium channel of presynaptic sites are effected causing decrease release of Ach which does not respond to anticholinesterase but responds to 3,4 diaminopyridine (3,4, DAP).

Acute Anticholinesterase Poisoning (Accidental, Suicidal or Homicidal)

Symptoms are due to muscarinic and nicotinic receptor stimulation, *viz.* lacrymation, sali-vations, sweating, miosis, breathlessness, urination, hypotension, tachycardia, arrhythmia, excitement, convulsion, coma (muscarinic effect), muscle fasciculation and respiratory muscle paralysis (nicotinic effect).

Treatment

- Termination of further exposure (fresh air, washing of skin and mucous membrane by soap).
- Maintain patent airway and positive pressure respiration.
- Supportive measures—maintain BP, hydration, control convulsion with diazepam.

- Specific antidote is **atropine**.
- Cholinesterase reactivators (Pralidoxime is effective as antidote to organophosphorus; other oximes are diacetylmonoxime, obi-doxime). Pralidoxime (Neopam) 500 mg/ 20 mL IV slowly up to 1–2 gm. Diacetyl monoxime crosses BBB, but pralidoxime and obidoxime cannot. These are effective in reversing neuromuscular block by organo-phosphorus. Toxicity by oximes are local irritation, drowsiness, giddiness, blurred vision, diplopia, tachycardia, hypotension. Pralidoxime possesses some anti-ChE activity so contraindicated in treatment of overdose of physostigmine or neostigmine.

Pralidoxime has quarternary nitrogen attaches to anionic site of the enzyme and remains unoccupied. In the presence of organophos-phorus, it reacts to phosphorus atom of esteric site which diffuses away by leaving reactivated cholinesterase. It is not effective for carbamate anticholinesterase when anionic site is not free.

Treatment with oximes should be started at early as possible before the phosphorylated enzyme undergoes ageing and becomes resistant to hydrolysis.

Chronic organophosphrus poisoning due to repeated exposure causes neuritis, weakness, tenderness, decreased tendon reflex, LMN paralysis, spasticity and UMN paralysis starts gradually. Recovery takes long time. Mechanism of symptoms are not by cholinesterase inhibition. No specific treatment known.

28

Anticholinergic Drugs

Cholinergic blocking drugs conventionally block the action of acetylcholine, done through muscarinic receptors competitively.

Classification of Anticholinergic Drugs

1. **Natural alkaloids:** Atropine, Hyoscine.

2. **Semisynthetic compounds:** Homatropine, atropine methonitrate, hyoscine butylbromide, ipratropium bromide, tiotropium bromide.

3. **Synthetic compounds:**

   (a) Mydriatic: Tropicamide, cyclopentolate.

   (b) Anti-secretory antispasmodic:

   (i) Quarternary compounds:
   Propantheline, oxyphenonium, clidinium, pipenzolate methylbromide, isopropramide, glycopyrrolate.

   (ii) Tertiary amines:
   Dicyclomine, pirenzepine, telenzepine, valethamate.

   (c) Antiparkinsonian: Benzhexol, procyclidine, biperiden, benzatropine.

   (d) Vasicoselective: Flavoxate, oxybutynin, tolterodine.

Apart from this, some antihistaminics, phenothiazine and tricylic antidepressants have antimuscarinic actions.

Pharmacological Actions of Anticholinergic Drugs (Atropine as Prototype) (Fig. 28.1)

CNS : Stimulation; decreases tremor and rigidity of parkinsonism.

Eye : Mydriasis and cycloplegia, atropine has mild local anesthetic action on cornea.

Glands : Secretion of lacrimal, salivary and sweat glands decreases. Body temperature rises.

CVS : Tachycardia due to blockade of M_2 receptor on heart and unopposed sympathetic effect. Atropine and physostigmine should not be given simultaneously to terminate the effect of competitive neuromuscular blocking agent, rather should be given in some times apart because a

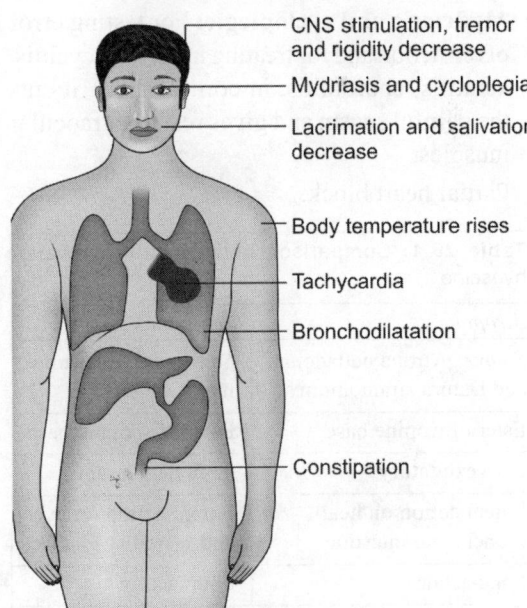

Fig. 28.1: Pharmacological action of anticholinergic drugs (atropine as prototype)

CNS stimulation, tremor and rigidity decrease

Mydriasis and cycloplegia

Lacrimation and salivation decrease

Body temperature rises

Tachycardia

Bronchodilatation

Constipation

transient bradycardia may occur with atropine due to central vagal stimulation and blockade of pre-synaptic (M1) receptor on ganglionic parasympathetic stimulation causing increase in ACh release.

Respiratory system: Bronchodilatation.

GI tract : Decreases gastric secretion and gut motility.

Therapeutic Uses of Anticholinergic Drugs

* Antisecretory: Atropine in preanesthetic medication to prevent laryngospasm by decreasing respiratory secretion.
* Peptic ulcer by decreasing gastric secretion of fasting and neurogenic phase.
* Pulmonary embolism.
* Salivation in parkinsonism.
* To decrease sweating.
* Antispasmodic of renal, abdominal cramps, pylorospasm, enuresis, dysmenorrhea, IBS, spastic constipation, urinary urgency.
* Bronchial asthma: COPD (ipratropium bromide by inhalation).
* **Mydriatic and cycloplegic:** For testing error of refraction and for treating iritis, iridocyclitis, keratitis, choroiditis, in corneal ulcer, it cuts the painful spasm and gives rest to intraocular muscles.
* Partial heart block.

Table 28.1: Comparison between atropine and hyoscine

Atropine	Hyoscine
Source: Atropa belladonna and Datura stramonium	Source: Hyoscyamus niger
Ester of tropine base	Ester of scopine base
CNS excitatory	CNS depressant
Potent action on heart, bronchi and intestine	Potent action on eye and secretory glands
Long-acting	Short acting
Not effective in motion sickness	Effective in motion sickness

Parkinsonism: Used in drug induced Parkinson's and as adjuvent to levodopa.
* Motion sickness (Hyoscine is used)
* Twilight sleep and amnesia during labor
* To treat muscarinic poisoning.

Contraindications and precautions of Atropinic Drugs: Narrow iridocorneal angle; prostatic hypertrophy. Congestive cardiac failure with tachycardia, pyloric obstruction.

Pharmacokinetics: Atropine and hyoscine are rapidly absorbed from GIT and cornea, metabolized in liver and excreted in urine. Hyoscine enters blood-brain barrier better. Rabbit contains atropinase, an enzyme degrading atropine.

Individual Anticholinergic Drugs

* Hyoscine butyl bromide used for GIT spasm. Dose 10–40 mg oral, IM, SC, IV; Buscopan 10 mg tab or 20 mg/mL amp.
* Atropine methonitrate 2.5–10 mg orally for GI colics or acidity.
* Homatropine methyl bromide 2.5–10 mg orally or IM for antispasmodic.
* Hyoscine methyl bromide 2.5 mg oral or IM as anticolic and anti-secretion
* Ipratropium bromide (Ipravent) 20–40 μg by inhalation in bronchial asthma 2 puffs TDS or QDS. Ipranase Aq (0.084%) as nasal spray in common cold 42 μg per actuation 1–2 spray TDS or QDS.
* Tiotropium bromide (Tiova 18 μg/rotacap) congener of ipratropium bromide used in asthma. 1 rotacap by inhalation daily. It has high bronchial selective action. OD dose.
* **Propantheline** (Probanthine 15 mg tab) 15–30 mg for peptic ulcer.
* **Oxyphenonium** (Antrenyl 5–10 mg tab) for peptic ulcer and for gastrointestinal hyper-motility.
* **Clidinium** 2.5–5 mg orally. Generally, available as the combination with chlordiazepoxide (spasril) or dicyclomine (normaxin). Used in irritable bowel syndrome.
* **Pipenzolate** methylbromide 5–10 mg orally in infantile colic, flatulent dyspepsia.
* **Mepenzolate** (30 mg/mL) orally for colics.

- **Isopropamide** (5 mg orally) available in combination with trifluoperazine (stelabid) used for hyperacidity, irritable bowel syndrome, nervous dyspepsia.
- **Glycopyrrolate** (glyco-p 0.2 mg/mL amp) 0.1–0.3 mg IM or 1–2 mg orally for preanesthetic medication.
- **Dicyclomine** 10 mg tab; 10 mg/mL amp given orally or IM as antispasmodic.
- **Valethamate** (valamate 8 mg/mL inj. or epidosin 10 mg tab or 8 mg/mL inj.) used to dilate cervix during labor or visceral antispasmodic.
- **Pirenzepine**: 100–150 mg/day. MI selective, 30% absorbed, brain penetration is less, excreted with urine unchanged. **Telenzepine** is also M1 selective used in peptic ulcer.
- **Homatropine** (eyedrops) used for mydriasis lasting for 1–3 days (homide 1–2%)
- **Cyclopentolate** (cyclomid eye 0.5–1%) mydriasis and cycloplegia occur in ½ to 1 hour and last for a day. May produce behavioral change.
- **Tropicamide** (0.5–1% eyedrops) quick-acting, perferred for refraction testing (tromide 0.5–1% eyedrops).
- **Benzhexol**, procyclidine, benztropine, *etc.* are dealt in antiparkinsonism chapter.
- **Oxybutynin** (oxybutin 2.5–5 mg tab) used for detrusor instability and urge incontinence, neurogenic bladder, nocturnal enuresis. Dose 5 mg BD or TDS. It is also used in transdermal system.
- **Tolterodine** (torq 1–2 mg/OD) M3 selective antagonist, used for urinary frequency and urgency. Metabolized by CYP450D$_6$4 should be used with caution in patient receiving Fluoxetine.
- **Flavoxate** (urispas 200 mg indicated for urinary frequency, urgency, dysuria). Dose 1 tab TDS.
- **Drotaverine** (drotin 40–80 mg tab; 40 mg/ 2 mL inj.) 1 tab TDS indicated in IBS; gastrointestinal, renal or biliary colic). It inhibits phosphodiesterase-4, selective to produce muscle relaxation. **Fenoverine** is similar to its action.
- **Solifenacin** and **Darifenacin** are M3 blockers useful for irritable bowel syndrome and overactive bladder (oxybutynin is also used urinary tract overactivity). The other effective drugs are as follows:
  (a) Trospium 20–40 mg/day
  (b) Tolterodine 2–4 mg/day
  (c) Solifenacin 5–10 mg/day
  (d) Darifenacin 7.5–15 mg/day
  (e) Fesoterodine 4–8 mg/day

Fesoterodine is a prodrug hydrolyzed to tolterodine. Dose adjustment for trospium is required in renal imparied patient because it is eliminated *via* kidney. Solifenacin is metabolized by CYP3A4 and Tolterodine by CYP2D6. Flavoxate has direct sympatholytic action on smooth muscle of urinary tract and is used to treat dysuria, urgency and nocturia associated with cystitis, prostatitis, urethritis. Duloxetine is useful in stress incontinence acts centrally by influencing 5HT and NAd level.

Mirabegron: This Beta-3 adrenergic agonist causes relaxation of detrusor muscle to increase bladder capacity, used for overactive bladder. It may cause dizziness, tachycardia, raise BP, urinary retention and gi symptoms.

Onabotulinum toxin A : Single intradetrusor injection used to treat overactive bladder.

Urinary retention in female after menopause may be treated with topical application and oral oestrogen because distal urethral epithelium has oestrogen receptors which are degenerated after menopause.

Urinary retention is treated by bethanecol, neostigmine if there is no BPH.

DATURA POISONING OR BELLADONNA POISONING

Presents with:

- Dry mouth
- Flushed hot skin specially over face

- Dilated pupil
- Rash
- Hypotension
- Fever
- Convulsion
- Photophobia
- Palpitation
- Hallucination, ataxia
- Scarlet rash
- Sluggish bowel sound
- Blurred vision
- Rapid pulse
- Cardiovascular collapse
- Respiratory depressions.

It is diagnosed by methacholine 5 mg or neostigmine 1 mg SC which fails to produce muscarinic effect.

Treatment of Datura Poisoning

- Gastric lavage with tannic acid; $KMNO_4$ not effective to oxidize atropine.
- Keep patient in dark and quite room.
- Cold sponging to reduce body temperature.
- Physostigmine 1–3 mg SC or IV to antagonize central and peripheral affects, but may produce hypotension or arrhythmia.
- General measures like artificial respiration, blood volume maintenance and treatment of convulsion with diazepam.

29

Sympathomimetic (Adrenergic) Drugs

Noradrenaline transmission is restricted to sympathetic division of ANS. Three closely related endogenous catecholamines which act as neurotransmitters in sympathetic system are adrenaline, noradrenaline and dopamine. β-phenyl ethylamine is a benzene ring with ethylamine side chain, is the parent structure of sympathomimetic amine. 3–4 positions of benzene ring is hydroxylated in catecholamine.

The catecholamine (NAd) is a neurotransmitter in postganglionic sympathetic sites except in sweat glands, hair follicles, vasodilatation fibers and some areas of the brain. Adrenaline (Ad) has role as neurotransmitter in the brain and secreted by adrenal medulla. Dopamine (DA) has limited action as neurotransmitter in periphery but is an important transmitter in basal ganglia, limbic system and chemoreceptor trigger zone (CTZ).

Synthesis of Catecholamine (CA) (Fig. 29.1)

The enzyme systems are synthesized in perinuclear of the nerve cells, but terminal axons are the important sites for catecholamine synthesis from where they are transported by axonal transports.

The starting point for synthesis of CA is essential amino acid phenylalanine. Phenylalanine is converted to tyrosine by phenylalanine hydroxylase. Tyrosine hydroxylase catalyzes the addition of 2-hydroxy group to tyrosine and converts it into dihydroxyphenylalanine (DOPA), a catechol ring. Both tyrosine hydroxylase and phenylalanine hydroxylase act on L-isomer and loosely attached to endoplasmic reticulum synthesized in cell body. This increased activity of tyrosine hydroxylase is inhibited by puromycin, cycloheximide and actinomycin D.

Tyrosine hydroxylase is inhibited by metyrosine, used in the treatment of pheochromocytoma.

DOPA decarboxylase: Converts DOPA to dopamine. DOPA is given in high doses in treatment of parkinsonism. Conversion of DOPA to dopamine is inhibited by methyldopa, carbidopa and benserazide.

- Dopamine β-hydroxylase: Catalyzes the conversion of dopamine to noradrenaline, requires copper and ascorbic acid.

- Storage of catecholamine: NAd is stored in synaptic vesicles. DA is actively taken up by granules and converted to NAd from dopamine. β-hydroxylase is stored as complex with ATP.

Releasing of Catecholamine from Granular Vesicle and Restoration to Storage

The release is modulated by α2 inhibitory control. Other cotransmitters Y2; NPY; ATP inhibit transmitter release. Besides these; dopaminergic, serotonergic, muscarinic and PGE2 inhibit and β2 adrenoceptor; AT1, and nicotine receptor enhance noradrenaline release. The events are as follows (Fig. 29.2).

- **Uptake of CA:** This is very efficient mechanism to recapture and terminate the actions of CA. Uptake-I—Axonal uptake blocked by drugs like cocaine, desipramine, and many H_1 blockers. Extraneuronal uptake by other cells are called uptake-II. The other uptake is a vesicular uptake. Uptake-I is an active amine pump (NET) at neuronal membrane transports NAd by Na^+ coupled mechanism. Uptake-II is carried out by extraneuronal amine transporter (ENT) or organic cation transporter (OCT3) uptakes Ad faster. The membrane of

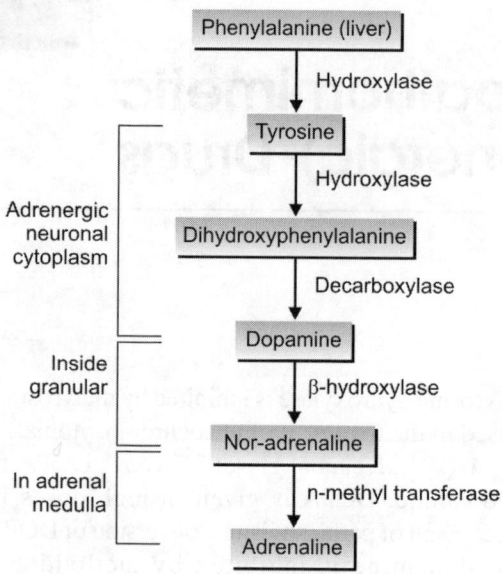

Fig. 29.1: Synthesis of adrenaline

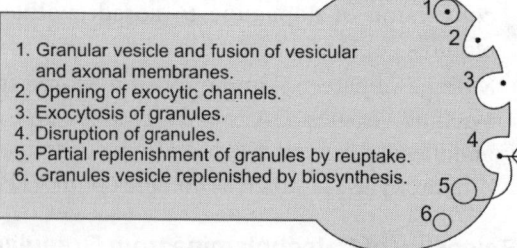

1. Granular vesicle and fusion of vesicular and axonal membranes.
2. Opening of exocytic channels.
3. Exocytosis of granules.
4. Disruption of granules.
5. Partial replenishment of granules by reuptake.
6. Granules vesicle replenished by biosynthesis.

Fig. 29.2: Release of noradrenaline

intracellular vesicles contains vesicular mono-amine transporter (VMAT-2) from cytoplasm to vesicles exchanging with H^+ ion. It can be inhibited by reserpine and causes depletion of catecholamine.

Uptake-II can be blocked by glucocorticoids, normetanephrine, phenoxybenzamine.

- **Metabolism of CA:** The portion of CA reuptaken is acted upon by MAO and the portion diffuses into circulation is acted upon by catechol-orthomethyltransferase (COMT) in liver and other tissues and metabolized which is mentioned in Fig. 29.3.

The sympathomimetic may be direct-acting which directly acts on receptors or indirectly acting, which releases catecholamines from presynaptic nerve terminals (like amphetamine, ephedriner, *etc.*). The indirectly acting sympatho-mimetic produces tachyphylaxis, *i.e.* quick protection on quick successive use (Fig. 29.5).

Some Drugs which Modify the Action of Adrenergic Neurons (Effecting Syntheses, Storage and Uptake)

- Supplying amine precursor, levodopa in parkinsonisn.
- By blocking uptakes, potentiate actions of adrenergic nerves: Imipramine, cocaine, *etc.* (Fig. 29.4).

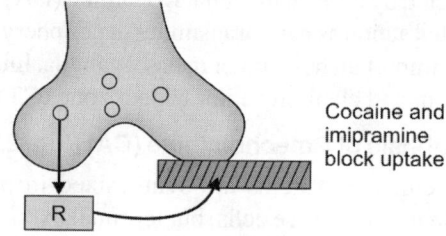

Cocaine and imipramine block uptake

Fig. 29.4

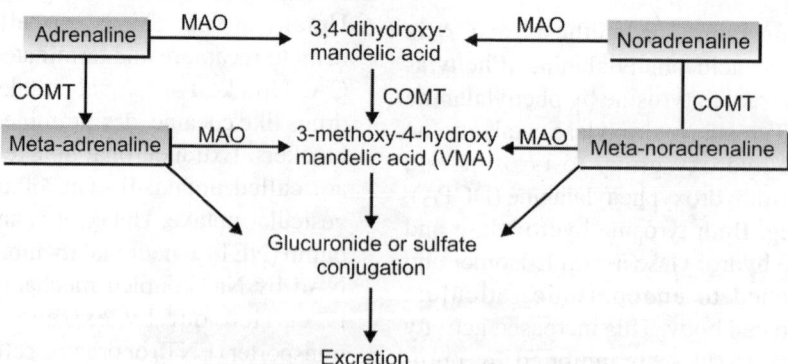

Fig. 29.3: Metabolism of catecholamine

- Indirectly acting drugs release noradrenaline from storage sites. May be responsible for cheese reaction with tyramine. They produce tachyphylaxis (Fig. 29.5).

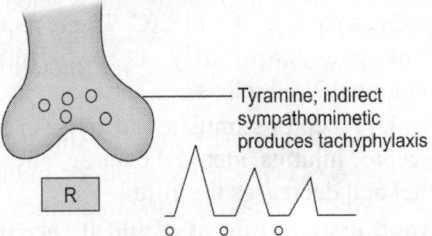

Tyramine; indirect sympathomimetic produces tachyphylaxis

Fig. 29.5

- Modifying storage leading to depletion like reserpine and tetrabenzine (Fig. 29.6).

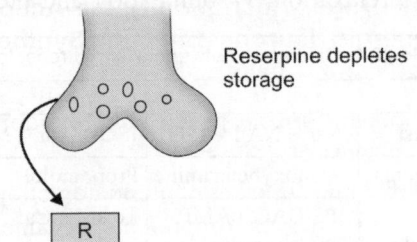

Reserpine depletes storage

Fig. 29.6

- Blocking release—guanethidine (Fig. 29.7).

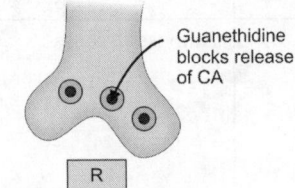

Guanethidine blocks release of CA

Fig. 29.7

- Synthesizing false transmitter—methyldopa (Fig. 29.8).

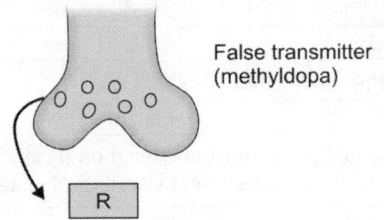

False transmitter (methyldopa)

Fig. 29.8

- By blocking postsynaptoreceptor (α and β blockers) (Fig. 29.9).

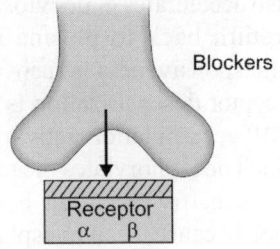

Blockers

Receptor
α   β

Fig. 29.9

- By blocking intraneuronal breakdown after uptake of MAO inhibitors (Fig. 29.10).

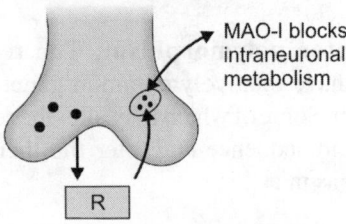

MAO-I blocks intraneuronal metabolism

Fig. 29.10

Supersensitivity

Interruption of nerve supply to effector organs make it more sensitive to exogenous neurotransmitters, may be due to disappearance of enzymes normally inactivating neurotransmitter or rise in number of postsynaptic receptors. Prolong use of blocking agent may also cause supersensitivity.

Regulation of Adrenoceptors

Responses of adrenoceptors are not fixed and static. They are regulated by catecholamine, other hormones, drugs, age, disease states, *etc.*

The cells may be less sensitive to agonist, exposed for a period of time called desensitization (also called tolerance, refractoriness, tachyphylaxis) limiting its therapeutic response. The mechanism involved in desensitization includes phosphorylation of amino acid residues of receptor or rechange in their substrate location. The G-protein coupled receptors may be desensitized homologously, *i.e.* receptor is exposed to same drug repeatedly or for prolonged time. Heterology desensitized receptors are not exposed to drug on question. Phosphorylation of the receptor increases the affinity of the receptor for β-arrestin and decreases its response.

β-arrestin also accelerates endocytosis of receptor which return back to plasma membrane receptor and responsiveness is recovered.

β-adrenoceptor desensitization is also mediated by cAMP accumulation activating protein kinase A, which phosphorylates the receptor and decreases its sensitivity called heterologous desensitization because it can phosphorylate any structurally similar receptor.

The other mechanisms which contribute desensitization operate at transcription, translation and protein synthesis levels which take place slowly.

Receptor polymorphism: The receptors α and β have relatively common genetic polymorphism. Some of which may alter the receptors amino acid sequence and alter the therapeutic response as in asthma.

Adrenergic Receptors

Receptors: These are membrane-bound G-protein coupled receptors act by production of second messenger cAMP or IP3/DAG. In some cases, G-protein itself produces prostaglandin or operates K^+ or Ca^{2+} channel.

Ahlquist classified adrenoceptors as stimulatory (α) and inhibitory (β) receptors, which are further classified into α_1, α_2, β_1, β_2 and β_3 depending upon agonistic activity. α_1 is further cloned into α_1A, α_1B, α_1D and α_2 into three subtypes as α_2A, α_2B and α_2C. The α receptor present presynaptically is α_2, inhibits prejunctional NAd release.

The D_1 receptor stimulates adenylyl cyclase. D_2 receptor inhibits adenylyl cyclase, opens K^+ channel and decreases Ca influx.

Broad distribution of α and β receptors: The α receptors are excitatory except in GI tract and β receptors are inhibitory except in heart. β_1 receptors are responsible for myocardial stimulation and lypolysis. β_2 for bronchial smooth muscle relaxation, vasodilatation and uterine

Table 29.1: Difference between α and β receptors

	α	β
Agonist	Adr > NAd > ISO	ISO > Adr > NAd
Antagonist	Phenoxybenzamine	Propranolol
Acts through	IP3/DAG, cAMP, $\downarrow K^+$ channel	$\uparrow$cAMP, $Ca^{2+}\uparrow$

Table 29.2: Difference amongst β_1, β_2 and β_3 receptors

	β_1	β_2	β_3
Site	• Heart • JG cells of kidney	• Bronchi • Blood vessels • Uterus • Liver • GI tract • Urinary tract • Eye	Adipose tissues
Agonist	Dobutamine	• Salbutamol • Terbutaline	BRL 37344
Antagonist	Metoprolol	ICI 118557	CGP 20712A

Table 29.3: Difference between α_1 and α_2 receptors

	α_1	α_2
Location	Postjunctional	Prejunctioal (α_2A), postjunctional on β cells of pancreas, brain, some blood vessels and platelets
Agonist	Phenylephrine	Clonidine
Antagonist	Prazosin	Yohimbine
Pathway	IP3/DAG$\uparrow$, PG release, phospholipase A2$\uparrow$	cAMP$\downarrow$, K^+ channel$\uparrow$, Ca channel$\downarrow$ or $\uparrow$, IP3/DAG$\uparrow$

relaxation. α_1 receptors present in vascular smooth muscle, α_2 receptors are responsible for inhibition of renin release from kidney and for central adrenergically blood pressure depression.

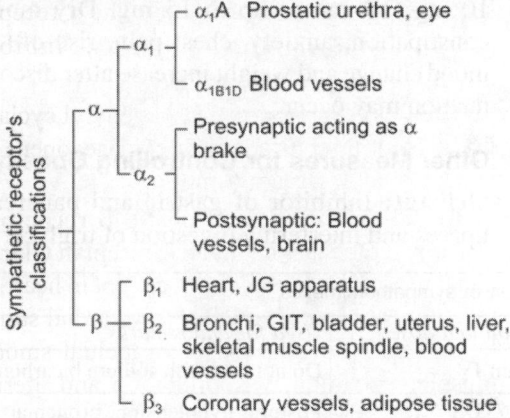

Dale's vasomotor reversal (Fig. 29.11): Adrenaline acts on both α and β receptors, but more on β. By stimulating α, it raises BP and stimulating β, decreases BP which is more prolonged, *i.e.* it produces biphasic response. Dale noticed prior administration of ergot (an α blocker) produces only depressor response. The phenomenon is known as Dale's vasomotor reversal. If pretreatment is done by β blocker then only hypertensive effect is noted.

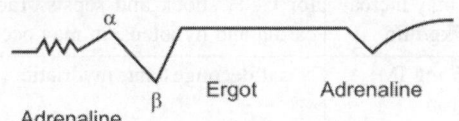

Fig. 29.11 Dale's vasomotor reversed

Adrenergic agonist may be also classified as:
- **Direct acting (acting on receptors):** Their actions are not reduced by prior reserpine.
  - (a) Selective α_2 = clonidine, β_1 = dobutamine
  - (b) Non-selective α_1 and α_2-oxymetazoline; α_1-, α_2-, β_1-, β_2-epinephrine. They act directly and indircetly.
- **Indirect acting:** Release noradrenaline and their action decreases with prior reserpine, *viz.* amphetamine and tyramine.
- **Mixed acting:** Response decreases with reserpine prior treatment, *e.g.* ephedrine, releases noradrenaline and acts on α_1, α_2, β_1 and β_2 receptors.

- **Uptake inhibitors:** *viz.* cocaine, TCA, MAO or COMT inhibitors, pargyline, entacapone respectively are also indirect acting sympathomimetric.

PHARMACOLOGICAL ACTION OF SYMPATHOMIMETICS

1. **Heart:** Increases rate, force of contraction and cardiac outputs, conduction velocity and oxygen consumption of heart. Refractory period of all cardiac cells is decreased. Actions on heart is mediated by β receptors.

2. **Blood vessels:** Produce cutaneous vessels constriction. Adrenaline dilates skeletal muscle vessels. Adrenaline increases systolic BP and decreases diastolic BP (Fig. 29.12).

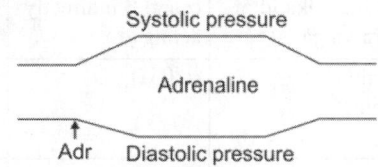

Fig. 29.12

3. **Skeletal muscle:** Facilitates neuromuscular transmission.

4. **Smooth muscles:** Bronchi dilates (β_2), uterus relaxes to Adr in last trimester otherwise it is stimulated, gut relaxes and pilomotor muscles contract. Detrusor is relaxed (β) and trigone is constricted (α) hindering micturation.

5. **Eye:** Mydriasis, due to contraction of radial muscles (α_1) of iris. Vasoconstriction by α_1 receptor reduces aqueous humor formation. β_2 enhances secretory activity. It increases uveoscleral outflow. Overall effect is decreased aqueous formation and increased outflow.

6. **Respiration:** IV Adr produces apnea; toxic doses of Adr may produce pulmonary edema by shifting systemic blood to pulmonary circuits.

7. **CNS:** IV or intracarotid CA produces stupor, excitement, vomiting and coma.

8. **Metabolism:** Increases blood sugar by glucogenolysis and FFA, hyperlactacidemia, **hyperkalemia. Augments glucagon (β_2) and inhibits insulin (α_2) secretion.**

Miscellaneous: Viscid secretions of parotid, leukocytosis and platelet aggregation.

Other Anorectics Drug

Non-adrenergic drugs: Phenteramine, phenyl pronolamine, diethypropion, Mazindol

Serotonergic drugs: Fenfluramine and dexfenfluramine. They enhance serotonergic transmission in hypothalamus. Phenteramine and fenfluramine combination may cause valvular defects, pulmonary hypertension and sudden death.

Non-adrenergic/serotonergic agent: Sibutramine. It inhibits uptake of noradrenaline and 5HT and indirectly activate β_3 in adipose tissue causing thermogenesis. Used as antiobesity. Marketed as obestat 5 and 10 mg cap. Dose 10 mg OD raised up to 15 mg. Dry mouth, constipation, anxiety, chest pain, rise of BP, mood change and weight increase after discontinuation may occur.

Other Measures for Controlling Obesity

Orlistat: Inhibitor of gastric and pancreatic lipases and interfering digestion of triglyceride.

Table 29.4: Classification of sympathomimetics			
Drugs pressor agents	*Acting on receptor*	*Preparation and dose*	*Used for and remarks*
Noradrenaline	α	2–4 µg/min IV	Do not mix with sodium bicarbonate
Ephedrine (alkalid of ephedra vulgaris)	α and β indirectly acting	15–30 mg/TDS	Postural hypotension, bronchial asthma
Dopamine (intropin)	α, β, D_1, D_2	0.2–1 mg/min	It is a substrate for MAO and COMT so orally inactive. Used for CHF and cardiogenic shock and septic shock.
Fenoldopam	D_1 and α	10 mg/mL	Used for severe hypertension because of vasodilatory property. Not given orally because of first pass effect. Headache, flushing, dizziness, tachycardia or bradycardia may occur.
Dopexamine	D_1, D_2, β_2	0.5– 1 µg/kg/min *via* caval catheter may increases up to 6 µg/kg/min	Inhibits catecholamine uptake used for CCF, shock and sepsis. Tachycardia and hypotension may occur.
Phenylephrine (Frenin)	α_1 agonist	0.5 mg IV, 2–5 mg IM 0.25% nasal drop 5–10% eyedrop	Nasal decongestant, mydriatic
Methoxamine (Vasoxine)	α_1	20 mg/mL inj.	Pressor agent given IM or slow IV
Adrenaline	β	0.5–1 mg/mL 1:1000 adrenaline 0.2–0.5 mg SC or IM	Allergic reaction, bronchial asthma, cardiac arrest, control of hemorrhage, to prolong action of local anesthesia. Adrenaline unstable in alkaline solution. When exposed to light it turns pink (adrenochrome formation) and then brown due to polymer formation so antioxidant or acid is included.
Isoprenaline	β	20 mg sublingual, 50–10 µg IV per min, 400 µg/meter dose inhaler	Bronchial asthma, Stokes-Adams syndrome, shock
Dobutamine	α_1, β_1	2.5–10 µg/kg/min IV	Used for cardiac shock and cardiac surgery, myocardial infarction, CCF

Table 29.5: Selective adrenergic agonist (α_2)

Drugs	Receptor	Used and remarks
Clonidine	α_2	Hypertension, diabetic, autoneuropathy, withdrawal of drug, menopausal hot flush (transdermal patch is used)
Apraclonidine	α_2	Typically used for glaucoma
Brimonidine	Clonidine derivatives α_2 agonist	Decreases aqueous humor production and outflow
Dexmedetomidine	α_2 agonist with sedative properties	Used for anesthetic adjunct for sedation and anxiolysis
Guanfacine	α_2 agonist	Hypertension, withdrawal syndrome may occur.
Guanabenz	α_2 agonist	Hypertension
α-methyldopa	Activate α_2 receptor	Blood pressure
Tizanidine	α_2 agonist	Possesses skeletal muscle relaxant properties. Used for spasticity associated with cerebral and spinal disease

Fat-soluble vitamin absorption is also impaired. Loose motion, steatorrhea, flatulence and vitamin deficiency may occur.

Olestra: It is used in cooking medium in place of fat. It is a sucrose polyester.

Leptin, and neruropeptide Y antagonist under investigational level.

Rimonabant: Selective cannabinoid (CB-1) receptor antagonist, decreases appetite. Also tried for smoking cessation. Withdrawn from market due to suicidal tendency.

Sibutaramine: Inhibit 5HT, NAd and DA uptake used as appetite suppressants. Mechanism of different antiobesity drugs are dealt in Chapter 21.

Phenylpropanolamine: Similar to ephedrine pharmacologically causing vasoconstriction. Included in many cold preparation. It is also used to reduce weight. It may precipitate hemorrhagic stroke or behavioral or psychiatric changes. Therefore, phenylpropanolamine containing products are either withdrawn or marketed with caution level. In India it is still available as OTC drug.

Therapeutic Uses of Drugs

1. **Vascular uses**
   - Hypotensive states (shocks, spinal anesthesia, hypotensive drugs)
   - Along with LA to increase duration. Adrenaline 1 : 20,000 to 1,00,000 dilution with LA is infiltered.
   - To control bleeding locally of epistaxis, skin and mucous membrane (adrenaline 1 : 10000, phenylephrine or ephedrine 1%)
   - Nasal decongestant: Ephedrine 0.5%; xylometazoline 0.1%, oxymetazoline 0.05%. Other nasal decongestants are tuamino heptane sulfate (%), propylhexedrine by inhalation (Benzedrex) which causes less CNS stimulation.

   An ideal nasal decongestant should produce prompt and prolong reliable effect without tachyphylaxis, local irritation and no damage to nasal cilia.
   - **Midorine:** A prodrug used for postural hypotensions.

2. **Cardiac uses**
   - Cardiac arrest (adrenaline IV) due to drowning, electrocaution, Stokes-Adams syndrome).
   - Partial or complete heart block isoprenaline is used.

   Congestive: Cardiac failure (Dopamine/Dobutamine is used).

   Noradrenaline 0.2% solution administered i.v. diluted with 500 ml of 5% dextrose making concentration 4 microgram / ml. Initial response with 2 to 3 ml rest is administered with close observation of BP. Noradrenaline is unstable with neutral pH so vitamin-C 500-1000 mg is administered if infused with normal saline.

Table 29.6: Bronchodilators

Direct pressor agent	Acting on receptor	Preparation and dose	Used for and remarks
Orciprenaline not acted COMT (Alupent)	β_2	20 mg oral, 0.5–1 mg IM or SC, 0.65–1.3 mg by inhalation	Bronchial asthma
Salbutamol (Asthalin)	β_2	2–4 mg TDS, 2 mg/5 mL syr, 100 mg metered dose inhaler	Used for bronchial asthma, palpitation tremor, ankle edema may occur.
Terbutaline (Bricarex)	β_2	2.5–5 mg orally, 0.5 mg/mL, 100–250 mg metered dose, 3 mg/5 mL syr, 10 mg/mL nebulizing solution	Similar to salbutamol used for long-term treatment of COPD
Salmeterol (Serobid)	β_2 showing acting	25 µg metered dose inhaler, 2 puff BD	Long-acting, used for nocturnal asthma
Isoetharine	β_2	Used by inhalation because it is a substitute COMT.	Used in acute episode of bronchoconstriction
Pirbuterol	β_2 selective	Used by inhalation every 4–6 hours	Structurally releated salbutamol
Bitoterol	β_2, agonist	Given by inhalation	Prodrug. Activated to colterol by esterase of lung
Fenoterol	β_2 selective	Given by inhalation	Prompt action. A report of New Zealand showing increase death rate with it, is controversial
Formoterol	β_2 high efficiency	Given by inhalation 12 µg rotocap, dose 12–24 µg twice daily	Long-acting used for nocturnal asthma, prophylactic to exercise induced asthma and COPD
Procaterol	β_2	Given by inhalation	Prompt action lasting for 5 hours
Bambuterol (Betaday)	β_2	10 mg, 20 mg tab, 5 mg/5 mL oral susp. single evening dose	Prodrug of terbutaline, hydrolyzed in lung by pseudo-cholinesterase used for chronic bronchial asthma
Anorectics			
Amphetamine use not justifiable	Acts on NA/DA pathways	5–10 mg orally	Narcolepsy, obesity, petit mal epilepsy. Dextroamphetamine used for hyperactive disorder
Fenfluramine	Increases serotonergic transmission	20–40 mg BD or TDS	Tranquilizing. USFDA has withdrawn it.
Mazindol	Acts on Na and DA pathways	1 mg **BD intermittently** used	Anorectic, increases metabolic rate. Stimulation and drowsiness both occur.

Contd...

Table 29.6: Bronchodilators (*Contd...*)

Direct pressor agent	Acting on receptor	Preparation and dose	Used for and remarks
Uterine relaxants			
Isoxsuprine (Duvadilan) Dysmenorrhea	β	5–10 mg BD or QDS orally or IM	Threatend abortion
Ritodrine (Ritodine)	β₂	10 mg/mL or 10 mg tab. Start with 50 mg/min IV and increase gradually	–
Others			
Methylphenidate	–	–	Used for narcolepsy, attention deficit, hyperactive disorder controlled drug
Dexmethylphenidate	–	–	Attention deficit, hyperactive disorder controlled
Pemoline	–	–	Used for attention deficit, hyperactive children, controlled drug. Liver failure may occur.
Nasal decongestants			
Xylometazoline (Otrivin)	α₂	0.05 to 1% drops	Should be used with caution in hypertensive and patient getting MAO inhibitors.
Oymetazoline (Nasivion)	α₂	0.025 to 0.5% drops	–
Naphazoline (Privine)	α₂	0.1% drops	–

3. **Bronchial asthma:** β₂ stimulants.
4. **Allergic disorder:** Adrenaline being physiological antagonist is used.
5. **Mydriatic:** Phenylephrine and dipivefrine (2nd choice for open angle glaucoma, phenylephrine also used for fundal examination.)
6. **CNS uses:** Hypokinetic children (amphetamine is used.)
   Narcolepsy: Amphetamine and imipramine (1st choice).
   Epilepsy: Amphetamine is used as an adjuvant and improves mood and rigidity.
   Parkinsonism: Amphetamine as adjuvants. Improves mood and rigidity.
7. **Obesity:** Anorectics
8. **Nocturnal enuresis in children:** Amphetamine benefits.
9. **Uterine relaxants:** Isoxuprine; ritodine IV.
10. **Insulin hypoglycemia:** Used as expedient measure, but glucose should be given earliest.
11. **Clonidine and** a-methyl dopa, a2 agonist used for hypertension.
12. **Apraclonidine and brimonidine** are used for glaucoma.
13. **Tizanidine is** a2 agonist used as centrally acting muscle relaxant.

Adverse Effects of Adrenergic Agonists

Adrenaline may cause restlessness; tremor, palpitation, throbbing headache which subsides with rest, cerebral hemorrhage, BP may rise, cardiac arrhythmia, angina. It should not be used in patient on non-selective β blocker because of sharp rise of BP due to α_1 action.

Before DA is administered in shock, hypovolemia should be corrected. Extravasation of DA may cause necrosis and sloughing.

Dobutamine may precipitate ventricular tachycardia by facilitating AV condition so digoxin should be kept in hand. It may increase infarct.

α-Adrenoceptor Blocking Agents

Dale first shown the blocking of function of adrenaline and noradrenaline by ergots.

Most of the α receptor blockers are competitive, except haloalkylamines produce non-competitive antagonism. The alpha (α) blocking agents can be chemically classified into:

1. **Non-equilibrium type**
   - **Beta-haloalkylamine**—dibenamine, phenoxybenzamine.
2. **Equilibrium competitive type**
   - **Natural ergot alkaloids**—ergotamine, ergotoxine.
   - **Imidazoline**—phenotolamine, tolazoline.

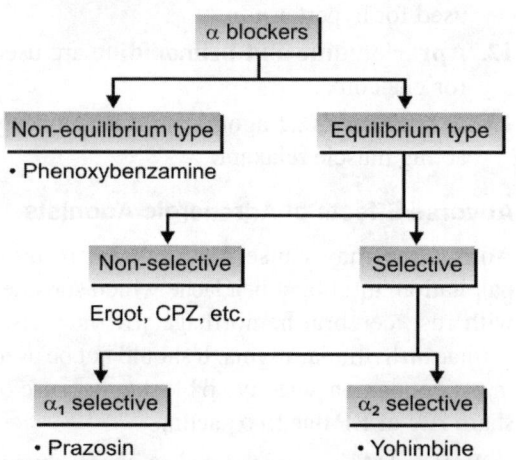

- **Miscellaneous**—chlorpromazine, ketanserin.
3. **α₁ selective**
   - Prazosin, terazosin, doxazosin, alfuzosin, tamsulosin
4. **α₂ selective yohimbine**

General Effects of α blocker

- Fall in BP due to reduction of peripheral resistance (α_1 and α_2).
- Abolish pressure effect of adrenaline, phenylephrine.
- Reflex tachycardia due to fall of arterial pressure and increases release of noradrenaline due to α_2 blockade.
- The first drug effect of fall of BP can be minimized by decreasing less dose and start at night.
- Nasal stuffiness
- Miosis
- Diarrhea
- Hypotension causes decreased GFR leading to Na retention and increased blood volume.
- Bladder trigone and sphincter tone decrease and improve urinary flow in BPH patient.
- α blocker inhibits ejaculation and may cause impotence.

Therapeutic Uses of α-adrenergic Blockers

- Pheochromocytoma—phentolamine or phenoxybenzamine is used.

- **Phentolamine test:** IV 5 mg is injected over 1 minute and fall in BP more than 35 mmHg systolic or 25 mmHg diastolic is suggestive of pheochromocytoma. Provocative test with histamine or glucagon or methacholone is dangerous to produce rise in BP, phentolamine should be kept in hand.
- Hypertension (prazosin) phenoxybenzamine or phentolamine is used for clonidine withdrawal. Cheese reaction with MAO-inhibitors. Indoramine or urapidill is used as antihypertensive in some countries.
- Secondary shock by counteracting reflex vasoconstriction and improving perfusion.
- Peripheral vascular disease, Raynaud's phenomenon and intermittent claudication (tolazoline, prazosin, phenoxybenzamine)
- CHF (prazosin)
- Prazosin is also used in some conditions of scorpion sting.
- Benign hypertrophy of prostate (prazosin, terazosin, doxazosin; tamsulosin; alfuzosin). Terazosin and doxazosin apart from α_1 blocking, have apoptosis effect on prostate smooth muscle cells which further lessen the symptoms of BPH. Tamsulosin is $\alpha_1 A$ and $\alpha_1 D$ subtype specific and has little effect on blood pressure. It produces floppy iris syndrome during cataract surgery.
- Migraine (ergotamine)
- Papaverine 3–20 mg with or without phentolamine 0.5–1 mg injection in corpus cavernosum induces penile erection in impotence.

Robert Furchgott; Ferid Murad; Louis Ignarro got Noble Prize for their work on nitric oxide.

- **Erectile dysfunction**

Here male is unable to maintain erection of penis for sufficient period to permit satisfactory intercourse. Cyclic GMP form by action of NO is metabolized by PDE-5. Sildenafil inhibits PDE-5 leading to increased cyclic GMP level to produce sufficient erection. Difficulty in color vision (blue color) may occur due to simultaneous inhibition of PDE-VI. It is also effective in the management of pulmonary hypertension. It should act coordinately with parasympathetic system (S_2–S_4). Other drugs useful for this disorder are:

i. Used orally; (a) Sildenafil; Verdenafil; Tadalafil (should not be prescribed with patient liking nitrates). Other orally effective drugs are: Dopamine agonist, apomorphine and antidepressant, trazodone.

ii. Alprostadil PGE_1 analogue; Phentolamine injected into corpora cavernosa.

Papaverine can be used alone (3–20 mg) or with phentolamine (0.5–1 mg) injected in corpora cavernosa called PIPE therapy. Aviptadil is an analogue of vasoactive intestinal peptide causes smooth muscle relaxation. Ketanserin $5HT_2$ and a receptor blocker used in combination with Alprostadil. Thymoxamine α blocker used as an injection in corpora cavernosa. Naltrexone has also been tried. Some herbal drugs like Ginseng, Gingko, *etc.* are also claimed to be effective in erectile dysfunction.

Drugs which may cause errectile dysfunction: β blockers, clonidine, α-methyldopa, thiazides, MAO-inhibitors, benzodiazepines, alcohol, antiandrogen.

β-Adrenoceptor Blocking Agents (β Blockers)

Based on their action, β receptors are classified as β_1, found in heart and adipose tissue and β_2, predominating in vascular and bronchial smooth muscle and pancreas.

Ideal β blockers for cardiovascular disorders
- Selective cardiac β_1 antagonism
- No β_2 blockade in lungs and peripheral vasculature
- Peripheral vasodilator activity
- Intrinsic cardiac stimulatory activity
- Long pharmacodynamic half-life.

Therapeutic Uses of β blockers

Cardiac
- Hypertension
- Angina
- Arrhythmia
- Silent ischemia
- Hypertropic obstructive cardiomyopathy
- Mitral valve prolapse
- Dissecting aneurysm
- Fallot tetralogy
- QT interval prolongation syndrome
- LVH regression
- Syncope

Non-cardiac
- Glaucoma (carteolol; betaxolol; levobunodol; metoprolol; timolol; levobetaxolol are used).
- Thyrotoxicosis
- Migraine (propranolol, timolol and metaprolol are effective)
- Essential tremor
- Bleeding esophageal varices (propranolol and nadolol are efficacious)
- Anxiety
- Alcohol withdrawal

Classification of β blockers			
1st generation	• Propanolol • Nadolol • Sotalol	• Pindolol • Penbutolol • Timolol • Alprenalol	Non-selective β_1 and β_2. Used in hypertension and angina. Adverse effects are bronchospasm, metabolic and peripheral vascular effects.
2nd generation	• Atenolol • Bisoprolol • Acebutolol*	• Metoprolol** • Oxprenolol* • Esmolol	Relatively selective for β_1. No vaso- or bronchial constriction.
3rd generation	• Labetalol • Carteolol • Nebivolol	• Carvedilol • Bucindolol	With additional α blocking and vasodilator property
β_1 selective	• Betaxolol	• Celiprolol 3rd generation	β_1 selective, β blocker with additional actions.

*Possesses ISA activity. **Possesses membrane stabilization action in higher doses.

3rd generation β blockers with some additional features producing vasodilatations

- **Producing NO:** Celiprolol, nebivolol, carteolol, bopindolol, nipradilol.
- **α_1 receptor antagonism:** Carvedilol, bucindolol, bevantolol, nipradilol, labetalol.
- **Blocking voltage gated Ca^{2+} channel:** Carvedilol, betaxolol, bevantolol.
- **K^+ channel opening:** Tilisolol.
- **Beta receptor agonism:** Celiprolol, carteolol, bopindolol.
- **With antioxidant property:** Carvedilol.
- Labetalol is a α_1 and β receptors competitive antagonist. Its response to different isomers varies.

NO production have the following advantages for system.

1. Inhibits platelet aggregation and adhesion.
2. Decreases LDL oxidation and smooth muscle cell proliferation.

Adverse effects and contraindications of β blockers

1. CHF
2. Bradycardia
3. COPD may be worsened
4. Exacerbate prinzmetal angina
5. Carbohydrate intolerance
6. Alters plasma lipid profile
7. Propranolol withdrawal should be gradual otherwise rebound hypertension may occur.
8. Contraindicated in complete heart block
- Safety in pregnancy limited. May cause fetal bradycardia.

PRECISE (**P**rospective **R**andomised **E**valuation of **C**arvedilol on **S**ymptoms and **E**xercise) and **MOCHA**, (**M**ulticentre **O**ral **C**arvedilol **H**eart failure **A**ssessment) studies: Have shown carvedilol improved patient symptoms, ejection fraction and mortality reduction in heart failure patients.

β blockers and drug interactions

1.	Aluminum hydroxide	Decrease absorption
2.	Aminophyline	Mutual inhibition
3.	Amiodarone	Cardiac arrest
4.	Antidiabetic	Masking of hypoglycemic effect. Enhanced hypoglycemia and hypotension.
5.	Cimetedine	Prolong t½ of Propranolol, Metoprolol and Labetolol— use it with caution.
6.	Clonidine	Hypertension during clonidine withdrawal
7.	Digitalis	Potentiation of bradycardia
8.	Epinephrine	Hypertension, bradycardia
9.	Ergot	Vasoconstriction
10.	Glucagon	Inhibition of hyperglycemia
11.	Indomethacin	Inhibition of antihypertensive response
12.	Isoprenaline	Mutual inhibition
13.	Levodopa	Antagonism of levodopa, hypertensive and positive inotropic response.
14.	Lignocaine	Propranolol pretreatment increases lignocaine blood level, use lower doses.
15.	Methyldopa	Hypertension during stress
16.	MAO-I	Uncertain, theoretical
17.	Phenothiazine	Additive hypotensive effect
18.	Phenyl propylamine	Severe hypertension effect
19.	Phenytoin	Additive cardiac depressant effect
20.	Quinidine	Additive cardiac depressant effect
21.	Reserpine	Excessive sympathetic blockade
22.	Tricyclic anti-depressants	Inhibits negative inotropic and chronotropic effects.

INDIVIDUAL β BLOCKER DRUGS

Propranolol (Inderal): 10 to 160 mg. Used for systemic hypertension, myocardial infarction, arrhythmia, pheochromocytoma, migraine prophylactically, parkinsonism, akathisia by antipsychotic drugs, variceal bleeding, anxiety and essential tremor.

Sotalol (sotagard): 40 to 80 mg tab, used in class III antiarrhythmic.

Timolol, betaxolol, levobundol, cartilolol, metipranolol are used for topical application in glaucoma.

Pindolol 5 mg tab (visken): Possesses intrinsic sympathomimetic action (ISA).

Oxprenolol: With partial agonist activity.

Alprenolol: Similar to pindolol.

Metoprolol: 50 to 100 mg tab, 5 mg/mL used in myocardial infarction (metolar; betaloc). S(–) is an active enantiomer, effective in half doses.

Atenolol: β_1 selective, low lipid solubility and 50–100 mg daily. S(–) atenolol is an active enatiomer. Used in half dose.

Acebutolol: Cardioselective, partial agonist, membrane stabilizing (sectral 200–400 mg; 10 mg/2 mL IV used for arrhythmia).

Bisoprolol (Concor 5 mg OD): Used for angina and hypertension.

Esmolol: Ultrashort acting β_1 blocker used in auricular fibrillation, SVT, to control BP during surgery, myocardial infarction (miniblock) 100 mg/10 mL.

Nebivolol (nodon 5 mg): NO donating β_1 blocker reverses endothelial dysfunction and prevents atherosclerosis.

Celiprolol: β_1 blocker with β_2 agonist (celipres 100–200 mg tabs).

Carvedilol (Carvi 3.125 mg): $\beta_1 + \beta_2 + \alpha_1$ receptor blocker, causes vasodilation. It has calcium channel blocker and antioxidant properties.

- **Nadolol:** Long-acting with equal affinity for β_1 and β_2 receptors, used for hypertension and angina.

- **Bucindolol (sandonorm):** β and α receptor blockers with β_2 and β_3 agonists action. Decreases afterload and increases HDL, but no effect in triglyceride.

Adrenergic Neuron Blocking Drugs

These groups of drug impair the functioning of peripheral sympathetic nerves. They do not block adrenoceptor. They were formerly used in the treatment of hypertension because of their lack of effect on parasympathetic system. Prototypes of this group of drug are bretylium and guanethidine.

Difference between antiadrenergic drugs and adrenergic neuron blocking drugs		
	Antiadrenergic drugs	*Adrenergic neuron blocking drugs*
Acts on	Adrenergic receptors are blocked	Adrenergic neurons or contents are blocked
Adrenergic nerve stimulation	Less completely blocked	More completely blocked
Effect of injected adrenaline	Blocked	Not blocked
Type of effect blocked	Either α or β (Labetolol blocks both)	Sympathetic function decreased
Example	α=Phentolamine; ergot, β=Propranolol α + β=Labetalol	Reserpine, guanethidine, bretylium, α-methyl-p-tyrosine

Drugs Acting on Autonomic Ganglia

Acetylcholine is a primary excitatory neurotransmitter in both sympathetic and parasympathetic ganglia.

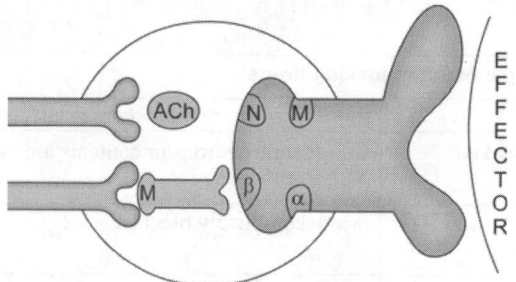

Fig. 33.1

Ganglionic Stimulant

Selective nicotinic agonist

- Nicotine, lobeline
- Dimethyl phenyl piperazinium (DMPP)
- Tetramethyl ammonium (TMA).
- Vareniciline

Non-selective muscarinic agonist

- ACh; carbachol, pilocarpine; MCN 343 a nicotine transdermal (nicotinell TTS) 10; 20; 30 cm^2 is used to treat nicotine dependence. Vareniciline is a nicotinic N_N receptor's partial agonist controls craving of nicotine withdrawal.

Ganglion Blocker

a. **Competitive blocker:** Hexamethonium, pentolinium, mecamylamine, pempidine, trimethaphan, are rarely used to control hypertension.

Mecamylamine is used for smoking cesation and Trimethaphan used in treatment of controlling hypertension. Otherwise ganglion blocker has no clinical reliance.

b. **Persistent depolarizers** like large dose of nicotine and anticholinesterases can block the ganglion of autonomic nervous system.

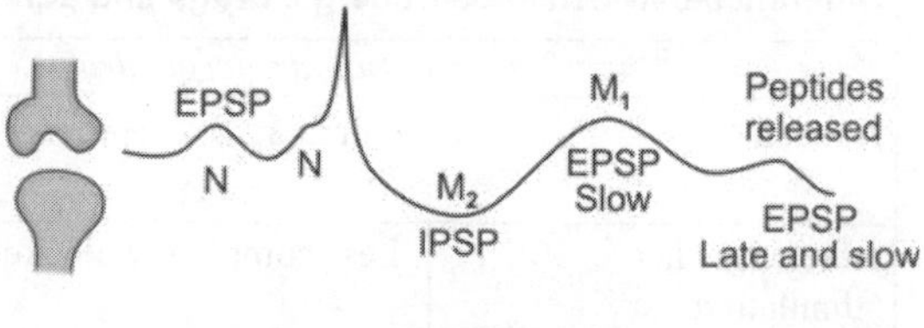

Fig. 33.2

Postsynaptic regulation of ganglion transmission: In ganglion transmission, postganglionic autonomic cells are depolarized by binding neuronal (N_N) receptor of ACh causing fast excitatory postsynaptic potential (EPSP) followed by slow inhibitory postsynaptic potential (IPSP) by long-lasting hyperpolarization after potential by M2 receptor opening potassium channels. IPSP is followed by slow EPSP due to closing of potassium channel linked in M1 cholinoceptor. Very slow EPSP is due to peptides released by other fiber and modulates responsiveness of postsynaptic cells. (Fig. 33.2)

Antismoking Drugs

(a) **Vareniciline:** Direct acting N_N receptor agonist having selectivity for $\alpha_4\beta_2$ isoform of N_N receptor. Used orally, t½ is 14–20 hours ADR. Headache, nausea and sleep disturbances.

(b) **Transdermal nicotine patch** effective in 18–20% of cases.

(c) **Bupropion:** Inhibits the uptake of 5HT, NE and DA, basically antidepressant used for cessation of smoking. It may cause CNS stimulation and seizure also known as amfebutamonel its generic name.

(d) **Rimonabant** is an antagonist to cannabinoid (CB_1) receptor causing rise in 5HT and DA levels ADR: Nausea, vomiting, suicidal tendency (depression) and anxiety may occur.

(e) **Clonidine:** α_2 agonist decreases craving for nicotine. It is also useful for insomnia. It is better than nicotine chewing gum as it can be used in cardiac patients also.

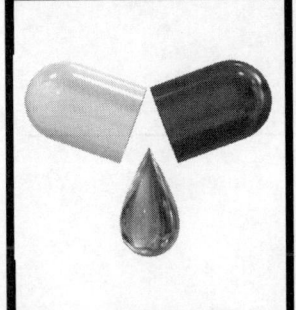
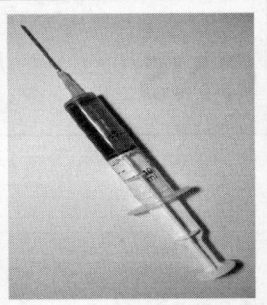
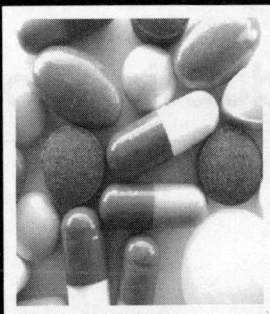
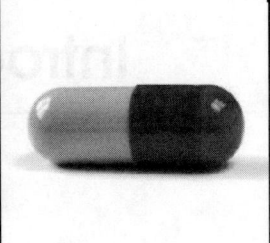

SECTION 4

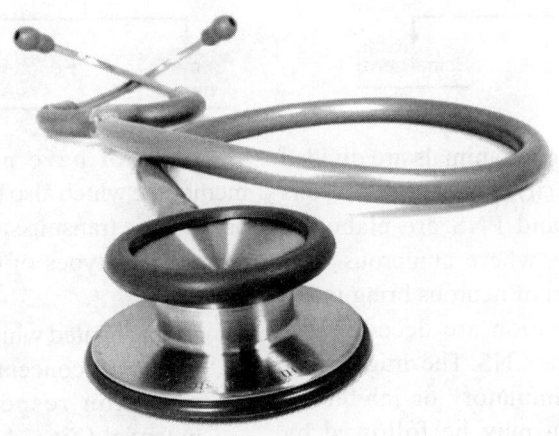

CENTRAL NERVOUS SYSTEM

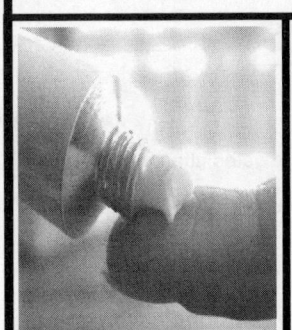
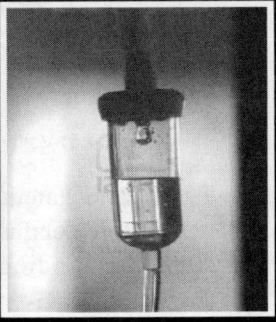
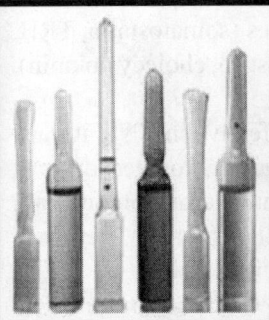
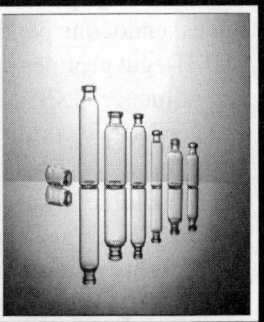

34

Introduction to CNS

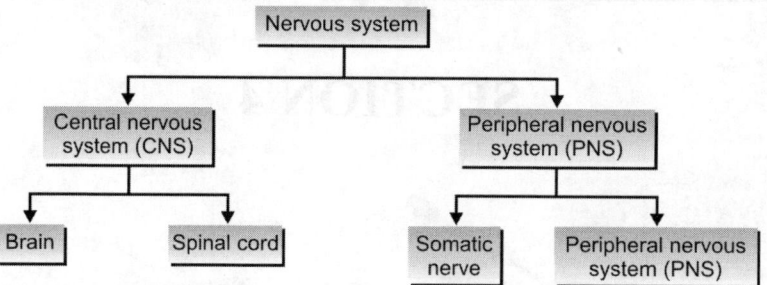

Nervous systems of higher animals are divided into: (i) Central and (ii) Peripheral nervous systems. Both CNS and PNS are elaborate systems of telegraphy, where numerous wire connections in the form of neurons bring information. These information are decoded and decisions are taken in the CNS. The drugs acting on CNS are either stimulatory or inhibitory. Excessive stimulation may be followed by inhibition. Like CNS, PNS contains numerous excitatory or inhibitory neurotransmitters. The inhibition may be postsynaptic or presynaptic (reducing quantum of release of neurotransmitters). Apart from neurotransmitter, several endogenous peptides like enkephalins, endorphins, endocrine peptides (somatostatin, TRH, LHRH), gut peptides (gastrin, cholecystokinin), *etc.* influence CNS.

In order to be drug effective in CNS, it must cross the blood-brain barrier. Ionized drug or lipid-insoluble drug cannot cross blood-brain barrier. Meningeal inflammation increases permeability of the drug into CNS.

All drugs acting on CNS act on specific receptors except a few like general anesthetics and alcohol have non-specific actions on membrane which also have demonstrable actions on synaptic transmission. The nerve membranes contain two types of channels which are open and close.

i. Voltage gated which responds to membrane potential, concentrated on initial segment and axon responsible for fast action potential (Fig. 34.1).

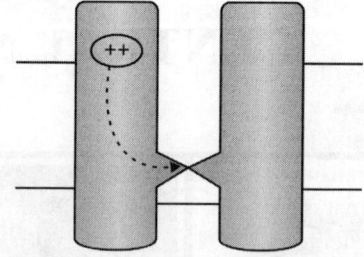

Fig. 34.1: Voltage gated channel

ii. The ligand gated or ionotropic receptor responsible for fast synaptic transmission opens by binding neurotransmitters. It also binds to G-protein coupled receptors (metabotropic receptors through which they modulate voltage gated channels). Metabotropic channel may modulate second messenger, *viz.* β receptors producing cAMP (Figs 34.2 and 34.3).

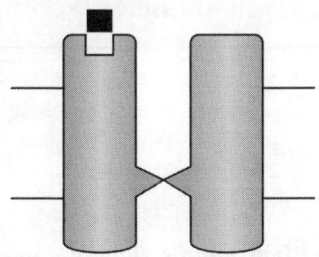

Fig. 34.2: Ligand gated channel

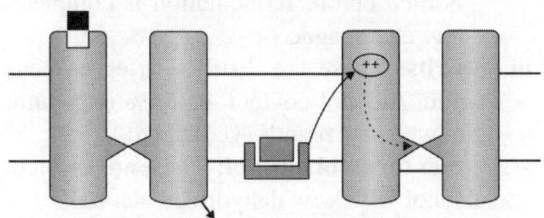

Fig. 34.3: Metabotropic channel

The ionotropic receptors for glutamate can be further divided into three subtypes based on the action of selective agonist: (a) α-amino-3-hydroxy-5-methyl-4-isoxazole-proprionic acid (AMPA), (b) kainic acid (KA) and (c) N-methyl-D-aspartate (NMDA). All of these receptors are composed of four subunits.

The communication between neurons in CNS occurs at synapse. Most drugs produce their actions in some steps of chemical synaptic trasnsmission, which may be presynaptic (like synthesis, storage metabolism and release of neurotransmitters) or postsynaptic (drugs acting as agonist or antagonist).

The neuronal system of CNS may be divided into: (i) Hierarchical system including all pathways of sensory perception and motor control. The excitatory transmitter released here is mostly glutamate and local circuit of smaller neurons are inhibitory, releasing either glycine or GABA. Their neurons are myelinated, and (ii) nonspecific neuronal systems contain monoamines like NAd, DA, 5HT or some peptides. Their neurons are unmyelinated.

Some Central neurotransmitters
In the CNS, following neurotransmitters are known to produce their effects.
- **Amino acids:** Glutamate, GABA, glycine and aspartic acid.
- **Acetylcholine**
- **Monoamines** like DA, NAd and 5HT.
- **Peptides:** Opioid peptides (enkephalin and endorphin), neurotensin, substance P, vasoactive intestinal peptide, neuropeptide Y, *etc.*
- **Nitric oxide**
- **Endocannabinoids**
- **Gut hormones:** Cholecystokinin, gastrin pancreatic polypeptide.
- **Hormones:** Angiotensin, calcitonin, glucagon, insulin.
- **Pituitary peptides:** ACTH, growth hormone, α-melanocyte-stimulating hormone (α-MSH), oxytocin, vasopressin.
- **Hypothalamic releasing hormones:** Corticotropin-releasing hormone (CRH), luteinizing hormone-releasing hormone (LHRH), somatostatin, thyrotropin-releasing hormone (TRH).
- **Miscellaneous peptides:** Bombesin, bradykinin, neurotensin, prolactin, substance K, carnosine, Orexin.
- **Other signaling substances:** Endocannabinoids nitric oxide, purines (*viz.* Adenosine, ATP, UTP; UDP).

Earlier it was thought that each neuron uses one neurotransmitter, but now it is established that many neurons have more than one neurotransmitters for cotransmission, *i.e.* neuron uses polypharmacy of its own.

35

Alcohol

Aliphatic alcohol contains hydroxy (–OH) group on aliphatic hydrocarbon. It is manufactured by fermentation of sugars.

$$C_6H_{12}O_6 \xrightarrow[\text{in yeast}]{\text{Zymase}} 2C_2H_5OH + 2CO_2$$

Starchy cereals are soaked to produce malt, which is fermented by yeast to produce alcohol. Commercial alcohol is obtained from mollases.

Classification

- Monohydroxy: Ethyl, methyl and propyl alcohols.
- Dihydroxy (glycol): Ethylene glycol, propylene glycol.
- Trihydroxy: Glycerol
- Polyhydroxy: Mannitol, sorbitol.

Alcohols are not important therapeutically, but its social significance is very important. History of alcohol consumption is as old as civilization. In ancient Indian literature, it is mentioned as *Somrash*.

Some Commonly Consumed Alcoholic Beverages

i. **Malted liquors** produced by fermentation of germinating cereals are undistilled alcohol. Alcohol content is 3–6% low, *e.g.* beers, stout. Strong beers content is up to 10% of alcohol.

ii. **Wines** produced by fermenting sugars of grapes are undistilled.
- **Light wine's** alcohol content is 9–12% (claret, cider).

- **Fortified wine's** alcohol content is 16–22% (port, sherry).
- **Effervescent wine's** 12–16% alcohol bottled before fermentation is complete, *e.g.* champagne.

iii. **Spirits:** These are distilled after fermentation. Alcohol content 40–55% (*e.g.* rum, gin, whiskey, brandy, vodka, *etc.*)

iv. **Other forms of alcohol:** These are absolute alcohol 99% w/w dehydrated alcohol.

v. **Rectified spirit** 90% w/w ethyl alcohol from mollases by distillation.

vi. **Proof spirit** 57% v/v alcohol. Whisky is poured in gun powder and ignited to explode. If water is mixed then there will be no ignition.

vii. **Methylated spirit** is used as antiseptic and astringent. It is not fit for consumption and so colored blue.

Pharmacological Actions (Ethyl alcohol)

Local action: It depends upon the concentration of alcohol. Since it evaporates quickly it is refreshing and its cooling is used for reduction of temperature in fever. Higher strength alcohols are astringent (precipitates surface proteins) irritant, germicidal and antiseptic. 100% alcohol is poor antiseptic, but dehydrating. It does not kill spores of the bacteria.

CNS: Alcohol depresses the CNS in a descending order. In small doses, it causes euphoria, freedom from anxiety and worry, improves communication. Alcohol causes generalized membrane action by altering the state of membrane lipids.

- Promotes $GABA_A$ mediated synaptic inhibition.
- Inhibits NMDA type excitatory receptor.
- Augments actions of 5HT on $5HT_3$ inhibitory autoreceptors.
- Reduces neurotransmitter release by inhibiting voltage sensitive Ca^{2+} channel. Blocks adenosine uptake.
- Turnover of NAd in brain increases through opioid receptor dependent mechanism.
- Activity on Na/K^+-ATPase and adenylyl cyclase is altered.
- Alcohol affects alteration of phosphorylation of protein kinase C (PKC) and protein kinase A of (PKA) in the membrane.

Alcohol induces sleep during its action on brain. It is anticonvulsant, but it is followed by epileptic fits. It raises pain threshold, but not an analgesic. Its chronic abuse damages brain neurons.

CVS: Small doses produce vasodilatation, there may be conjunctival injection, moderate doses produce tachycardia, large doses cause cardiac arrhythmia and fall in BP. Chronic alcoholism produces cardiomyopathy and conduction defects. Regular intake of moderate amount of alcohol raises HDL and lowers LDL which are beneficial for CAD. called "J Shaped" relationship. The antioxidant of red wine increases production of endogenous anticoagulant, tissue plasminogen activator (tPA) and inhibiting some inflammatory process also helps preventing atherosclerosis. It can produce cardiac arrhythmia due to QT prolongation.

Blood: Megaloblastic anemia may occur due to its interference in folate metabolism.

Body temperature: Raises temporarily due to vasodilatations. Large doses suppress temperature regulating center.

Respiration: May be stimulated by stimulating buccal and pharyngeal mucosa, but overall action of alcohol is respiratory depression.

Endocrine system: It increases adrenaline release, when taken in moderately causing hyperglycemia, but acute intoxication depletes hepatic glycogen due to inhibition of gluconeogenesis causing hypoglycemia.

Liver: Mobilizes peripheral fat and increases fat synthesis in liver. Acetaldehyde produced by its metabolism damages hepatocytes. Vitamin deficiencies also take place. Chronic alcoholism causes hepatic cell necrosis and fibrosis. Increased lipid peroxidation and glutathione depletion occur. It impairs gluconeogenesis, reduces synthesis of albumins and transferrin, and induces microsomal enzymes on chronic intake.

Gastrointestinal tract: 10% alcohol increase gastric secretion (specially acid) and higher concentration induces vomiting and gastritis. It lowers the tone of lower esophageal sphincters. Pancreatitis may occur.

Kidney: Acts as diuretics as it inhibits ADH secretion.

Skeletal muscles: Myopathy occurs in chronic alcoholism. Fatigue may be allayed by small dose of alcohol.

Sex: It increases desire, but decreases performance. Chronic alcoholism leads to impotence, sterility, gynecomastia, prostatic congestion leading to urinary retention, stimulating ACTH release may produce pseudo-Cushing's syndrome. Drinking during pregnancy has damaging effect on fetus (fetal alcohol syndrome), uterine contraction is suppressed.

Fetal alcohol syndrome: Alcohol abuse during pregnancy causes mental retardation, flattened face, microcephaly, mild joint anomaly.

Pharmacokinetics: Rate of absorption from stomach of alcohol depends upon concentration and presence of foods. Intestinal absorption is very fast. Gets distributed in the body Vd = 0.7 L/kg. Crosses blood-brain barrier and placental barrier efficiently. Oxidized in liver 98%. Metabolism follows zero order kinetics, *i.e.* constant amount of 8–12 mL/hour is degraded. Excretion occurs *via* kidney and lungs, 0.05% of blood concentration in exhaled air is utilized for medicolegal determination of drunken state by measuring alcohol by breath analyzer.

Alcohol is not a food though it provides energy (1 gm = 7.1 Cal) as because it is:

- Inadequate to maintain basal metabolism
- Addiction liability
- Contained no nitrogen.
- Rather chronic alcoholics produce dietary deficiencies.

The energy produced by alcohol cannot be stored.

Alcohol Metabolism (Fig. 35.1)

Alcohol is metabolized to acetaldehyde by two major pathways which is then oxidized by third metabolic process.

(a) **Alcohol dehydrogenase pathway:** Cytoplasmic alcohol dehydrogenase (ADH) enzyme converts alcohol to aldehyde. The enzyme is found in stomach, brain and liver. It requires NAD. It is blocked by fomepizole. (Fig. 35.1)

(b) **Microsomal ethanol oxidizing system (MEOS):** This enzyme system operates when large amount of ethanol is consumed or in chronic alcoholism, it is induced.

(c) **Acetaldehyde metabolism:** Acetaldehyde formed from alcohol oxidized in liver by NAD dependent aldehyde dehydrogenase (ALDH) and can be blocked by disulfiram; metronidazole; cafotetan; trimethoprim.

A person deficient in ALDH enzyme may show high aldehyde concentration, if consumes alcohol with features of antabuse reaction.

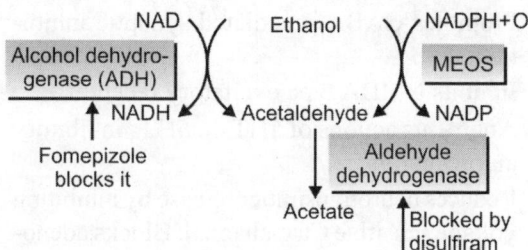

Fig. 35.1: Metabolism of alcohol

Therapeutic uses of alcohol

- Symptomatic cooling of surface temperature, *i.e.* fever.
- Prevents bedsores.
- Antiseptic 70% w/v.
- To wash phenol in accidental skin contamination.
- To destroy nerve in trigeminal neuralgia
- Systematically as appetizer and carminative 10% (30–50 mL)
- Methanol poisoning.
- As rubefacient in sprains; joint pain as after-shaving lotion.

Alcohol Use Disorder

According to Jellinek, there are five species of alcohol dependence. (Table 35.1)

Physical dependence occurs to round the clock drinking leading to nutritional deficiencies (food neglect, malabsorption), polyneuritis, pellagra, tremor, seizure, Wernicke's encephalopathy, Korsakoff's psychosis, megaloblastic anemia, cirrhosis, cardiomyopathy, pancreatitis,

Table 35.1: Alcohol dependence

α-*alcoholism*	β-*alcoholism*	γ-*alcoholism*	δ-*alcoholism*	ε-*alcoholism (malignant alcoholism)*
• Excessive and inappropriate drinking to relief pain (physical and mental) • No loss of control • Ability to abstain present	• Excessive and inappropriate drinking • Physical complications (cirrhosis, gastritis, neuritis) • No dependence	• Progressive course • Physical dependence with tolerance and withdrawal symptoms • Psychological dependence with inability to control drinking	• Inability to abstain • Tolerance • Withdrawal symptoms • The amount of alcohol consumed can be controlled • Social disruption is minimal	• Dipsomania (compulsive drinking) • Spree drinking

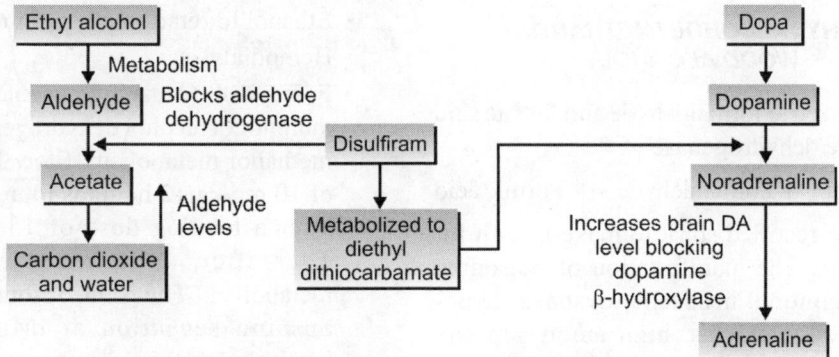

Fig. 35.2: Mechanism of action of disulfiram

CCF, arrhythmia, gynecomastia, infertility, myopathy, malignancy (hepatic, oral).

Treatment of Alcohol Dependence

i. Behavior therapy
ii. Deterrent agents (antabuse).

It has been observed that workers of rubber industry developed unpleasant response to alcohol intake due to accidental absorption of antioxidant, disulfiram (Tetramethylthiuram disulfide).

Contraindications of antabuse therapy

• First trimester of pregnancy
• CAD
• CRF
• Liver failure
• Neuropathy
• History of psychosis in past
• Uncontrolled diabetes mellitus.

Treatment should be undertaken in patient department. DER (disulfiram ethanol reaction) can be very severe and life-threatening due to one or more of the following: shock, myocardial infarction, convulsion and coma. The general reactions to disulfiram are facial flushing, nausea, vomiting, dizziness and headache.

Preparation

Antabuse disulfiram (250 g) tab.

Other aldehyde dehydrogenase inhibitors like citrated calcium carbamide is short-lasting.

Drug interactions of alcohol

• CNS depressant effect with tranquilizers, antidepressant, antihistamine, hypnotics.

• Sulfonylurea, cephalosporin, metronidazole produce antabuse reaction.
• Insulin enhances hypoglycemia.
• Aspirin causes gastric bleeding.

Guidelines for safe drinking

• 1–2 drinks are safe, but no more than 3 drinks in one occasion.
• Do not take alcohol with interacting drugs or with any contraindication.
• Do not drink or engaged in hazardous activities.

Withdrawal syndrome of alcohol: It produces anxiety, sweating, tremor, sleep distribution, hallucination, convulsion and collapse.

Treatment

a. Psychological
b. Medical supportives like:

• Diazepam or chlordiazoxide. Short acting drugs like lorazapam or oxazepam with patient of liver disease as they do not accumulate.
• Naltrexone (opioid antagonists) helps to prevent relapse of alcoholism.
• **Acamprosate:** It is a weak NMDA receptor antagonist and $GABA_A$ receptor agonist reduces relapse of drinking behavior used in Europe.
• Ondansetron $5HT_3$ antagonist decreases alcohol craving.
• Antiepileptic topiramate shows promising result in treating alcoholism.
• Spasmolytic drug baclofen.

METHYL ALCOHOL / METHANOL / WOOD ALCOHOL

Metabolized to formaldehyde and formic acid by aldehyde dehydrogenase.

Methanol $\longrightarrow$ Formaldehyde $\longrightarrow$ Formic acid

Added to rectified spirit to make it unfit for consumption. The manifestation of poisoning includes vomiting, headache, dyspnea, hypotension, lactic acidosis, high anion gap and retinal damage. Visual damage described as snow storm which can cause blindness. It follows zero order kinetics. Methanol poisoning generally occurs with unscientifically made country liqours and is responsible for several casualties every year.

NB: By the term anion gap means sum of $[Na^{\oplus} + K^{\oplus}]$ – sum of $[Cl^- + HCO_3^-]$. Normally, it is 12–17 mmol/L.

- Na^+ normal range is 136–146 mmol/L and average is 140 mmol/L.
- K^+ normal range is 2–5 mmol/L and average is 3 mmol/L.
- Cl^- normal range is 93–103 mmol/L and average is 98 mmol/L.
- HCO_3^- normal range is 24–32 mmol/L and average is 28 mmol/L.

$\therefore$ $(140 + 3) - (98 + 28)$ = Anion gap
$143 - 126 = 17$ mmol/L.

Treatment of methanol poisoning

The principles of treatment of methyl alcohol treatment are:

i. Suppressing its metabolism either with ethyl alcohol or fomepizole.

ii. Hemodialysis

iii. Alkalization to combat acidosis.

- Keep patient in quiet darkroom, protect eyes.
- Gastric lavage with sodium bicarbonate.
- Acidosis treated with sodium bicarbonate infusion.
- KCl infusion to treat hypokalemia of alkali therapy.

- Ethanol to retard methanol metabolism.
- Hemodialysis.
- Fomepizole (4-methylpyrazole)—specific inhibitor of alcohol dehydrogenase retards methanol metabolism. Slow IV infusion of 10 mg/kg/12 hours is found to be safe after a loading dose of 15 mg/kg IV. Thereafter, as it increases its own metabolism. The ADR of fomepizole are burning sensation at infusion site, headache, nausea, dizzines.
- Folate therapy—calcium leucovorin injected repeatedly reduces blood formate level with promising results. 50 mg injected every six hourly.

Ethylene glycol ($CH_2OH–CH_2OH$): Polyhydric alcohol, ethylene glycol used as an industrial solvent and a heat exchanger. May produce three stages of overdose manifestations. In the first stage, there is CNS excitation followed by depression. After 4–12 hours, there is severe acidosis due to lactate accumulation and in last stage renal insufficiency occurs with deposition of oxalate in renal tubules.

Diagnosis of ethylene glycol poisoning: Anion gap, osmolar gap and oxalate crystals in urine.

Metabolism of ethylene glycol

Glycoaldehyde $\longrightarrow$ Glycolic acid $\longrightarrow$ Glyoxylic acid $\longrightarrow$ Oxalic acid in stepwise.

Treatment: The orphan drug fomepizole is used to retard its metabolism like methanol poisoning.

The adverse effects of fomepizole are headache, nausea, dizziness, allergic reaction, burning sensation at infusion site. It rapidly induces its own metabolism.

- Ethyl alcohol is used as an alternative.
- Hemodialysis.

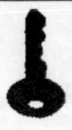 *Some common drugs causing antabuse like reaction are: Metronidazole, Chlorpropamide, Furazolidone, Procarbazine, Phenylbutazone, Griseofulvin, Moxalactam, Cefamandole, Cefoperazone.*

36

Sedative and Hypnotics

Nearly one-third of our life is spent in sleep. We go to bed voluntarily and transit into state of easily reversible relative unresponsiveness and tranquility which repeats regularly. The duration and pattern of sleep can be divided into two different phases, based on EEG. EMG and electro oculogram NREM (Non rapid eye movement) sleep starts while falling asleep when para sympathetic activity predominates with decrease in metabolic rate heart rate, cardiac output and peripheral vascular resistance. Dreams are rare. After 90–120 minutes of NREM sleep REM sleep occur lasting 5–30 minutes in which sympathetic activity predominates dreams are vivid, sexual errection may occur.

The EEG (electroencephalogram) recording of waking state shows a wave of 8–12 sec. Onset of sleep is characterized by disappearance of α-activity.

State 0 (Awake)

- From lying down to falling sleep.
- EEG shows α-activity when eyes are closed and β-activity when eyes are open.
- Eye movements are slowly rolling or irregular.
- 1–2% of total sleep.

Stage 1 (Dozing)

- Eye movements are reduced. There is relaxation of neck muscle.
- α-waves are interspersed with θ-waves.
- 3–6% of total sleep.

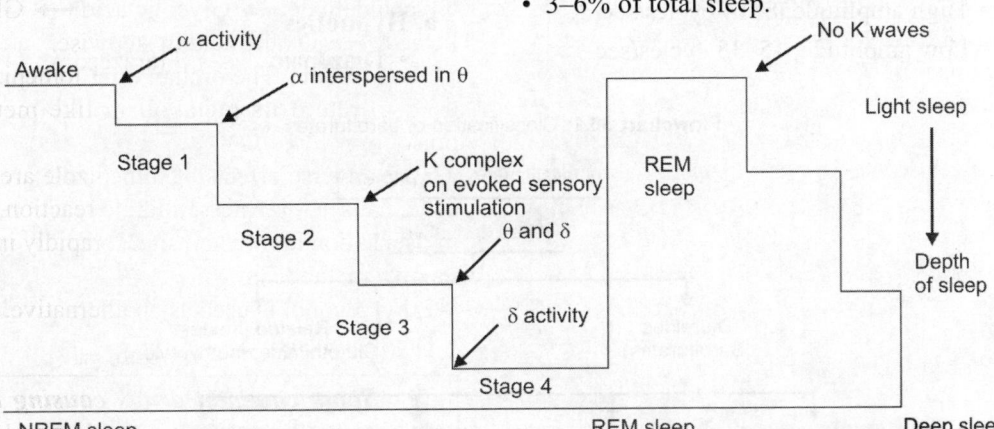

D sleep (desynchronized sleep or dreaming or REM or active or paradoxical sleep).
S sleep (synchronized, NREM, quiet or orthodox sleep which further divided into four stages).

Fig. 36.1: Sleep cycle

Stage 2 (Unequivocal Sleep)

- Within few minutes goes on to stage 2.
- Characterized by sleep spindles interspersed in waves, K complex present intermittently.
- 40–50% of sleeping period.
- Easily arousable.

Stage 3 (Deep Sleep Transition)

- EEG shows θ-, δ- and spindle activities.
- K complexes are evoked by strong stimulation.
- Subjects are not easily arousable, 5–8% of sleep time.

Stage 4 (Cerebral Sleep)

- δ-activity predominates in EEG.
- K complex cannot be evoked.
- Night terror might occur, comprises 10–20% of sleep time.

REM sleep (paradoxical sleep): EEG shows all types of waves except K complexes. Irregular darting eye movements, dreams, nightmares, stages 0–4 and REM recur over period of 80–100 minutes in cyclic ways. Most important central determinant of sicep is biological clock and melatonin production of pineal gland.

EEG Waves

α = High amplitude, 8–14 cycles/sec

β = Low amplitude, 15–35 cycles/sec

θ = Low amplitude, 4–7 cycles/sec

δ = High amplitude, 0.5–3 cycles/sec

K complex is deep negative wave followed by positive wave and some spindles.

Sedative: The drugs which reduce excitement and calm the subject.

Hypnotics: Drugs which produce sleep resembling natural sleep (Flowchart 36.1).

Hypnosis: Is a trans like state where subject becomes passive.

Both sedative and hypnotics are generalized CNS depressants. Generally, quicker in onset with shorter duration with steeper dose response curve gives better hypnotics whereas slow acting drugs with flattened dose response curve is preferred as sedative. In general anesthesia, there is further CNS depression. Hypnotics and sedatives are generally used for insomnia.

Alcohol and opium are oldest hypnotics. Then came bromides (1857), chloral hydrate (1869) and paraldehyde (1882).

Classification of drugs of sedative and hypnotics:

i. **Barbiturates** (Classification on Flow chart 36.1)

ii. **Benzodiazepines:** (divided according to therapeutic uses)

    a. Hypnotics

      - Diazepam   • Flurazepam

Flowchart 36.1: Classification of barbiturates

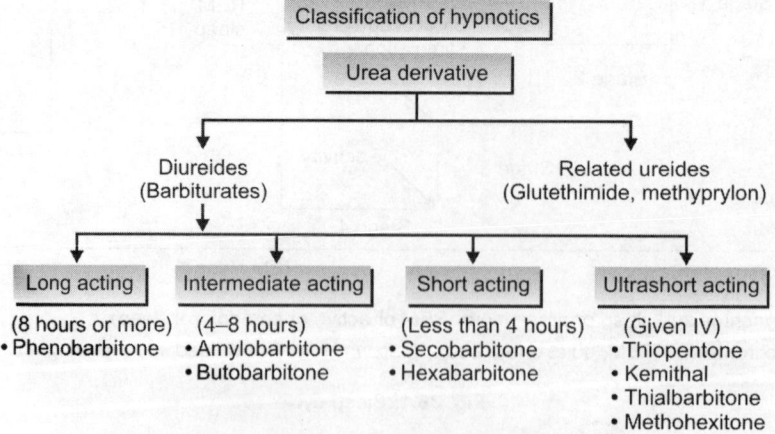

- Nitrazepam
- Temazepam
- Midazolam
- Triazolam
- Alprazolam

b. **Antianxiety**

- Diazepam
- Oxazepam
- Alparazolam
- Chlordiazepoxide
- Lorazepam

c. **Anticonvulsant**

- Diazepam
- Clobazam
- Clonazepam
- Lorazepam

iii. **Alcohol:** Choralhydrate

iv. **Aldehydes:** Paraldehyde

v. **Acetylated carbinols:** Ethinamate

vi. **Miscellaneous:** Meprobamate, methaqualone, antihistaminics (promethazine diphenhydramine), hyoscine, scopolamine, triclofos, antidepressants (amitryptyline).

vii. **Inorganic ions:** Bromides

viii. **Newer non-benzodiazepines:** Zopiclone, zolpidem and zaleplon.

Morphine and pethidine besides analgesic action, also possess hypnotic property so they are grouped as anodyne hypnotics.

BARBITURATES

Urea derivative barbiturates are common hypnotics till 1960, now they are prototypes to CNS depressants. Barbituric acid is produced when malonic acid condense with urea. Barbiturates are introduced by Fisher and von Mering in 1903.

$$O = C \underset{NH_2}{\overset{NH_2}{<}} \quad + \quad HOOC \underset{HOOC}{\overset{H}{>}} C \underset{H}{\overset{H}{<}}$$

Urea   Malonic acid

$$O = C_2 \quad \begin{matrix} H \\ | \\ N - C = O \\ {}^1 \quad {}^6 \\ {}_3 \quad {}^5 CH_2 + H_2O \\ N - C = O \\ | \\ H \end{matrix}$$

Barbituric acid

Structure–Action Relations

Barbituric acid is a six-membered ring structure. Barbituric acid itself is devoid of hypnotic activity. When hydrogen atom attached to C_5 is replaced by alkyl of aryl group, it gets hypnotic activity. An increase in length of side chain attached to C_5 increases solubility, shortens period of action (hexobarbitone). Introduction of phenyl group at C_5 produces phenobarbitone which is more anticonvulsant. Replacement of 0 at position 2 by sulfur produces thiobarbiturate which is an intravenous anesthetic.

Mechanism of action of barbiturates

- Depress polysynaptic responses and delay synaptic recovery. They primarily act on GABA. BZD receptor Cl^+ channel. Potentiate GABA-ergic inhibition by increasing the lifetime of Cl^+ channel opening induced by GABA.

- They react to picrotoxin sensitive site of BZD, but do not to BZD receptor.

- Also enhance BZD binding to receptor. At higher doses, directly increase Cl^- conductance (GABA mimetic contrast to BZD which is a GABA facilitatory).

- Voltage sensitive Na^+ and K^+ channels are depressed at high doses.

- They depress glutamate induced neuronal depolarization through AMPA receptors.

Pharmacokinetics

Well-absorbed by oral and intramuscular routes. They are weak acids, therefore, absorbed in acid pH of stomach, after absorption they are bound to plasma proteins. Readily cross placental barrier and excreted in milk. Activity mainly terminated by redistribution, metabolized by liver and renal excreted by route. Barbiturates inactivated in liver are conjugated to glucuronic acid and excreted through urine. Alkalinization of urine increases ionization and thereby increases renal excretion. Barbiturates induce hepatic microsomal enzymes and as a consequence they increase the rate of their own metabolism and many other drugs.

Therapeutic uses of barbiturates

- Sedative hypnotic (largely replaced by benzo-diazepine and phenothiazine)
- Anticonvulsant
- Preanesthetic medication
- Anesthetic (thiopentone)
- Neonatal jaundice
- Congenital nonhemolytic jaundice
- Kernicterus, it hastens glucuronic acid conjugation of bilirubin to hasten excretion
- Psychiatric use of amylo- and pentobarbitone (IV) to produce sleep.

Adverse effects of barbiturates

- Hangover
- Idiosyncrasy—elderly may produce excitement instead of hypnosis.
- Hypersensitivity—in atopic patient (rash, swelling of lips)

- Tolerance and dependence (cellular and pharmacokinetics)
- Withdrawal symptoms like excitement, hallucination, delirium.

ACUTE BARBITURATE POISONING

Mostly suicidal, may be accidental inspite of rare availability due to **drug automatism.** Lethal dose 2–3 gm for fat-soluble barbiturate and 5–10 gm for less fat-insoluble phenobrabitone. Signs and symptoms, comatose, failing respiration, BP and cardiovascular collapse (all due to excess pharmacological action).

Treatment of acute barbiturate poisoning

- Gastric lavage with activated charcoal.
- Cardiorespiratory support.
- Alkaline diuresis with sodium bicarbonate and diuresis with mannitol or furosemide.

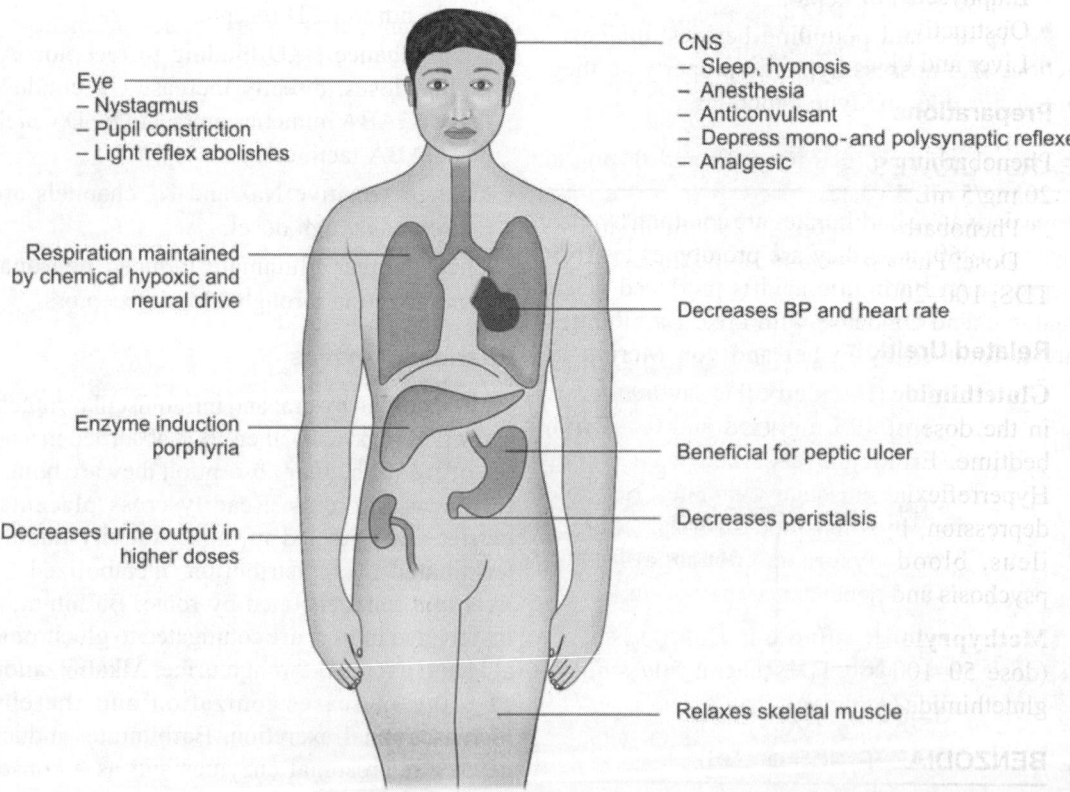

Eye
– Nystagmus
– Pupil constriction
– Light reflex abolishes

Respiration maintained by chemical hypoxic and neural drive

Enzyme induction porphyria

Decreases urine output in higher doses

CNS
– Sleep, hypnosis
– Anesthesia
– Anticonvulsant
– Depress mono- and polysynaptic reflexes
– Analgesic

Decreases BP and heart rate

Beneficial for peptic ulcer

Decreases peristalsis

Relaxes skeletal muscle

Fig. 36.2: Pharmacological action of barbiturates

- Dopamine infusion for vasopressor and renal vasodilation.
- IV fluid and forced alkaline diuresis.
- Hemodialysis through column of activated charcoal adsorbents.
- Metrazol or bemegride is used to awaken patient, but may lead to convulsion.
- Prophylactic antibiotics, if tracheostomy or catheterization.

Drug interaction of barbiturates

- Since it induces hepatic enzymes, reduces effectiveness of warfarin, OCP, tolbutamide, griseofulvin, theophylline.
- With alcohol, opioids and antihistaminics additive effect of CNS depression.
- Griseofulvin's absorption is decreased.

Contraindications of barbiturates

- Acute intermittent porphyria
- Emphysema or COPD
- Obstructive sleep apnea
- Liver and kidney diseases

Preparations

Phenobarbitone (Gardenal 30 and 60 mg/tab, 20 mg/5 mL 5 year)

Phenobarbitone sodium 200 mg/ml inj.

Dose: Phenobarbitone 30–60 mg orally OD-TDS; 100–200 mg IM or IV.

Related Ureides

Glutethimide (Doriden): It is daytime sedative in the dose of 125 mg TDS and 0.5–1 gm at bedtime. Erratically absorbed from GI tract. Hyperreflexia, muscular twitching, respiratory depression, hypotension, mydriasis, paralytic ileus, blood dyscrasia, neuropathy, toxic psychosis and dependence may occur.

Methyprylon (Noludar): Daytime sedative (dose 50–100 mg TDS) chemically similar to glutethimide. Addiction may occur.

BENZODIAZEPINES (BZDS)

Benzodiazepines are group of drugs cause sedation, hypnosis (shortens time spend in stage 4 and REM sleep, but increases the total sleep time and sleep produced by it is more refreshing) and decrease anxiety. Muscle relaxation and some of them possess anticonvulsant properties. They are popular because they have high therapeutic index about 20 times of hypnotic doses are tolerated, less depressant action on respiration and CNS (fall in BP is due to less cardiac output, but with flunitrazepam and midazolam, it is due to decrease in peripheral resistance). Enzyme induction is less. They are less likely to produce physical and psychological dependence and withdrawal symptoms. Flumazenil is its specific antagonistic which is available to treat poisoning of BZDs.

Site and mechanism of action

- Acts on reticular activating formation of midbrain maintaining wakefullness and limbic system maintaining the thought and mental functions. It decreases sleep latency when first used and time spent in stage 0; decreases stages 1, 2 and 3. REM sleep is shortened, but REM cycle is increased. Zolpidem and zaleplon suppress REM sleep. Nitrazepam increases REM sleep.
- BZD inhibits pre- and postsynaptic BZD receptors, the integral part of GABA$_A$ receptor Cl$^-$ channel. The subunits of this complex form of transmembrane anion channel gated by GABA (primary ligand). BZD ligand modulate it (secondary ligand). The binding for GABA is located on β-subunits, while the α-subunits contain BZD binding site (Fig. 36.3).

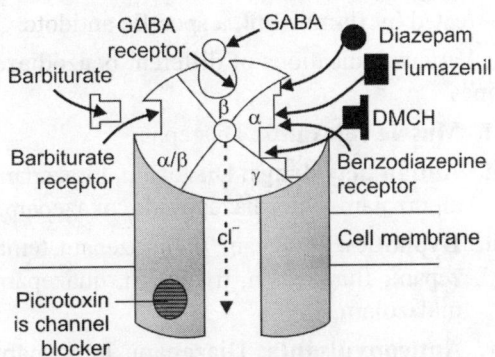

Fig. 36.3: GABA-BZD receptor complex

- It potentitates the depressant action of adenosine in higher concentration by blocking its uptake, which can be antagonized by theophylline.

GABA$_A$: BZD receptor Cl⁻ channel is a complex structure composed of five subunits α, β, γ pentamer. α_1 subunits are involved in sedation, hypnotic, amnesis and anticonvulsant action. α_2 subunits are involved in anxiolytic and muscle relaxant actions. Benzodiazepines appear to act on α_1, α_2, α_3 or α_5 subunits, therefore, has broad-spectrum of action. These studies are based on genetically mutated mice. Zaleplon and zolpidem have high affinity for α_1 subunits of BZD receptor, therefore, have less muscle relaxants effect and anticonvulsant action.

The chloride channel as shown in Fig. 36.3, is gated by GABA$_A$ receptor located on β subunits. Benzodiazepine receptor present on α and γ subunits modulates GABA$_A$ receptor, *viz.* agonist diazepam facilitates, inverse agonist DMCM hinders GABA$_A$-mediated Cl⁻ channel and BZD receptor antagonist flumazenil blocks the both. Barbiturate receptor located on either α or β subunit also facilitates GABA. GABA$_A$ receptor blocker is bicuculline. Cl⁻ channel is blocked by picrotoxin directly.

Benzodiazepines are preferred over bartiturates because of:

- High therapeutic index
- Produces less hangover and less distortion of sleep pattern
- Less abuse liability and drug interactions
- Also produces analgesia. Its poisoning can be treated by **flumazenil,** a specific antidote.

Various indications of different benzodiazepines.

  i. Muscle relaxants: Diazepam.

  ii. Antianxiety drugs: Diazepam, lorazepam, alprazolam, chlordiazepoxide, oxazepam.

  iii. Hypnotics: Diazepam, flunitrazepam, temazepam, flurazepam, triazolam, quazepam, midazolam.

  iv. Anticonvulsants: Diazepam, lorazepam, clonazepam, clobazam.

DRUGS AFFECTING GABA LINKED CHLORIDE CHANNELS

GABA$_A$: BZD–Cl⁻ channel complex as depicted in Fig. 36.3, which on opening increases conductance of chloride ions resulting depression of CNS. Several compounds can modulate this channel.

- **Endogenous GABA$_A$ receptor agonist** increases Cl⁻ influx.
- **Muscimol:** Agonist at GABA$_A$.
- **Bicuculline:** Competitive antagonist at GABA$_A$ receptor.
- **Picrotoxin:** Blocks Cl⁻ channel noncompetitively acting on picrotoxin sensitive site.
- **Barbiturates:** Agonist at allosteric picrotoxin and prolong GABA action.
- **Alcohol:** Opens Cl⁻ channel directly and allosteric facilitation of GABA.
- **β-carboline:** Inverse agonist at BZD receptor and impedes GABA action.
- **Flumazenil:** Competitive antagonist of BZD site.
- **Benzodiazepines:** Agonist at allosteric BZD site, facilitate GABA action.
- **Inhalation anesthetics:** Open Cl⁻ channel directly.
- **Pharmacokinetics:** BZDs are adequately absorbed from GI tract, but their phamacokinetic properties differ considerably and protein binding also differs depending upon compounds.
  › Flurazepam t½ = 40–00 hours
  › Diazepam t½ = 25–60 hours
  › Nitrazepam t½ = 25–30 hours
  › Lorazepam t½ = 10–20 hours
  › Oxazolam/triazolam t½ = 4–5 hours
  › Chloradiazepoxide t½ = 15–40 hours in young and up to 36 hours in 80 years old.

INDIVIDUAL DRUGS

- **Flurazepam:** Produces active metabolite having long t½, residual and cumulative effects are likely on daily ingestion. Prescribed

Flowchart 36.2: Diagram of biotransformations in different benzodiazepines

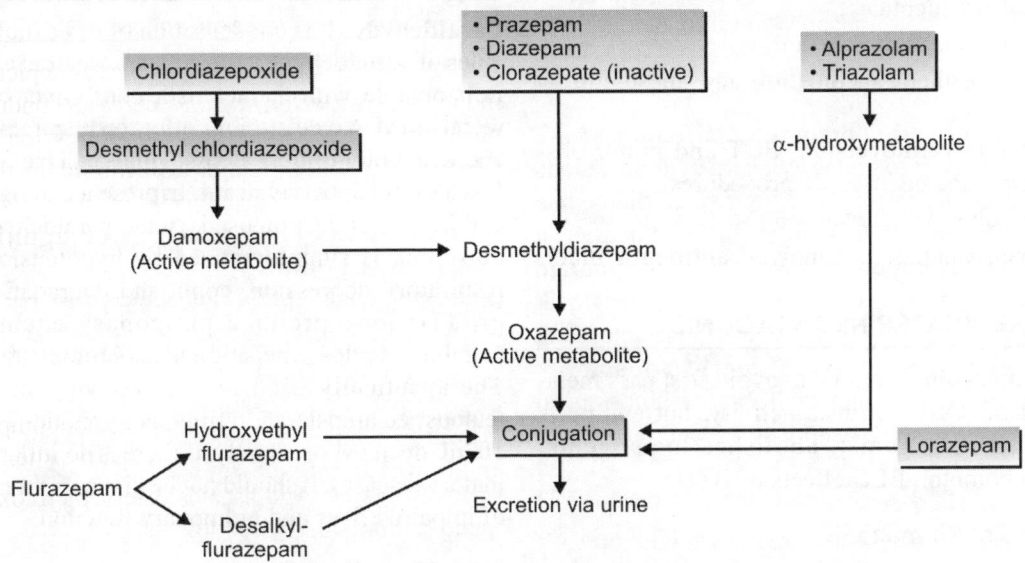

to those complaining frequent nocturnal awakening and daytime sedation is acceptable (Nindral 15 mg cap).

- **Diazepam:** Converted to desmethyl diazepam, oxazepam. Used frequently. Produce cumulation; good anxiolytic (valium; Calmpose 2, 5 and 10 mg tabs or 10 mg/2 mL inj, 2 mg/5 mL syrp).
- **Nitrazepam:** Used in patient of frequent nocturnal awakening (Hypnotex or nitravet 5, 10 mg tabs).
- **Flunitrazepam:** More potent, rapidly absorbed, markedly redistributed.
- **Temazepam:** Absorption fast with gelatin capsule than with tablets. Good for patient of sleep onset difficulty.
- **Triazolam:** Not marketed in India, good for sleep induction, but poor to maintain it. Rebound insomnia, higher doses alter sleep pattern, antegrade amnesia and anxiety, paranoia may occur. Potent with peak effect within 1 hour.
- **Midazolam:** Peak effect within 20 minutes because of rapid absorption. In elderly may produce ataxia and blackouts.
- **Zopiclone:** Hypnotic action resembles BZD, does not alter REM sleep, but prolongs stages 3 and 4. No disturbance of sleep architecture,

hangover or withdrawal. Used to wean off insomnia patient taking regularly BZD. Potentiate GABA. Side effects are metallic taste, impaired judgement, dry mouth, dependence rarely, psychological disturbance. It is cyclopyrrolone derivative (Zylop; Zopicon 7.5 mg at bedtime). Its S-isomer is **eszopeclone.**

- **Zolpidem:** Imidazopyridine, hypnotic, reduces sleep latency, but increases sleep duration, does not act on BZD receptor. Minimial daytime sedation and withdrawal symptoms (Nitrest 5–10 mg tab at bedtime).
- **Zaleplon (zaplon 5; 10 mg tabs):** Newer shortest acting hypnotic. It acts on α_1 subunits of BZD receptor. Oral bioavailability is 30% due to first pass effect. It is used for sleep onset insomnia.

Drug interactions of benzodiazepines

- CNS depressant and alcohol synergise.
- Concurrent use with sodium valporate provokes psychotic symptoms.
- Cimetidine, INH, OCP retard BZD metabolism.

Therapeutic uses of benzodiazepines

- Hypnotics
- Anxiolytic

- Anticonvulsant (for febrile convulsion or status epilepticus)
- Central muscle relaxant
- Preanesthetic medication and anesthetic by IV route
- Before cardioversion, ECT and minor obstetric and endoscopic procedures.
- Alcohol withdrawal.
- With analgesic, spasmolytic, antipeptic ulcer.

BENZODIAZEPINE ANTAGONIST

Flumazenil: Given IV to avoid first pass metabolism. Little intrinsic activity, but competes with BZD agonist, abolishes hypnogenic, psychomotor, EEG effects of BZD.

Uses of Flumazenil

- To reverse BZD anesthesia
- BZD overdose
- Hepatic coma
- Alcohol intoxication

   Adverse effects: Agitation, discomfort, anxiety, tearfulness, coldness and withdrawal of seizures may occur.

ALCOHOLS

Ethanol: Taken at bedtime may act as mild sedative, but not recommended. May produce excitement and addiction.

Chloral hydrate and trichloroethanol: Sedative dose 1 gm at bedtime, do not have significant anticonvulsant effect. Local application produces rubefacient action. It is satisfactorily absorbed from GI tract including rectum. It is converted to trichloroethanol (responsible for hypnotic effect), conjugated to glucuronic acid and from urochloralic acid may give false positive Benedict's test.

   Adverse effects: Nausea, vomiting, unpleasant taste. Toxic dose is more than 10 gm, causes loss of reflexes, pinpoint pupil. Break in tolerance may produce death. Withdrawal produces delirium, mania and convulsion. It is contraindicated in cardiac, hepatic and renal damages, peptic ulcer patient. Banned in India.

ALDEHYDES

Paraldehyde: It is condensation of three molecules of acetaldehyde, colorless, transparent and inflammable, with characteristic odor. Given per rectal or IM. No deleterious effect on respiratory and vasomotor centers. Crosses placental barrier. It is a useful anticonvulsant. In presence of light and heat, it is decomposed. Acute paraldehyde poisoning is symptomatized by hypotension, respiratory depression, coma and degradation product may produce pulmonary edema, metabolic acidosis, hepatic and nephrotoxicities. Therapeutically used to treat convulsion of tetanus; eclampsia and rarely as hypnotics (5–10 mL deep IM or rectally, if there is no inflammatory disease). It should not be given to patient of impaired liver and pulmonary function.

ACETYLATED CARBINOLS

Ethinamate (Valmid) used 0.5 gm orally to produce hypnotic effect. Rarely used because BZDs are available.

MISCELLANEOUS

Methaqualone: It is developed in India and has effect similar to short acting barbiturate, also has antitussive, local anesthetic, spasmolytic, weak antihistaminic properties. Addiction liability is there (available as 150–300 mg tabs as mandrex with diphenhydramine).

   Some antihistaminics like diphenhydramine, promethazine have hypnotic properties. Anticholinergic scopolamine has sedative property. Antianxiety drug meprobamate has sedative-hypnotic property like barbiturate. Tricyclic antidepressant and MAO-I also produce sleep in patient of depression.

   Bromides: Better hypnotics are available, so rarely used. Cumulative toxicity known as **bromism** characterized by dermatitis, conjunctivitis, headache, anorexia, constipation, tremor, motor in coordination and slurred speech.

IDEAL HYPNOTICS

- Should be effective orally with predictable sufficient long hypnotic action resembling normal sleep.

- Non-irritating, non-toxic and should not produce hangover.
- Tolerance, habituation and addiction should not be there.
- It should be cheap.
- Should not produce danger of suicide, if an overdose is taken.

Melatonin: N-acetyl-5-methoxytryptamine, the principal hormone of pineal gland secreted at night responsible for sleep wakefulness cycle with circadian rhythm. Low doses of melatonin (2–10 mg) does not depress CNS, but propensity of falling sleep increases. It reduces jet lag symptoms. It helps weaning of BZD users and elderly insomniac, also used for cluster headaches. Combination with pyridoxine 10 mg is available as eternex.

ADR: Lower seizure threshold, psychiatric change.

Ramelteon: Used for those patients who feel difficulty in falling sleep. It is MT1 and MT2 melatonin receptor agonsits located in suprachiasmatic nucleus of brain. It decreases latency of persistent sleep, rebound insomnia and there is no withdrawal symptoms with it. It is orally absorbed, forms active metabolite with longer t½. It is metabolized in liver by CYP_{1A2} so other drug metabolized by CYP_{1A2} like fluvoxamine should not be a co-prescription.

It causes dizziness, fatigue, somnolence, decreases testosterone secretion and increases prolactin secretion.

Parasomnia is sleepwalking, night terror and nightmare, idiopathic in nature in children may be benefited by diazepam or flurazepam.

In adult depression is major cause of insomnia treated by tricyclic antidepressant.

Some drugs which can cause insomnia are:

Ephedrine, amphetamine, nicotine, caffeine, bupropion, amantidine, MAO-I, nasal decongestants chloroquine, metronidazole, systemic corticosteroids levodopa.

37 Analgesics, Antipyretics and Nonsteroidal Anti-inflammatory Drugs (NSAIDs)

Inflammation process is the response of vascular tissue to a wide variety of noxious agents (infections, antibodies or physical injuries) which is essential for survival. It has three distinct phases. *1st acute phase* is vasodilatation with increased vascular permeability, the *2nd subacute phase* is leukocytic and phagocytic cells infiltration and *3rd phase* is tissue degeneration and fibrosis.

The adhesive interactions include selectins E, P, L; intercellular adhesion molecule 1 (ICAM-1); vascular cell adhesion molecule 1 (VCAM-1) and leukocyte integrins. Activation of endothelial cells by inflammatory noxious agents causes leukocyte adhesion recognized by L and P selectins. Some traditional NSAIDs interfere with cells adhesive molecule. Inflammatory cells at the site of injury liberate mediators like complement factors $C_5\alpha$, platelet activation factor, eicosanoid, cytokines like interleukin 1 (IL 1), tissue necrosis factor α (TNFα) are liberated from monocyte, macrophase, adipocyte in response to endotoxins. Cytokines and growth factors induce gene expression to synthesize protein to mediate and promote inflammation in variety of cells.

The non-narcotic analgesic not only relieves pain, but also reduce inflammation and raised body temperature. So they are also called non-narcotic, antipyretic analgesics. Since they are not steroid in nucleus, they are also known as nonsteroidal anti-inflammatory drugs (NSAIDs). The first drug synthesized in this group is obtained from hydrolysis of willow bark (salix alba) contains bitter glycosides and salicylic acid.

The NSAID group of drugs produced their action by inhibiting the synthesis of prostaglandin (PG). They are usually mild analgesics. The other mediators apart from PG which elicit pain are bradykinin, substance P and calcitonin gene- related protein (CGRP).

The PGs (eicosanoids) are widely distributed autacoids in the body and more or less cells are capable of synthesizing it by rate governing mechanism from membrane lipids arachidonic acid by appropriate stimuli-activating phospholipase A. The arachidonic acid, thus released is metabolized by two enzymes:

- Cyclooxygenase
- Lipoxygenase.

The cyclooxygenase (COX) produces ring structures [PG, thromboxane (Tx) and prostacycline, PGI_2] and lipoxygenase (LOX) produces open chain compounds (leukotrienes, LTs).

Cyclooxygenase (COX) exists in two isomers, COX-1 and COX-2. **COX-1** is a constitutive enzyme participates in physiological housekeeping, *viz.* production of gastric mucosa, hemostasis and kidney function. **COX-2** leads to inflammatory and pathological changes in inducible form.

PHARMACOLOGICAL ACTION OF PG SYNTHESIS INHIBITION

- Analgesia
- Antipyresis
- Anti-inflammatory

- Effective in dysmenorrhea
- Antiplatelet aggregation
- Closure of PDA
- Parturition is delayed
- Gastric mucosal damage
- Anaphylactic reactions

CLASSIFICATION OF NSAIDS

NSAIDs are chemically diverse organic acids and can be classified as follows:

a. Analgesic and Anti-inflammatory

i. Non-selective COX inhibitors or traditional NSAID

- **Salicylates:** Aspirin, salicylamide, diflunisal, benorylate
- **Pyrazolone derivatives:** Phenylbutazone, oxyphenbutazone
- **Indole derivatives:** Indomethacin, sulindac
- **Propionic acid derivatives:** Ibuprofen, naproxen, ketoprofen, flurbiprofen, fenoprofen
- **Anthranilic acid derivative:** Mefenamic acid
- **Oxicam derivatives:** Piroxicam, tenoxicam, lornoxicam
- **Pyrrolopyrrole derivatives:** Ketorolac
- **Arylacetic acid derivatives:** Diclofenac, tolmetin, aceclofenac.

ii. Preferential COX-2 inhibitors

Nimesulide, Meloxicam, Nabumetone

iii. Selective COX-2 inhibitors

Celecoxib, Etoricoxib, Parecoxib

b. Analgesic and Antipyretic with Poor Anti-inflammatory Action

- **Para-aminophenol derivative:** Paracetamol
- **Pyrazolone derivatives:** Metamizol, propyphenazone
- **Benzoxazocine derivative:** Nefopam

INDIVIDUAL DRUG

Aspirin as a Prototype of Salicylates

Aspirin is rapidly converted to salicylic acid in the body. The pharmacological effects are:

1. **Analgesic, antipyretic, anti-inflammatory actions.**
2. **Metabolic actions:** They are manifested in anti-inflammatory doses. Cellular metabolism is increased due to uncoupling of oxidative phosphorylation producing heat. Blood sugar decreases and liver glycogen is depleted due to increased metabolic need. Hyperglycemia may occur due to sympathetic and corticosteroid release. Chronic use of large doses causes negative nitrogen balance by neoglucogenesis. FFA in plasma decreases.
3. **Respirations:** Effect is dose dependent. In higher anti-inflammatory dose, respiration is stimulated by increased carbon dioxide production. If dose of salicylate is increased, further depression of respiration may lead to respiratory failure.

Acid–base balance: Initial anti-inflammatory doses stimulating respiration washes out carbon dioxide leading to respiratory alkalosis compensated by increased renal excretion of carbonate, sodium, potassium and water, causing compensated respiratory alkalosis.

Further increment in doses depresses respiration with excess CO_2 production producing respiratory acidosis. Dissociated salicylic acid as well as metabolic acids like lactic, pyruvic, acetoacetic acid all added to uncompensated metabolic acidosis with decrease in bicarbonate plasma. Dehydration occurs due to increased water loss in urine, sweating and hyperventilation.

CVS: Larger doses increase cardiac output to meet increased oxygen demand at periphery. Further rise in doses depresses vasomotor center, fall in BP, CCF due to sodium and water retention with low cardiac reserve.

GIT

- Irritates gastric mucosa
- Decreases mucus production

- Water is logged in gastric mucosal epithelial cells leading to hydropic degeneration of gastric mucosa → which sloughs ultimately producing peptic ulcer.

Soluble aspirin-containing calcium carbonate and citric acid buffered preparations are less likely to produce peptic ulceration.

Uric acid excretion: Effect is dose dependent < 2 gm/day, retention of uric acid, *i.e.* antagonisms of uricosuric drug.

| 2–5 gm/day | Variable |
| >5 gm/day | Uricosuric effect |

Therefore, it is not suitable for gout patient.

Blood: Aspirin in small doses inhibits TXA2 by platelets and increases bleeding time by interfering platelet aggregation. Long-term use with large doses decreases synthesis of clotting factors in liver, and bleeding may occur, which can be antagonized by vitamin K therapy.

Pharmacokinetics: Absorbed from stomach, rapidly deacetylated in gut wall, liver and other tissues. Salicylic acid and aspirin both are conjugated with glycine producing salicyluric acid and with glucuronic acid, which are excreted. The excretion of salicylic acid can be hasten by alkalization.

Adverse effects

- **Side effects:** Nausea, vomiting, diarrhea. Occult blood in stool due to gastritis in analgesic doses and abdominal pain.
- **Hypersensitivity:** Rash, angioedema, rhinorrhea, asthma, anaphylactoid reaction, urticaria, hypotension, shock and profuse gastric bleeding.
- **Anti-inflammatory** doses produce (3–6 gm/day) salicylism. Aspirin in children may increase serum transaminase in liver and may produce hepatic encephalopathy known as "Reye's syndrome" suffering viral diseases (varicella and influenza) if treated by aspirin.
- **Vascular:** Premature closure of PDA.
- **Renal:** Edema, salt and water retention, decreased action of antihypertensive, decreased

diuretic action, decreased urate excretion and hyperkalemia.

- **Pregnancy:** Prolongation of gestation and labor.
- **CNS:** Headache, dizziness, vertigo, lower seizure threshold, depression and hyperventilation.
- **Blood:** Bruise and risk of hemorrhage.

Contraindications and precautions of aspirin

- Peptic ulcer
- Chronic liver diseases
- Should be stopped before elective surgery
- Pregnancy
- Glucose-6PO$_4$ deficient individuals.

Interactions

- It displaces protein-bound drugs like warfarin, sulfonylureas, phenytoin, methotrexate from plasma proteins and increases their toxicities.
- Blunts diuretic action of thiazides and uricosuric effects of probenecid.

Therapeutic uses of aspirin

- Analgesics
- Antipyretic
- Antirheumatic
- Rheumatoid arthritis
- Osteoarthritis
- Postmyocardial infarction and strokes
- Pregnancy induced hypertension and preeclampsia
- To delay labor
- To close PDA and avoid surgery
- Niacin intolerability symptomised by intense flushing caused by niacin (cholesterol lowering agent) is due to PGD$_2$ release from skin, can be treated by aspirin.
- **Systemic mastocytosis:** Large amount of PGD$_2$ released in patient of systemic mastocytosis causing vasodilatation and hypotension can be treated by aspirin or ketoprofen and the mast cell degranulation caused by them should be prior treated with H$_1$ and H$_2$ receptor blockers.

• **Cancer chemoprevention:** Aspirin and NSAID decrease risk of colon cancer and are used in patient of familial adenomatous polyposis (FAP).

INDIVIDUAL ANALGESICS

Pyrazolone derivatives: Antipyrine and amidopyrine were first introduced for antipyretic and analgesic actions, withdrawn for side effects of agranulocytosis.

In selecting the individual NSAID, the merits and demerits and the pathological conditions like liver, kidney, cardiac diseases should be kept in mind.

The newer NSAIDs have fewer side effects.

Oxyphenbutazone is an active metabolite of phenylbutazone.

Metamizol is a prompt analgesic and antipyretic, but poor in anti-inflammatory action, may be given orally, IM or IV (may cause fall in BP withdrawn from the USA and Europe). Marketed as analgin or novalgin 500 mg tab, 0.5 gm/mL in 2 mL and 5 mL ampoule and vial.

Pyrazolone Derivatives			
Drug	Pharmacokinetics and pharmacodynamics	Side effects	Therapeutic uses
Phenylbutazone (Zolandin 100–200 mg tabs, 200 mg/mL injection)	• COX inhibitor more anti-inflammatory. • Completely absorbed orally • 90% protein-bound	Banned in some countries due to side effects of agranulocytosis.	• Rheumatic fever • Gout
Indole Derivatives			
Indomethacin (Idicin) 25–50 mg caps, 1–2 caps BD or TDS, Indoflam 1% eyedrop	• Anti-inflammatory • Relieves pain of tissue injury • PG synthesis suppressed and so neutrophil motility	• GI irritation • Dizziness • Agranulocytosis • Bleeding due to decreased platelet aggregation • Protein-bound so interacts with other protein-bound drug • Blunts action of diuretics.	• Ankylosing spondylitis • Rheumatoid arthritis • Psoriatic arthritis • To close PDA • Bratter's syndrome • Spondylitis
Sulindac	• Prodrug, weaker than indomethacin and less toxic	• Does not interfere with diuretic, β blockers and ACE inhibitors	
Etodolac	• COX-2 inhibitor, 200–400 mg	• Skin rashes • Neurological eyedrop	Used for rheumatoid and osteoarthritis
Propionic Acid Derivatives			
Ibuprofen (Brufen 200, 400) 600, 400–800 TDS, safest traditional NSAID	• Orally absorbed • Inhibits PG synthesis • 80–90% protein-bound NSAID	• GI discomfort • Headache • Dizziness • Blurred vision • Tinnitus • Drug interactions with protein-bound drugs	Used for • Analgesics • Antipyretic • Rheumatoid arthritis • Osteoarthritis • Dysmenorrhea

Contd...

Contd...

Drug	Pharmacokinetics and pharmacodynamics	Side effects	Therapeutic uses
		• Decrease efficiency of β blockers, diuretics and antihypertensive, crosses blood-brain barrier, synovial and placental membrane. Best tolerated with BD doses.	
Naproxen (Naprosyn 250 mg tab), 250 mg BD (Xenobid)	• Potent PG inhibitors amongst propionic acid derivatives • Inhibits leukocyte migration		More effective propionic acid derivatives. Used for same as ibuprofen, gout and ankylosing spondylitis.
Ketoprofen (Ketofen 50 and 100 mg tabs), 100 mg BD or TDS	• PG inhibition • Lysosome stabilization		More or less same as ibuprofen.
Carpofen	Is a new propionic acid derivative with t½ 10–16 hours indicated like other NSAID.		
Flubiprofen (Flurofen 50 and 100 mg). Dose 50 mg BD. Ocuflur 0.03% eyedrop	More effective	GI disturbance is also more.	More or less same as ibuprofen used as ocular anti-inflammatory also.

Tiaprofen is recemic propionic acid derivative, undergoes stereoconversion used orally or IM. It inhibits renal uric acid absorption.

Anthranilic Acid Derivatives

Mephenamic acid (Meftal; ponstan, 250–500 mg tab cap. 50 mg/5 mL syr). Dose 250–500 mg	Inhibits PG synthesis, orally absorbed, highly protein-bound. So displacement interaction can occur.	• Diarrhea • Epigastric distrubance • Hemolytic anemia • Skin rash • Dizziness, analgesic; antipyretic; but weak anti-inflammatory	• Used for muscle joint and soft tissue pain • Dysmenorrhea • Osteoarthritis • Rheumatoid arthritis

Aryl Acetic Acid Derivatives

Diclofenac sodium (Voveran diclofenac 50 mg). Dose 50 mg TDS. 25 mg/mL, 3 mL inj. Diclofenac 1% topical gel	• Inhibits PG synthesis • Orally absorbed • Highly protein-bound 100 mg SR tab	• Epigastric pain • Reversible elevation of serum aminotransferase • Raises plasma lithium and digoxin level	Used in • Rheumatoid arthritis • Osteoarthritis • Ankylosing spondy-litis
Dictofenac Potassium (ultra K, voltaflam)			• Dysmenorrhea • Postoperative pain • Traumatic pain

Contd...

Contd...

Drug	Pharmacokinetics and pharmacodynamics	Side effects	Therapeutic uses
			• Osteoarthritis • Ankylosing spondylitis
Aceclofenac (Aceclo 100 mg) Dose BD	Somewhat selective COX-2 congener of diclofenac. Chondroprotective because enhances glycosamino-glycan synthesis		Same as diclofenac
Tolmetin 400–600 mg TDS	Inhibits PG synthesis	Side effects of tolemetin are gastric, ulcer and vertigo and tinnitus but less.	• Used for arthritis • Soft tissue inflamma-tion
Oxicam Derivatives			
Piroxicam (Pirox 1–20 mg cap, 20 mg/mL inj). 20 mg BD × 2 days. Then 20 mg OD	Long acting PG inhibitor, analgesic and antipyretic, penetrates synovial memb-rane, prolongs bleeding time and decreases IgM production and platelet aggregation. Orally absorbed, protein-bound, metabolized in liver.	• Heart burn • Nausea rash • Pruritus • Reversible • Azotemea	• Rheumatoid and osteoarthritis • Spondylitis • Dentistry • Dysmenorrhea • Episiotomy • Musculoskeletal injuries
Tenoxicam (Tobitil 20 mg tab). 20 mg OD	Congener of piroxicam with similar use, but costiler than piroxicam		
Meloxicam (Mel–OD 7.5 mg and 15 mg tab)	Preferential inhibitor of COX-2	GI side effects are less	• Rheumatoid and osteoarthritis
Sulfonanilide Derivative			
Nimesulide (Nimulid; Nimodol 100 mg tab; 50 mg/5 mL syr). 100 mg BD	Weak PG inhibition selec-tive for COX-2 and reduces generation of superoxide, PAF synthesis, TNFα release, free radical scaven-ging; inhibits metalopro-teinase activity in cartilage. Orally absorbed, protein-bound, excreted in urine.	GI upset (ulceration, loose motion) rash, pruritus, somnolence and dizziness. Its use in children is banned.	Used for short lasting painful conditions like: • Sports injury, ENT pain • Dental surgery • Low back pain • Dysmenorrhea • Antipyretic
Alkanones			
Nabumetone (Nabuflam 500 mg tab OD)	• It is a non-acid NSAID prodrug produces active metabolite 6-MNA. • Inhibits COX-2	Low incidence of gastric irritation, pseudopor-phyria, photosensitivity may occur.	Used for • Osteoarthritis and • Muscle pain

Contd...

Contd...			
Drug	Pharmacokinetics and pharmacodynamics	Side effects	Therapeutic uses
Pyrrolopyrrole Derivative			
Ketorolac (Ketanov 10 mg tab, 30 mg/mL). Dose 10–20 mg 6 hourly by IM route. Should not be used continuously for more than 5 days.	Potent analgesic, anti-inflammatory. Inhibits PG synthesis. Orally absorbed, may be given IM, highly plasma-bound. Metabolized by glucuronidation in liver and excreted in urine.	Nausea, vomiting, nervousness, pruritus, fluid retention, rise in serum transaminase	Pain of muscles, skeletal and postoperative. But should not be used for obstetric pain and preanesthetic.

Propyphenazone (300–600 mg TDS with paracetamol, Saridon): Better tolerated with less chance of agranulocytosis.

Azapropazone is less likely to cause agranulocytosis.

Para-amino Phenol Derivatives

Phenacetin: This is an extensively used analgesic banned in many countries including India because of abuse nephropathy.

Paracetamol: It is deethylated active metabolite of phenacetin, has negligible anti-inflammatory action. Poor inhibition of PG at periphery, but more on brain, may be due to peroxide at the site of inflammation. It does not stimulate respiration or effect acid–base balance, orally absorbed, distributed in body, conjugated with glucuronic acid and sulfate and excreted in urine. In antipyretic doses, it is safe. Nausea, rash, leukopenia may occur occasionally. After heavy ingestion; produces papillary necrosis, tubular atrophy and renal fibrosis. Urine concentrating power is lost and kidney shrinks.

Acute paracetamol poisoning occurs, if large doses (150 gm/kg or more than 10 gm) are taken which has low hepatic glucuronide conjugating capacity. Manifestations are nausea, vomiting, liver tenderness, centrilobular hepatic necrosis, renal tubular necrosis, hypoglycemia all may progress to coma. Jaundice may appear in 2 days.

Mechanism of toxicity: N-acetyl-p-benzoquinone imine (NAPQI) is a highly reactive metabolite of paracetamol, detoxified by conjugating with glutathione which is depleted and minor metabolite produced binds to liver cells and renal tubules causing necrosis. It is earlier in alcoholics and premature babies.

Treatmemt of paracetamol poisoning

- Induced vomiting or gastric lavage.
- Activated charcoal to prevent further absorption.
- N-acetyl cysteine 150 mg/kg IV over 15 minutes, to be repeated after 20 hours or 75 mg/kg orally in every 4–6 hours for 2–3 days, replenishes glutathione, stores and prevents metabolite induced hepatic and renal damages. Earlier the treatment started better is the result, ineffective, if used after 16 hours of paracetamol ingestion.

Preparations, doses and therapeutic uses of paracetamol

- It is an OTC drug (crocin/calpol/fepanil).
- Ultragin 500 mg tab, 125 mg/5 mL syrup. Febrinil 300 mg/2 mL inj used for
  › Headache
  › Dysmenorrhea
  › Musculoskeletal pain
  › Antipyresis

One of the best drugs for children as antipyretic because of no risk of Reye's syndrome, however it should not be prescribed in premature infants below 2 kg of body weight.

Benzoxazocine Derivatives

Nefopam (Nefomax 30 mg tab, 1 tab TDS or 20 mg/mL ampule): This non-opioid NSAID does not inhibit PG. It has anticholinergic action (dry mouth, urinary retention, blurred vision and sympathomimetic action, tachycardia, nervousness) and contraindicated to epileptic. Used for short lasting musculoskeletal pain.

Newer Drugs: Celecoxib, rofecoxib, parecoxib, lumiracoxib, valdecoxibs, etoricoxib all inhibit COX-2 isoenzymes, exert potent, anti-inflammatory, antipyretic, analgesic actions. The celecoxib slowly absorbed, 97% plasma protein-bound and metabolized by liver used for osteoarthritis and rheumatoid arthritis. Dose—celecoxib (celact 100 mg cap. 1 BD Revebra).

Rofecoxib (robivax 12.5; 25 and 50 mg/tab) **OD Valedecoxib** (valed 20 and 40 mg); used for postoperative pain, osteoarthritis, rheumatoid arthritis, dysmenorrhea. **Etoricoxib** (nucoxia 60 mg) orally absorbed, protein-bound, metabolized in liver, excreted with urine as metabolite.

The valdecoxib and rofecoxib are withdrawn due to increased cardiovascular risk (increased incidence of myocardial infarctions). Lumiracoxib is marketed in Europe. Parecoxib is a prodrug of valdecoxib given by injection in postoperative pain.

Topical NSAIDs: Many NSAIDs as gel formulation are available for muscle and joint pains of osteoarthritis, sprain, sports injuries, spondylitis, tenosynovitis to avoid first pass effect and GI side effects. Its local concentration is high up to dermis, but below 25 mm depth, its concentration is low.

It casts doubt about its contribution to produce beneficial effect.

Different preparations are

Diclofenac	1 % gel	Voveran emulgel
Ibuprofen	10% gel	Ribufen gel
Naproxen	10% gel	Naprosyn gel
Ketoprofen	2.5% gel	Rhofenid gel
Flubiprofen	5% gel	Froben gel
Nimesulide	1% gel	Nimegesic T. gel
Piroxicam	0.5% gel	Pirox gel

Fixed drug contribution of NSAID with hypotics/anxiolytic or sedatives are banned in India to avoid misuse and producing dependence.

Zaltoprofen (Zalto 80 mg): This is a new propionic acid derivative NSAID, preferentially acts on COX2 inhibition and other proposed mechanisms are bradykinin induced nociceptive inhibition by blocking β_2 receptor and also inhibits bradykinin induced 12-lipoxygenase (12-LOX) activity.

Used for rheumatoid arthritis, lumbago, periarthritis, cervicobrachial syndrome, dental extraction, post-trauma. Dose 80 mg BD to TDS. Should not be used in lactating mothers.

Diacerein: This NSAID inhibits interleukin 1 implicated for osteoarthritis. It also does not inhibit PG.

38

Social Pharmacology

As far as back history is concerned, every societies have used drugs to produce effects on moods, thoughts and feelings. There were always groups who disgraced the customs with respect to the line in which these drugs were to be used. Thus the problem of non-medical use of drugs is as old as civilization.

Drug abuse refers by self-administration of any drug, which deviates from approved medical and social patterns within a given culture. The term conveys due to social disapproval. Non-medical drug use may be:
• Experimental curiosity
• Recreational
• Casual

Sources of Abused Drugs

• Permissive   • Prescriptive
• Proscriptive

Variables of Drug Abusers

The variables which operate in influencing drug abuse may be grouped as follows:

Agent, i.e. drug
• Greater reinforcing drugs are more likely to produce addiction.
• Availability
• Cost, if cheaper
• Mode of administration
• Speed of termination of effects

Host, i.e. user
• Heredity
• Metabolism

• Prior experience
• Psychiatric symptoms
• Risk-taking attitude

Environment
• Social setting
• Educational background
• Community attitude

COMPULSIVE DRUG USE

The drugs used to alter mood and feeling may eventually develop dependence and the patient continues to take it in absence of medical indications, and the intensity may vary from mild desire to craving or compulsion. The dependence is not necessarily the cause of concern, if the drug is relatively inexpensive and low in toxicity. Compulsive drug use is generally associated with:

1. Tolerance
2. Physical dependence

Tolerance

When increased amount of drug is required for desired effect after repeated drug administration. It may be:
i. **Innate** (pre-existing sensitivity)
ii. **Acquired:** The acquired tolerance may be:
   • Pharmacokinetics or pharmacodynamics
   • Learned tolerance (behavioral and conditional)
   • Acute tolerance

- Reverse tolerance or sensitization, *i.e.* shifting of dose response curve to left.
- Cross-tolerance with same group of drugs.

Tolerance mechanism

- **Dispositional:** When there is increased metabolism of the drug.
- **Pharmacodynamic:** Adaptive changes in the target tissues.
- **Behavioral:** When increased amount is required to get an award.
- **Immune:** Due to formation of antibodies.

Tachyphylaxis (Tachy = quick; phylaxis = protection): It is an acute tolerance after repeated drug administration in quick succession.

Theories of tachyphylaxis

- Depletion of stores of neurotransmitter.
- Prior occupation of the receptors.

Drug addiction

It is a state of periodic and chronic intoxication produced by repeated consumption of a drug (natural and synthetic) characterized by:
- An overpowering desire or need (compulsion) to continue for taking the drug and to obtain it by any means.

- Tendency to increase dose.
- Psychic and physical dependence to the effect of the drug.
- Detrimental effect on individual and society.

Drug habituation: This condition arises on repeated consumptions of drug characterized by:
- Desire, but not compulsion to continue the drug for the sense of improved well-being.
- Little tendency to increase the dose.
- Some degree of psychic dependence, but no physical dependence.
- Detrimental effect, if any individual taking it not on society.

Drugs which can produce dependence or habituations are categorized into following groups:
- Alcohol
- Opioids
- General CNS depressants
- CNS sympathomimetic
- Nicotine and tobacco
- Cannabinoids
- Psychedelics
- Cocaine
- Other stimulants (caffeine)

Table 38.1: Withdrawal syndrome					
Alcohol	*Benzodiazepines*	*Nicotine*	*Opioid*	*Cocaine*	*Marijuana*
• Craving • Tremor • Nausea • Sleep disturbance • Irritability • Tachycardia • Hypertension • Sweating • Visual or tactile hallucination • Seizure • Delirium tremens • Fever • Dilated pupil • Diarrhea	• Anxiety • Agitation • Paranesthesia • Sensitivity to light or sound • Muscle cramp • Sleep disturbance • Dizziness • Seizure • Delirium	• Irritation • Anxiety • Depression • Dificulty in concentration • Restlessness • Decreased heart rate • Weight gain • Increased appetite	• Craving • Restlessness • Irritation • Increased pain sensitivity • Nausea • Muscle cramps • Dysphoria • Anxiety • Pupil dilated • Sweating • Goose flesh due to piloerection • Tachycardia • Fever • Yawning • Vomiting and diarrhea	• Dysphonia • Depression • Craving • Sleepiness • Bradycardia	• Restlessness • Irritation • Insomnia • Nausea • Cramp

THEORIES OF PHYSICAL DEPENDENCE

- **Counteradaptation theory:** Counteradaptation to agonist results in the development of latent hyperactivity in neural system affected by the drug which manifests as overshoot phenomenon when drugs are stopped or displaced by antagonist.

- **Martin redundancy model:** Proposes opening of redundant pathways, when primary pathway is blocked by the drugs. When drugs are withdrawn action of primary pathway restores, with continued action of redundant pathway.

- **Disuse supersensitivities** like denervation type supersensitivity.

- **Enzyme induction theory:** Drugs decrease enzyme that synthesizes a product important for cellular activity (neurotransmitters) and the level of the enzyme itself is regulated by its product, the neurotransmitters. The drug effect is due to decrease in transmitter, which induce enzyme, and a new steady state of neurotransmitter is restored. When drugs are withdrawn this induced enzyme produces excess transmitters producing rebound effect, *e.g.* opioids decrease adenyl cyclase in cultured neuronal cells. After some days concentration of 3', 5'-cAMP returns to control value in spite of the presence of adenyl cyclase and rise in intracellular concentration of 3', 5'-cAMP .

- **Receptor theories:** Drugs increase number of receptors active or silent. The increase in receptor for transmitters is responsible for tolerance.

Neurotransmitter Theories

a. Depletion of 5HT, interferes with development of tolerance to opioid and ethanol.

b. Decreased noradrenaline results tolerance to barbiturates.

c. Decreased catecholamine causes increase withdrawal syndrome of alcohol.

d. Increased GABA level has got ameliorative effects.

39

Antiepileptic Drugs

The epilepsies are the group of disorders characterized by chronic, recurrent and paroxysmal changes in neurological function caused by abnormalities in the electric activity of the brain. It is a common neurological disorder where 0.5 to 2% of world population suffer from it. **Seizure** is paroxysmal abnormal discharge from aggregate of neurons of cerebral cortex. **Convulsion** is the violent prolonged spasmodic contraction of skeletal muscle.

Anticonvulsants abolish seizure whereas **antiepileptic drugs** used prophylactically to prevent seizure.

Classification of Antiepileptic Drugs

- **Hydantoins:** Phenytoin, methoin, ethotoin, fosphenytoin
- **Barbiturates:** Phenobarbitone, mephobarbitone, metharbitone
- **Deoxybarbiturate:** Primidone
- **Iminostilbenes:** Carbamazepine, oxcarbazepine
- **Acetylurea:** Phenacemide
- **Succinimides:** Phensuximide, ethosuximide, methsuximide
- **Aliphatic carboxylic acids:** Sodium valproate, divalproex
- **Oxazolidinediones:** Trimethadione, paramethadione
- **Benzodiazepines:** Clonazepam, clobazam, diazepam, midazolam, lorazepam.
- **Newer drugs:** Lamotrigine, gabapentin, vigabatrin, topiramate, xonisamide, levetiracetam, felbamate, eslicarbazine.
- **Miscellaneous:** Bromide, acetazolamide, sulthiame, pheneturide, amphetamine, lacosamide, rufinamide, retigabine, stiripentol.

Trimethadione, phenacetamide, bromide, suthiame, phaneturide and acetazolamide are rarely used as anticonvulsants because of their toxicities.

The antiseizure drugs generally give adequate control in majority of the patient, but drug resistance may be observed from the onset or

Flowchart 39.1

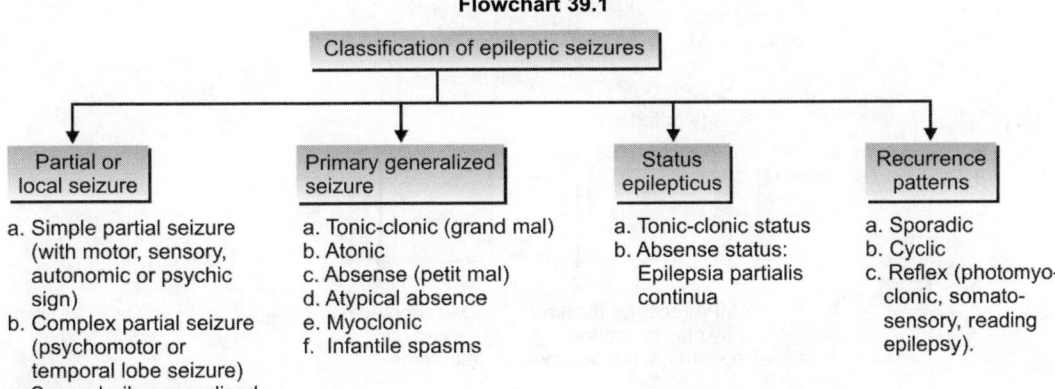

may develop thereafter either due to impaired access of the drug to the target or insensitivity to the target molecule. Some focal seizures are refractory in adults.

Glutamate
GABA
Increasing release (Gabapentin) (Pregabalin)
• Barbiturates
• Benzo-diazepine
GAT-1 inhibited by tiagabine
GABA transaminase
GABA
Inactive
GABA$_A$
GABA$_B$
Inhibited by vigabatrin

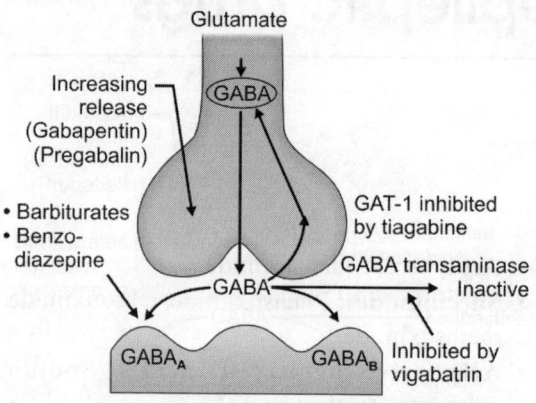

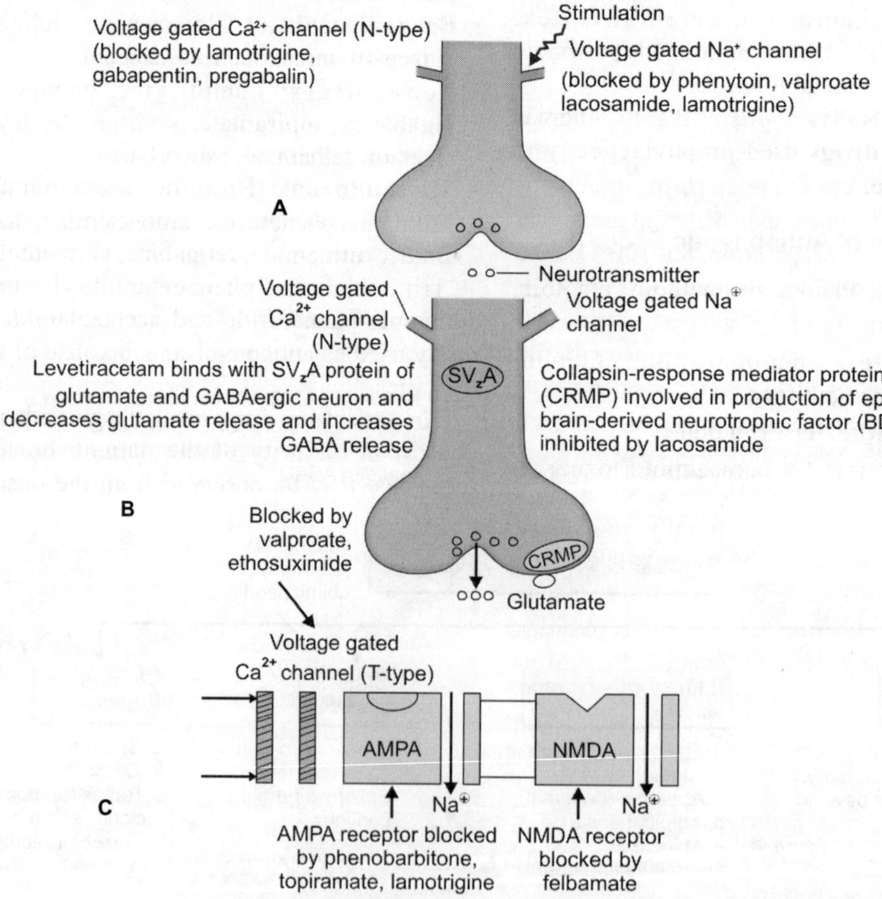

Fig. 39.1: Mechanisms of action of antiepileptic drugs

Some drug resistance patients respond to vagus nerve stimulation in partial seizures. Temporal lobe epilepsy is also treated by surgical resection. Other non-pharmacological method is responsive neurostimulator and deep brain stimulation device.

INDIVIDUAL DRUGS

Phenytoin: First introduced in 1908, but its anticonvulsant activity was discovered by Merritt and Putnam in 1938.

Phenytoin is not CNS depressant, rather in toxic doses produce excitation. It stabilizes neuronal membrane and prevents repeatitive detonation of normal brain cells (Figs 39.2A to C and Flowchart 39.2).

Voltage gated Ca^{2+} channel (N-type) (blocked by lamotrigine, gabapentin, pregabalin)
Stimulation
Voltage gated Na^+ channel (blocked by phenytoin, valproate lacosamide, lamotrigine)
A
Neurotransmitter
Voltage gated Ca^{2+} channel (N-type)
Voltage gated Na^+ channel
Levetiracetam binds with SV$_2$A protein of glutamate and GABAergic neuron and decreases glutamate release and increases GABA release
SV$_2$A
Collapsin-response mediator protein (CRMP) involved in production of epileptogenic brain-derived neurotrophic factor (BDNF) inhibited by lacosamide
B
Blocked by valproate, ethosuximide
CRMP
Glutamate
Voltage gated Ca^{2+} channel (T-type)
AMPA
NMDA
Na^+
Na^+
C
AMPA receptor blocked by phenobarbitone, topiramate, lamotrigine
NMDA receptor blocked by felbamate

Figs 39.2A to C: Mechanisms of action of some antiepileptic drugs

Flowchart 39.2

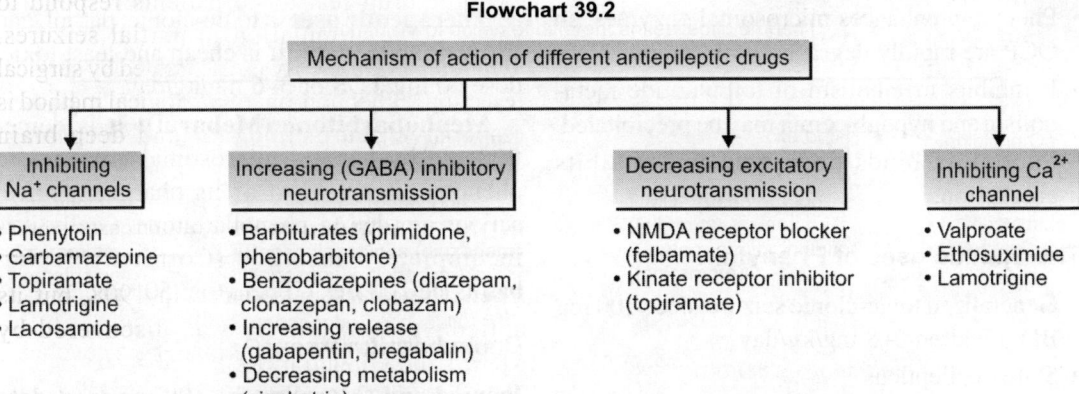

Mechanism of action of different antiepileptic drugs			
Inhibiting Na$^+$ channels	**Increasing (GABA) inhibitory neurotransmission**	**Decreasing excitatory neurotransmission**	**Inhibiting Ca^{2+} channel**
• Phenytoin • Carbamazepine • Topiramate • Lamotrigine • Lacosamide	• Barbiturates (primidone, phenobarbitone) • Benzodiazepines (diazepam, clonazepan, clobazam) • Increasing release (gabapentin, pregabalin) • Decreasing metabolism (vigabatrin) • Inhibiting reuptakes of GABA (tiagabine)	• NMDA receptor blocker (felbamate) • Kinate receptor inhibitor (topiramate)	• Valproate • Ethosuximide • Lamotrigine

- It has been observed to prolong inactive state of voltage-sensitive Na$^+$ channel.
- It decreases influx of calcium ions as such or as a consequence of reduced intracellular concentration of sodium (Fig. 39.2).
- Inhibition of glutamate and facilitation of GABA response occur at higher concentration.

Pharmacokinetics of phenytoin: Its absorption from GIT depends upon different incipients used in the market preparation. 80–100% of the drugs reach circulation. The drug level in CSF is proportional to plasma level. After IM, absorption is unpredictable because of its precipitation in muscle. **Fosphenytoin** is a prodrug, converted to phenytoin which is used for parenteral use. Distributed widely in the body and is plasma protein-bound. The concentration in CSF is equal to unbound fraction in plasma. It is metabolized in liver by hydroxylation and glucuronide conjugation. Its elimination capacity is limited, changes from first order to zero order. It has also some genetic influences. Most of its drug interactions are due to binding of protein and metabolism (since it induces microsomal enzymes).

Adverse effects of phenytoin

At therapeutic level
- Gum hypertrophy
- Hirsutism

- Hypersensitivity, rash, DLE, lymphadenopathy, neutropenia.
- Megaloblastic anemia (due to decreased folic acid absorption and increased excretion)
- Osteomalacia due to desensitization of target tissue to vitamin D interfering absorption of calcium.
- Hyperglycemia due to decrease in insulin release. Used during pregnancy can produce fetal hydantoin syndrome (hypoplastic phalanges, cleft lip, cleft palate, microcephaly)
- Acne (troublesome for young girls).

Dose-related toxicity

- Ataxia
- Vertigo
- Diplopia
- Nystagmus
- Drowsiness
- Behavioral alteration
- Hallucination
- Nausea
- Vomiting
- Epigastric pain
- Decrease in BP
- Arrhythmia
- IV injection may cause local vascular injury

Drug interactions of phenytoin

- Carbamazepine and phenytoin mutually enhance each others metabolism.
- Sodium valproate displaces protein-bound phenytoins so plasma level of free phenytoin increases.
- Chloramphenicol, INH and cimetidine inhibit phenytoin metabolism and can precipitate phenytoin toxicity.

- Phenytoin enhances microsomal enzymes, so OCP are rapidly degraded with failure.
- It inhibits metabolism of tolbutamide metabolism and hypoglycemia may be precipitated.
- Sucralfate binds phenytoin and inhibits absorption.

Therapeutic uses of Phenytoin

- Generalized tonic-clonic seizure, dose 100 mg BD, children 5–8 mg/kg/day.
- Status epilepticus
- Trigeminal neuralgia
- Cardiac arrhythmia
- To enhance wound healing

Preparation: Dilantin, epsolin 100 mg cap; 100 mg/4 mL; susp 100 mg/2 mL inj.

Ethotoin (Peganone): Pharmacological spectrum same as phenytoin, but of low efficacy so occasionally used. Available as 250 and 500 mg tabs. Dose 2–3 gm daily. It is recommended for patient sensitive to phenytoin, but larger is the dose requirement.

Mephenytion: It is metabolized 5, 5-ethylphenylhydantoin which has got antiseizure action.

Barbiturates

Phenobarbitone: It is an antiepileptic though its GABA receptor mediated synaptic inhibition. It has GABA facilitatory, GABA-mimetic, antiglutamate and it decreases Ca^{2+} influx within neuronal cells, raises seizure threshold with wide spectrum of antiepileptic properties. (Fig. 39.1 and Flowchart 39.2)

Pharmacokinetics: It is completely and slowly absorbed from GIT. Steady plasma concentrations are reached after 2–3 weeks, excreted with urine in pH dependent manner, unchanged or inactivated by liver to parahydroxyphenyl derivative with glucuronide conjugation. It is 40–60% plasma protein-bound and its plasma $t\frac{1}{2}$ is 80–120 hours.

Adverse effects: Sedation, decrease intelligence, impairment of learning and memory, rashes, megaloblastic anemia, osteomalacia.

Therapeutic uses in tonic-clonic, partial, and in status epilepticus. It is cheap and least toxic; dose 60 mg TDS or 3–6 mg/kg/day.

Mephobarbitone (Mebaral): It is demethylated by hepatic microsomal enzymes to phenobarbitone. Most of its pharmacological actions are due to phenobarbitone. Orally it is incompletely absorbed (Cornital: Mephobarbitone 100 mg + Phenytoin 50 mg).

Deoxybarbiturates

Primodione (Mysoline 50–100 mg tabs, dose 250–500 mg BD, children 10–20 mg/kg/day) is a congener of phenobarbitone, uniformly and completely absorbed from GIT. After absorption converted to phenobarbitone and phenylethyl malonamide (PEMA) in liver and all are active against seizure. 60–80% excreted in urine within 24 hours.

Used for grand mal, psychomotor, myoclonic, and petit mal epilepsies, essential tremor resistant propranolol.

ADR: Sedation, vertigo, dizziness, nausea, vomiting, ataxia, maculopapular or morbilliform rash, leukopenia, SLE, lymphadenopathy are the side effects.

Iminostilbenes

Carbamazepine: This compound is chemically related to antidepressant imipramine.

Carbamazepine is used for

- Complex partial seizure
- Generalized tonic-clonic seizure
- Simple partial seizure
- Neuralgia
- Mania depressive illness as an alternative to lithium
- Cranial diabetes insipidus by enhancing ADH action

Its mechanism of action on Na channel is like phenytoin (prolonging inactivated state). It also acts presynaptically to decrease synaptic transmission. It also combines with glycine receptor, but its significance is not known.

It is absorbed completely, but relatively slowly. The conventional and chewable tablets yield mean peak plasma concentrations of 12 hours and 6 hours respectively. Ingestion of food does not interfere with its absorption. Steady plasma concentration is attained within 1–2 weeks. It is bound to plasma protein 70–80%. The concentration of unchanged substance in CSF and saliva reflects nonprotein-bound portion of plasma. Apparent volume of distribution is 0.8 to 1.9 L/kg. Elimination $t\frac{1}{2}$ is 20–36 hours. It is autoinducer of hepatic enzyme system. One of its metabolites carbamazepine-10, 11-epoxide has anticonvulsant activity. In pregnancy, it increases the chances of malformation. Folic acid deficiency is aggravated. It passes in breast milk. Mother on carbamazepine can breastfeed their infant, provided infant is observed for possible adverse effects like somnolence, skin reactions.

Adverse effects: Dizziness, headache, diplopia, jaundice, erythematous, skin rash, thrombocytopenia, aplastic anemia, water retention and hyponatremia in elderly.

Interactions: Cytochrome $P4503_{A4}$ ($CYP3_{A4}$) is the main enzyme catalyzing formation of carbamazepine-10, 11-epoxide. Coadministration of inhibitors of $CYP3_{A4}$ may result in increased concentration which could increase adverse reactions.

The agents that may raise plasma carbamazepine level are INH, verapamil, diltiazem, dextropropoxyphene, danazol, macrolide antibiotics, cimetidine, terfenadine, ketoconazole and loratidine. Agents that may decrease carbamazepine may be phenobarbitone, phenytoin, primidone, theophylline, phensuximide, methsuximde.

Preparation: Tegretol, carbatol, mazetol 100, 200, 400 mg tabs; 100 mg/5 mg susp. Dose 200–400 mg TDS, 15–30 mg/kg/day.

Oxcarbazepine: This antiseizure drug is closely related to carbamazepine $t\frac{1}{2}$ of 1–2 hours. It is excreted as glucuronide conjugation after conversion of 10-hydroxymetabolite. It induces hepatic enzyme less, but hyponatremia is common. Dose to dose for carbamazepine, is

1½ times less potent. Available as 150, 300 and 600 mg tabs (oxetol and oxcarb). Dose 900–2400 mg/day or 30–45 mg/kg for children in 2 divided doses.

Eslicarbazine: This prodrug is rapidly converted to active product used for adjunctive therapy in adults with partial onset seizure, once dosing 400–1200 mg/day.

SUCCINIMIDES

Ethosuximide (Zarontin 250 mg cap or 250 mg/ 5 mL). Effective in petit mal epilepsy, primary action appears to be on thalamocortical system. Thalamic neurons exhibit prominent T transient current which is low threshold Ca^{2+} current due to inflow of Ca^{2+} through T-type Ca^{2+} channels, that amplify repeatitive spikes. Ethosuximide selectivity suppresses T current without affecting other types of Ca^{2+} or Na^+ current. It does not potentiate GABA in therapeutic level. (Fig. 39.2)

It is slowly and completely absorbed from GIT, not protein-bound, largely metabolized in liver by hydroxylation and glucuronidation and excreted via urine.

Adverse reactions: Nausea, vomiting, drowsiness, mood changes, parkinsonism, skin rashes and blood dyscrasia, occasionally SLE may occur. Dose 750–1250 mg/day or 20–40 mg/day in 2–4 divided doses.

Methsuximide (celontin 500 mg tabs): Pharmacologically similar as ethosuximide used in temporal lobe epilepsy with other drugs.

Aliphatic Carboxylic Acid

Sodium Valproate

Aliphatic branched chain carboxylic acid used in Europe since 1960, but launched in India since 1980. It is broad-spectrum antiepileptic.

Mechanism of action (Figs 39.1 and 39.2))

- Frequency dependent prolongation of Na channels inactivation
- Attenuation of Ca^{2+} mediated T current suppression like ethosuximide

- Augmentation of release of inhibitory transmitter GABA by inhibiting its degradation by GABA transaminase and probably by increasing its synthesis.

Pharmacokinetics: Orally absorbed, 90% plasma protein-bound, metabolized by liver by oxidation and glucuronide conjugation, excreted through urine. Plasma t½ is 10–15 hours.

Adverse effects: Indian tolerate it less. It may produce anorexia, vomiting, drowsiness, ataxia, tremor, alopecia, curling of hair, increased blood ammonia level. Rise in transaminase and fulminant hepatitis are serious toxic effects. Should be used with caution in pregnancy as it can produce neural tube defect and spina bifida in fetus. Long-term use in young girl may produce polycystic ovary and menstrual irregularities.

Dose: 200 mg TDS, 15–30 mg/kg/day (Valparin 200 mg tab, 200 mg/5 mL liquid, 100 mg/mL injection).

Therapeutic uses of valproate

- Grand mal
- Simple partial seizure
- Complex partial seizure
- In myoclonic and atonic seizures, control is incomplete, but it is drug of choice.
- In mania and bipolar illness, it is alternative to lithium.
- Has some prophylacitc effect on migraine.

Interactions of valproate

- It increases plasma level of phenobarbitone by inhibiting its metabolism.
- Increases phenytoin by displacing it from protein binding.
- Mutually induces metabolisms of carbamazepine.
- Concurrent use with clonazepam may precipitate absence status.

Divalproex (Semisodium valproate)

This coordination compound of valproic acid with sodium valproate 1:1, is slowly absorbed orally with better gastric tolerance and equally bioavailable to sodium valproate (valance 125, 250, 500 mg tabs).

OXAZOLIDINEDIONES

Trimethadione (Troxidone 300 mg cap): Effective in absence seizure. Action is like succinimide derivative. It is rarely used because of its high toxicity, hemeralopia (inability to tolerate bright light). Kidney and liver toxicities, exfoliative dermatitis and blood dyscrasia may occur.

Paramethadione (Paradione) is similar in toxicity and use of trimethadione.

BENZODIAZEPINES

1. **Clonazepam (Revotrial):** This benzodiazepine potentiates GABA induced Cl⁻ influx to produce sedation and is used for its anticonvulsant properties. Oral absorption is good, bound to plasma proteins, metabolized in liver, excreted in urine. (Fig. 39.1)

   ADR: Lack of concentration, irritability, behavioral abnormalities may occur in children, motor disturbance and ataxia occur at higher doses. Salivation and increased respiratory secretion may occur (lonzep 0.5, 2 mg tab, dose 0.5 to 4 mg TDS). Children 0.02 to 0.2 mg/kg/day.

   Clonazepam is used for:
   - Absence seizure
   - Akinetic epilepsy
   - Myoclonic epilepsy
   - Infantile spasm

   Tolerance develops within six months.

2. **Clobazam (Frisium 10 mg cap, dose at HS):** Used as adjuvant for:
   - Partial
   - Generalized tonic-clonic
   - Myoclonic, and
   - Atonic seizures.

   Sedation and psychomotor disturbance are less, oral bioavailability is 90%, produces active metabolite, used as adjuvant to phenytoin, carbamazepine, valproate, phenobarbitone. These drugs also lower plasma concentration of clobazam.

3. **Diazepam:** Used for all emergency conditions of convulsions, *viz.* status epilepticus, tetanus, eclampsia, convulsant poisoning. Long-term use may produce tolerance of these effects, dose 0.2–0.5 mg/kg/slow IV.

   ADR: Respiratory depressions, hypotension may occur. Rectal instillation is preferred for febrile convulsion of children.

4. **Lorazepam** is an alternative to diazepam 0.1 mg/kg IV is given in a rate of 2 mg/min for status epilepticus or to control convulsion. It is longer acting than diazepam.

5. **Midazolam:** Used as anticonvulsant in status epilepticus.

Miscellaneous and Newer Drugs

1. **Lamotrigine (lamitor; lamidus 25 mg tab, dose 50 mg/day increase up to 300 mg/ day):** Orally absorbed, metabolized in liver, used in refractory cases of partial and generalized epilepsies. It blocks voltage-sensitive Na^+ channel at presynaptic membrane to release excitatory neurotransmitter, glutamate or aspartate. It does not block NMDA type glutamate receptor.

   ADR: Sleepiness, dizziness, diplopia, ataxia, vomiting, rash may be severe requiring durg withdrawal.

2. **Gabapentin (Neurontin 300 mg cap):** Dose 900–2400 mg in 3–4 divided doses. This lipophilic GABA derivative crosses blood-brain barriers to enhance GABA release. It reduces seizure frequency, when added to first drug. Orally absorbed and excreted, unchanged in urine t½ of 6 hours.

   ADR: Sedation, dizziness, tiredness may occur.

   It is also used for diabetic neuropathy, postherpetic neuralgia and migraine.

3. **Pregabalin:** Modify synaptic release of GABA. Binds to $\alpha_2\delta$ subunit of voltage gated Ca^{2+} channel and decreases Ca^{2+} entry, also decreases synaptic release of glutamate. More than one dose required for

short t½. Available as 25, 50, 75, 100, 150, 250 and 300 mg capsules.

4. **Vigabatrin:** Inhibits GABA transaminase which degrades GABA, and increases synaptic GABA concentration. Orally absorbed and excreted, unchanged in urine, dose 2–4 gm/day. Children 40–100 mg/kg/ day. Depression, psychosis and visual field contraction may develop. Chemically it is sulfamate substitute monosaccharide.

5. **Topiramate (Topex 25, 50 and 100 mg tabs, dose 200–400/day)** is a broad-spectrum antiepileptic. Its action is due to:
   • Prolong Na^+ channel reactivation
   • GABA potentiation
   • Glutamate antagonism
   • Activates hyperpolarizing K^+ current.
   • It has weak carbonic anhydrase inhibition activity.

   It is used with primary drug for simple partial, complex partial, generalized tonic-clonic seizures as monotherapy. It is also used for prophylaxis to migraine. May produce renal stone.

6. **Tiagabine:** Dose 32–56 mg/day in 2–4 divided doses. It is nipecotic acid derivative depresses GABA transporter I. Used as add-on therapy. Sedation, nervousness, amnesia, pain in abdomen may occur. Marketed as Gabitril.

7. **Zonisamide (Zonegram, dose 200 mg/day in 2–4 divided doses):** It has carbonic anhydrase inhibitory action, sulfonamide derivative with carbon. Prolongs Na^+ channel inactivation. Used as add-on therapy for refractory cases of partial seizures.

   ADR: Somnolence, ataxia, anorexia, skin rash, nervousness may occur as adverse effects.

8. **Rufinamide:** Triazole derivative, may be useful in difficult to treat epileptic syndrome and Lennox-Gastaut syndrome.

9. **Levetiracetam (Keppra, 1000–3000 mg/ day in 2 divided doses):** Used as adjuvant medication of refractory cases of partial

seizures. It decreases synaptic release of glutamate by binding with SV_2A synaptic protein.

ADR: Sedation, fatigue, incoordination, psychosis, anemia, leukopenia are important ADRs.

10. **Felbamate:** Blocks NMDA receptor, potentiates $GABA_A$ receptor response. Increases valproate and phenytoin level, but decreases carbamazepine level. Dose 2000–3600 mg/day used for partial seizure and Lennox-Gastaut syndrome's seizure. It may cause aplastic anemia and hepatitis.

11. **Acetyl urea derivative phenacemide:** Broad-spectrum antiepileptic is disreputed because of personality changes, suicidal tendencies, hepatitis, aplastic anemia.

12. **Acetazolamide (Diamox):** Carbonic anhydrase inhibitor increases brain CO_2 level, decreases Na^+ influx of neurons, is weak anticonvulsant, used for adjuvant in absence seizures.

13. **Sulthiame (Ospolot):** Sulfonamide derivative, orally absorbed, effective in temporal lobe and to a some extent in grand mal and myoclonic seizure. Dose100–600 mg/day as adjuvant to other antiepileptic drugs. It is carbonic anhydrase inhibitor.

14. **Bromides:** Useful in grand mal epilepsy, full effect develops after 2–3 weeks.

    ADR: May produce cumulative toxicity characterized by drowsiness, psychotic changes, skin rashes called **bromism**.

15. **Pheneturide:** Given in the dose of 200–1000 mg daily. It is less toxic.

16. **Amphetamine:** Adjuvant therapy for epilepsy of grand and petit mal. Decreases drowsiness produced by phenobarbitone. It sedates mentally retarded children with hyperkinetic epilepsy.

17. **Lacosamide:** Studied for pain syndrome and for partial seizure. It inhibits collapsin response mediator protein 2 which produces and releases brain-derived neurotropic factor (BDNF) having role in epilepsy.

18. **Stiripentol:** Used with clobazam and valproate in refractory cases of severe myoclonic epilepsy of infancy. It inhibits CYP2A4 and CYP1A2. Concomitant drug should be reduced and it is started as 10 mg/kg/day and increased gradually.

19. **Retigabine (Ezogabine):** It is a potassium channel facilator with minimal drug interaction potentialities used in the dose of 600–1200 mg/day. Used for partial onset seizures. Dizziness, somnolence, bladder dysfunction, dysarthria may occur.

20. **Clorazapate dipotassium:** Used in the dose of 45 mg/day for complex partial seizure.

21. **Perampanel:** This drug is approved for use in partial seizure. Orally active, long acting, plasma protein bound, acts as AMPA antagonist.

TREATMENT OF EPILEPSY

Start antiepileptic as early as possible after diagnosis. Start with single drug at low dose and increase the dose gradually till control is achieved or add second drug or substitute. Try monotherapy. Dose monitoring is required. If drug withdrawal is required, it should be done gradually (except in case of toxicity).

- **Generalized tonic-clonic and simple partial seizures:** Carbamazepine and phenytoin are the 1st choice then phenobarbitone and lastly primidone. Phenobarbitone and valproate are used in head injury patient to control epilepsy. Other add-on drugs are gabapentin, lamotrigine, topiramate.

- **Complex partial seizure:** Carbamazepine is a preferred drug, valproate or phenytoin may be added. Phenobarbitone, primidone, clobazam, lamotrigine, gabapentin, vigabatrin, zonisamide, topiramate, tiagabine may be added.

- **Absence seizure:** Ethosuximide and valproate are preferred drugs. Clonazepam is second alternative, clobazam or lomotrigine may be added.

- **Atonic seizure:** Valproate, primidone, clonazepam are preferred drugs. Lomotrigine may be added.

- **Febrile convulsion:** Diazepam 0.5 mg/kg rectally. Intermittent prophylaxis with diazepam. Chronic prophylaxis with phenobarbitone is not preferred because of behavioral changes.
- **Infantile spasm:** Corticosteroid gives symptomatic relief. Valproate and clonazepam are good adjuvants.
- **Status epilepticus:** Diazepam 10 mg IV bolus followed by slow infusion, clonazepam 1–2 mg IV is alternative or phenobarbitone 100–200 mg IM or IV or phenytoin 25 mg/min IV. Fosphenytoin IV or general anesthetics (midazolam/propofol/thiopentone).

  Maintain airways, oxygenation, BP control, fluid and electrolytic balance, cardiac and blood sugar monitor.

Ideal antiepileptic should be

- Quick acting
- Effective for all varieties of epileptics and acts on epileptogenic focus.
- Less toxic, non-addicting
- Long acting
- Orally effective and cheap

Some special issues related to women and epilepsy

- Women during menses, if develops epilepsy then acetazolamide may be effective, if started 7–10 days before menstruation.
- Women taking OCP, if takes enzyme inducer antiepileptic, *viz.* phenobarbitone, phenytoin may antagonize OCP's action. Should be considered as an alternative method of contraception.

- **Breastfeeding:** Mother breastfeeding her child may be encouraged because of lack of evidence of long-term harm to infants, however if drug effects like lethargy, poor feeding, *etc.* develop it should be reconsidered.
- Pregnant women should be given lowest possible dose because of drug's side effects on baby. Enzymes inducing drugs may cause deficiency in vitamin K dependent clotting factors and mother should get vitamin K in last weeks of pregnancy.

- **Withdrawal of antiseizure durgs:** Withdrawal of non-epileptic patient does not cause seizure, if not above therapeutic level otherwise it may cause seizure with increased frequency and severity. Anti-absence seizure drug withdrawal is easier. Benzodiazepines and barbiturates should be withdrawn gradually in weeks to months. A seizure free period of 3–4 years, gradual withdrawal may be trialed.

Suicidality: The ratio of patient taking antiepileptic drugs and with suicidality is not very clear.

Psychopharmacology

Psychiatric illness can brodly be divided into—
(i) **Neurosis**—where insight is present, *viz.* OCD, phobia, anxiety, posttraumatic stress disorder and (ii) **Psychosis**—where insight is absent, *viz.* schizophrenic affective disorders (mania, depression, bipolar disorder).

In the past, psychiatric disorders were treated in institution and those treatments now seem to be ridiculous or fantastic or both. Psychopharmacology is oriented not only towards discovering new drugs and its action on CNS but also oriented towards understanding diseases of the CNS by altering them through drugs of known action.

Earliest recorded psychopharmacology except in the use of alcohol, opiates and other dependence producing drugs were used for mentally ill since antiquity. Then came chloral hydrate (1869); paraldehyde (1882); barbiturates (1903). Malarial treatment for general paralysis for insane by von Jauregg 1917, received Nobel Prize. The first successful treatment of psychosis came from India by Ganesh Sen and Kartik Bose 1931, used *Rauwolfia serpentina* extract, reserpine got recognition in 1958 when Kline confirmed the finding. During last 50 years, psychiatric patients and doctors have witnessed major changes due to advent of newer drugs. Jean Delay and Pierre Deniker introduced chlorpromazine and transformed the life of schizophrenics into productive life, tricyclic antidepressant and MAO inhibitors (1957–58) covered another group of patients. Meprobamate in 1954 shown hope for anti-anxiety drugs without producing sedation. Chlordiazepoxide (1957), benzodiazepines (1960) and bupropinone are recent additions.

Code1949 described effectiveness of lithium but its wide use started after 1960. Antiepileptic, carbamazepine shown promise for mania and bipolar disorders.

The term tranquilization is used synonymously with peace of mind. It was originally designed to produce peace of mind produced by reserpine and chlorpromazine without sedation. The drugs, which selectively modify behavior pattern, are known as psychoactive or psychotropic drugs. Most of the mental illnesses are treated empirically because little is known about pathology. During last two decades, many drugs have come up in market. The psychotropic drugs excluding the drugs of dependence are classified as follows:

- Antipsychotic
- Mood stabilizing
- Antidepressant
- Antianxiety drugs

Dopamine Hypothesis for Schizophrenia

Neurotransmitter dopamine is involved in the genesis of schizophrenia is developed by following circumstantial evidences:

- Most of the antipsychotic drugs block postsynaptic D_2 receptor in mesolimbic system of CNS.
- Dopaminergic drugs (levodopa, amphetamine) aggravate schizophrenia. However, antagonist of NMDA receptor, phencyclidine also produces schizophrenia like symptoms. ACh and GABA are also involved in schizophrenia.
- Dopamine receptors density of schizophrenia not treated by antipsychotic as evident postmortomly or by positron emission tomography (PET) in schizophrenia are increased.

- Schizophrenia treated by antipsychotic, the amount of homovanillic acid (metabolite of DA) is changed in CSF, plasma or urine.

Serotonin hypothesis of schizophrenia

- $5HT_{2A}$ receptor stimulation has hallucinatory effects.
- $5HT_{2A}$ receptor blockers is one of the key mechanisms of typical antipsychotic, *viz.* clozapine and quetiapine are inverse agonists of $5HT_{2A}$ receptor. $5HT_{2A}$ stimulation depolarizes glutamate and stabilizes NMDA recpetor.

Glutamate hypothesis of schizophrenia

- Glutamate is a major excitatory neurotransmitter.
- Inhibition of NMDA receptor by phencyclidine and ketamine exacerbates schizophrenia.

Types of Dopamine Receptors and Effects

Till now five DA receptors are known and grouped into two families like D_1 and D_2.

D_1 receptor family

- Coded on chromosome 5.
- Increases cAMP by activation of adenylyl cyclase.

D_2 receptor

- Coded on chromosome 11
- Decreases cAMP by inhibiting adenyl cyclases, inhibiting Ca channel and opens K channel.

It is really difficult to define what constitutes psyche or mind which carry out three functions:

- Reception of environmental stimuli (cognition)
- Analyzing the information received and reaction pattern (affect)
- Actual behavior response (conation)

Antipsychotics are those psychoactive drugs which are used for the treatment of major psychosis. They are also known as major tranquilizer, neuroleptic, antischizophrenic drugs and D_2 (dopamine) blockers, but anti-psychotics are most appropriate.

Pharmacokinetics: Antipsychotic drugs are readily absorbed (some are incompletely absorbed), some undergo 1st pass metabolism so their bioavailability vary. They are lipid-soluble and protein-bound and have high affinity for selected neurotransmitter receptors in the CNS and their metabolites may be excreted in urine even after last dose of chronically administered drug. Some antipsychotic drugs are metabolized and some of the products of metabolism mesoridazine in case of thioridazine retain activity. Excretion occurs *via* kidneys.

Pharmacological actions: Differ in normal and psychotic patients. In normal individuals it produces neuroleptic syndrome characterized by indifference to surroundings, emotional quietening, spontaneous movements are minimized. In psychotic patient, it reduces psychotic symptomatology, aggressive behavior, agitation, disturbed thought, behavior, hallucination, delusions, hyperactivity are suppressed gradually.

Mechanism of action: All antipsychotics except clozapine are potent dopamine D_2 receptor blockers. Phenothiazines and thioxanthine also block D_1, D_3 and D_4. Clozapine is a weak D_2 blocker, but it has effect on $5HT_2$ and α_1 blockers.

Pharmacological actions of antipsychotic drugs

- **Actions on ANS:** Neuroleptics have varying degree of α-adrenergic blockade causing orthostatic hypotension, impotence, failure to ejaculate. Their blocking properties are graded below:

  CPZ = Triflupromazine > Thioridazine > Fluphenazine > Haloperidol > Trifluoperazine > Clozapine > Pimozide.

  Anticholinergic properties are graded below:

  Thioridazine > chloropromazine > Triflupromazine > Trifluperazine = Haloperidol. Producing dry mouth, difficulties in micturitions, constipation, loss of accommodation. Phenothiazines have weak H_1 blockers and 5HT blocking activities.

- **Local anesthetic:** CPZ has LA action as procaine, but its irritant nature makes it useless.

- **CVS:** Postural hypotension, reflex tachycardia, but tolerance develops after chronic use may be explained by α-blocking properties. Higher doses of CPZ prolong QT interval, it has antiarrhythmic properties because of membrane stabilization, but arrhythmia may occur with thioridazine.

- **Skeletal muscle:** It does not alter spinal reflexes, but muscle spasticity reduced by its action on basal ganglia or medulla oblongata.

- **Endocrine:** Increases prolactin release by blocking inhibitory action of DA on lactotropes, resulting in galactorrhea and gynecomastia. Reduces gonadotropin secretion, but amenorrhea and infertility are rare. ACTH release and corticoids level fail to increase. GH release is also decreased, but it is not beneficial for acromegaly.

    ADH secretion decreases leading to increase in urine volume.

- **Weight gain:** Possible due to H_1 and $5HT_2$ blockade effects.

- **CNS:** Antipsychotic; lowers seizure threshold and can precipitate epilepsy. Loss of temperature control, antiemetics *via* CTZ. It blocks conditional avoidance response (CAR).

- **Tolerance and dependence:** Occurs to sedative action within a week, but antipsychotic and extrapyramidal effects of DA antagonism remain unchanged.

- **Use in pregnancy:** It is better to avoid antipsychotic in pregnancy because it may effect neurodevelopment.

Special Features of Individual Drugs

- **Triflupromazine:** This aliphatic side chain phenothiazine is more potent than CPZ. Marked as Siquil. Produces muscle dystonia in children used as antiemetic.

- **Thioridazine (Melleril):** Lowest incidence of extrapyramidal effect, low potency phenothiazines with marked central anticholinergic action. Eye damage, cardiac arrhythmia and male sexual dysfunction may occur.

- **Trifluoperazine (Espazine):** 1, 5 mg tabs, 1 mg/mL inj.

- **Fluphenazine (Anatensol):** 1 mg tab. High potency piperazine side chain phenothiazine with minimum autonomic, hypotensive and sedative actions. Less likely to produce jaundice and epileptic seizure, but extrapyramidal effect is severe. The Atanesol decanoate is depot preparation of fluphenazine given IM in every 2–4 weeks.

- **Thioproperazine (Majeptil):** 5 mg tab

- **Haloperidol (Serenace):** Potent antipsychotic with few autonomic, less epileptogenic, does not cause weight gain and jaundice is rare. Used for schizophrenia, Huntington's disease and Gilles de la Tourette's syndrome. Dose 2–20 mg/day. Available as 2.5, 10, 20 mg tabs; 5 mg/mL inj.

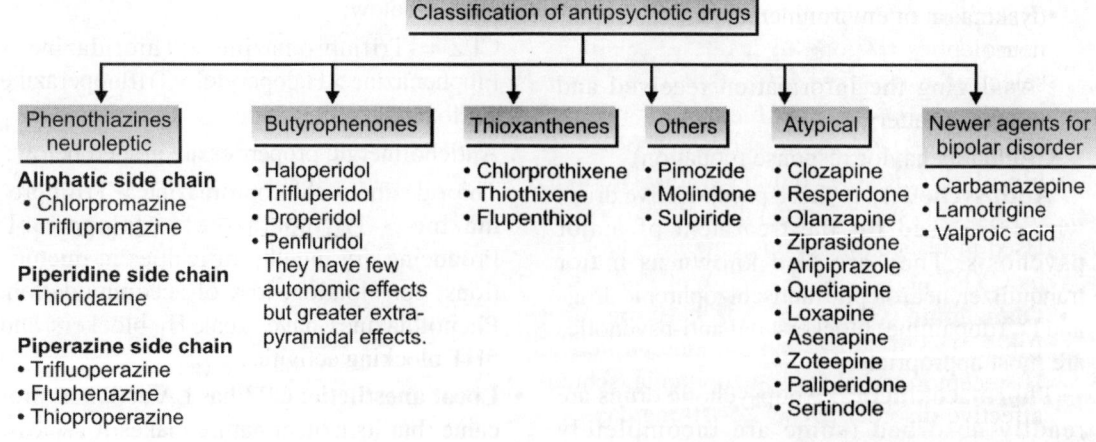

- **Trifluperidol:** More potent than haloperidol (Triperidol 0.5 mg tab; 2.5 mg/mL inj.)
- **Droperidol:** 2.5 mg inj short acting neuroleptics used in anesthesia.
- **Penfluridol (semap; flumap 20 mg tab, dose 20–60 mg weekly):** Given weekly exceptionally long acting neuroleptics used for chronic schizophrenia, withdrawal and social maladjustment patient.
- **Chlorprothixene (Taractan):** It is thioxanthene analogue of CPZ low potency antipsychotics.
- **Flupenthixol (Fluanxol 0.5, 1, 3 mg tab):** Less sedating. Indicated for schizophrenia, psychosis. Dose 1–3 mg/day.
- **Pimozide (Orap):** Specific DA antagonist with little α-adrenergic or anticholinergic effect. Good for maintenance therapy. Orally used, because of long duration of action without psychomotor agitation. Dystonia is less, but increases action potential duration of cardiac muscle, may produce arrhythmia. Used particularly for Gilles de la Tourette's syndrome and ticks.
- **Molindone (Moban):** Indole derivative with less marked antidopaminergic and sedative actions.
- **Loxapine (Loxapac):** Dibenzoxazepine derivative blocks DA receptor and antipsychotic. Quick acting. Neuro and cardiac toxicties are more on overdose. Dose 20–100 mg/day.
- **Clozapine (Lozapine 10, 25, 50 mg tab; dose 25–300 mg/day):** Weak D_2 blocker with less extrapyramidal symptoms and tardive dyskinasia, many patients refractory to typical neuroleptics respond to it due to relatively selective for D_4 receptors (sparse in basal ganglia). $5HT_2$ and α_1 blockade, antimuscarinic and H_1 blocking activity. It produces blood dyscrasia, urinary incontinence, myocarditis start like flu, but death may occur. Used in resistant schizophrenia. Metabolized by CYP3A4.
- **Olanzapine (Olace 2.5, 5, 7.5, 10 mg tab):** Blocks D_2, $5HT_2$, α_1 and α_2; muscarinic and H_1 receptors, used for schizophrenia, schizoaffective disorder. Dose 2.5–10 mg/day.

- **Risperidone:** Blocks D_2, $5HT_2$, H_1 with high affinity to α_1 and α_2 blockades. Resembles clozapine with few extrapyramidal side effect and tardive dyskinesia in low dose (<6 mg/day) sedation and hypotension are rare. It may increase the risk of stroke in elderly. Dose 2–12 mg/day. Available as risperidone 1, 2, 3 and 4 mg tabs.
- **Sulpiride (Dolmatil):** Selective D_2 receptor blockade. In lower doses alerts apathetic, withdrawn schizophrenic and in higher doses controls florid schizophrenia. Dose 200–400 mg BD.
- **Reserpine (Serpasil):** Depletes DA, 5HT and NAd, mental depression, suicidal tendency prominent with antipsychotic doses. It is rarely used as antipsychotic. It has only historical importance now.
- **Ziprasidone:** Causes QT prolongation and carries risk of arrhythmia, dose 40 mg/day. Available as azona 20, 40 mg tabs.
- **Quetiapine:** Short half-life, dose 50–400 mg/day metabolized by $CYP3A_4$ so can interact with macrolide and antifungal. Can cause cataract formation.
- **Aripiprazole:** Partial agonist at $5HT_{1A}$; D_2 and antagonist on $5HT_{2A}$ receptor also known as dopamine-serotonin stabilizer. Dose 5–30 mg/day. Available as anibra 10 and 15 mg/day.
- **Adverse effects of neuroleptics:** It is based on dose-related pharmacological effect otherwise they are safe.
- **CNS:** Drowsiness, lethargy, confusion, tolerance, increased appetite, weight gain.
- **α bockade:** Postural hypotension, palpitation, ejaculation defect (thioridazine)
- **Endocrine:** Amenorrhea, infertility, gynecomastia, lactorrhea
- **Anticholinergic:** Dry mouth, blurred vision, constipation, urinary hesitancy
- **Extrapyramidal disturbances**
  a. **Parkinsonism**
  b. **Acute muscular dystonia:** Bizzare muscle spasm generally in face and tongue

muscles producing grimacing, torticollis, tongue thrusting, locked jaw. Central anticholinergic promathazine or hydroxyzine is given IM to treat it.

c. **Akathisia (restlessness, agitated):** Central anticholinergic alprazolam or propranolol is used to treat it.

d. **Malignant neuroleptic syndrome (rigidity, immobility, semiconsciousness, fever, fluctuating BP and HR):** Myoglobin in blood.

   Treatment: Stop neuroleptics and treat symptomatically. Bromocriptine in large doses is helpful. Dantrolene IV is also used.

e. **Tardive dyskinesia:** Purposeless involuntary facial and limb movements, chewing, pouting, puffing of cheeks, lips licking, choreoathetoid movements occur late in therapy. Temporarily suppressed by higher doses of neuroleptics, less common with clozapine and risperidone.

- **Blue pigmentation of skin:** Corneas and lenticular opacities, retinal degeneration with thioridazone.

- **Hypersensitivity:** Cholestatic jaundice, skin rashes, urticaria, contact dermatitis, photosensitivity, agranulocytosis.

Drug interactions

- Blunts action of levodopa in parkinsonian patient.

- Potentiates CNS depressants like hypnotics, anxiolytic, alcohol, opioids, analgesic.

- Enzyme inducers like phenobarbitones reduce plasma level of neuroleptics.

Therapeutic uses of antipsychotic drugs

- Schizophrenia
- Schizoaffective disorder
- Mania with lithium and carbamazepine
- Organic psychiatric disorder (in low doses)
- Gilles de la Tourette's syndrome (haloperidol)
- Infantile autism (haloperidol)
- Agitated depression (with antidepressants)
- Severe intractable anxiety in low doses
- Major depression with psychotic feature (antidepression)
- Attention deficit when stimulant medicines are contraindicated
- Hiccough
- Nausea, vomiting
- Huntington's chorea
- Neuroleptanesthesia (droperidol with fentanyl)
- Tetanus-CPZ is secondary drug to skeletal muscle relaxation.
- To potentiate hypnotics, analgesics.
- Tourette's syndrome.
- Behavior disturbance in Alzheimer's disease.

Choice of drug is highly empirical with associated feature and mood state

- Agitated, combative violent—CPZ, triflupromazine,
- Withdrawn and apathic—trifluperazine, fluphenazine.
- Patient with mainly negative symptoms and resistant cases—clozapine.
- Mood elevation and hypomania—haloperidol, thioproperazine.
- To avoid extrapyramidal side effect—thioridazone, risperidone, clozapine.

Antidepressants
(Mood Elevators/Thymoleptics)

Mania and depression are two extremes of diseases and the drugs used are antimaniac (mood stabilizer and antidepressant).

Mitochondiral enzyme MAO oxidatively deaminates biological amines (Adr, NAd, DA, 5HT). There are two isoenzymes MAO-A and MAO-B. MAO-A deaminates NAd and 5HT inhibited by clorgyline and moclobemide present in peripheral adrenergic nerve ending, intestinal mucosa and placenta.

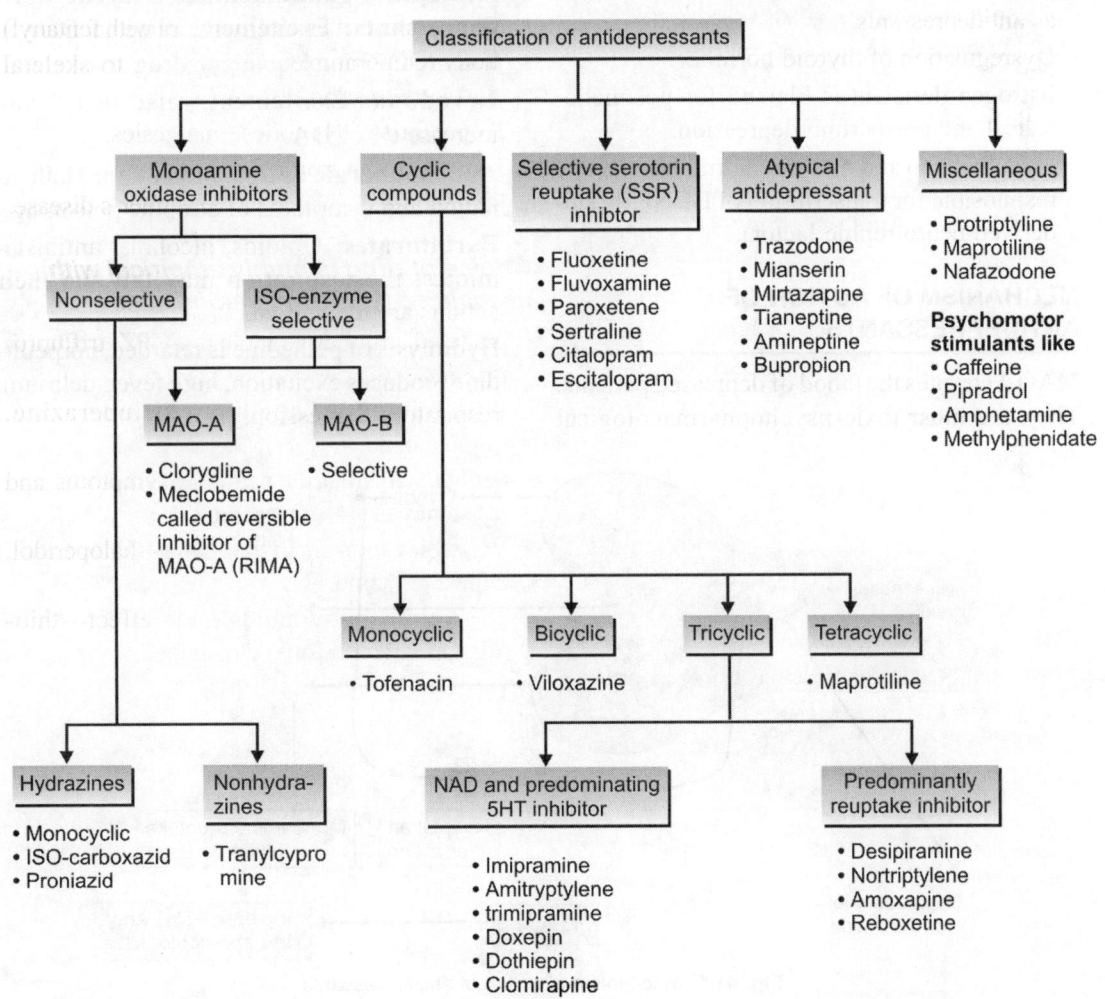

Classification of antidepressants

Monoamine oxidase inhibitors
- Nonselective
- ISO-enzyme selective

MAO-A
- Clorygline
- Meclobemide called reversible inhibitor of MAO-A (RIMA)

MAO-B
- Selective

Hydrazines
- Monocyclic
- ISO-carboxazid
- Proniazid

Nonhydra-zines
- Tranylcypromine

Cyclic compounds
- Monocyclic
  - Tofenacin
- Bicyclic
  - Viloxazine
- Tricyclic
- Tetracyclic
  - Maprotiline

NAD and predominating 5HT inhibitor
- Imipramine
- Amitryptylene
- trimipramine
- Doxepin
- Dothiepin
- Clomirapine

Predominantly reuptake inhibitor
- Desipiramine
- Nortriptylene
- Amoxapine
- Reboxetine

Selective serotorin reuptake (SSR) inhibtor
- Fluoxetine
- Fluvoxamine
- Paroxetine
- Sertraline
- Citalopram
- Escitalopram

Atypical antidepressant
- Trazodone
- Mianserin
- Mirtazapine
- Tianeptine
- Amineptine
- Bupropion

Miscellaneous
- Protriptyline
- Maprotiline
- Nafazodone

Psychomotor stimulants like
- Caffeine
- Pipradrol
- Amphetamine
- Methylphenidate

MAO-B deaminates phenylethylamine, is inhibited by selegiline. MAO-B is present in platelets and brain.

Liver contains both MAO-A and MAO-B. DA is a substrate for both MAO-A and MAO-B.

Pathophysiology of depression

- Deficit of monoamine (NAd, 5HT, DA) in central brain (monoamine hypothesis)
- Drop in brain-derived neurotrophic factor (BDNF), which is responsible for neural plasticity, resilence and neurogenesis.
- Integration of hypothalamus–pituitary axis and steroid abnormalities are normalized by BDNF.
- Glutamate antagonist, melatonin agonist and glucocorticoid specific agents have also role as antidepressants.
- Dysregulation of thyroid hormone.
- Estrogen deficient is blamed for postmeno-pausal and postpartum depression.
- Hypothalamo and pituitary hormones may be responsible for transcription of BDNF (brain-derived neurotrophic factor).

MECHANISM OF ACTION OF ANTIDEPRESSANTS

MAO-I elevates the mood of depressed patients. They are most toxic psychopharmacological agents. Side effects are fatigue, irritability, insomnia, postural hypotension (due to decreased sympathetic outflow, interferes with ganglionic transmission), peripheral neuropathy due to B_6 deficiency. Hepatocellular failure, overdose may produce sweating, agitation, confusion, hallucination and mania.

Drug Interaction of Antidepressants

- **Cheese reaction:** Cheese, beer, wines, pickled meat, *etc.* contain large quantity of indirectly acting sympathomimetics which are meta-bolized by MAO and their inhibition leads hypertensive crisis and CVA.
- **Cold and cough remedies** containing ephe-drine does the same hypertensive crisis.
- **Reserpine, guanethedine, tricyclic anti-depressants:** Excitement, raise in BP and body temperature.
- **Levodopa:** Excitement, raise in BP and increase t½ of DA.
- **Anticholinergic antiparkinsonian:** Halluci-nation and symptoms of atropine poisoning.
- **Barbiturates:** Opioids, alcohols, antihista-minics, the respiration may fail and their actions are intensified.
- Hydrolysis of pethedine is retarded, norpethi-dine produces excitation, high fever, delirium, respiratory depression.

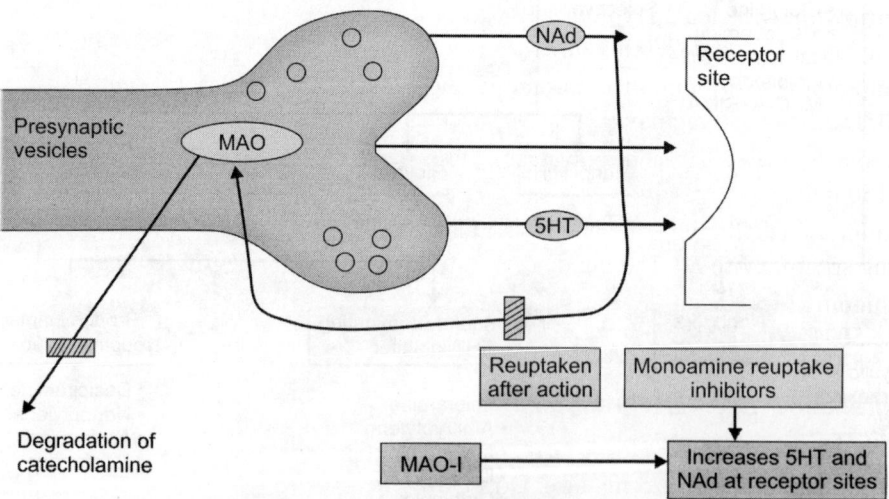

Fig. 41.1: Mechanism of action of antidepressants

MAO-I rarely used. Uses are restricted to patient not responding to tricyclic antidepressant or ECT is refused or contraindicated. Phobic and obsessive compulsive disorders or narcolepsy respond well with MAO-I. They are hit and run drugs, *i.e.* their action persists for 2–3 weeks after their discontinuation.

Serotonin syndrome: This is a serious pharmacodynamic drug interaction of MAO-I and serotonergic agents like SSRIs and SNRIs. The symptoms are tachycardia, raised BP, delirium, coma, myoclonus, hyperreflexia, tremor. SSRI should be withdrawn two weeks before MAO-I and SNRI administration. For fluoxetine this period is 4–5 weeks.

Moclobemide (Rimarex 150–300 mg tab): Selective reversible inhibitor of MAO-A (RIMA), cheese reaction rare. Lack anticholinergic, sedative, cardiovascular effect emerging as the alternative to tricyclic antidepressants. 1 tab BD to TDS.

ADR: Nausea, headache, dizziness, insomnia, excitement and liver damage.

Tricyclic and Related Antidepressants Classification

Noradrenaline and 5HT reuptake inhibitors

- Imipramine (Depsonil, Antidep 25 mg tab; 75 mg sr cap). Dose 50–200 mg/day.
- Amitriptyline (Serotena, Tryptomer 10, 25 and 75 mg tabs). Dose 50–200 mg/day.
- Trimipramine (Surmontil 10, 25 and 75 mg tabs). Dose 50–150 mg/day.
- Doxepin (Spectra 10, 25 and 75 mg tabs). Dose 50–150 mg/day.
- Clomipramine (Clonil 10, 25 and 50 mg tabs; 75 mg sr tab). Dose 50–150 mg/day.
- Dothiepin (Prothiaden 25 and 75 mg tabs). Dose 50–150 mg/day.

Noradrenaline (NA > 5HT) reuptake inhibitors

- Nortriptyline (Sensival 25 mg tab). Dose 50–150 mg/day.

- Desipramine (Norpramin). Dose 75–300 mg/day.
- Protriptyline (Vivactil). Dose 20–40 mg/day.
- Amoxapine (Demolox 50–100 mg tab). Dose 100–300 mg/day.

Selective 5HT Serotonin reuptake inhibitors (SSRIs)

- Fluoxetine (Fludac 20 mg cap). Dose 20–50 mg/day. Bicyclic compound, slow onset but long acting SSRI antidepressant. May be used in, children above 7 years if psychotherapy fails. Less suitable for patient requiring rapid effect.
- Fluvoxamine (Fluvoxin 50 and 100 mg tabs). Dose 50–200 mg/day. It is CYP3A4 inhibitor. Short acting SSRI used in hospitalized patient or for anxiety disorder or OCD patient. Nausea and agitation may occur.
- Paroxetine (Xet 10, 20, 30 and 40 mg tabs). Dose 20–50 mg/day. Short acting SSRI with higher GI side effect. (Serlin 50; 100 mg tab; Dosa 50–200 mg)
- Sertraline (Serlin 50 and 100 mg tabs). Dose 50–200 mg/day. Less dropout due to less side effects and less drug interaction due to CYP isoenzyme inhibition. Produces long acting active metabolite.
- Citalopram (Celica 10, 20 and 40 mg tabs). Dose 20–40 mg/day. $5HTI_A$ partial agonist have either lower binding capacity at receptor or having a typical properties. The older TCA inhibit monoamine uptake and react with variety of receptors a-adrenergic, muscarinic, H_1 receptor, $5HT_1$ and $5HT_2$ and occasionally D_2 receptors. The newer selective serotonin reuptake inhibitors (SSRI) act on fewer receptors and have limited side effects. Should be avoided in patient of sucidal tendencies. $S^{(+)}$ enantiomer is Escitalopram (Esdap 5, 10 and 20 mg). Here less dose is required.
- Escitalopram (Esdep 5, 10 and 20 mg tabs). Dose 10–20 mg/day. It is S(+) enantiomer of citalopram.

Atypical antidepressants

- **Tarzodone** (Trazodac 25 and 50 mg tabs). Dose 50–200 mg/day. It is CYP3A4 inhibitor so chances of drug interaction is there.

- **Bupropion** (Smoquit 150 mg tab). Noradrenergic and dopaminergic reuptake inhibitor (NDRI). Metabolized to amphetamine like compound. Dose 150–300 mg/day. Also use for smoking abstinence. Insomnia, agitation, dry mouth and seizure may occur in high doses.

- **Mianserin** (Tetradep 10, 20 and 30 mg tabs). Dose 30–100 mg/day. It blocks presynaptic α_2.

- **Duloxetin** (Delok 20, 30 and 40 mg caps) serotonin–noradrenaline reuptake inhibitor. It is also used for stress incontinence of urine.

- **St. John's wort:** This natural substance contains hypericin and hyperforin which are used as natural antidepressants.

Newer Compounds

Tianeptin (Stablon 12.5 mg tab, dose 12.5 mg BD and TDS): It increases 5HT uptake, neither sedative or stimulant useful for anxiety and depressive psychosomatic and endogenous depression. Dry mouth, epigastric pain, insomnia, tremor may occur.

Amineptin (Survector 100 mg tab, dose 100 mg BD): Enhances 5HT uptake. Tachycardia, delirium, confusion, conduction disturbance, postural hypotension may occur with heart disease patient.

Venlafaxine (Ventor 25, 37.5 and 75 mg tabs): Serotonin and noradrenaline reuptake inhibitor (SNRI). Dose 75–150 mg/day.

Mirtazapine (Mirt 15, 30 and 45 mg tabs): Noradrenergic and specific serotonergic antidepressant (NaSSA).

It blocks α_2-auto on NAd neurons and 5HT heteroreceptors enhancing the release of both NAd and 5HT release. It blocks H_1 receptor, but no anticholinergic or antidopaminergic action. Dose 15–45 mg.

Nefazodone: Serotonin 2 receptor antagonist reuptake inhibitor (SARI).

Amoxapine: Tetracyclic compound, blocks D_2 receptor and inhibits NAd uptake, has antidepressant and neuroleptic properties used for psychotic depression. Extrapyramidal side effects and status epilepticus may occur in overdose.

Reboxetine (Narebox 4 and 8 mg tabs, dose 4–8 mg BD): Selective NAd reuptake blocker with less side effects even in overdose. Insomnia, dry mouth, constipation, sexual distress and urinary symptoms may occur as side effects.

Most of the SSRI and some TCA delays or inhibits ejaculation. Dapoxetine a SSRI is taken 60 mg tablet one hour before intercourse is projected as delaying ejaculation.

SELECTIVE SEROTONIN REUPTAKE INHIBITORS (SSRIs)

- SSRIs selectively inhibit SERT and because of their better acceptability they are now used for phobia, depression and anxiety.
- Little sedation, no anticholinergic, α-adrenergic blocking, no seizure precipitating propensity or overdose arrhythmia problem or weight gain problem.

It may produce nausea ($5HT_3$ stimulation) and interferes with ejaculation. Restlessness, insomnia anorexia, dyskinesia, headache, diarrhea, epistaxis or ecchymosis may occur.

SSRIs inhibit cytochromes $CYP2D_6$ and $CYP3A_4$ and increase the plasma level of many drugs. Serotonin syndrome may be precipitated, patient simultaneously taking SSRI and serotonergic drugs manifest as agitation, restlessness, sweating, twitching, convulsion.

Mechanism of Action of Tricyclic Antidepressant (TCA)

TCA inhibits reuptake of biogenic amines NAd and 5HT, but does not inhibit the reuptake of DA except bupropion which causes increased concentration of amines in CNS and peripheral synaptic cleft which is associated with antidepressant actions. Initially presynaptic α_2 and $5HT_1$ autoreceptors are stimulated by increasing NAd and 5HT causing decreased firing of locus coeruleus by NAd and raphe by 5HT, but long-term administration desensitize α_2 and $5HT_{1A}$ and $5HT_{1D}$ autoreceptors resulting in enhanced NAd and 5HT turnover in brain.

Pharmacological Actions of TCA

CNS: In normal individual: Clumsy feeling, lightheadedness, concentration difficulties, gait unsteady.

In depressed patient: Sedation, mood elevates after 2–3 weeks of continuous treatment, suppress REM sleep, seizure threshold is lowered.

ANS: TCA by virtue of anticholinergic effect produces dry mouth, constipation, blurred vision, urinary hesitancy.

CVS: Tachycardia, postural hypotension (α_1 blocked), cardiac arrhythmia may occur.

Tolerance and dependence to anticholinergic action and hypotension develop gradually though antidepressant action is sustained. Psychological dependence rare, though some physical dependences like feeling of malaise, chills, muscle pain which requires gradual withdrawal. Does not have abuse potential.

Pharmacokinetics: TCAs are absorbed orally, bound to plasma and tissue protein, metabolized in liver by oxidation and glucuronide conjugation and excreted through urine. Imipramine, amitriptyline, nortriptyline show unusual therapeutic window, below and above this range their beneficial effect is low. The dose need titration because of individual variability of plasma concentration.

Adverse effects: Sedation, mental confusion, weakness, increased appetite and weight gain (with TCA and tarzodone), but not with SSRI and bupropion. Dry mouth, constipation, urinary retention, palpitation, blurred vision (anticholinergic effect) or mania may occur in bipolar illness/sweating and fine tremor/seizure may be precipitated (desmipramine and SSRI are safer). Postural hypotension rare with SSRI. Cardiac

arrhythmia in patient with IHD and jaundice due to hypersensitivity may occur.

Drug Interaction of Antidepressants

TCAs potentiate sympathomimetic amine, abolish antihypertensive action of guanethedine and clonidine by preventing their transport.

Potentiate CNS depressant of alcohol, antihistaminics. The protein-bound drugs are displaced (phenytoin, PBZ, aspirin) causing their toxicity.

Phenobarbitone competitively inhibits imipramine metabolism and induces it with MAO-I produces hypertensive crisis.

Uses of Antidepressants

- **Endogenous depression:** Meclobemide.
- **Obsessive-compulsive disorders and phobic states:** SSRI is a drug of choice. TCA, specially clomipramine effective for OCD and panic.
- **Antianxiety:** SSRI may be used with BZD.
- **Neuropathic pain:** Amitriptyline for post-herpetic neuralgia pain and diabetic pain.
- **Attention deficit and hyperactive disorder of children:** Amoxapine, imipramine, nortriptyline are used.
- **Enuresis:** Imipramine may be used.
- **Migraine:** Amitriptyline has got prophylactic role.
- **Pruritus:** Topical doxepin to relive itching of atopic dermatitis.

For compulsive buying, kleptomania, eating disorder, school phobia, menstrual dysphoria; fluoxetine is used.

Refractory depression: 35% of patients do not respond to antidepression because (i) poor drug compliance, (ii) inadequate doses, (iii) insufficient treatment duration and (iv) low plasma level of antidepressants.

Sudden antidepressant changing or stopping should not be done. The dose of new drug is gradually increased and the older drug is gradually withdrawn the process of cross-tapering.

LITHIUM AND OTHER MOOD STABILIZING DRUGS

Lithium is the smallest alkali ion element with atomic number 3 and atomic mass 7. Arfuedson in 1817 discovered it, since then it was used for gout and salt replacement in cardiac disease, but its use was restricted because of fatal toxicity. Established indications of lithium are:

- Acute mania
- Prophylaxis of bipolar mood disorder
- Schizoaffective disorders
- Acute depression
- Chronic alcoholism with depressive symptoms
- Cluster headache
- Hyperthyroidism
- Kleine-Levin syndrome
- Huntington's chorea
- Neutropenia
- Inappropriate ADH secretion syndrome to counter water retention.

Pharmacokinetics: Rapidly absorbed from GI tract, not metabolized, excreted entirely by kidney, depletes Na, results in retention of Li. Plasma concentration for maintenance of Li therapy for bipolar disorder is 0.5 and 0.8 mEq/L and for acute mania 0.8–1.2 mEq/L.

Mechanism of Action of Lithium

Decreasing CA Activity

- Affects Na^+/K^+-ATPase, and accumulates lithium intracellularly.
- Inhibits adenyl cyclase, thus decreases cAMP second messenger intracellularly.
- Accelerates presynaptic destruction of catecholamine.
- Inhibits release of CA at synapse.
- Decreases the postsynaptic receptor sensitivity.

The second messenger for α-adrenergic and muscarinic transmission are IP_3 and DAG which are produced by Gq-protein coupled phospholipase C (PLC). PLC hydrolyzes PIP_2 to IP_3 which being water-soluble enters cytoplasm to release

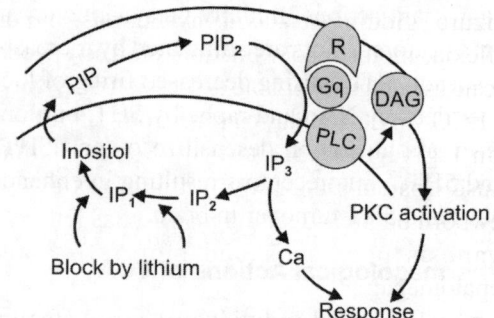

Fig. 41.2: Mechanism of action of lithium

PIP_2	Phosphatidyl inositol biphosphate
PIP	Phosphatidyl inositol phosphate
IP_3	Inositol triphosphate
IP_2	Inositol diphosphate
IP_1	Inositol monophosphate
DAG	Diacyl glycerol
R	Receptor for neurotransmitter
Gq	G coupling protein
PLC	Phospholipase C
PKC	Protein kinase C

Ca^{2+}, IP_3 is inactivated to IP_2, IP_1, and inositol which is precursor for PIP_2.

Lithium inhibits hydrolysis of inositol diphosphate by inositol phosphatase as a consequence source of IP_3 and diacyl glycerol is reduced and hyperactive neurons are preferentially inhibited because supply of inositol from external source is negligible and selectively dampens signal transduction in hyperactive neurons.

It uncouples receptors from G-protein. Polyuria and hypothyroidism due to lithium is due to uncoupling of vasopressin and TSH from G-proteins.

Other Actions

- Li inhibits action of ADH on distal tubules and causes diabetes insipidus like state. Lithium induced diabetes insipidus responds to amiloride, but resistant to vasopressin.
- It has insulin-like action on metabolism.
- Leukocyte count is increased by Li therapy.
- It reduces thyroxine synthesis interfering with thyroxine.

Adverse effects: Nausea, vomiting, diarrhea, thirst and polyuria, edema, fine tremor, rarely seizure, giddiness, ataxia, nystagmus, hyper-reflexia, motor incoordination, slurred speech. It causes benign reversible depression of T wave in ECG. Toxic symptoms start from 1.5 mEq/L don't give to expectant mother as it may cause Ebstein's anomaly. Lithium toxicity in newborn on breastfeeding manifest as lethargy, cyanosis poor suck and mororeflex and hepatomegaly.

Treatment: Osmotic diuresis and sodium bicarbonate infusion promote Li excretion. Hemodialysis, if serum level above 4 mEq/L. It is contraindicated in pregnancy and in sick sinus syndrome.

Interactions: Diuretics increase plasma Li level, so does tetracyclines, indomethacin and ACE inhibitors. It reduces pressor response of NA. It enhances insulin and sulfonyl urea induced hypoglycemia. Succinyl choline and pancuronium produce prolong paralysis with lithium. Neuroleptic action is potentiated by Li.

Alternative of Lithium for Mania and Bipolar Disorder

- Carbamazepine
- Sodium valproate
- Clonidine and verapamil are also investigated for substitute to Li.
- Lamotrigine
- Topiramate
- Gabapentin

Availability of Lithium

It is available as carbonate and citrate because these are less hygroscopic. Dose 300–600 mg TDS to maintain plasma level as 0.6 mEq/L (lowest) to 0.9 mEq/L.

ANTIANXIETY DRUGS

Some degrees of anxiety is a part of normal life and helps in solving problems, but when this emotional state is unpleasant in nature associated with unpleasant discomfort and concerns fear about some undefined future threats, it requires treatment.

Classification of antianxiety drugs

- **Benzodiazepines:** Diazepam, chlordiazepoxide, oxazepam, lorazepam, alprazolam.
- **Azapirones:** Buspirone, gepirone, ispapirone
- **Miscellaneous**
  (a) **Carbamates:** Meprobamate (Equanil) not used because of abuse and dependence.
  (b) **Piperidinedione:** Glutethimide (dependence producing)
  (c) **Alcohol:** Ethanol and chloralhydrate (dependence producing)
  (d) **Quinazoline:** Methaquolone (Mandrax) become street drug because of dependence.
  (e) **Antihistaminics:** Diphenhydramine (Benadryl) and promethazine (Phenargan) may be used as hypnotics.
  (f) **Cyclic ethers:** Paraldehyde not very effective.
  (g) **Antipsychotic:** Thioridazone
  (h) **Antidepressant:** Doxepin
  (i) **β blockers:** Propranolol role is still investigational.

Benzodiazepines: At antianxiety doses, CVS and respiratory depression is less and little effect on other body systems, lower dependence producing and relatively safe because of long half-life. Adverse effects are sedation, lightheadedness, vertigo, confusion in elderly, increased appetite and weight gain, altered sexual function.

Chlordiazepoxide (Librium and Equilibrium 10 mg tabs, dose 20–100 mg): Preferred in chronic anxiety state.

Diazepam (Calmpose 5, 10 mg tabs; 2 mg/ Srnl syr): Preferred for acute panic associated with organic disease.

Oxazepam (Serepax 15, 30 mg tabs; dose 30–60 mg in BD or TDS): Slowly absorbed and slow duration of action preferred for elderly and in those with hepatic disease.

Lorazepam (Ativan 1–2 mg tab, 4 mg/2 mL inj, dose 1–6 mg): Preferred for short-lived anxiety states, tension syndrome, obsessive-compulsive neurosis. It produces amnesia. This is the only benzodiazepine may be given IM.

Alprazolam (Alzolam 0.25–0.5 mg, dose 0.25–1 mg TDS up to 6 gm/day): In addition to antianxiety has some mood elevations. It produces less drowsiness, but some experiences anxiety in between doses.

Buspirone is a azapirone (buspine 5 and 10 mg tabs, dose 5–15 mg up to TDS), distinct from BZD as it does not interact with BZD receptors, no significant sedation/cognitive/functional impairment. No tolerance or physical dependence or withdrawal symptoms. No muscle relaxation or anticonvulsant property.

It is a partial agonist of $5HT_{1A}$ and has weak dopamine D_2 blocking action, mood elevation may be due to facilitation of central non-adrenergic system. Patient of buspirone should be cautioned of driving vehicle or machine though they remain alert.

Hydroxyzine (Atarax l0–25 mg tab, 25 mg/ 2 mL inj and 10 mg/2 mL syr, dose 50–200 mg daily): H_1 antihistaminics with antiemetic, antimuscarinic, sedative, spasmolytic properties claimed to have anxiolytic with marked sedation. It is used for pruritis and urticaria also. Dose 50–200 mg.

β blockers: It relieves many anxiety symptoms due to sympathetic activities, *viz.* rise in BP, shaking, tremor, *etc.* Dealt in ANS chapter.

Fixed dose combinations of tranquilizers with vitamins are banned in India.

- Zopiclone, Zolpidem and Zaleplon are used as antianxiety drugs discussed in the chapter of sedative and hypnotics.
- Newer drugs—Suriclone (a cyclopyrrolone derivative), bretazenil and imidazenil are anxiolytic, rapid acting. These are partial benzodiazepine agonists. Abecarni is an anticonvulsant and anxiolytic. Alpidem is used as anxiolytic.

Psychotogenic Drugs

A drug capable of producing a state by maladaptive behavior in which an individual reacts inappropriately to his environment, changes mood, varieties of effects on memory and learned behavior. They are also known as hallucinogens.

Drugs are

- **Lysergic acid diethylamide (LSD):** Most potent, psychedelic with central sympathetic stimulation and also involves 5HT neurons of brain.
- **Lysergic acid amide:** Close to LSD, but less potent, found in morning glory seeds.
- **Psilocybin:** Found in Mexican mushroom used by Red Indians in festivals.
- **Harmine:** Brazilian natives use it as snuff.
- **Bufotenin:** Isolated from toad skin.
- **Mescaline:** It is a phenylalkylamine derivative used by Native Americans during rituals, has no sympathomimetic effect.
- **Ecstasy:** Methylenedioxymethamphetamine (MDMA) used by college students as a recreational euphoriant drug. It is neurotoxic. Acute effects are dose dependent with feeling of energy, altered sense of time, enhanced perception. The negtive effects are tachycardia, dry mouth, muscleache, jaw clenching. In higher doses visual hallucination, panic, hyperthermia, agitation may occur.
- **Phencyclidine:** Anticholinergic, causes disorientation, distortion of body image, hallucination, anesthesia like ketamines. It became a drug of abuse in 1970 as oral or as smoke

50 µg/kg produces bizzare response to projective thinking, emotional withdrawal, catatonic posturing, hostile or assaultive behavior, with increase of dose anesthetic effect starts and stupor, coma, rhabdomyolysis, hyperthermia may occur. It blocks NDMA type glutamate receptors. Overdose is treated with life support as there is no antagonist and known way for excretion.

- **Dimethoxymethyl amphetamine and methylene dioxyamphetamine** (MDA) have hallucinogenic properties.
- **Tetrahydrocannabinol:** It is an active principle of *Cannabis indica* which is a popular recreational and ritualistic intoxicant. The pharmacological effect varies with dose, route and prior experience of the user. Intoxicity causes mood changes, impairment of coordination, tracking behavior, increased hunger, giddiness and acute psychosis. The evidence of brain damage is not known, some beneficial effects are also known such as antinauseating, muscle relaxing, decrease in intraocular tension, anticonvulsant, increased FEV_1 in bronchial asthma patient, but rarely used because these are at the cost of addiction liability.

Withdrawal symptoms are restlessness, irritability, agitation, insomnia, nausea, cramps.

The dried leaves are **Bhang**, female influorescence (smoked) are **Ganja**. The resinous flowering extract from flowering top (**Charas**) and leaves smoked with tobacco is **Hashish**. All are potent hallucinogens.

CNS Stimulants

These drugs stimulate specific brain functions. They generally produce generalized action results in convulsion in higher doses.

Classification of CNS Stimulants

- **Convulsants:** Strychnine, picrotoxin, bicuculline, pentylenetetrazole
- **Analeptics:** Doxapram, ethyl and propyl butanamide, nikethamide.
- **Psychostimulants:** Amphetamine, methyl phenidate, pemoline, cocaine, methylxanthines (caffeine, theophylline), modafinil.

CONVULSANTS

Strychnine: Alkaloid obtained from seeds of *Strychnos nux-vomica,* acts by blocking postsynaptic inhibition produced by inhibitory transmitter glycine in Renshaw cells. Its therapeutic use is banned in India. It is only of toxicological importance.

Picrotoxin: It blocks presynaptic inhibition mediated through GABA and prevents Cl⁻ channel opening. Obtained from fish berry of *Anamirta cocculus.* Potent convulsant, accompanied by vasomotor and respiratory stimulation and vomiting. No therapeutic use. Diazepam is a drug of choice for its poisoning.

Bicuculline: Competitive $GABA_A$ receptor antagonist, used for research only.

Pentylenetetrazole: Directly depolarizes central neuron. Low doses cause excitation, large doses produce convulsion. It was used for respiratory paralysis, circulatory failure, mental improvement in dementia patient or depression in the past. It has been shown to interfere GABAergic inhibition like picrotoxin.

ANALEPTICS (Stimulate Respiration)

Uses of Analeptics

- As an expedient measure of hypnotic drug poisoning
- Suffocation on drowning
- Apnea in premature infants
- Failure to ventilate spontaneously after GA
- Respiratory failure, but their role is doubtful.

Individual Analeptic Drugs

Doxapram: (Caropram 20 mg/mL in 5 mL amp, dose 40–80 mg IV, IM or 0.5–2 mg/kg/hour as infusion). At low doses selective for respiratory center than other analeptics. Rarely used. It stimulates respiration by carotid and aortic chemoreceptors.

Nikethamide: Less selective than doxapram and rarely used.

Ethyl and propyl butanamide: Used in postoperative pulmonary complications, ventilatory insufficiency, suffocation and drowning, contains equal amount of two solutions (Restimulen 150 mg/mL oral drop or 250 mg/1.5 mL injection).

Reflex: Stimulation by a drop of alcohol in nose or smelling ammonia is used in hysterical patients.

Psychostimulants

Pharmacologically, their psychic effects are more important than their actions on medullary center.

Amphetamine: Central indirectly acting sympathomimetics. They stimulate mental status more than motor activity.

Methylphenidate (Retalin 5 mg tab): Used for hyperkinetic and attention deficit children, indirectly acting sympathomimetics, less likely to cause tachycardia, absorbed orally, may produce anorexia, insomnia, abdominal discomfort. It releases NAd and DA in brain.

Pemoline: Therapeutic effect develops gradually, activates dopaminergic mechanism of brain used for attention deficit hyperkinetic children, narcolepsy, daytime sleepiness. It is hepatotoxic, therapeutic benefit develops after 3–4 weeks.

Cocaine: Inhibits catecholamine uptake, addiction liability is there.

Methylxanthine and caffeine: They are CNS stimulants, irregularly absorbed form GI tract, completely metabolized in liver by demethylation and oxidation and excreted in urine. Tonics with caffeine is banned in India.

Caffeine is used in analgesic mixture, migraine and apnea in premature infants as alternative to theophylline.

Side effects: GI irritation, vomiting, nervousness, insomnia, agitation, muscle twitching, tachycardia, extrasystole.

Modafinil: Used for nightshift workers (working in call center) to keep awake in daytime. Narcolepsy, sleep apnea syndrome, cocaine induced dizziness, confusion, amnesia, personality disorder, tremor, hypertension, dependence may occur (Modalert 100–200 mg tab). Dose 100–200 mg at morning and afternoon for daytime sleepiness.

Atomoxetine: This is a selective NAd uptake inhibitor improves attention span in ADHD. In children should not be given with MAO-inhibitors. Dose 0.5 mg/kg/day.

Caffeine: Used as

i. In analgesic mixture

ii. Migraine in combination with ergotamine.

iii. Apnea in infants as alternative to theophylline.

Cognition Enhancer

Used in dementia and other cerebral disorders. Therapeutic indications are:

- Senile dementia of Alzheimer's disease and multiinfarct dementia
- TIA
- Learning defect in children
- Organic diseases of brain like head injury, ECT, brain surgery. They enhance cerebral blood flow, cerebral neuronal metabolism and increase memory.
- Dizziness and memory disturbances of elderly.

They probably act by global or regional cerebral blood flow supporting neurons metabolism, improving memory and enhancing neurotransmission.

Classification

- Nootropic: Piracetam
- Metabolic enhancer: Dihydroergotoxine, nicergoline, piribedil.
- Cholinergic activator: Tacrine, rivastigmine, donepezil, galantamine.
- Vasoactive cerebral protector: Pyritinol, ginkgo biloba.
- Glutamate antagonist: Memantine.

Piracetam: Cyclic GABA derivative enhances memory, synaptic transmission and interhemisphere information transfer. It is not a vasodilator, but reduce blood viscosity (available as normabrain 400–800 mg caps, 500 mg/5 mL syr). Side effects are excitement, gastric discomfort, insomnia and skin rash.

Dihydroergotoxine: Adrenergic blocking agent claim to increase cerebral blood flow. (Hydergine 1 mg tab; 0.3 mg/mL, Cereloid 1 mg tab, dose 1.5 mg TDS oral or sublingual or 0.3 mg IM OD). Side effects are flushing, headache, hypotension.

Nicergoline (Sermion 30 mg tab) is a synthetic ergot derivative.

Piribedil (Trivastal 50 mg tab): It is a dopamine agonist, improves memory, concentration and vigilance. Giddiness, GI upset are common mild side effects. Dose 50 mg OD to BD.

Tacrine: Centrally acting reversible anticholinesterase used for Alzheimer's disease. It improves memory, attention, language, reason and praxis. Side effects are diarrhea, nausea, abdominal cramps, polyuria, hepatitis.

Rivastigmine: Inhibits true and pseudo cholinesterase G_1 isoform more specifically present in certain areas of brain. Peripheral side effect of cholinergic system is less and does not damage liver, used for AD (Exelon 1.5, 3, 4.5 and 6 mg caps). Dose 1.5 mg BD increases gradually to 6 mg BD.

Donepezil (Dopezil 5–10 mg tab): Cerebroselective reversible anti-ACE. Elevates ACh level in surviving neurons in the cortex. Cholinergic side effects are less. Used once daily. Dose 5 mg at HS used for AD.

Galantamine (Galamer 4, 8 and 12 mg tabs; dose 4 mg BD to 12 mg BD): This natural alkaloid selectively inhibits cerebral AChE and has some agonistic actions on nicotinic receptor. Improves cognitive and behavior of AD. It is better tolerated.

Memantine: NMDA antagonist slows the functional decline of AD. Beneficial to parkinsonism also. It blocks glutamate transmitter noncompetitively. Better tolerated to anti-ACE. Constipation, tiredness, headache, drowsiness may occur (Admenta 5 and 10 mg tabs, starts with 5 mg OD and increases up to 10 mg BD).

Pyritinol: Two pyridoxine molecules joined by disulfide bridge activate cerebral metabolism and cholinergic transmission and improve cerebral circulation (Encephebol 100 and 200 mg tab, 100 mg/5 mL suspension). GI upset, rash, itching, taste disturbance may occur. Used for cerebral hypoxia due to cardiac arrest, anesthesia, brain operation, stroke. Dose 100–200 mg TDS, withdrawn from some countries.

Ginkgo biloba (Ginkocer 40 mg TDS for 1 month): Dried extract of Chinese herb contains ginkgo flavone glycosides having platelet activating factor antagonist activity, improve microcirculation of hypoxic brain, but beneficial effect not proved. Side effect includes mild GI upset. IV infusion may cause fever, shock, arrhythmia.

Citicoline (Citinova 500 mg, tab or 500 mg/ 2 mL): Derived from choline, involved in the synthesis of lecithin. It increases cerebral blood flow to enhance metabolism, short-term improvement in memory in CVA patient is observed. Used in ischemic strokes, head injury, parkinsonism. Dose 200–600 mg orally or IM or IV in divided doses.

46

Opioid Analgesics and Antagonist

Pain is ill-defined, unpleasant sensation, usually evoked by an external or internal noxious stimulation which is very much subjective. Pain may be:

- Superficial/cutaneous
- Deep muscle, joints, ligaments, bone
- Visceral
- Referred
- Psychogenic

Varieties of naturally occurring compounds are capable of producing pain, *viz.* histamine, 5HT, ACh, bradykinin, *etc.*

The pain carrying fibers are of two types—(i) Aδ and (ii) C. The Aδ fibers are thicker, myelinated to conduct faster sharp, localized pain, but the C fibers are non-myelinated, thin and conduct slow pain of diffuse sensation. The neurotransmitter of Aδ and C fibers with substantia gelatinosa are glutamate and substance P respectively. Substantia gelatinosa at times partially opened or closed controlling as a gate to control pain.

Pain from its sites of orgin is carried by Aδ and C fibers and their cell bodies are in dorsal root ganglion and terminate in substantia gelatinosa of rolando. From substantia gelatinosa second order neuron starts which cross the opposite side and moves up in the white matter of spinal cord as spinothalamic tract, to terminate in thalamus. The third order neuron strats from there to terminate in cerebral cortex in somatosensory areas of I and II.

Analgesics are group of drugs which relief pain by acting on CNS or peripheral mechanism without alerting consciousness.

Analgesics are of two types

- Opioid/Narcotic/Morphine causes CNS depression, and acts on opioid receptors.
- Non-opioid/Non-narcotic/Anti-inflammatory antipyretic. The term narcotic is derived from the Greek word for 'stupor', but now it is associated with opioid.

Opium Alkaloids

Opium is a milky exudate obtained from unripe capsule of poppy plant *(Papaver somniferum)*. The pharmacologically active alkaloids of opium are:

1.   Phenanthrene group
(Morphine, codeine, thebaine*)

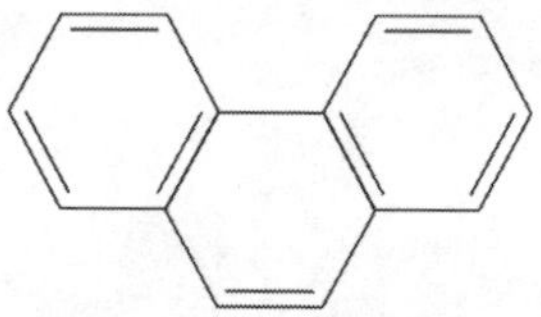

Phenanthrene nucleus

2.   Benzyl isoquinoline group
(Papaverine*, noscapine*, narcine*)

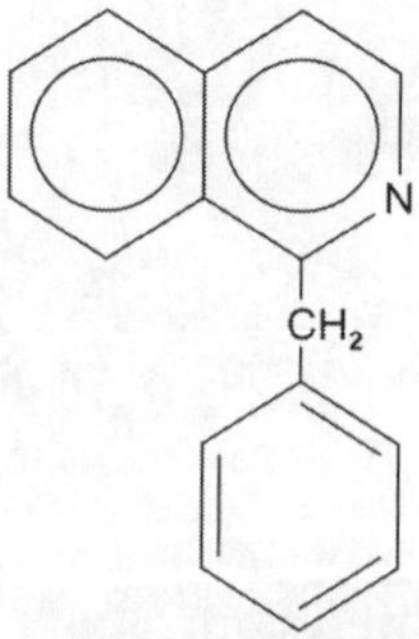

These are non-analgesics

Benzyl isoquinoline nucleus

i. Phenanthrene derivative.

ii. Benzyl-isoquinoline derivative.

PHARMACOLOGICAL ACTIONS OF MORPHINE (Morphine the prototype opioid acts on μ, K and δ receptors as agonists)

1. **CNS**

   A. **Stimulates**
   - CTZ-vomiting
   - Vagal and center bradycardia
   - Muscle rigidity and convulsion
   - Edinger westphal nucleus stimulated producing miosis.

   B. **Depresses**
   - Analgesia, sedation, mood changes, euphoria
   - Respiration (center depression and CO_2 retention)
   - Thermoregulation. Center depression and hypothermia may occur in cold surroundings.

2. **CVS:** Cardiac output decreases, vasodilatation (decreases tone, histamine release and depression of vasomotor center)

3. **GIT:** Segmentation due to increase tone, decreases peristalsis, spasm of ileocecal junction, decreases GI secretion and increases absorption: Straub's sign in mice (*i.e.* erection of tail)

4. **Respiration:** Bronchospasm due to histamine release, respiratory centre depresses.

5. **Uterus:** Prolong labor

6. **Urinary bladder:** Tone of detursor and bladder sphincter increase, causisng urinary urgency with difficulty.

7. **Biliary system:** Spasm (treat with atropine, nitrates or naloxone, theophylline)

8. **Neuroendocrine**
   - **Decreases:** FSH, LH and ACTH release
   - **Increases:** Prolactin and GH level.

9. **It has weak anticholinergic action:** Produces hyperglycemia central, sympathetic stimulation.

Pharmacokinetics

Oral absorption of morphine is unreliable because of first pass metabolism, therefore, parenteral administration preferred. 30% bound to plasma proteins, freely crosses placenta and secreted with milk, effects fetus. Morphine is primarily metabolized in liver by glucuronide conjugation. Morphine-6-glucuronide is an active metabolite, small amount may persist in enterohepatic circulation after elimination in 24 hours. Plasma t½ 2–3 hours. It can be given by oral, rectal, IV, IM, intrathecal or epidural route.

Pethedine is metabolized by MAO, metabolized to meperidinic acid and little is demethylated to norpethidine which has cumulative and seizure inducing properties (particularly in renal failure and patient receiving MAO-inhibitors). Both meperidinic acid and norpethidine are conjugated with glucuronic acid for excretion with urine.

Adverse effects of morphine

Side effects

- Sedation
- Lethargy

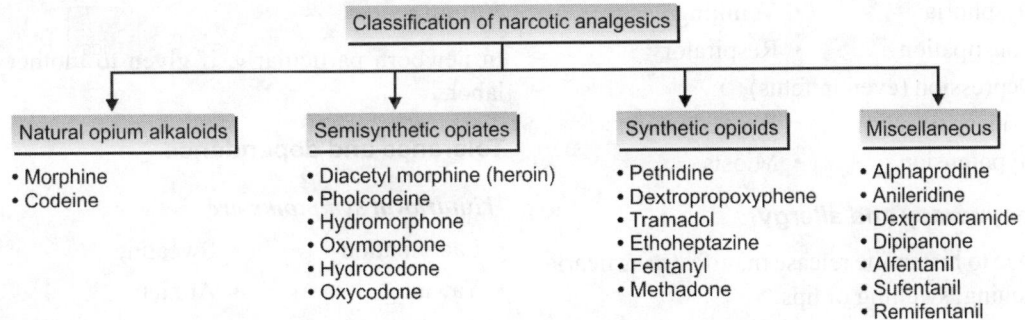

Classification of narcotic analgesics			
Natural opium alkaloids	**Semisynthetic opiates**	**Synthetic opioids**	**Miscellaneous**
• Morphine • Codeine	• Diacetyl morphine (heroin) • Pholcodeine • Hydromorphone • Oxymorphone • Hydrocodone • Oxycodone	• Pethidine • Dextropropoxyphene • Tramadol • Ethoheptazine • Fentanyl • Methadone	• Alphaprodine • Anileridine • Dextromoramide • Dipipanone • Alfentanil • Sufentanil • Remifentanil

Table 46.1: Some important narcotic analgesics

Drugs with trade name	Preparation and doses	Uses	Remarks
Codeine		Diarrhea, cough	Orally active, less potent analgesic, abuse liability low
Pholcodeine	10–15 mg (Ethnine 5 mg/ 5 mL)	Cough	Less constipating
Diacetyl-morphine	Heroin		Banned in most countries because of euphoriant action and addiction.
Pethidine	Pethidine HCl 100 mg/2 mL inj and 50 and 100 mg tabs. Dose 50–100 mg IM, orally or IV	Analgesics and preanesthetics. Reduce shivering of anesthesia	Completely metabolized in liver by hydrolysis and de-methylation and conjugated with glucuronic acid. May produce seizures.
Fentanyl	Fentanyl citrate 50 mg/mL, 2 mL amp and 10 mL/vial	Neuroleptanalgesic with droperidol. Transdermal fentanyl as analgesia.	80–100 times potent than morphine
Methadone	Physeptone 10 mg inj, 2 mg/5 mL linctus	Substitution for opioid dependence, analgesic	Does not give kick. It is a long acting opioid, can be given oral, IV, SC, per rectal. It blocks (μ) NMDA receptors and uptake of morphine.
Dextropropoxyphene	Parvodex 60 mg cap	Oral analgesic	Less constipating
Tramadol	Domadol, contramal 50 mg cap, 50 mg/mL inj and 1 and 2 mL amp. Dose 50–100 mg orally/IM, IV (slow)	Used for short lasting pain, diagnostic procedure, injury, surgery, chronic pain of cancer.	Low abuse and dose rising potential
Ethoheptazine	75–150 mg in combination with aspirin (Equagesic)	Low efficacy, orally active analgesic	Used in combination with analgesic

Lipid-soluble fentanyl, alfentanil and sufentanil are used as adjuncts to other anesthetic agents whereas morphine is used as preanesthetic agent.

- Dysphoria
- Constipation
- Depression (even in fetus)
- Urinary retention
- Hypotension

- Vomiting
- Respiratory
- Blurred vision
- Miosis

Apnea

In newborn particularly, if given to mother in labor.

Tolerance and dependence

Idiosyncracy and allergy

- Due to histamine release manifest as urticaria, itching, swelling of lips.

Withdrawal symptoms are

- Lacrymation
- Yawning
- Sweating
- Anxiety

- Fear
- Gooseflesh
- Diarrhea
- Weight loss

- Restless
- Mydriasis
- Abdominal colic

Tolerance is due to

- Pharmacokinetics (enhanced rate of metabolism)
- Pharmacodynamics (cellular)

Drug interactions: Phenothiazines, tricyclic antidepressants, MAO-I, amphetamine and neostigmine potentiate opioids. Morphine retards absorption of many drugs by delaying gastric emptying.

Dose: 10–15 mg IM or SC or 2–6 mg IV, 2–3 mg epidural intrathecal, 10–50 mg oral.

Preparation: Morphine sulfate 10, 15 and 20 mg injections. Morcontin 10, 30, 60 and 100 mg continuous release tablets for cancer pain.

Morphine's Precaution and Contraindication

- Extremes of age (infants and elderly) susceptible to respiratory depression.
- In bronchial asthma, emphysema, corpulmonale sudden death may occur.
- Head injury because it retains CO_2, increases intracranial tension and causes vomiting and respiratory depression.
- Undiagnosed acute abdomen.
- Hypothyroid, liver and kidney disease patients are more susceptible.
- Addiction liability.
- Elderly patients may develop urinary retention.

Therapeutic Uses of Morphine and its Congener

1. **Analgesic**
2. **Preanesthetic medications**
3. **Balanced anesthesia and neuroleptalgesia** (fentanyl, alfentanil, sufentanil, morphine, pethidine are used.)
4. **Relief of anxiety and apprehension** (in myocardial infarction, internal bleeding. It is not routine anxiolytic to induce sleep.)

5. **Cardiac asthma** (acute left ventricular failure. It helps by):
   - Reduces preload on heart by vasodilatation.
   - Shifts blood to systemic circulation from pulmonary circuit and reducing pulmonary edema.
   - Cuts sympathetic stimulation by calming patient.
   - Depress respiratory center, cuts air hunger.
6. **Cough** (codeine)
7. **Diarrhea** (diphenoxylate; loperamide)

Opioid Receptors

Opioids produce their action by action on specific receptors in CNS and periphery. Three types of opioid receptors μ (mu), κ (kappa), and δ (delta) are identified and different agonists, partial agonists or antagonists are also available.

A. μ (Mu) receptor

High affinity for morphine and its endogenous ligand is endorphin. Enkephalin and dynorphins bind with μ receptor with lower affinity. μ receptor is detected in periaquiductal gray, thalamus, tractus solitarious nucleus, area prostrema, nucleus ambigus.

μ (Mu) receptor activation in presynaptic neuron decreases Ca^{2+} influx to incoming action potential causing decrease in release of glutamate, an excitatory neurotransmitter and in postsynaptic opioid receptor increases K^+ influx to decrease postsynaptic response to excitatory neurotransmitter.

Types of μ receptors (two types)

$μ_1$: Blocked by naloxonazine. High affinity for morphine, mediates supraspinal analgesic.

$μ_2$: Low affinity for morphine produces spinal analgesia, respiratory depression, constipation.

B. κ (Kappa) receptor

$κ_1$ and $κ_3$: High affinity for dynorphin A, ketocyclazocine. Norbinaltorphimine is a selective κ antagonist. Analgesia caused by $κ_1$ agonist is spinal, $κ_3$ produces lower ceiling supraspinal analgesia.

C. δ (delta) receptor

High affinity for Leu/Met enkephalin. Analgesic produced by it is spinal. Myoenteric plexus contains high population of δ receptors, reduces GI motility. Naltrindole is selective δ antagonist.

Actions mediated by μ, κ, δ receptors

μ = Sedation, analgesic, constipation, euphoria, respiration, depression, miosis.

κ = Dysphoria, analgesia, constipation.

δ = Spinal analgesia, modulation of hormone release.

OPIOIDS AGONIST AND ANTAGONIST

I. *Agonist/antagonist (Agonist of one opioid receptor and antagonist to other)*
  a. *Used as analgesics*
    • Pentazocine (Fortwin κ agonist, μ antagonist)
    • Nalorphine
    • Meptazinol (not available in India)
    • Dezocine (not available in India)
  b. Not used as analgesics
    • Nalorphine (κ agonist, μ antagonist)
    • Levallorphan (not available in India)

II. *Partial or weak μ agonist + κ antagonist*
  • Buprenorphine
  • Butorphanol

III. *Pure antagonist*
  • Naloxone
  • Naltrexone
  • Nalmefene

INDIVIDUAL DRUGS

Nalorphine (Lethidrone 1 mg/mL): Agonist and antagonist of morphine. Agonist by κ receptor activation depresses respiration, miosis, hypothermia.

Antagonizes μ receptor promptly reverses respiratory depression, precipitates morphine withdrawal symptoms.

Use: Opioid poisoning, 3–5 mg IV or IM.

Neonatal dose 0.1–0.2 mg in cord. Not effective orally because of first pass metabolism.

Pentazocine: Used for analgesic in post-operative and cancer patient ($κ_1$) produce compulsive abusers. Produce tachycardia, rise of BP (better avoid in ischemia and myocardial infarction due to sympathetic stimulation) less biliary spasm, vomiting (Fortwin 25 mg tab, 30 mg/mL injection).

Nalbuphine: Agonist-antagonist with μ receptor. Not available in India. The USA approved it for postoperative pain, myocardial infarction and labor.

Buprenorphine: It is a synthetic thebaine congener, 25 times potent than morphine, can be given sublingually, resistant to naloxone reversal because dissociates slowly from μ (mu) receptor.

Dose 0.3–0.6 mg IM, SC or slow IV, 0.2 mg sublingual (norphine, tidigesic 0.3 mg/mL or 0.2 sublingually).

Used for postoperative pain, myocardial infarction.

Butorphanol: κ analgesic, but more potent than pentazocine. Abuse potential is low. Very low interaction with μ receptor, used for post-operative pain, short lasting pain (*viz.* renalcolic). Available as 1 mg/mL inj. Dose 1–4 mg IM or IV.

PURE OPIOID ANTAGONIST

Naloxone: Competitive antagonist for all opioid receptors (μ, κ, δ). It promptly antagonizes all actions of morphine if given IV. It blocks placebo, acupuncture and stress-induced analgesic, mediated by endorphin. It is not effective orally because of first pass metabolism, given IV (narcotan 0.4 mg/mL for adult or 0.04 mg/2 mL for infant).

Use of Naloxone

• Morphine poisoning
• Diagnosis of opioid dependence
• Alcohol intoxication
• Increase BP in endotoxic and hypovolemic shock, stroke and spinal injury.

Naltrexone: Pure opioid antagonist, orally active, used in post-addict. Marketed in India (naltima 50 mg tabs). Higher dose is hepatotoxic.

Nalmefene is opioid antagonist, orally effective, not hepatotoxic.

ENDOGENOUS OPIOID PEPTIDES

The important peptides having opioid-like actions are found in mammalian brain, pituitary, spinal cord, GI tract called endogenous opioid peptides, *viz.* three opioid families are known— enkephalin, endorphin and dynorphin derived from distinct precursor proteins prepro-opiomelanocortin, preproenkephalin and preprodynorphin respectively.

* **Endorphin** (μ action) with 31 amino acids, derived from pro-opiomelanocortin (POMC), endorphin which also produces γ-MSH; ACTH and Lipotropins. Endorphins I and II possess many properties of opioid peptides.
* **Enkephalin** (μ and δ actions) (met-ENK has affinity for μ and δ, L-ENK acts on δ receptor). These are pentapeptides, obtained from precursor proenkephalin.
* **Dynorphin** (κ, μ and δ actions) with 8–17 amino acids derived from prodynorphins.

Endogenous peptides and their actions on receptors

Endorphin on μ (mu) receptor, dynorphin on κ (kappa) receptor, enkephalin on δ (delta) receptor and nociception on orphanin FQ (N/OFQ) receptors.

The wide distribution and short t½ of enkephalin and dynorphin suggest that they act as neuromodulators or neurotransmitters.

Recently homologous to opioid peptides nociception or orphanin FQ (N/OFQ) have been isolated from mammalian brain believing role in stress, reward, reinforce learning and memory. The N/OFQ is also called orphanin opioid receptor like-I (ORL-I). In some N/OFQ can act as anti-opioid through ORL-I. Its endogenous ligand is called nociceptin or orphanin FQ by different groups. Nociceptin is structurally similar to dynorphin without N terminal tyrosine, acts on ORL-I receptor mediated analgesia, modulates drug reward reinforcement, learning and memory. It is present in CNS and periphery.

Transducer machanism of opioid receptor

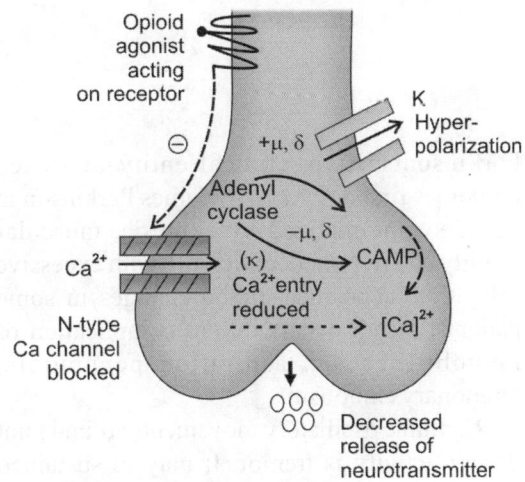

Fig. 46.1

All opioid receptors are G-protein coupled receptors generally on prejunctional neurons to produce inhibition by decreasing release of NAd, DA, 5HT. GABA and glutamate are also involved. Opioid receptor decreases CAMP, opens K channel *via* μ and δ receptors. N-type Ca^{2+} channel is blocked and the cells become hyperpolarized resulting to decrease in neurotransmitter release.

OPIOID DEADDICTION

Opioid on chronic administration produces physical and phychological dependence and on withdrawal produces symptoms which may be lifethreatening. Short duration of addiction is treated with β blockers or clonidine. Long duration addiction should be treated with methadone which stimulates opioid receptors but less addictive. Methadone is tapered off gradually to stop. The addiction relapse is prevented by naltrexone which prevents euphoria blocking μ (mu) receptor.

47

Drugs for Parkinsonism and Movement Disorders

Parkinsonism is a clinical entity of varied etiologies first described by James Parkinson in 1817, symptomatized by akinesia, muscular rigidity and tremor, occasionally with excessive salivation, seborrhea, mood changes in some patients. Death occurs due to complication of immobilities *viz.* aspiration penumonia, pulmonary embolism.

Rhythmic oscillatory movements around joint during activity is tremor. It may in sustained posture (postural **tremor**) or during movement (intention tremor). Postural tremor is familial, intention tremor occurs in lesions of brain stem cerebellum, superior cerebellar peduncle. Tremor at rest is characteristic of parkinsonism.

Chorea is irregular, involuntary, unpredictable, muscle jerks in different parts of body. It may hereditary or acquired. Slow and writing movement is **athetosis**. It occurs in perinatal brain damage with focal or generalized cerebral lesion. *Tics* are sudden coordinated repeatitive abnormal movement generaly around face and head. Gilles de la Tourette's syndrome is chronic multiple tics.

Pathogenesis of Parkinsonism

In parkinsonism there is oxidative stress, mito-chondrial damage, impaired protein degradation, accumulation of proteins and inflammation and apoptosis of the cells. Genetic factors are also implicated. Mutation of α-synuclein gene at 4q21 occurs or there is duplication or triplication of normal synuclein gene occurs in parkinsonism, mutation of parkin gene is responsible for early onset parkinsonism.

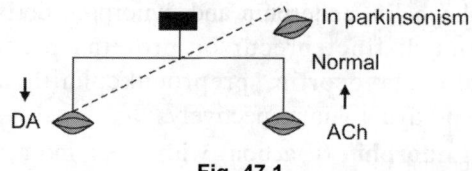

Fig. 47.1

In parkinsonism degeneration occurs in substantia nigra, the depigmented neurons make efferent connections to putamen, globus and caudate nucleus. Since these neurons are dopaminergic, loss of dopamine and as a consequence cholinergic predominance have been established in its causation. Pharmacologically, dopamine deficit responsible for akinesia and cholinergic predominance responsible for tremor and rigidity.

The catecholamine dopamine is synthesized in dopaminergic neuron, from tyrosine as mentioned in Chapter, Sympathomimetic Drugs. It is stored and released and after producing its action, it is being metabolized. The dopamine acts *via* dopamine receptor which is a G-protein coupled receptor in heptahelical structure.

Pathophysiologically, dopaminergic neurons in substantia nigra normally inhibit the output of GABAergic cells of corpus striatum are lost. In parkinsonism there is selective loss of dopaminergic neurons (Fig. 47.2).

In Huntington's chorea, some cholinergic neurons are lost, but more GABAergic neurons.

Aims of treatment in Parkinsonism
- Relief of symptoms (akinesia, rigidity and tremor)
- Correction of mood changes.
- Treatment of symptoms of salivation and seborrhea.

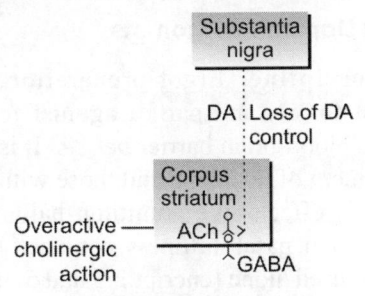

Fig. 47.2

- Correction of possible cause if any, say if drug induced stop the drug.

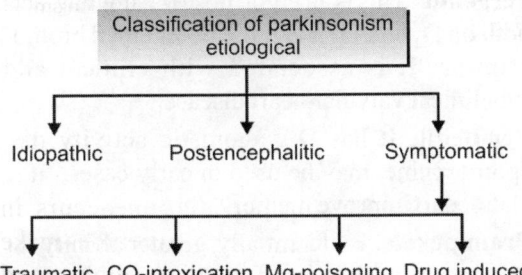

CLASSIFICATION OF ANTIPARKINSONIAN DRUGS

Affecting Brain Dopaminergic System

- **Dopamine precursor** (Levodopa)
- **Dopamine agonist** (Bromocriptine, Lisuride, Pergolide, Peribedil, Pramipexole; Ropinirole; Apomorphine, Rotigotine)
- **Dopamine transmission facilitator** (Amantadine)
- **Peripheral decarboxylase inhibitor** (Carbidopa, Benserazide)
- **MAO-B inhibitor:** Selegiline, Rasagiline
- **COMT inhibitor:** Entacapone, Tolcapone

Affecting Central Cholinergic System

- **Central anticholinergics** (Trihexyphenidyl, Procyclidine, Biperiden)
- **Antihistaminics** (Orphenadrine, Promethazine)

MAO-Inhibitors

- **Non-selective:** Isocarboxazid; Phenelzine; Tranylcypromine
- **MAO-A inhibitors:** Meclebemide
- **MAO-B inhibitors:** Selegeline; Rasagiline

Individual Drugs

Levodopa is precursor of dopamine and is

$$Levodopa \xrightarrow{Decarboxylase} Dopamine \xrightarrow{MAO} NAd$$

$$DOPAC \xrightarrow{COMT} HVA$$

inactive to produce any central pharmacological effect. It can pass through blood-brain barrier whereas dopamine cannot.

It after being absorbed from intestine by carrier-mediated active transport process. Amino acids of food compete for the same carrier. It undergoes first pass metabolism and about 1% of drugs enters brain with the help of carrier-mediated active transport. The symptoms of akinesia respond first, followed by rigidity and tremor, seborrhea, mood improvement. Drug-induced parkinsonism does not improve with it. At times symptoms of akinesia, rigidity and tremor increase transiently and passes of spontaneously called "on-off phenomenon". The off period akinesia alternate over the course of hours with on period of improved motility, but with marked dyskinesia. This phenomenon occurs in those patients who repsonded to treatment initially, unresponsive to on-off patient, subcutaneous apomorphine provides temporary benefit. Levodopa is also used to treat heart failure (since it increases cardiac contractility and reduces arterial pressure) and hepatic coma.

Drug holiday (Discontinuance of drug for 3–21 days): Temporarily improves responsiveness to levodopa and decreases its adverse effects but no help to on-off phenomenon. It is now not recommended because it may cause aspiration pneumonia, venous thrombosis, embolism and depression.

Dopamine receptors: Originally, two types of receptors are described, D_1 and D_2 later three more receptors D_3, D_4 and D_5 have been isolated and cloned, all are of G protein coupled receptors and placed in two families.

D_1 receptor family	D_2 receptor family
D_1 and D_5 are excitatory, act by increasing cAMP formation and PIP_2 hydrolysis increasing intracellular Ca^+ and activating protein kinase C *via* IP_3 and DAG.	D_2, D_3, D_4 are inhibitory, act by inhibiting adenylyl cyclase/opening K^+ channels, depressing voltage sensitive Ca^+ channel.

Other Actions of Levodopa

By acting on CTZ, it produces nausea and vomiting. It acts on pituitary mammotroph to inhibit prolactin and somatotropes to increase GH release which cannot be noted in parkinsonism patient. It acts on β-adrenergic receptors to produce tachycardia, and fall in BP (postural hypotension).

Side Effects

Nausea, vomiting, postural hypotension, cardiac arrhythmia, aggravation of symptoms of angina. After prolong administration, choreoathetoid movements and tics appear which can be prevented by vitamin B_6 (responsible for conversion of levodopa to DA which can only penetrate to brain). The insomnia though common in parkinsonism are not complained by the patient because they are more bothered of their symptoms. Depression, anxiety, agitation, somnolence, confusion, delusion, hallucination, nightmare, euphoria, mood change may occur with patient taking levodopa and carbidopa. Clozapine, olanzapine, quetiapine, resperidone, *etc.* are used to treat these behavioral changes.

Positive Coomb test, BUN and SGOT, cholesterol may rise and impaired carbohydrate tolerance may occur.

Available as 0.50 gm tab. Start with 0.25 gm BD and increases gradually till symptoms subsides.

Important Drug Interaction of Levodopa

• Pyridoxine—decreases effects of levodopa
• MAO inhibitors—hypertensive crisis.
• Anticholinergic—synergism for antiparkinsonism effect.

Direct Dopamine Agonists

Bromocriptine: Ergot preparation, potent agonist for D_2 and partial agonist for D_1. It crosses blood-brain barrier *per se*. It is used as supplement of levodopa and those with intolerable side effects like vomiting, hallucination, hypotension, nasal stuffiness, conjunctival injections, if used alone (encript 2.5 and 5 mg).

Lisuride: D_2 and 5HT agonists and D_1 antagonist. Dose up to 5 mg/day improves parkinsonism and on-off phenomenon of levodopa.

Pergolide: This is an ergot, dose 0.2 mg/day, acts both on D_1 and D_2 and more potent than bromocriptine. It is associated with clinical and subclinical valvular heart disease.

Peribedil: It has DA agonistic activity like apomorphine, may be used in early cases. It is claimed to improve memory.

Pramipexole: Preferentially, greater affinity for D_3 receptor. It is used to decrease dose of levodopa or as monotherapy for early PD cases. Start with 0.125 mg TDS and increase up to 0.5–1.5 mg TDS.

Apomorphine: Subcutaneous apomorphine 3–6 mg TDS helps to relief off period of PD. Nausea caused by it may be treated by trimethobenzamide 300 mg TDS, 3 days before starting apomorphine. It has high affinity for D_4 receptor; moderate affinity for D_2, D_3, D_5 and adrenergic $α_1D$, $α_2B$, and $α_2C$; and low affinity for D_1 receptors. It is used as resume therapy during 'off' period of PD on dopaminergic therapy. Don't give 5HT antagonist as antiemetic. It should be administered, if monitoring is possible.

Ropinirole (Ropitor 0.25, 0.5, 1 and 2 mg tabs, dose 0.25 TDS and increase gradually): D_2 receptor agonist used as monotherapy and patient on levodopa to smooth its response. Orally absorbed, 40% protein-bound. Metabolized by CYPIA2. It is also used for restless legs syndrome.

Nausea, vomiting, hallucination, postural hypotension, daytime sleeping may occur.

Rotigotine: DA agonist, used as patch for PD, but product was recalled for crystal formation in patch.

Dopamine Facilitators

Amantadine: Anti-influenzal A_2 prophylactic antiviral found to be effective in parkinsonism, releases DA from presynaptic nerve terminals, not useful in drug-induced parkinsonism. Also has anticholinergic property and blocks NMDA glutamate receptor. It antagonizes adenosine A_{2A} receptor which blocks the action of D_2 funciton. Amantadine marketed as (symmetrel or amantral 100 mg tabs) given 100 mg OD and increased to BD depending upon side effects of insomnia, dizziness, confusion, nightmare, hallucination, livedo reticularis, ankle edema due to local release of catecholamine.

Selegiline: MAO-B inhibitor acts on DA in human brain and platelets. *Per se* does not have antiparkinsonial effect but effective with levodopa and carbidopa. Diminishes weaning-off phenomenon. It may delay progression of early parkinsonism. Available as 5 mg tab (selgin; selmax), 1 tab twice daily with levodopa or carbidopa or both. Contraindicated in convulsive disorders. Postural hypotension, nausea, confusion, psychosis are common.

Metabolites of selegiline include amphetamine and methamphetamine which may cause anxiety and insomnia.

Rasagiline: Another MAO-B inhibitor, potent than selegiline. Doses 0.5 mg/day prevents MPTP-induced parkinsonism. It is effective in early and advanced PD.

COMT inhibitor (Entacapone and tolcapone): These are potent selective reversible COMT inhibitors, used to prolong and therapeutic effect of levodopa and caridopa but they worsen the side effects too. Used for late PD cases. Dose, entacopone 200 mg with each levodopa and carbidopa dose.

Tolcapone 200 mg TDS. Apart from this, it may cause diarrhea, yellow orange urine. Tolcapone causes hepatitis, rhabdomyolysis. Stalevo contains levodopa + carbidopa + entacapone.

Peripheral Decarboxylase Inhibitors

Carbidopa and benserazide do not penetrate the blood-brain barrier, act to inhibit conversion of levodopa to dopamine at periphery, thereby increase dopamine concentration in dopaminergic neurons in the brain. The advantages of their use are prolong plasma t½ of levodopa and reduce systemic toxicities of levodopa, *viz.* nausea, vomiting, cardiac arrhythmia, on-off phenomenon are less with the degree of improvement with less dose. They do not affect pyridoxine reversal of levodopa effect.

But disadvantages are involuntary movement, behavioral changes, postural hypotension. Combination of levodopa with decarboxylase inhibitors is called co-careldopa.

	Carbidopa		Levodopa tabs
Tidomet LS	10 mg	+	100 mg
Tidomet plus	25 mg	+	100 mg

Start with lower doses and increase gradually.

Central anticholinergics: They act by decreasing hypercholinergic action in CNS occurring in parkinsonion patient. It improves tremor more than rigidity and hypokinesia. They have less side effects. Their side effects are those of antimuscarinic drugs. Dyskinesia occurs rarely. Suppurative parotitis may occur due to dry mouth. Effective in drug-induced parkinsonism.

Some antihistamines have antiparkinsonian effect by virtue of their anticholinergic effects like orphanadrine, promethezine. The commonly available central anticholinergic drugs:

Drugs	Dose
Procyclidine (Kemadrin)	5–10 mg/day
Trihexyphenidyl (Pacitane)	2–12 mg/day
Biperiden (Dyskinon)	2–10 mg/day
Benztropine	1–6 mg/day
Orphenadrine (Disipal)	100–300 mg/day
Promethazine (Phenergan)	25–75 mg/day

Surgery for parkinsonism: Done in patient poorly responding to pharmacotherapy. Following surgeries are done:
- Low thalamotomy or posteroventral pallidotomy for tremor
- Thalamic stimulation by implanted electrode stimulation to improve tremor

- Subthalamic or globus pallidus stimulation for advanced parkinsonism
- Transplantation of foetal substantia nigra tissue (dopaminergic tissue) offers benefit to PD, but results are controversial.

Gene therapy has scope for PD.

Drug-induced parkinsonism: Drugs depleting biogenic amines from storage site (reserpine, tetrabenzine), blocking dopamine receptors (halloperidol, phenothiazine) or narcotic durgs related to meperidine may produce parkinsonism.

MPTP and Parkinsonism: 1-methyl-4 phenyl-1, 2, 3, 6-tetrahydropyridine (MPTP) is a protoxin unwitingly taken by persons, attempt to support opioid habbit by mepevirdine. MPTP is converted by MAO-B to N-methyl-4-phenyl-pyridinium (MPP+). MPP+ is taken up by dopaminergic cells and inhibits mitochondrial complex-1 and thereby inhibits oxidative phosphorylation and causing cells death and strial dopamine depletion. Environmental toxins may be responsible for spontaneous PD.

Pretreatment of animals exposed to MPTP with MAO-B inhibitor like selegiline protects it from PD as it prevents conversion of MPTP to MPP+.

Neuroprotective therapy: Antioxidants, antiapoptotic, glutamate antagonist, glial derived neurotropic factors, anti-inflammatory drugs may slow the disease process of PD are under investigational lebel.

Treatment of other movement disorder

1. **Essential tremor**
   - Metoprolol or propranolol (β blockers)
   - Primidone 250 mg TDS
   - Topiramate 400 mg OD
   - Gabapentin 100–200 mg/day
   - Alprazolam 3 mg daily
   - Diazapam, Chlordiazepoxide, mephenesin
   - Intramuscular botulinum toxin
   - Thalamic stimulation

2. **Huntington's chorea**

   It is an autosomal dominant disorder characterized by gradual onset motor incoordination and cognitive decline from mid life, manifest as jerky movement of extremites, trunk, face with deterioration of personality. Here there is loss of GABA neurons leading to dopamine over activity.
   - Reserpine 0.25 mg/day or tetrabenzine (depletor of dopamine).
   - Haloparidol or olanzapine or perphenazine to block dopamine receptor.

3. **Drug-induced chorea:** Withdraw the offending drugs.

4. **Ballismus:** Halloperidol, perphenazine or other dopamine blockers are used, though its pharmacological basis not known.

5. **Athetosis and dystonia:** Diazepam, amantadine, antimuscarinic high dose, levodopa, beclofan, carbamazepine, halloperidol, phenothiazines are given. Pharmacological basis not known. Focal dystonia responds to botulinum toxin injection into hyperactive muscle.

6. **TICS:** Gilles de la Tourette's syndrome, halloperidol, pimozide are effective. Other drugs are flufephenazine clonazepam, clonidine, carbamazepine or injection of botulinum toxin A to site of problematic tics. Guanfacine, an α agonist is also used.

7. **Drug-induced dyskinesia:** Antimuscarinic benztronine 2 mg IV or diphenhydramine 50 mg IV or biperiden 2–5 mg IV or IM is helpful. Diazepam 10 mg IV alternates abnormal movements.

8. **Tardive dyskinesia:** DA blockers, dopamine depletors are given. It occurs to person taking long-term neuroleptics.

9. **Restless leg syndrome:** Cause not known, correct the coexisting iron deficiency and dopamine agonists like levodopa, diazepam, clonazepam or opiates, pramipexole, ropinirole.

10. **Wilson's disease:** Symptoms and signs include tremor, chorea, rigidity, brady-kinesia, dysphagia, dysarthria, hepatic and

neurodysfunction. It occurs due to increased concentration of copper in brain and viscera.

Drugs used are

- *Penicillamine* 500 mg TDS (copper chelator) or trientine 1–1.5 gm.

  Vomiting, nephrotic syndrome may occur. Therefore, urine analysis should be done along with blood count, SLE, pemphigus, myastheria are also reported. It is also used for rheumatoid arthritis.

- **Potassium disulfide** 20 mg to reduce copper absorption or zinc sulfate 200 mg/day.

- **Trientine hydrochloride** and **tetrathiomolybdate** are other copper chelators.

- **Zinc acetate** to increase fecal excretion of copper as maintenance therapy. Liver transplantation or gene therapy has scope in therapy.

- To control neurological symptoms levodopa or trihexyphenydyl is given.

11. **Amyotrophic lateral sclerosis:** Here ventral motor neurons and cortical neurons providing afferent neurons are diseased with progressive muscle weakness, muscle atrophy, fasiculation, spasticity, dysarthria, dysphagia (oculomotor neurons are spared).
   It may be familial or sporadic

- Clonazepam is used to treat spasticity, but may cause respiratory depression.

Drugs used are

- Riluzole which inhibits glutamate release, blocks postsynaptic NMDA and kainate type glutamate receptor and inhibits voltage dependent Na^+ channel. Given 50 mg BD, 1 hour before or 2 hours after meal. May cause nausea or diarrhea or raise hepatic transaminase.

- $GABA_B$ receptor agonist, baclofen 5–10 mg/day, but may be increased up to 200 mg/day.

- Tizanidine α_2 receptor agonist of CNS in the dose of 2–4 mg at bedtime reduces muscle spasticity.

12. **Multiple sclerosis:** Autoimmune disease causing demyelination of neurons. Spasticity decreases with beclofen or tizanidine. Monoclonal antibody natalizumab is tried.

13. **Rabit syndrome:** Produced by neuroleptics, presents with rhythmic vertical movements around mouth, may be treated by anticholinergics.

Drugs for Gout

48

Hyperuricemia/gout is a metabolic disorder characterized by deposition of uric acid (a product of purine metabolism) in joints, kidney and subcutaneous tissues. In gouty arthritis, synoviocytes phagocytose urate crystals to secrete mediators which attract leukocyte and macrophage which liberate further inflammatory mediators. Normal uric acid level is 3–6 mg/dL and it is low soluble in water in low pH.

Hyperuricemia may be secondary to leukemia, lymphoma, polycythemia, drug induced (thiazide, frusemide, ethacrynic acid, pyrazinamide, ethambutol, *etc.*) by decreasing uric acid excretion.

Uric acid is synthesized by oxidation of exogenous and endogenous purines and is a normal excretory product in man.

PATHOPHYSIOLOGY OF GOUT

Synoviocytes phagocytose uric acid and secretes inflammatory mediators causing attraction of leukocyte, polymorphonuclear (PMN) leukocyte and mononuclear phagocyte (MNP).

Antigout drugs inhibit crystal phagocytosis and release inflammatory mediators (Fig. 48.1).

The treatment of gout aims at to

- Give immediate symptomatic relief by colchicine, phenylbutazone, indomethacin, corticosteroids.
- Decrease uric acid level by metabolic inhibitors: Allopurinol or as uricosuric drug: Probenecid; sulphinpyrazone.

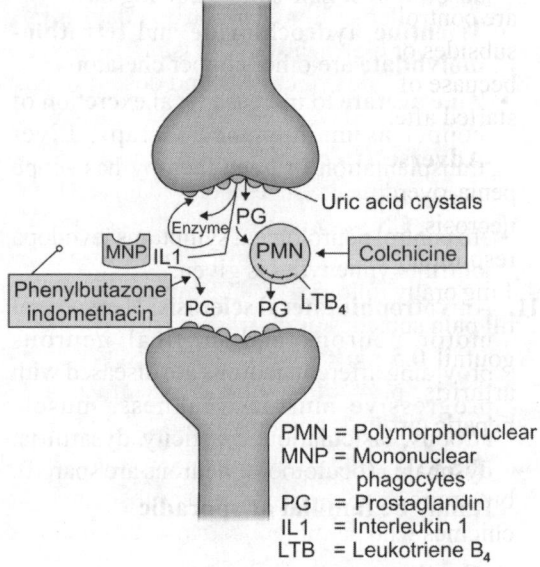

Fig. 48.1: Pathophysiology of gout

PMN = Polymorphonuclear
MNP = Mononuclear
phagocytes
PG = Prostaglandin
IL1 = Interleukin 1
LTB = Leukotriene B_4

Colchicine (goutnil 0.5 mg tab): An alkaloid known since 1763 obtained from *Colchicum autumnale* is neither analgesic nor anti-inflammatory, nor metabolic inhibitor, nor uricosuric agent, but inhibits specifically gouty inflammation. Uric acid deposition precipitated in synovial fluid starts inflammatory response, chemotactic factors are produced, migration of granulocyte starts in joint place to phagocytose urate crystals which release glycoprotein aggravating inflammation by:

- Producing lactic acid
- Releasing lyposomal enzymes causing joint destruction.

Colchicine Inhibits

- Release of glycoproteins
- Granulocyte migration
- Inhibits formation of LTB$_4$

Other functions: Colchicine arrests cell division in metaphase and increases gut motility.

Pharmacokinetics: It is absorbed orally, metabolized in liver, excreted in bile, undergone enterohepatic circulation, ultimately excreted in feces and urine.

Dose: 0.25 mg every 1–3 hourly till attacks are controlled or upto 6 mg in 3–4 days till pain subsides or diarrhea starts. It is rarely used now becuase of side effects. Second dose if required started after 7 days.

Adverse effects: GI upset, anemia, leukopenia, overdose produces kidney damage, hepatic necrosis, CNS depression. Death may be due to respiratory failure and muscular paralysis. Dose 1 mg orally followed by 0.25 mg every 1–3 hours till pain subsides or diarrhea starts. Available as goutnil 0.5 mg tab. It is also used for sarcoid arthritis, prevention of mediterranean fever, hepatic cirrhosis and amyloidosis.

NSAID (indomethacin, naproxen, phenylbutazone or piroxicam) has substituted colchicines who are not able to tolerate colchicine.

Corticosteroids: Used in refractory cases or not able to tolerate NSAID or colchicine. Given intra-articularly or prednisolone 40–60 mg may be given orally which is tapered gradually over a few weeks.

URICOSURIC AGENTS

Probenecid (Benenid 0.5 mg TDS) competitively blocks active transport of uric acid at all sites. At lower doses, decreases distal tubular secretion of uric acid and at higher doses, increases excretion by blocking tubular resorption of uric acid. Drug is non-toxic, well-tolerated, and should not be used in combination with phenylbutazone or salicylates.

Drug interaction: Inhibits excretion of penicillin, cephalosporin, sulfonamide methotrexate, indomethacin. Inhibits biliary excretion of rifampicin.

It is orally absorbed. 90% protein-bound, excreted with kidney. Generally; well-tolerated, may produce dispepsia, used with caution in peptic ulcer patient.

Therapeutic uses of probenecid

- Gout (primary and secondary)
- To prolong the action of penicillin, cephalosporin, *etc.*
- Lesch-Nyhan syndrome

Benzbromarone (Dose 40–80 mg/day): It is a reversible inhibitor of urate anion exchanger, used in Europe. It is effective in patient of renal insufficiency and patient allergic to other drugs of gout. Allopurinol and benziobromarone decrease uric acid level efficiently.

Etebenecid: Close to probenecid in all aspects except cost of therapy.

Sulfinpyrazone (anturane, artiran 200 mg caps, 100–200 mg BD up to 800 mg/day): Uricosuric, inhibits platelet aggregation, orally absorbed, protein-bound, excretion is fairly rapid by secretion. Inhibits metabolism or warfarin, sulfonylurea. Common adverse effect is peptic ulcer.

The uricosuric drugs are ineffective in impaired renal function.

Uric Acid Synthesis Inhibitors

Allopurinol (zyloric 100 and 300 mg): This hypoxanthine analogue was proposed for antineoplastic drug, but came out as xanthine oxidase inhibitor, responsible for uric acid synthesis. Allopurinol is short acting competitive inhibitor of xanthine oxidase and its major metabolite alloxanthine is long acting noncompetitive inhibitor. It is well-tolerated, occasionally produces nausea, vomiting, diarrhea, leukopenia, hepatic damage. Hemosiderosis is rare, but dangerous complication. It can be combined with uricosuric drugs and used in secondary gouts. It is also used for kala-azar.

Febuxostat: It is a new non-purine xanthine oxidase inhibitor. Orally absorbed, protein-bound, oxidized and conjugated with glucuronide in liver before excreted via kidney. Liver function test should be done during therapy as it damages liver. Interacts with theophylline mercaptopurine, azathioprine. Dose 80–120 mg. It is metabolized in liver.

Rasburicase (elitek): This recombinant urate oxidase catalyzes oxidation of uric acid into soluble inactive metabolite and lowers urate level used in patient of leukemia, lymphoma or solid tumors with anticancer durgs. Dose 0.15–0.2 mg/kg OD × 5 days with chemotherapy. Produced from *Saccharomyces cerevisiae* by genetic modification. May produce antibodies against it. Hemolysis, renal failure, methemoglobinemia may occur in Glu 6-PD deficient patient. Other ADRs are vomiting, fever, pain in abdomen, headache, constipation, diarrhea.

Anakinra: Targets interleukin-1, has potential benefit for gout, but it is not recommended for gout. Dose 100 mg/day SC. Chest infection, local reaction may occur. Other drugs are rilonacept, canakinumab.

Pegloticase: Used for refractory chronic gout given by infusion intravenously.

49

Drugs for Rheumatoid Arthritis

The etiology of the disease, rheumatoid arthritis is not known and natural course varies from person to person. Treatment is empirical, aims at:
• Relief pain and control inflammation
• Improvement and maintenance of function
• Prevention of deformity.

Drugs used are
• **Anti-inflammatory analgesics** like NSAIDs (discussed with NSAIDs)
• Anti-inflammatory without analgesics like glucocorticoids, ACTH
• **Disease-modifying antirheumatic** drugs: (DMARDs)
  a. Chloroquine, gold salts, penicillamine cyclosporine.
  b. Immunosuppressants: Azathioprine/methotraxate/cyclophosphamide/chlorambucil.
  c. TNFα-blocking agent: Adalimumab, infliximab, etanercept, golimumab, tofacitinib.
  d. Abatacept
  e. Rituximab, Tocilizumab. (IL - 6 antagonist)
  f. Leflunomide
  g. Interleukin antagonist: Anakinra, canakinumab, rolinacept, belimumab
• **TNFα blocking agents:** TNFα is an important cytokines for inflammatory process, affects cellular function *via* TNF receptors (TNFR1 and TNFR2). Drugs interfering TNFα is approved for treatment of RA. Drugs are:

Adalimumab: It complexes with TNFα to prevent interaction with p55 and p75 cell surface receptors resulting downregulation of macrophage and T cells function. It is given subcutaneously 40 mg/2 weeks used for RA, ankylosing spondylitis, psoriatic arthritis. Opportunistic infection may flare.

Infliximab: Given 3–5 mg/kg every 2 months by intravenous infusion. It is chimeric (25% mouse, 75% human). Used for RA, ankylosing spondylitis, psoriatic arthritis, Wegener's granulomatosis, sarcoidosis, giant cell arthritis.

ADR: URTl, nausea, headache, sinusitis, rash, opportunistic infection, demyelination of multiple sclerosis patient, activation of hepatitis, leukopenia may occur as ADR.

Etanercept: It is a recombinant fusion protein consisting of two soluble TNF p75 moieties linked to Fc portion of IgG. It also inhibits lymphotoxin α. Dose 25 mg biweekly subcutaneous; used for RA, psoriasis or psoriactic arthritis, juvenile chronic arthritis, ankylosing spondylitis.

ADR: Opportunistic infection, lymphoma, positive antinuclear antibodies may occur.

Tyrosine kinase inhibitor, tofacitinib: Orally effective given to patient intolerant to methotrexate.

Abatacept: It inhibits activation of T cells. It is given first on two weeks apart and then monthly by IV infusion of 500 mg, if body weight is less than 60 kg. It improves the signs and symptoms of RA and slows its radiographic progression. It may cause infection, hypersensitivity.

Rituximab: This chimeric monoclonal antibody targets CD20 B lymphocyte used in RA refractory to anti-TNF agents. Given IV infusion 1000 mg seperated by two weeks, may be repeated every 6–9 months.

Anakinra: It is a recombinant human interleukin antagonist. Dose 100 mg SC used as DMARD. Chest infection may occur. Other monoclonal antibodies used for RA are tocilizumab and certolizumed.

Leflunomide: Converted to active metabolite

in intestine and plasma which inhibits dihydrofolate dehydrogenase causing decrease RNA synthesis and arrest cell in G1 phase of growth. It also decreases T cell proliferation and TNFα. Diarrhea and rise of liver enzymes, alopecia, leukopenia and thrombocytopenia, weight gain, raise of blood pressure may occur. Should not be used in pregnancy.

Dietary modification: Use of eicosapentaenoic acid 2–4 gm/day instead of eicosatetraenoic acid derivative. Arachidonic acid which produces PG and several inflammatory mediators *via* cyclo- and lipoxygenase pathways.

Immunoabsorption apheresis: Through columns of silica matrix and highly purified staphylococcal protein A, weekly for 3 months in patient of multiple therapy failure. Joint pain, hypotension, sepsis, pulmonary embolism may occur.

Gold Salts: Reduces:
• Chemotaxis
• Phagocytosis
• Macrophage and lysosomal activity
• Monocyte differentiation
• Inhibits CMI, RA level and ESR is lowered; but exact mechanism not known.
    Indicated in rapidly progressing RA with NSAID. Aurothiomate Na contains 50% gold, start 10 mg IM/week and increased gradually till remission occurs up to 50 mg/kg. Bound to plasma protein and fixed in kidney. High toxicity like vasodilatations, hypotension, dermatitis, rash, exfoliative dermatitis, albuminuria, hepatitis, neuritis, encephalopathy, pulmonary fibrosis, eosinophilia, bone marrow depression may occur. Should not be given in kidney, liver, skin disease, colitis, pregnancy and lactating mother.
    Auranofin (ridaura, 3 mg cap (goldar) 6 mg/day) is orally active, less toxic. Adverse effects are diarrhea, abdominal cramps.

d-penicillamine (Artamin 150, 250 mg caps): Mechanism not known, not a favored drug because of toxicity (similar to gold). Urine should be tested periodically for albumin.

Chloroquine and hydroxychloroquine: Antimalarial, produces remission up to 50%. Exact mechanism of its action is not known. Following mechanisms are proposed:
• Suppresses T lymphocyte response to mitogen.
• Stabilizes lysosome

• Decreases leukocyte chemotaxis
• Inhibits DNA and RNA syntheses
• Traps free radicals.
    May produce cumulative toxicity, retinal damage and corneal opacity, graying of hair, myopathy, neuropathy. Dose of hydroxychloroquine 400 mg/day for 4 weeks followed by 200 mg/day as maintenance.

Cyclosporine: Peptide antobiotic is non biologic (DMARD) inhibits gene transcription of IL - 1 and 2 receptor used in RA.

Sulfasalazine: Basically, anti-inflammatory drug used for ulcerative colitis, efficacy similar to chloroquine, better tolerated than gold and penicillamine. Dose 1–3 gm in 2–3 divided doses. It is metabolized to sulfapyridine and 5-aminosalicylic acid. Sulfapyridine is an active moiety treating rheumatoid arthritis along with sulfasalazine, the parent compound. It decreases IgA and IgM rheumatoid factors production.

Immunosuppressants: Discussed in anticancer. Drugs used are azathioprine, cyclophosphamide, cyclosporine methotrexate, mycophenolate mofetil.

Mycophenolate mofetil: Prodrug converted to mycophenolic acid, inhibits T cell lymphocyte proliferation and interferes with leukocyte adhesion to endothelial cells. Occasionally used in RA in the dose of 2 gm/day (efficacy doubtful). Its other uses are SLE, vasculitis and Wegener's granulomatosis.

Corticosteroids: Dealt with steroid hormones. It is used for extra-articular manifestation of RA, *viz.* pericarditis or eye involvement. Delayed—release predinisone given at 9–10 pm releases prednisone after 4–6 hours used for morning stiffness in RA at 3–6 mg dose, does not inhibit adrenal pituitary axis.
    Newer monoclonal antibody used for rheumatiod arthritis are:
  i. Golimumab.
 ii. Tofacitinib
iii. Canakinumab (Used for systemic Juvenile idioopathic arthritis).
 iv. Rolinacept
  v. Tocilizumab
 vi. Adalimumab
vii. Certolizumab
viii. Belimumab

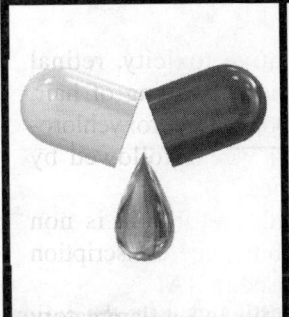
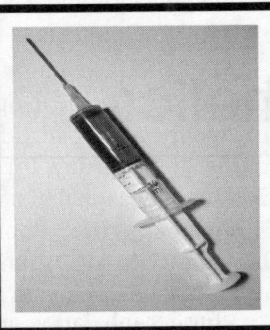
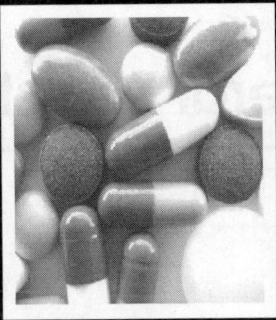
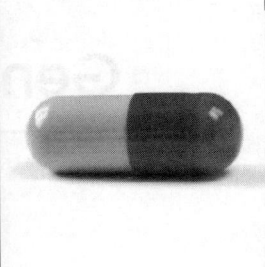

SECTION 5

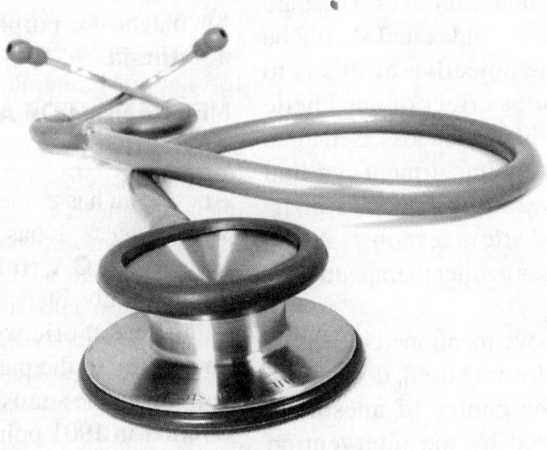

DRUGS USED IN ANESTHESIA

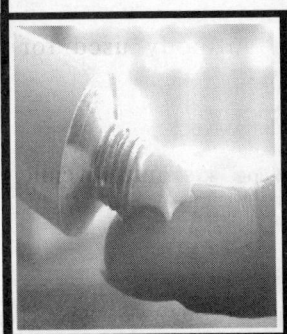
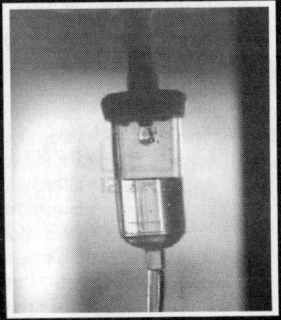
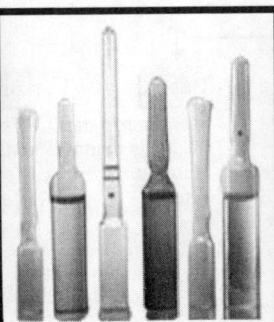
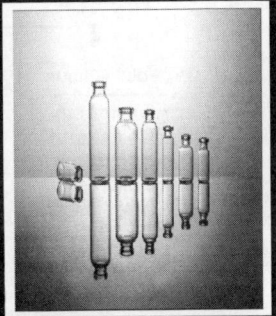

50

General Anesthetics

General Anesthetics

General anesthetics (GAs) are the agents which produce surmountable loss of all sensations and consciousness. The other cardinal features of GA are muscle relaxation, abolition of reflexes, amnesia and loss of autonomic reflexes. These are drugs with low therapeutic index and should be used with care and the objective of this is to minimize the deleterious effect of anesthetic agents and hemostasis (like blood loss, ischemia, fluid balance, coagulation impairment and flud shift) during surgery, and to improve post-operative outcome and stress response. Anesthesia in most of the cases neither therapeutic nor diagnostic.

The extent of the above mentioned effects of the GA depends upon the drug used, dosage and clinical situations. The choice of anesthetic technique is determined by the intervention required. *viz.* (diagnostic, therepeutic or surgical procedure).

Earlier inhalation anesthetics were the major procedures but now intravenous anesthesia are commonly used or combination of intravenous and inhaled drugs are used (balanced anesthesia techniques) to reduce adverse affects.

Oral or perenteral sedatives are generally used for diagnostic purposes are called **monitored anesthesia.**

MECHANISM OF ACTION OF GENERAL ANESTHESIA

Anesthesia has come up with a new specialized science *per se*. It has a low margin of safety. The potency of GA (inhalation) is measured by minimum alveolar potency (MAC). The MAC of an anesthetic agent that produces 50% immobility to the patient or animals exposed to it, given at one atmospheric pressure. Mayer and Overton in 1901 pointed out lipid/water coefficient of GA and anesthetic potency. Anesthetics act on synapse. Presynaptically they act on

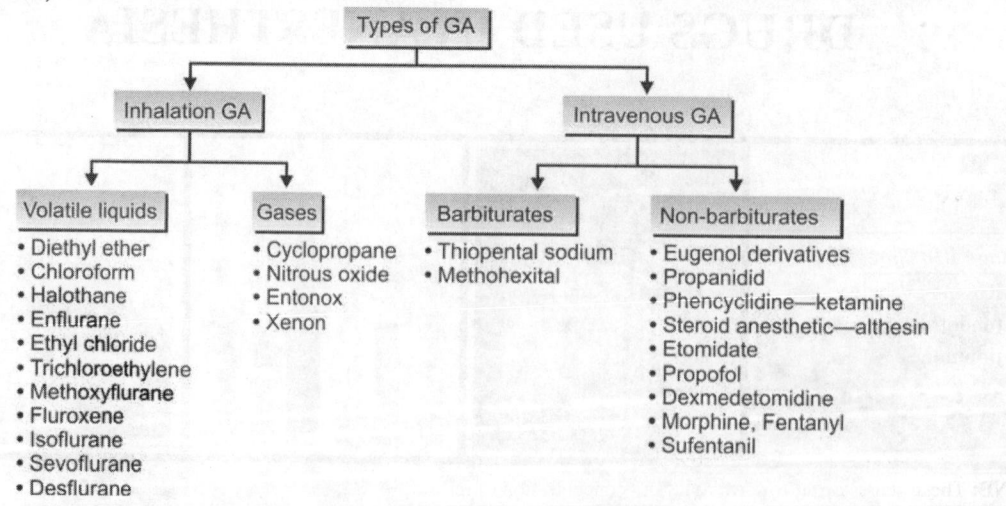

neurotransmitter release and postsynaptically alter frequency of amplitude so that excitatory transmission is impaired and inhibitory ion channels are target of anesthetic agents.

The factors which control the transfer of anesthetic agents to alveoli to tissue via blood are

- Solubility of the agent in the blood.
- Rate of blood flow through lungs and tissues.
- The partial pressure of the agent in arterial and mixed venous blood.

GA by dissolving in the membrane lipids, changes the structure favoring gel liquid transition (fluidization) which secondarily affects the state of membrane-bound functional proteins expanding it and closing the ion channels.

Different GAs act through different mechanisms

Barbiturates and propofol potentiate the action of GABA$_A$ receptor. Ketamine inhibits excitatory N-methyl-D-aspartate (NMDA) receptor type of glutamate receptor. Some GAs inhibit neuronal

Flowchart 50.1: Criteria for an ideal GA			
For patient	*For surgeon*	*For anesthetic*	*For manufacturer*
• It should be pleasant and non-irritating. • Without nausea and vomiting	• Should provide adequate muscle relaxation. • Analgesia • Immobility • Non-toxic • Non-inflammable • It should not react with rubber tubing or soda lime.	• Margin of safety should be high. • Oxygenation of patient should not suffer. • Adjustment of depth of anesthesia possible.	• Cost of production should be low. • There should not be storage problem.
NB: None GA fulfills the above criteria except cyclopropane and ether are closer to these requirement.			

Flowchart 50.2: Stages of anesthesia			
Stage I *(Analgesia stage)*	*Stage II* *(D)elirium stage*	*Stage III* *(Anesthesia stage)*	*Stage IV* *(Respiratory and medullary paralysis stage)*
• Patient can hear • Sees a dream • Reflexes normal	• Shout • Struggle • Hold his breath • Jaws are tightly closed • Breathing jerky • Vomiting • Micturates or defecates • Pupil dilate • BP raises This stage can be cut short by premedication.		• Cesation of breathing • Muscle flabby • Pupil dilate • BP down
Stage III (Plane 1)	*Stage III (Plane 2)*	*Stage III (Plane 3)*	*Stage III (Plane 4)*
• Roving eyeballs (endotracheal intubation done)	• Loss of corneal and laryngeal reflexes • BP falls • Heart rate increases • Respiration decreases in depth.	• Pupil starts dilating • Light reflex losts	• Intercoastal paralysis • Muscle tone decreases.
NB: These stages differ for different GAs concentration of inhalation. GA exceeding 1.2 MAC rarely used.			

cation channel gated by nicotinic, cholinergic receptors. It acts by depressing synaptic transmission. Strychinine sensitive glycine receptor is an another ligand gated ion channal may be target for some inhaled anesthetics.

Stages of anesthesia

Guedel in 1920 described four stages of GA produced by ether. The stage three divided into 4 planes is mentioned in the Flowchart 50.2.

Methods of Administering GA

1. **Open Method:** By Schimmelbusch mask (6–10 layers of gauze). Used for cheap GAs like ether, because the method is wasteful.

2. **Semi-open method:** The GA is prevented to be diluted by using masks like Ogston's mask or layers of gauze between the face and the mask.

3. **Semi-closed method:** Allows some re-breathing of the anesthetic drug with the help of a reservoir, but in addition, part of the volume of each succeeding inspiration is a new portion from anesthetic agent. It accumulates and rebreaths carbon dioxide.

4. **Closed method:** It employs a chemical agent (soda lime) to reabsorb the carbon dioxide present in expired air. It requires the use of a complicated apparatus, but is useful when anesthetic agent is potentially explosive.

Factors controlling uptake of anaesthetics
  i. Partial pressure
 ii. Alveolar concentration
iii. Solubility
 iv. Cardiac out put
    Alveolar to venous pressure difference.
    Factors determining elimination of anesthetics.
  i. Period of exposure
 ii. Ventilation
iii. Metabolism

INDIVIDUAL GENERAL ANESTHETIC AGENTS

Anesthetic potency is determined by Minimal Aveolar Concentration (MAC)

Pharmacodynamics of anesthetics:
  i. CNS: Decreases metabolic rate, blood flow, cerebral vasodilatation.
 ii. CVS: Depress cardiac contractility.
iii. Respiratory system: Irritation, bronchodilatation.
 iv. Kidney: Decreases GFR and renal blood flow.
  v. Liver : Decreases portal vein blood flow but hepatic artery flow may increases.
 vi. Smooth muscle: Halogeneted anesthetics are uterine muscle relaxant so used for uterine fetal manipulation or manual extraction of placenta but chances of bleeding is increased.

- **Ether**
Colorless, volatile liquid with odor and boiling point 35 °C. Marketed in amber colored bottles, covered with black paper to prevent conversion of either peroxide or acetic aldehyde. 10–15% of ether in inspired air required for induction and 4–5% for maintenance. Mainly excreted through lungs, crosses placental barrier.

Advantages
Surgical anesthesia may be produced without premedication. Satisfactory muscle relaxation, BP control, does not interfere with uterine contractility, not nephrotoxic. Not hepatotoxic and does not sensitize heart to adrenaline.

Disadvantages
Induction is slow with excitement, increases salivary and bronchial secretion. Not suitable for cautery, becaue of its inflammable nature. Nausea and vomiting may occur. Alcoholics are tolerants.

- **Chloroform**
Rarely used now because of hepatic and cardiotoxicity. May cause hyperglycemia.

- **Halothane (Fluothane)**
Fluronated, volatile, heavy, colorless, sweet odor. Supplied in amber colored bottles. Stable in presence of alkalies. Induction in concentration of 2–3% with O_2 and maintained with 1–2% with O_2 and N_2O.

Advantages

Non-inflammable and does not irritate respiratory passage, potent anesthetics, induction and recovery quick. Tracheal intubation easier. Does not produce bronchospasm, so preferred for asthmatic patient. May be used for bloodless field in plastic surgery. Relaxes uterus, so can be used for internal version and may be used in children.

Disadvantages

Muscle relaxation is poor. Depresses respiratory center, if concentration goes above 2%. Cardiac arrhythmia may occur. Recovery takes much time and shivering is common during recovery. Hepatic damaging, expensive, requires special apparatus. Poor analgesic supplemented with N_2O or opioids. Sensitizes heart to catecholamine. Don't use in PPH because it is difficult to control bleeding because of poor uterine contraction. May produce malignant hyperthermia, postoperative chills and shieving treated by pethedine.

- **Enflurane (Ethrane)**

Produced as a substitute of halothane. Muscular relaxation excellent, trachypnea rare, liver damaging effect less. It appears to be superior to halothane when repeat anesthesia is required. Contraindicated in epilepsy, inflammable, not a good analgesic.

- **Ethyl chloride**

Non-irritating, volatile, inflammable, boiling point 12 °C, vapor has characteristic odor. Used for induction of GA. While sprayed over skin rapidly evaporates and cools skin and transient paralysis of cutaneous sensory nerve occurs. It produces anesthesia within 1–2 minutes which recovers within 2–3 minutes of discontinuation. Maintenance of steady depth of anesthesic is difficult, with low margin of safety, inadequate muscle relaxation. May produce arrhythmia and liver damage.

- **Trichloroethylene**

Clear, colorless, non-irritant, non-inflammable with characteristic smell, potent analgesic with rapid onset of action, myocardium sensitized to adrenaline. Used as self-medication anesthetic during labor as intermittent inhalation.

Use restricted as supplement of $N_2O–O_2$ combination to obtain better analgesia. Muscle relaxation poor, should not be used in close circuit because with soda lime produce phosgene, which is responsible to produce acute respiratory distress syndrome and dichloroacetylene is neurotoxic to Vth and VIIth cranical nerves.

- **Methoxyflurane (Penthrane)**

Non-irritating, non-inflammable, boils at 105 °C, stable in air, light, alkali or moisture, potentiates muscle relaxation, sensitizes heart to catecholamine. It is nephrotoxic. Reacts with rubber tube used in close circuit.

- **Fluroxene (Fluromar)**

Colorless, volatile liquid, boils at 43 °C, inflammable, but non-irritant. Induction and recovery from quick anesthesia, muscle relaxation not satisfactory. Cardiac arrhythmia may occur.

- **Isoflurane**

Non-inflammable liquid related to enflurane. It has much less action on heart, uptake and excretion rapid than halothane, but less toxic. Used in day-care surgery of neuro or cardiac surgery.

- **Desflurane**

Less potent than isoflurane, irritates air passage to induce cough. Respiratory depression, vasodilatation, fall in BP, lack of seizure provoking potential, arrhythmogenic property hepato and renal toxicities similar to isoflurane. Postoperative cognitive and motor impairment is short lasting. Used for day-care surgery. Induces quickly.

- **Sevoflurane**

Polyfluorinated anesthetic with properties intermediate between isoflurane and desflurane. Acceptability good even for pediatric patient. Sevoflurane dose not cause sympathetic stimulation. Fall in BP, little effect on cardiac contractility. Degraded by soda lime, so not recommended for close method. Does not provoke seizure. Cognitive function quickly returns. Unlike desflurane there is no problem in its induction. Agent of choice for induction in children, good muscle relaxant, but poor analgesic. With close circuits it may produce nephrotoxic metabolite.

- **Xenon**

Expensive, potent inhalational ansthetic. Acts as agonist of 2 pore K^+ channel and non-competitive antagonist of NMDA receptor.

GASEOUS ANESTHETICS

- **Cyclopropane**

Colorless gas with sweet odor, available as liquid under pressure. Administered in closed circuit. 1–2% produces analgesia, 20% produces surgical anesthesia eliminated by exhalation. Color of cylinder is orange.

Advantages

Potent, quick induction in 2–3 minutes. Irritation to respiratory passage is rare so also of salivary secretion. BP and cardiac contractility well-anesthesia maintained, muscle relaxation is good, no visceral damage.

Disadvantages

Inflammable and explosive may produce laryngospasm, danger of overdose should be watched, sensitizes myocardia, depresses respiratory center. Sudden fall of BP with collapse (cyclopropane shock). Required complicated apparatus and trained anesthetics, increases capillary oozing, expensive. Mixture with oxygen is explosive.

- **Nitrous oxide**

Colorless, inorganic, non-inflammable, non-irritating gas marketed in steel cylinders at 650–800 lb/sq inch pressure. It produces excitment, delirium and amnesia, therefore, called laughing gas. Analgesia occurs in concentration of 35–40% and loss of consciousness at 65–70%. It is rapidly eliminated through lungs. It is used to measure cerebral and coronary blood flow by Fick's principle. Also used as carrier gas for inhalation agent, *viz.* halothane.

Advantages

Non-irritating, non-inflammable, produces rapid induction and recovery. Because of its analgesic action, it is used for tooth extraction and obstetric analgesic, changing dressing of burns. It is used with oxygen to induce anesthesia. Safest anesthetics with no remarkable effect on circulation, respiration. Nausea and vomiting are rare. Liver and kidney are not affected.

Disadvantages

Preanesthetics and muscle relaxant required. Excitement may be violent. CO_2 accumulation and hypoxia may develop, special apparatus required. May produce methemoglobinemia and laryngospasm due to impurities like NO and NO_2. Don't use in pnemothorax or volvulus.

Entonox is a mixture of 50% N_2O and 50% oxygen available in cylinders with blue body and with white shoulder whereas nitrous oxide is available in blue cylinders.

Color coding of some inhalation agents' cylinders: • Nitrous oxide—blue; • Cyclopropane—orange; • Air—grey body with white shoulders; • Oxygen—black body with white shoulders; • Carbondioxide—grey; • Helium—brown; • Entomox—blue body with white shoulders.

NON-VOLATILE ANESTHETICS WITH ULTRASHORT ACTING

- **Thiopentone sodium (Pentothal 0.5, 1 gm powder dissolved fresh):** Ultrashort acting thiobarbiturates, highly soluble in water yielding alkaline solution, prepared freshly before use. Injected IV 3–5 mg/kg as 2.5% solution. Produces unconsciousness within 15–20 seconds. Brain gets large amount. Fats and muscles also take up the drug. Consciousness regained in 10–20 minutes. Repeated doses produce cumulation. Poor analgesic, painful procedure can be done with opioids and N_2O, otherwise patient may struggle, changes in BP and respiration occurs. Weak muscle relaxant, does not irritate air passage, but respiratory depression can be severe, if more than therapeutic dose is used. Cardiovascular collapse may occur. Possesses anticonvulsant action.

Laryngospasm can be prevented by atropine. Succinyl choline reacts chemically with thiopentone, so should not be mixed in same syringe. Postanesthetic nausea and vomiting is not that common. May precipitate porphyria. Intra-arterial infection accidentally may cause ischemia and gangrene, if the needle is kept *in situ*. Dilutes with saline and injects heparin and papaverine. Steroid, vasodilator urokinase are other drugs.

Occasionally used to control convulsion, narcoanalysis, or to facilitate verbal communication with psychiatric patients.

Available as pentothal or intraval sodium 0.5–1 gm powder with injectable solution.

- **Methohexitone sodium**

  3 times more potent than thiopental, excitement during induction and recovery is more common as hiccough and cough. Rapidly metabolized. May induce seizure. Used for electroconvulsive therapy.

- **Propofol (Propovan 10 mg/mL in 10 mL vial)**

  Oily liquid used as 1% emulsion for IV induction and short duration anesthesia. Unconsciousness occurs after 15–45 seconds and lasts for 15 minutes. Used for out patient ambulatory surgery, prolonged sedation in critical care surgery. Postoperative nausea and vomiting are less. Induction apnea lasting for 1 minute is common. Pain during injection can be minimized, if given with lidocaine. Produces dose-dependent respiratory depression and pain during injection. Fospropofol drug containing aqua solution is less painful and used for sedation in diagnostic procedure. No muscle relaxation. Anesthetic choice for malignant hyperthermia, used with oxygen for total intravenous anesthesia. Myoclonic jerks may occur.

Dose

2 mg/kg bolus IV for induction 9 mg/kg/hr for maintenance. Fospropofol water soluble pro drug of propofol.

- **Etomidate (Hypomidate)**

  New induction anesthetics with brief duration of action for 5–10 minutes. Produce less cardiovascular or respiratory depression. Motor restlessness and rigidity are prominent. Diazepam suppresses these symptoms. It suppresses production of steroids, if continuously used. Poor analgesic, so opioids are required. Agent of choice for aneurism surgery. Vitamin C deficiency can develop with its use.

- **Propanidid**

  Less potent than thiopentone, oily liquid, produces involuntary movement and twitching, rarely used as IV anesthetics.

Short Acting

- **Benzodiazepines**

  Apart from their use in preanesthetic medications, they are frequently used for inducing, maintaining and supplementing anesthesia. It does not depress much respiratory and cardiac action, but in presence of opioids these functions are compromised. It is preferred for endoscopies, cardiac catheterization, angiography, fracture setting, *etc*. Its anesthetic action can be reversed by flumazenil 0.5–2 mg IV (available as valium, calmpose 10 mg/2 mL, dose 0.2–0.5 mg/kg slowly).

- **Lorazepam**

  Slow acting, less irritating and three times more potent than diazepam. Amnesia is common. Calmese 4 mg/2 mL as injection.

- **Midazolam**

  Water-soluble, nonirritating and three times more potent than diazepam. Used for sedation of intubated, mechanically ventilated patient. 1–2.5 mg IV for other critical care. 0.02–0.1 mg/kg/hour continuous IV infusion (available as mezolam, shortal 1 mg/mL or 5 mg/mL injection).

- **Ketamine**

Pharmacologically related to hallucinogens, phencyclidines, produces **dissociation anesthesia**. Featured by profound analgesia, immobility, amnesia, light sleep. Acts on cortex and subcortical area not reticular activating system. Respiration is not depressed and reflexes are not abolished. It blocks NMDA receptor of glutamate to produce its action.

Heart rate, BP, cardiac output increase due to sympathetic stimulation. It increases intraocular and intracranial pressures, so contraindicated for glaucoma and head injury. 1–4 mg/kg IV or 6.5–13 mg/kg IM produces above effects within minutes and recovery starts after 10–15 minutes. Children tolerate ketamine better. Used for head and neck operations, burn dressing, angiographies, cardiac catheterization. May be dangerous for hypertensions and in ischemic heart disease. 50 mg/mL in 2 mL ampoule or 10 mL vial injection.

- **Althesin (CT 1341)**

Steroid anesthetics combination of two pregenandione derivative alphaxolone and alphadolone. Given IV it produces analgesia. Muscle twitching, involuntary movements, hiccough may occur. BP and respiration not much affected. Duration of action is in between propanidid and methohexitone. May be used in place for thiopentone. May cause allergy and anaphylaxis. It is not used in practice.

COMPLICATIONS OF GENERAL ANESTHETICS (Fig 50.1)

During anesthesia: • Respiratory depression; • hypercarbia; • salivation; • respiratory secretion; • cardiac arrhythmia; • asystole; • fall of BP; • aspiration pneumonia; • laryngospasm; • asphyxia; • delirium; • convulsion; • fire explosion.

After anesthesia: • Nausea; • vomiting; • sedation; • pneumonia; • atelectases; • kidneys and liver damage; • Nerve paralysis.

Drug interactions: Patients on antihypertensive + GA: BP may fall. Neurolepics, opioids, clonidine, MAO-I-potentiate GA.

Halothane sensitizes heart to adrenaline. If patient is on corticosteroid, give 100 mg corticosteroid intraoperatively because anesthesia is a stress leading to adrenal insufficiency and cardiovascular collapse. Switch over to insulin and adjust dose in diabetic patient.

NEUROLEPTANALGESIA

Neuroleptics (antipsychotics) are a group of drugs which induce a state of apathy and mental detachment in which the patient is mildly sedated not caring for his surroundings. Neuroleptanalgesia is a method of intravenous anesthesia which combines the use of a neuroleptics with narcotic analgesic drug which relieve pain and produce a state in which patient cooperates. Droperidol (neuroleptics) and fentanyl (analgesic) are commonly used (related to pethidine).

Alfentanil and sufentanil, remifentanil are shorter acting may also be used in place of fentanyl. Droperidol blocks D_2 receptor so can produce extrapyramidal action.

PREANESTHETIC MEDICATION

The Purpose of Preanesthetic Medications

- To make anesthesia pleasant and safer
- To relief anxiety and facilitate smooth induction.
- Amnesia from pre- and postperative events.
- Supplement analgesic action and potentiate them.
- Decrease secretion and vagal stimulation.
- Antiemetics.
- To decrease acid volumes to reduce gastric aspiration.

Drugs used for Preanesthetic Medications

- **Opioids**—pethidine (100 mg) or morphine (10 mg) IM for analgesia (with thiopentone, halothane and N_2O).

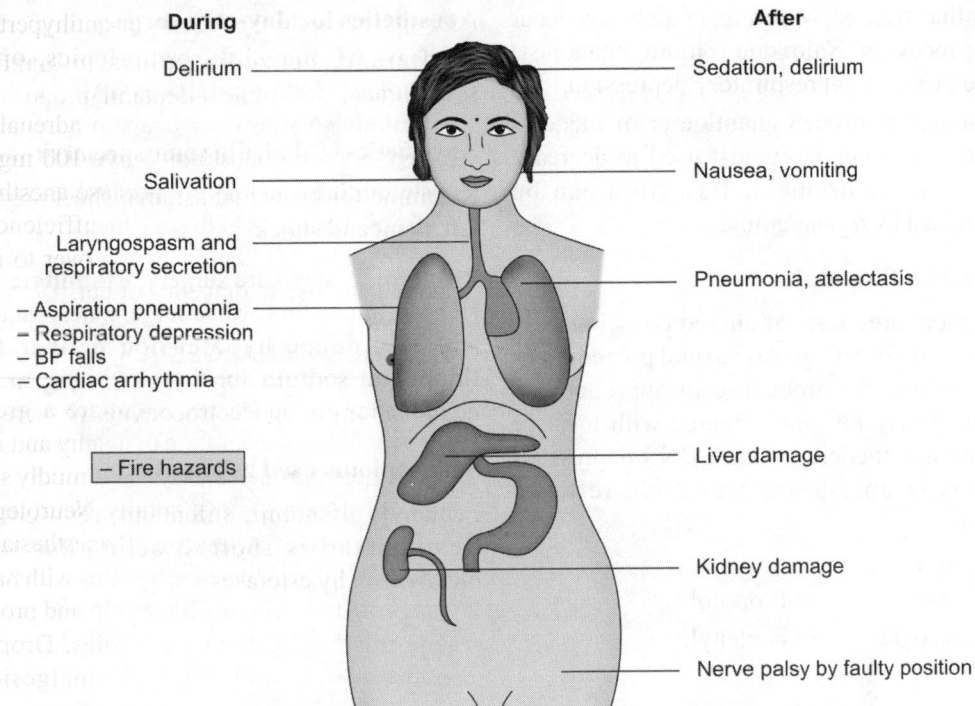

During

Delirium

Salivation

Laryngospasm and
respiratory secretion

- Aspiration pneumonia
- Respiratory depression
- BP falls
- Cardiac arrhythmia

- Fire hazards

After

Sedation, delirium

Nausea, vomiting

Pneumonia, atelectasis

Liver damage

Kidney damage

Nerve palsy by faulty position

Fig. 50.1: Complications and hazards of anesthesia

- **Antianxiety**—diazepam, lorazepam, mida-zolam.
- **Sedative hypnotics**—phenobarbitone (100 mg) or 100 mg secobarbitone or promethazine (50 mg IM) is antihistaminic, sedative, antiemetic, anticholinergic.
- **Anticholinergics** like atropine 0.6 mg IM or hyoscine, glycopyrrolate 0.1–0.3 mg IM is longer acting atropine substitute with anti-secretory and antibradycardiac drugs.
- **Neuroleptics** like chlorpromazine 25 mg or haloperidol 2–4 mg IM or triflupromazine 10 mg.
- **H₂ blockers and proton pump inhibitors** to reduce gastric secretion.
- **Antiemetics**—metoclopramide, domperidon, selective 5HT₃ blocker ondansetron (4–8 mg).

Toxicities of Anesthetics

Hepatotoxicity: Halothane may produce life-threatening hepatotoxicity, if exposed for second time in small group of patients. It may be due to reactive metabolism (free radicals or by immune-mediated response).

Nephrotoxicity: By metabolites of methoxy-fluraone, enthorane, servoflurane containing fluoride ions.

Malignant hyperthermia: Autosomal dominant genetic disorder of skeletal muscle occurs in susceptible individuals undergoing general anesthesia and with halothane or ether, muscle relaxant succinyl choline presents with serious hyperthermic crisis.

Chronic toxicity: Nitrous oxide may cause megaloblastic anemia in OT staff by decreasing methionine synthase activity, mutagenicity and carcinogenicity has not reported.

Fentanyl (Fent 50 µg/mL in 2 mL amp or 10 mL vial): This opioid analgesic related to pethidine used for paniful surgical procedure or for supplementing anesthetics for better hemodynamic stability. Often combined with benzodiazepines for endoscopy or angiographies or burn dressing in poor risk patient. Dose 2–4 mg/kg. Muscle relaxant may require to decrease chest muscle tone. It decreases heart rate by stimulating vagus, but it does not sensitize to adrenaline. Nausea, vomiting, itching may occur during recovery. Naloxone (opioid antagonist) may require to treat respiratory depression.

Dexmedetomidine: S-enantiomer of medetomidine α_2 adrenergic agonist used to decrease anesthetic requirement. Its action can be antagonised by α_2 antagonist.

Conscious Sedation

It is a monitored state of altered consciousness done to carry out diagnostic dental procedure or short therapeutic procedure in apprehensive patient. It may be supplemented with local or regional anesthetics. It caues CNS depression whereas in anesthesia protective reflexes are lost.

Drugs used are
- Diazepam
- Nitrous oxide
- Propofol
- Fentanyl.

Anesthetics for day-care surgery

Desflurane, benzodiazepines, midazolam sevoflurane, isoflurane, alfentanil, propofol.

Anesthetics of choice in some special situations

Ketamine for bronchial asthma, shock, right to left shunt and shock.

Propofol for day-care surgery, **Etomidate** for 1 HD; isoflurane for cardiac surgery, neurosurgery and to produce hypotension deliberately, **thiopental sodium** for thyrotoxicosis, methohexitone for giving electroconvulsive therapy.

Some opioids used as anesthetics

Fentanyl, alfentanil, sufentanil, remifentanil. Remifentanil is shortest acting due to its metabolism by esterases.

51

Local Anesthetics

Local anesthetics (LA) are drugs which on topical application or local injection produce surmountable loss of sensation specially pain. They reversibly block impulse conduction along nerve axons and excitable membranes which utilize Na^+ channels meant for action potential generation.

The local anesthetics act on peripheral nerves on restricted area without change in consciousness, may be used for poor health patient, generally used for minor surgery where patient is cooperative and care of the vital function is not that essential. In clinical practice, they are also used to block sympathetic vasoconstrictor, impulse to specific areas of the body.

Local anesthesia can be produced by local application of ice, CO_2 snow or ethyl chloride spray.

Lipoidal solubility is essential for migration of LA into neuronal fibers. Generally, nomenclature of local anesthetic ends with suffix (-aine). It generally consists of three parts (chemically):

- Hydrophilic amino group
- Intermediate chain
- Lipophilic aromatic group

Majority of chemically useful local anesthetics are nitrogen containing compounds as esters (cocaine, procaine, chloroprocaine, benzocaine, tetracaine) or amides (lidocaine, bupivacaine, ropivacaine).

The amide-containing local anesthetics are long acting not hydrolized by plasma esterase, binds α_1 acid glycoprotein in plasma.

Nerve fibers differ significantly to susceptibility to LA. Small fibers are preferentially blocked. Two or three nodes of Raniver should be blocked to inhibit impulse propagation. Preganglionic myelinated fibers blocked before smaller unmyelinated fibers are of pain transmission. High frequency depolarization are blocked earlier. In extremities, sensory blockade occurs first, but in trunk motor blockade occurs earlier, because of the location of nerve fibers.

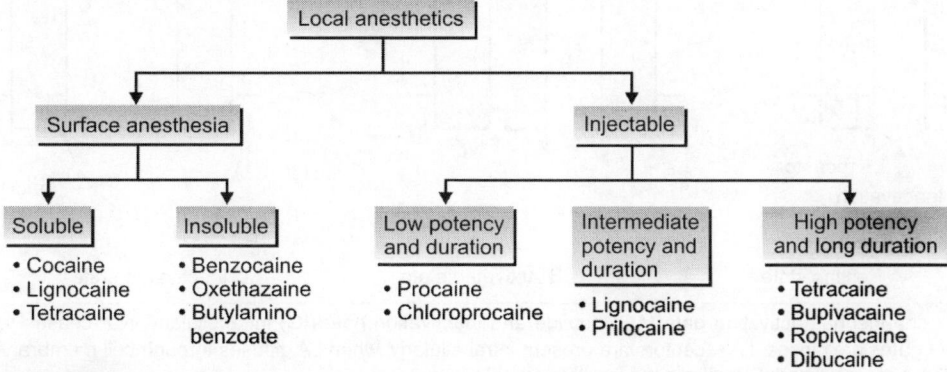

Mepivacaine, etidocaine, cyclomethycaine, dyclonine, proparacaine, benoxinate are occasionally used as local anesthetics in some countries.

Mechanism of Action

The local anesthetics decrease permeability of Na^+ ion in neurons thereby decreasing nerve conduction and impulse generation. Calcium is also involved in the action of local anesthetics. Smaller fibers of ANS are blocked first followed by sensory fibers conducting pain, touch, temperature, pressure, vibration. Motor fibers are blocked last. Applied on tongue bitter taste sensation lost first followed by sweet, sour and salt. All LAs are vasodilator except cocaine.

Pharmacological Action

Apart form local anesthetic properties, it stimulates CNS followed by its depression. Cocaine in smaller doses produces euphoria and hallucinations (cocaine bug; tactile hallucination). Lidocaine causes drowsiness. The stimulation produced by LA initially due to inhibition of inhibitory neurons.

CVS

The LAs are cardiac depressants. Decrease automaticity, conductivity and increase ERP. Bupivacaine is more cardiotoxic. BP falls due to sympathetic blockade and direct relaxation of arteriolar smooth muscle. Cocaine by blocking uptake has sympathomimetic properties and is a vasoconstrictor. Lidocaine is used as anti-arrhythmic. LA reduces BP due to sympathetic blockade.

Pharmacokinetics

Absorption is rapid through trachea and pharynx, but poor through urinary bladder. The amide LAs are bound to α_1 acid glycoprotein and degraded by liver microsomes by dealkylation and hydrolysis. Oral ingestion of liquid lignocaine is not effective as antiarrhythmic because of rapid first pass metabolism. Ester linked LAs are hydrolyzed by plasma pseudocholinesterase and by esterase of liver.

Uses of local anesthetics (Fig. 51.2)

1. Surface anesthesia by topical application (Fig. 51.2A)
2. Infiltration anesthesia (Fig. 51.2B)
3. Conduction block injecting in plexus of nerves (Fig. 51.2C)

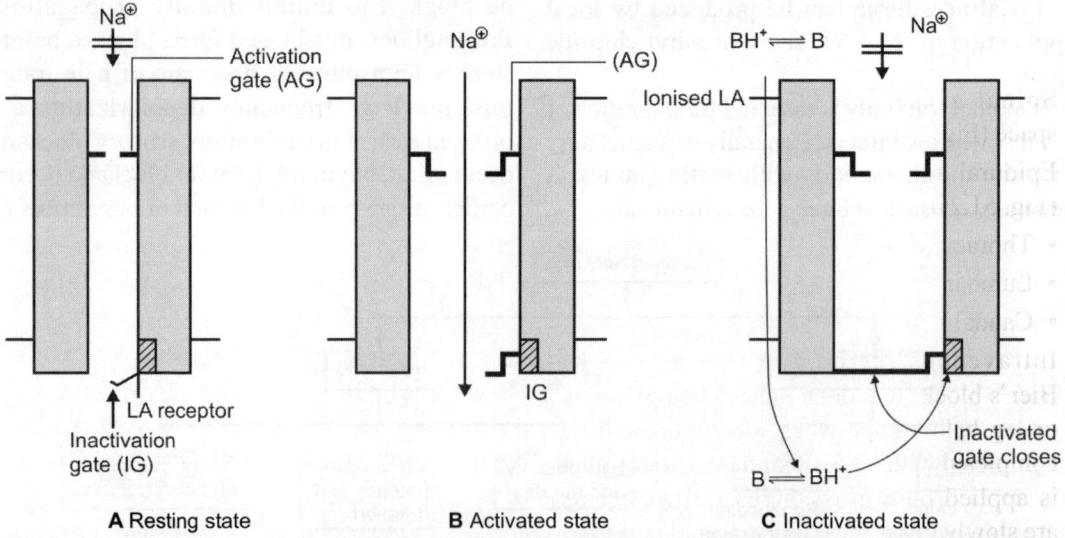

A Resting state   **B** Activated state   **C** Inactivated state

The Na channel has activation gate (AG) outside and inactivation gate (IG) intracellularly. Na⁺ ceases to flow when IG gates are closed. LA receptors are present intracellularly, when LA diffuses through cell membrane and binds to LA receptor and it stabilizes the inactivated gate.

Figs 51.1A to C: Mechanism of action of local anesthetics

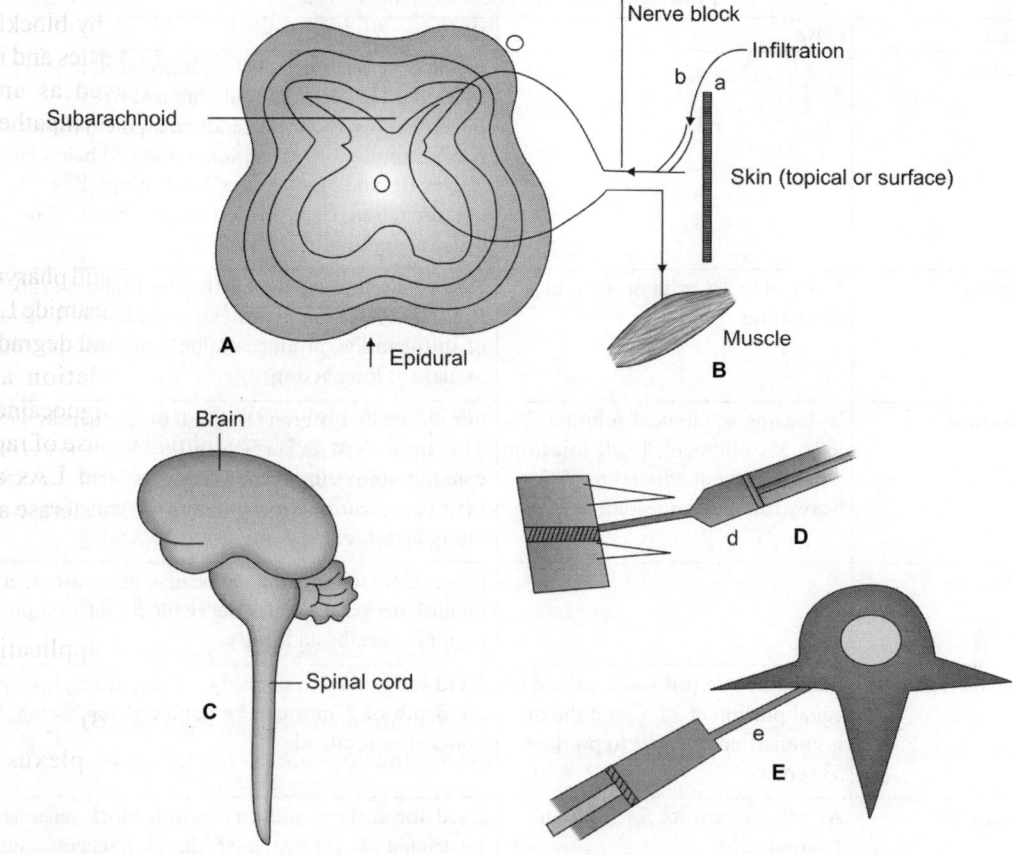

Figs 51.2A to E: Uses of local anesthetic

4. Spinal anesthesia injected in subdural space (Fig. 51.2D)
5. Epidural anesthesia (with Tuohy's needle) (Fig. 51.2D)
   • Thoracic
   • Lumbar
   • Caudal
6. Intravenous region anesthesia (IVRA) Bier's block: It is done on arm below elbow or leg below knee where operation will be completed within 45–60 minutes. Tourniquet is applied on arm or thigh and LA agents are slowly given through IV. Canula inserted in distal vein of the limb on which operation will occur. Pressure of tourniquet is kept above 50 mm of Hg of patient's systolic pressure. Preferred drug for this technique is prilocaine because it has large therapeutic index and least toxic. If lignocaine not available.

7. Infiltration block of autonomic sympathetic fibers to evaluate its role in peripheral vascular disease.

Addition of vasoconstrictor (adrenaline 1:50000–1:200000 or phenylephrine 1:20000 prolongs the action of LA and reduces toxicity, but it makes the tissues susceptible to edema and delays wound healing. BP may increase. The other methods to extent LA duration of actions are delivery system (polymers; suspensions) and transdermal local delivery system. Alternative to vasoconstrictor is felypressin can prolong the action duration of LA agent avoiding cardiovascular complication. Its onset can be

Flowchart 51.1: Individual local anesthetics

Drugs	Dose	Remarks
Cocaine		Isolated by Niehman (1860), introduced to practice by Koller (1894). Alkaloid obtained from *Erythroxylum coca*. Has addiction potentialities. (CNS stimulation, effects on mood and behavior). Raises BP and bradycardia. Inhibits uptake of noradrenaline. Used for ocular anesthesia. May cause sloughing of cornea.
Procaine	Novacaine 2% with or without adrenaline	First synthetic LA, synthesized by Einhorn (1905). Releases PABA on hydrolysis and can block action of sulfonamide, produces soluble salt with penicillin to make it long acting.
Lidocaine	Xylocaine 4% topical solution, 2% jelly, 5% ointment, 1–2% injection with or without adrenaline, 5% heavy for spinal anesthesia	Introduced by Lofgren (1943). It blocks nerves within 3 minutes. Used for surface, infiltration, nerve blocks, epidural, spinal, intravenous regional block. Overdose may cause cardiac arrhythmia, BP may fall, respiratory arrest, coma, convulsion, twitching.
Prilocaine		Lower CNS toxicity than lidocaine, but causes methemoglobinemia. Used for nerve block, infiltration, IV regional anesthesia locally.
Eutectic lidocaine/ prilocaine	Lidocaine and prilocaine mixed in equal portion at 25 °C and the oil is emulsified in water to produce 5% cream.	Used for occlusive dressing, skin grafting LA up to the depth of 5 mm can be achieved for lasting 1–2 hours after removal.
Tetracaine	Anesthetic powder for solution, 1% ointment	Used for surface and conduction block anesthetia. Restricted use for eye, nose, throat, tracheobronchial tree, it is PABA ester.
Bupivacaine	Marcaine 0.5–1% hyperbaric for spinal	Potent long acting amide LA. Used for infiltration, nerve block, epidural and spinal anesthesia. Used for obstetrics operation. Less likely to reach fetus from mother. Do not used IV ventricular tachycardia may develop.
Ropivacaine		It blocks pain transmission more completely. Continuous rapivacaine is used for relief of postoperative and labor pain.
Dibucaine	Nupercaine 0.5% injection, Nupercainal 1% ointment or drops	Potent, highly toxic, long acting LA. Used as surface anesthetic in anal canal and as spinal anesthetic.
Benzocaine and butylaminobenzoate	Proctoquinol 5% ointment of benzocaine	Slowly water-soluble, not absorbed from mucous membrane and abraded skin. PABA derivatives so, can antagonise sulfonamide, long acting without systemic effect, used as lozenges for stomatitis powder for wounds and ointment for anorectal lesions.
Oxethazaine	Component of mucaine gel	Potent topical anesthetics. Used to anesthetize gastric mucosa in acid peptic disease. Drowsiness may occur in dose above 100 mg/day.
Chlorprocaine		Shortest acting, contraindicated for spinal anesthesia.

acclerated by adding 1–2 mL of sodium bicarbonate. Tachyphylaxis can occur with repeated use due to extracellular acidosis.

Complications of local anesthetics

- Respiratory paralysis (due to respiratory and diaphragm paralysis)
- Hypotension (due to sympathetic blockade)
- Headache (due to seepage of CSF)
- Cauda equina syndrome (due to traumatic damage of nerve roots)
- Septic meningitis (due to infection)
- Nausea and vomiting
- Prilocaine as region anesthesia may cause methoglobinemia due to its metabolite o-toluidine.
- Esters in LA may cause allergic reaction.

Advantages of local anesthesia over general anesthesia

- Safer
- Produces good analgesia and muscle relaxation.
- Diabetic, heart, respiratory and kidney diseases patient tolerate it better.
- No loss of consciousness.

Contraindications of spinal anesthesia

- Not suitable for non-cooperative or mentally ill patient
- Hypotension; hypovolemia
- Infants
- Kyposis or lordosis
- Infection at the site of injection
- Raised intracranial tension
- Bleeding disorder on thrombolytic therapy
- **Relative contraindications:** Mitral and arotic stenosis, CNS disorder, recent MI, psychiatric disorder.

EMLA: (eutectic mixture of local anesthetics): Eutectic means the mixtures which on combination has lower melting point than its component, *viz.* lidocaine and prilocaine.

The prospect of LA will be towards sustained release formulation with less toxicity

Other local anesthetics are articaine, chloroprocaine, etidocaine, ropivacaine.

52

Skeletal Muscle Relaxants

Relaxation of the skeletal muscles are required in the following conditions

- Adjuvant to anesthesia, in orthopedic manipulation, abdominal surgery.
- In spastic disorders like tetanus, athetosis, status epilepticus.
- In electroconvulsive therapy (ECT)
- Centrally acting skeletal muscle relaxants—used for muscle spasm, torticollis, anxiety, spastic neurological disorder, orthopedic manipulation, tetanus, *etc.*

Centrally Acting Muscle Relaxants

(Acts on spinal and supraspinal polysynaptic internuncial neuron and block them). All drugs of this group cause sedation.

1. **Mephenasin (tolseram)** 500 mg tab. 1–3 gm/day.

2. **Carisoprodol (carisoma)** 350 mg tab. 1–2 tab TDS.

3. **Chlorzoxazone** (parafon 250 mg with paracetamol).

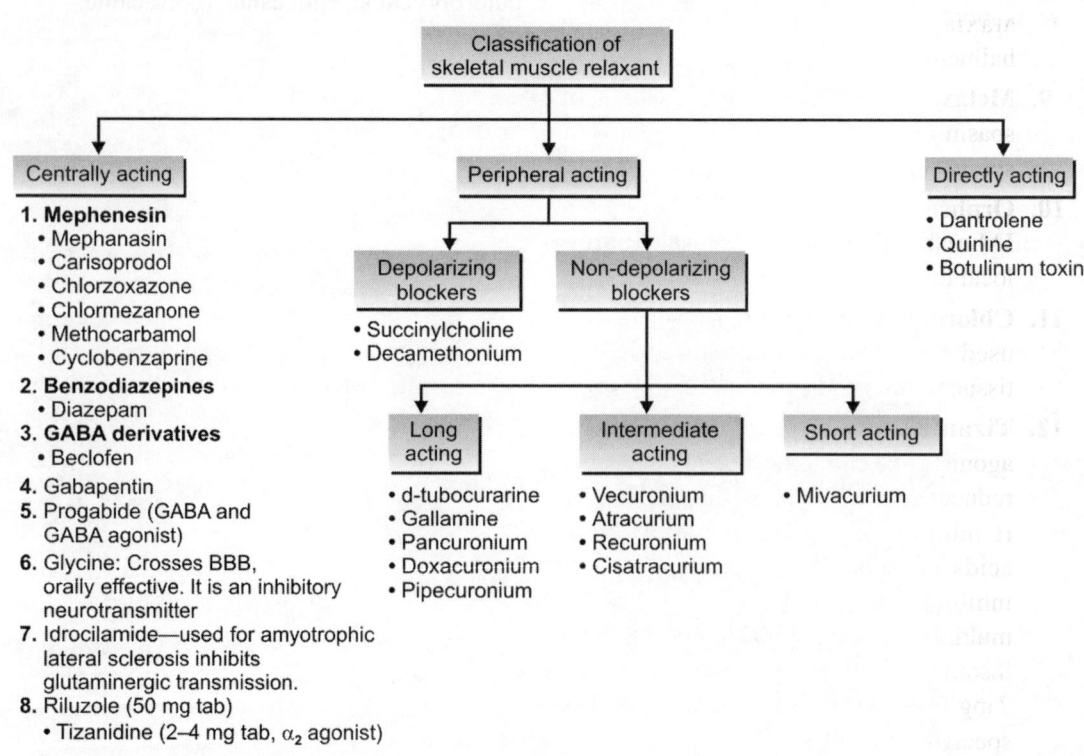

4. **Chlormezanone:** It has hypnotic and antianxiety actions as well (wintrac 100 mg tab, 1–2 tabs QID).

5. **Methocarbamol (robinax 500 mg tab, 1 tab TID):** 1 to 5 of this group of drugs are used for local muscle spasm due to sprain and spondylitis.

6. **Diazepam:** Enhances GABAergic transmission, acts on supraspinal region. Other benzodiazepine used as spasmolytic is midazolam used for tetanus.

7. **Cyclobenzaprine (Flexeril 10 mg):** Structurally related to tricyclic antidepressant, it has antimuscarinic effect, not effective in cerebral palsy or spinal cord injury. Dose 10–40 mg/day in divided doses. Used for injury related muscle spasm.

8. **Beclofen:** $GABA_B$ receptor agonist, increases K^+ conductance (lioresal 10 and 25 mg tabs, 10–25 mg BD or TDS) used for multiple sclerosis and spinal injuries, but not for cerebral palsy. Side effects are drowsiness, mental confusion, weakness, ataxia, sudden withdrawal may cause hallucination.

9. **Metaxalone (400 mg tab):** Used for muscle spasm caused by local tissue trauma and sprain.

10. **Orphenadrine (100 mg tab, 30 mg/mL for IM or IV use):** Used for muscle spasm of local tussue and sprain.

11. **Chlorophenasin (400 mg tab):** It is also used for muscle spasm caused by local tissue trauma and sprain.

12. **Tizanidine:** Congener of α_2 receptor agonists like clonidine, but no effect on BP, reduces spasticity in experimental animals. It inhibits release of excitatory amino acids in spinal interneurons. Facilitates inhibitory transmitter glycine. Used for multiple sclerosis, spinal injury, dry mouth, insomnia. Hallucination may occur. Dose 2 mg TDS. Do not use with antihypertensive specially, clonidine.

DIRECTLY ACTING MUSCLE RELAXANTS

• **Dantroline:** It reduces contraction of skeletal muscle by acting directly on excitation-relaxation coupling by decreasing calcium released from sarcoplasmic reticulum *via* calcium channel called ryanodine receptor (RyR) channel. Dantrolene binds to RyR channel and blocks its opening. The antigravity muscles are less affected compared to fast contracting muscles.

Side effects: Hepatotoxicity, sedation, euphoria, light headedness, dizziness.

Therapeutic uses: Spasticity in upper motor neuron disorders (in cerebral palsy, hemiplegia, paraplegia, multiple sclerosis). It is used from malignant hyperthermia which is due to persistent release of calcium from sarcoplasmic reticulum by fluorinated anesthesia and succinyl choline in genetically susceptible individual. Other supporting measures like discontinuation of anesthetic, O_2 inhalation, acid-base balance, *etc.* should be done (Dantrolene—25, 50, 100 mg caps or IV dose 1 mg/kg). It is also useful in case of neuroleptic malignant syndrome. Muscle weakness and hepatitis may occur.

• **Quinine:** Increases refractory period and decreases excitability at motor end plates, used for myotonia congenita. Dose 200–300 mg, also used for nocturnal leg cramps.

• **Botulinum toxin:** Used locally as short-term treatment for wrinkles around eyes by giving local injections. Local injections are also given for generalized spastic disorder (cerebral palsy), blepharospasm, dystonia, palmer hyperhydrosis. Both type A and type B botulinum toxins are available. Type B is used in those who are resistant to type A.

PERIPHERALLY ACTING MUSCLE RELAXANTS

Curare obtained from *Strychnos toxifera, Chondrodendron tomentosum* contains quarternary amonium containing active principle tubo-curarine and toxiferine which are not absorbed orally. Used as arrow poison by Amazon Basin of South American tribals. It acts by blocking nicotinic receptors (pentamer composed of four distinct subunits in stoichiometric ratio of $\alpha_2\beta\gamma\delta$), are arranged in a manner as to circumscribe in an internally located channel like a petal of lily). Curare acts as competitive blockers of nicotinic M receptor, surmountable by acetylcholine.

Two additional types of ACh receptor are associated with neuromuscular apparatus, one in presynaptic motor axon terminal which on activation mobilizes additional transmitter for subsequent release, the other variety of receptor is found on prejunctional cells released only in certain conditions (burn; prolonged immobilization) when they proliferate to affect subsequent neuromuscular transmission.

Larger muscles (abdominal, trunk paraspinal and diaphragm) are resisant to blockade and recover quickly than smaller muscles (hand, foot and face).

When small dose of non-depolarizing agents are used, they act on nicotinic receptor by competition blockade, but in higher doses it enters the pores of ion channel to further intense motor blockade. It also acts to block prejunction sodium channel and interferes with the mobilization of ACh at nerve ending.

Gallamine (Flexedil): Its actions are like d-tubocurarine, but rarely used.

Depolarizing blockers like decamethonium and succinylcholine have affinity for N_M receptor with submaximal intrinsic activity producing persistent depolarization (initial twitching and fasciculation followed by depolarization). The initial flaccid paralysis cannot be blocked by neostigmine called *phase I block* and prolong use converted to *phase II block* which can be reversed with anticholinesterase.

Succinylcholine preferred for endotracheal intubation.

Succinylcholine (SCh) is metabolized by pseudocholinesterase. Prolonged apnea on SCh may occur in some genetically determined persons due to atypical enzymes. The atypical enzyme activity can be assessed by dubicaine number. It may stimulate autonomic ganglia. It increases intracranial pressure and BP.

The depolarizing blockers have two quarternary N^+ atoms, but the molecule is long, slender and flexible termed *leptocurare*.

Pharmacological Actions of Skeletal Muscle Relaxants (SMR)

i. **Skeletal muscle**
   - Non-depolarizing paralyses of skeletal muscle.
   - Depolarizing blockers produce fasciculation followed by paralysis. (phase I depolarizing block). With continued exposure to succinylcholine, end plate depolarization decreased and repolarized, but because of desensitization cannot be depolarized again (phase II desensitization block).

ii. **Autonomic ganglion:** Some degrees of ganglion blocking produced by neuromuscular competitive blockers.

iii. **Histamine release:** By d-tubocurarine from mast cells.

iv. **CVS:** d-tubocurarine decreases BP by ganglion blockade, histamine release. Reduced venous return by muscle paralysis. Succinyl choline decreases heart rate, BP, may produce cardiac arrhythmia.

v. **GIT:** d-tubocurarine enhances paralytic ileus in postoperative patient of abdominal surgery.

vi. **CNS:** Does not cross blood-brain barrier so no effect. When given **ICV** produces strychnine like effect.

Toxicities of Skeletal Muscle Relaxants

- Respiratory paralysis
- Flushing with TC, atracurium, mivacurium
- Fall in BP and cardiac arrhythmia
- Precipitation of asthma by dTC by histamine release.

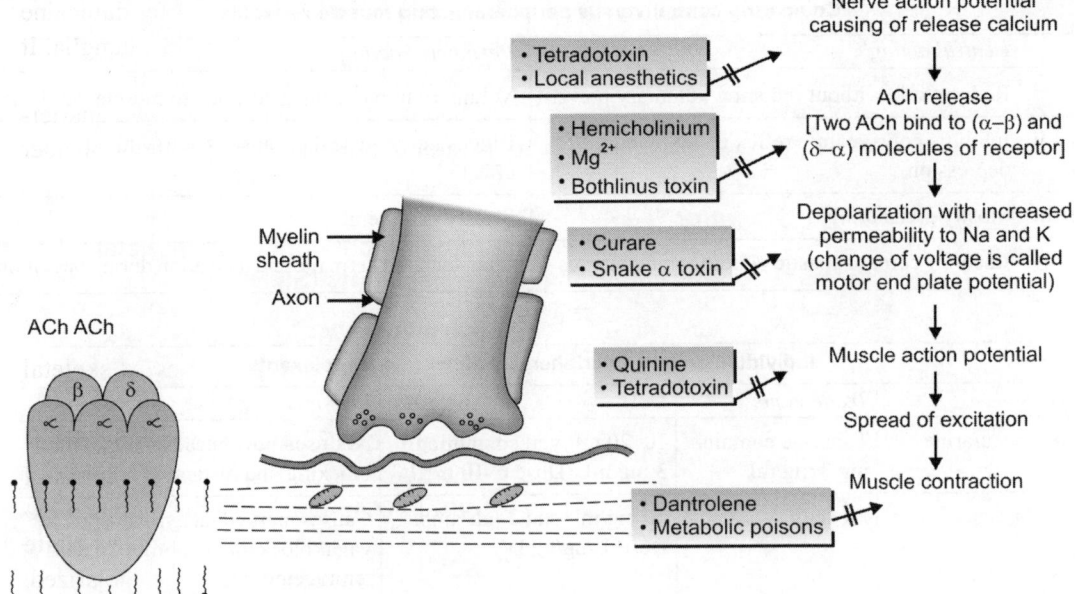

Fig. 52.1: Drugs interfering skeletal muscle contraction

Assessment of Neuromuscular Blockade

It is done by transdermal electrical stimulation of peripheral nerves of face or hand and to note twitched (evoked response by three commonly used patterns).

- Single twitch stimulation by supramaxial stimulation at peripheral nerves at frequencies 0.1 Hz to 1 Hz.
- Train of four, four successive supramaxial stimulation, 2Hz is given at 0.5 second interval.
- Titanic stimulation, 30–100 Hz is given for several seconds.
- Double brust stimulation used for those not responding to single twitch.

In case of d-tubocurarine there will be progressive decrease in twitch tension and restored by neostigmine. Succinylcholine first augments twitch followed by block which is not reversed rather worsened by neostigmine.

Adverse effects of depolarizing blockade

- Hyperkalemia particularly in head injury; burn or trauma patient.
- Can cause cardiac arrest.

- Raised intraocular tension
- Raised intragastric pressure
- Myalgia due to unsynchronized contraction of adjacent muscle fibres

Advantages of newer neuromuscular blockers over older ones

- Minimal ganglionic blockade
- Minimal cardiovascular effect
- Minimal histamine release
- They are easily reversible.

> Pancuronium; Vecuronium; Pipecuronium; Rocuronium; Rapacuronium are steroidal sketetal muscle relaxants.

Interactions of local anesthetics

- Thiopentine Na and succinylcholine react chemically.
- *General anesthetics:* Potentiate competitive blockers. Malignant hyperthermia produced by halothane is accentuated by succinylcholine.
- *Anticholinesterases:* Reverse the action of competitive neuromuscular blocker.

Comparing central *versus* peripheral acting muscle relaxants	
Central acting	*Peripheral acting*
i. Reduce tone without reducing voluntary power	Voluntary movements is lost due to muscle paralysis.
ii. Inhibitis polysynaptic reflex of CNS and CNS depression	Blocks neuromuscular transmission, without CNS effect
iii. Mostly given orally	Mostly parenteral
iv. Used for chronic spastic condition and tetanus	Used for short-term muscle relaxation during operation

Individual drugs of peripheral skeletal muscle relaxants			
Drug	*Trade name*	*Dose*	*Remarks*
d-tubocurarine	Tubarine containing 3 mg/mL	10–20 mL vial containing 3 mg/mL. Dose 6–10 mg IV	Not used now because of ganglion blocking and histamine release
Gallamine	Flexedil	40 mg/mL and 2 mL/amp. Dose 1 mg/kg IV	Causes marked tachycardia due to vagal blockade, nephrotoxic and teratogenic
Succinyl choline	Midarine	50 mg/mL and 2 mL amp.	Cardiac arrhythmia may occur. Used to pass tracheal tube.
Pancuronium	Pavulon	2 mg/mL and 2 mL amp.	Synthetic steroid 5 times potent to dTC. Rarely cause cardiac arrhythmia.
Vacuronium	Norcuron	4 mg amp dissolves in 1 mL of solvent. Recovery is spontaneous.	Close congener of pancuronium with short duration of action, without requiring neostigmine.
Atracurium	Tracrium	10 mg/mL in 2 mL vial.	Less potent than pancuronium, short acting. Non-enzymatic degradation (Hoffman elimination). Can be used in hepatic and renal insufficiencies. May produce seizure due to Laudonasine and its metabolite of cisatracurium is relatively safe.
Doxacurium			Longest acting, potent
Cisatracurium			R-cis enantiomer of atracurium. Four times more potent, slower onset.
Doxacurium			Long action, eliminated through kidney.
Pipecuronium	Arduan	4 mg/2 mL	Slow onset, long acting. Eliminated by liver and kidney.
Rocuronium 100 mg/10 mL vial	Coramid	50 mg/mL	Rapid onset, intermediate action without CVS changes. Generally used for intubation.
Mivacurium			Shortest acting competitive blockers. Prolonged paralysis in pseudocholinesterase deficient patients.

Comparing competitive and depolarizing variety of skeletal muscle relaxants	
Competitive block	*Depolarizing block*
Flaccid paralysis	Fasciculation then flaccid
Frog rectus (isolated), no contraction	Isolated frog rectus contracts
Neonates more sensitive	Less sensitive
Neostigmine blocks the action	No effect
Synergistic effect with ether	No effect
Low temperature reduces block	Intensifies block

Commonly used agents are neostigmine, pyridostigmine. Sygammadex is new and noval agents to reverse steroidal neuromuscular blockade.

- **Antibiotics:** Aminoglycoside reduces ACh release and potentiates the action competitive blockers. Tetracycline (chelates Ca^{2+}), peptide antibiotics, clindamycin, lincomycin synergize competitive blockers.
- Diuretic enhances competitive blockers by producing hypokalemia.
- Calcium channel blockers potentiate both competitive and non-competitive neuromuscular blockers.
- Diazepam, propranolol, quinidine intensify competitive blockers.
- Adrenaline, ephedrine reduce competitive block by increasing ACh release.

Dibucaine number

It identifies risk factors of patient receiving succinylcholine. It measures ability of the patient to metabolize succinylcholine. Dibucaine is a local anesthetic metabolized by atypical pseudo-cholinesterase (20%) and by normal enzymes 80%. Therefore for a normal person dibucaine number is 80. If it is less than 80 that means there is a rise in atypical enzyme.

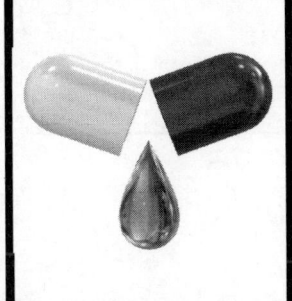
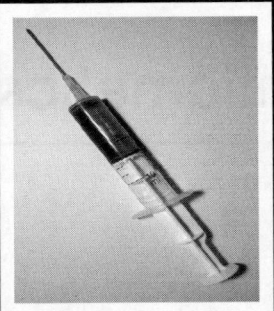
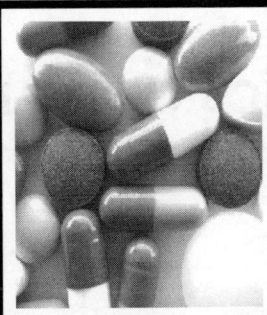
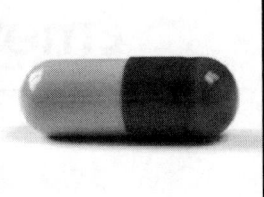

SECTION 6

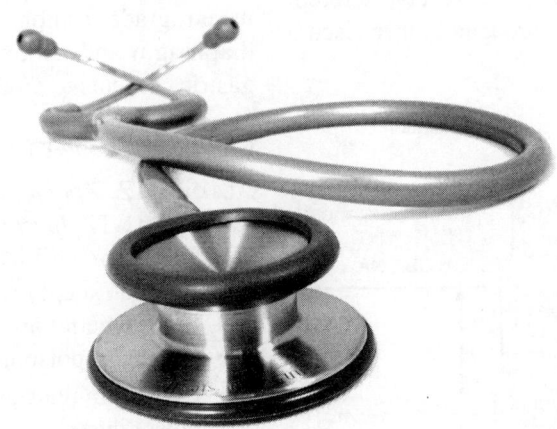

GASTROINTESTINAL SYSTEM

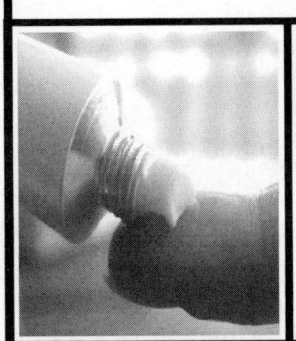
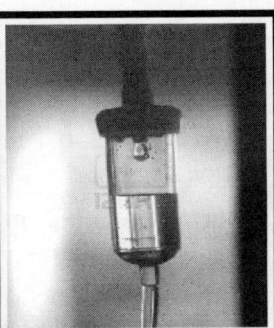
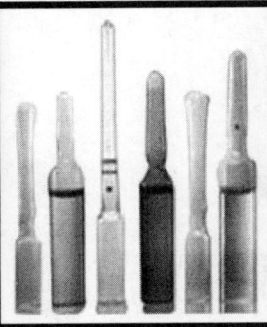
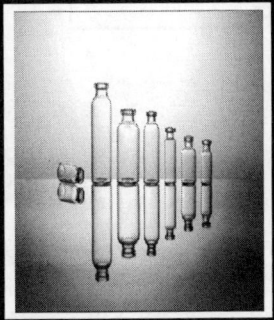

53

Emetics and Antiemetics

Emetics: Drugs Evoking Vomiting

Emetics: When vomiting center of medulla oblongata is stimulated vomiting is induced. Chemoreceptor trigger zone, area prostrema and nucleus tractus solitarii (NTS) receive afferent impulses from GI tract, throat and other viscera to induce vomiting.

Flowchart 53.1: Emetic stimulation

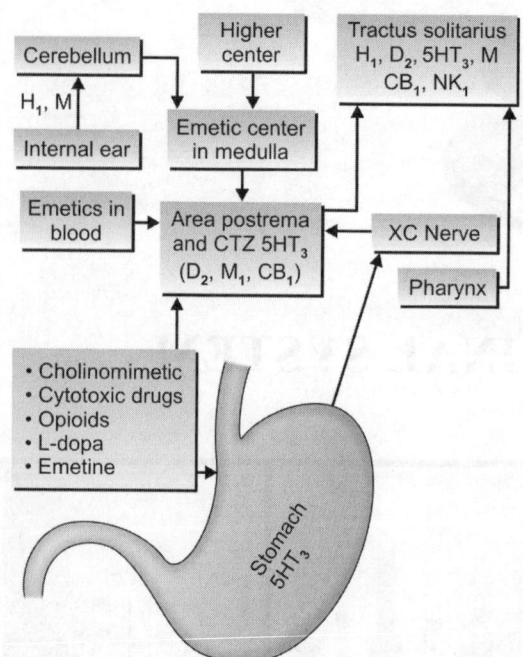

Variety of receptors, *e.g.* histamine (H_1), dopamine (D_2), serotonin ($5HT_3$), opioid (μ), muscarinic (M_1) produce vomiting when stimulated. Vestibular apparatus produces vomiting through

cholinergic M_1 and H_1 receptors present in cerebellum.

Nausea causes reduced in paristalsis and tone of stomach. In vomiting, esophageal sphincters relax, duodenum and pyloric sphincters contract in retrograde fashion. Rhythmic contraction of diaphragm and abdominal muscle propel out gastric contents to produce vomiting.

Emetics: Drugs Producing Vomiting

Act on CTZ, *Apomohine* 6 mg, IM or SC acts reflexly on CTZ, *Ipecauanha* 15–20 mL for adult and 5 mL for children. Vomiting is always discouraged except in poisoning.

Uses of emetics are contraindicated in
- Corrosive poisoning
- CNS stimulant and kerosene (petroleum poisoning)
- Unconscious patient. In morphone and phenothiazine poisoning, they are not effective.

Antiemetics: Antiemetics are drugs which prevent or suppress vomiting.

Classification of Antiemetics

Anticholinergics

Hyoscine: 0.2–0.4 mL oral, IM—used for motion sickness.

Dicyclomine: 10–20 mg orally used for motion and morning sickness.

H_1 blockers: Promethazine, diphenhydramine, dimenhydrinate. Used for motion sickness. Produce sedation and dry mouth. Promethazine theoclate (avomine 25 mg) used as antiementic. Cyclizine, meclizine used in seasickness.

Cinnarizine (cintigo, vertigon 25 mg): Used for vertigo and motion sickness. Inhibits Ca^{2+} influx into vestibular cells to mediate reflex.

Prochlorperazine (stemetil 5 and 25 mg tabs, 12.5 mg/mL): Used for vertigo and motion sickness.

Doxylamine: With pyridoxine is specifically promoted for morning sickness.

Neuroleptics: Halloperiodol is a broad spectrum antiemetics (act on D_2 receptor), used in post-anesthetic vomiting, disease-induced vomiting (GIT infection, migraine, uremia), cancer chemotherapy, radiation and morning sickness (except hyperemesis gravidarum). Not effective in motion sickness. Other drug is droperidol given IM or IV. Droperidol causes prolongation of QT interval.

They produce sedation and extrapyramidal side effects.

Prokinetics: Promote gastroduodenal peristalsis and gastric emptying. Acetylcholine is excitatory neurotransmitter in gastrointestinal tract. Neurons of cholinergic system contain $5HT_4$ excitation and $5HT_3$ and D_2 presynaptic inhibitory receptors. Therefore, agonist of $5HT_4$ and antagonist of D_2 and $5HT_3$ will stimulate GI motility. First drug of this group is metoclopramide, chemically related to procainamide. Increases gastric peristalsis, contracts lower esophageal sphincter (so gastroesophageal reflux is prevented), but no effect on gastric secretion, acts also on CTZ and prevents apomorphine-induced vomiting.

Mechanisms of action of prokinetics

- Dopamine D_2 antagonism
- Cholinomimetic
- $5HT_3$ antagonism action.

Physiology of Enteric Nervous System (ENS): The ganglion cells and nerve fibers mainly located in submucosa and in between circular and longitudinal muscles constitute enteric nervous system. The fibers from them connect with mucosa and deep muscles. Sympathetic and parasympathetic nerves project into these plexuses. ENS can independently regulate GI motility and secretion. The primary afferent neuron projects *via* dorsal root ganglion or vagus nerve to CNS. 5HT is released from intestinal mucosal enterochromaffin cells which stimulate $5HT_3$ receptor on extrinsic afferent nerves producing nausea, vomiting or abdominal pain. 5HT also stimulates 5HTIP receptor of intrinsic primary afferent nerve (IPAN) containing calcitonin gene-related peptide (CGRP). Presynaptic IPAN enhances the release of CGRP and ACh. Myoenteric interneurons control peristalsis. DA is an inhibitory neurotransmitter decreasing intensity of esophageal and gastric contraction.

Uses of prokinetics

- Antiemetic
- Dyspepsia
- Gastroesophageal reflux disease (GERD)

Other drugs for GERD

1. **$5HT_4$ agonist:** Cisapride, Mosapride, Renzapride, Prucalopride, Tegaserod, Itopride.

2. **Other prokinetics:** Levosulfide (l-isomer of sulfide antipsychotic drug with D_2 blocking activity)

3. **Loxiglumide:** CCKI receptor antagonist used for constipation of IBS.

4. **Motilin agonist macrolides:** Erythromycin used for diabetic gastroparesis, but it develops tolerance rapidly.

Domperidone: D_2 antagonist, extrapyramidal side effects are rare. Orally absorbed. Dose 10–40 mg.

Cisapride: Prokinetic, releases ACh in myoenteric plexus and $5HT_4$ antagonism. It is used for GERD, constipation, but not as antiemetic. Dose 10–20 mg TDS. Ventricular arrhythmia can occur with macrolide antibiotic and antifungal agents ketoconazole due to torsades de pointes. It has been withdrawn from market. It is metabolized by $CYP3A_4$ whereas itopride is metabolized by flavin mono oxygenase (FMO) so it is less prone to drug-drug interaction as FMO is neither induced or inhibited.

Mosapride: $5HT_4$ agonist, its metabolite has $5HT_3$ antagonist property. Orally active, used for GERD and heart burn. Dose 25 mg TDS. Tagaserod is a $5HT_4$ partial agonist.

$5HT_3$ antagonist: Ondansetron $5HT_3$ antagonist, used in cancer chemotherapy and radiation-induced vomiting (Emeset 4, 8 mg or 2 mg/mL or in 2 mL and 4 mL amp).

Granisetron: It is 10 times more potent to ondansetron. Used in cancer chemotherapy-induced vomiting.

$5HT_3$ antagonists used in chemotherapy-induced vomiting:

Drugs	Dose/IV
Ondansetron	0.15 mg/kg
Granisetron	10 µg/kg
Dolasetron	0.6–3 mg/kg
Palanosetron	0.25 mg
Ramosetron	300 µg/ kg

Adjuvants and Antiemetics

* **Corticosteroid** (Dexamethasone 8–20 mg IV) in cancer chemotherapy.
* **Benzodiazepines:** Adjuvant to ondansetron to reduce anxiety.
* **Cannabinoids:** Nabilone is a synthetic cannabinoid, inhibits chemotherapy-induced vomiting. Dronabinol by stimulating CB_1 receptor, obtained from marijuana plant, *Cannabis indica*. Dose 10 mg only singly for moderate chemotherapy-induced vomiting.

Neurokinin receptor antagonist: Aprepitant is a highly selective neurokinin NK_1 receptor antagonist crossing BBB, used with corticosteroid or $5HT_3$ antagonist in vomiting due to emetogenic chemotherapy. Orally 125 mg × 3 days, 1 hour before the chemotherapy followed by 80 mg/day after the chemotherapy on second and third days. It is metabolized by CYP3A4 so drug interactions may occur. Fosaprepitant is a prodrug of aprepitant used parenterally.

Substituted benzamides: Metoclopramide (also discussed with prokinetics) and trimethobenzamide block doapmine receptors. The later has week antihistamine actions too. Used for nausea and vomiting. Metoclopramide, dose is 10–20 mg orally or IV 6 hourly. Dose of trimethobenzamide 250 mg orally, 200 mg IM or by rectal route.

Carminatives

Carminative expulses gases from GIT and gives a feeling of comfort. Used for treatment of flatulent dyspepsia and regurgitation of milk in infants.

Sodium bicarbonate	1 gm
Aromatic spirit of ammonia	2 mL
Tinc cardamom	2 mL
Tinc ginger	0.5 mL
Camphor water	15 mL

Sodium bicarbonate reacts with HCl of gastric juice to produce CO_2 and brings out erructation. Ammonia, alcohol and volatile oil irritate the stomach and increase its peristalsis and help in evacuation of stomach used for flatulent dyspepsia.

Bitters: Bitters reflexly promote gastric secretion to increase appetite.

Compound 25% alcohol

Chirata infusion	2 mL
Mentha oil	0.1 mL
Chloroform water	15 mL

To be taken before meal. Mentha oil and chloroform water act as flavoring agent. Alkaloidal bitters quinine, strychnine are not justifiable to use as bitter appetizers.

Gallstone Dissolving Agents

Chenodeoxycholic acid (chenodiol) and urso-deoxycholic acid (ursodiol) decrease cholesterol content of bile, making it soluble from stone surface. The commonly used chenodiol and ursodiol are peptic ulcerogenics and contra-indicated in pregnancy.

Chenodiol

- Inhibits HMG CoA reductase.
- Raises LDL cholesterol.
- Reduces cholesterol secretion in bile after prolong use.
- Promotes micellar solubilization of cholesterol, dose 10–15 mg/kg/day.
- Side effects are:
  - Gastric ulcer,
  - Raised aminotransferase.

Ursodiol

- Inhibits cholesterol absorption form gut.
- Does not raise LDL cholesterol.
- Reduces cholesterol secretion in bile promptly.
- Promotes solubilization by liquid crystal formation. Dose 7–10 mg/kg/day.
- Side effects are diarrhea, hypertransaminemia, gastric ulcer. Contraindicated in pregnancy.

Uses of bile salts and bile acids

- Cholestasis
- Biliary fistula
- Hepatic disease

These are constituents of many combinations, but they should not be used because they are ineffective and harmful. Ursodiol is not hepato-toxic. So may be useful for cirrhosis or other hepatic disorder.

Drugs for Constipation

Laxative or Aperient: Evacuate bowels (milder action).

Purgative or Cathartic: Stronger action in evacuation of bowel.

Laxatives or Purgatives Act by

- Retaining water and electrolyte in intestinal lumen by osmotic action.
- Decreasing water reabsorption
- Increasing peristaltic activity
- Modifying fluid dynamics by following mechanisms:
  a. Inhibiting Na^+/K^+-ATPase and imparing water absorption.
  b. Stimulating adenylate cyclase and increasing water and electrolyte secretion.
  c. Enhancing PG synthesis which increases secretion of gut.
  d. Structural injury to absorbing intestinal mucosal cells.

Therapeutic uses of purgatives

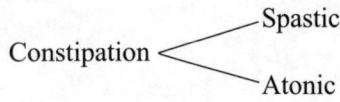

Constipation
- Spastic
- Atonic

- Bedridden patient
- To avoid straining of stool in bleeding piles, fissure in ano
- Preparation of bowel for surgery, colonoscopy, X-rays.
- With anthelmintics (with piperazine)
- Food poisoning

Purgative abuse may cause

- Flair intestinal pathology
- Electrolyte imbalance
- Malabsorption
- Spastic colitis
- Protein losing enteropathy.

Laxatives are contraindicated in

- Undiagnosed abdominal pain in colic
- Vomiting
- Secondary to intestinal obstruction
- Hypothyroidism
- Hypercalcemia
- Malignancies, with opioid, sedative, anticholinergic, antiparkinsonian, verapamil, iron- and clonidine-induced constipation.

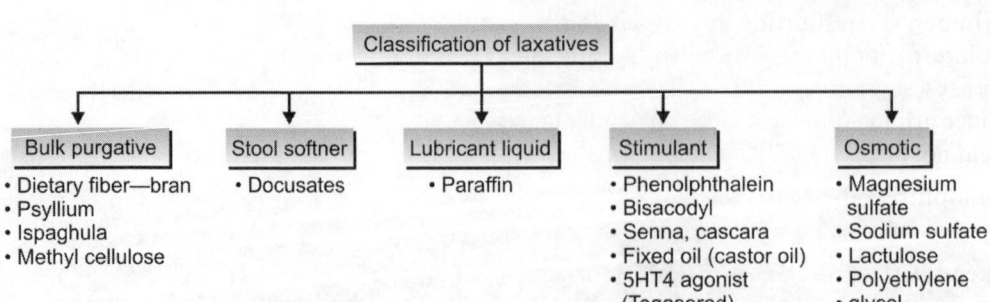

Classification of laxatives				
Bulk purgative	**Stool softner**	**Lubricant liquid**	**Stimulant**	**Osmotic**
• Dietary fiber—bran • Psyllium • Ispaghula • Methyl cellulose	• Docusates	• Paraffin	• Phenolphthalein • Bisacodyl • Senna, cascara • Fixed oil (castor oil) • 5HT4 agonist (Tegaserod)	• Magnesium sulfate • Sodium sulfate • Lactulose • Polyethylene • glycol

Individual Purgative

Dietary fiber: Supports bacterial mass, contribute to fecal mass. Degradation of cholesterol in liver is increased and plasma LDL cholesterol decreases. First line of treatment of constipation, takes 3–4 days to produce effects. No effects on impacted stool in rectum and not palatable.

Ispaghula

Produces colloidal mucilage mass by absorbing water. Should not be taken dry (may cause esophageal impaction), dose 3–12 gm/day.

Methyl cellulose

It is semisynthetic taken 4–6 gm/day with generous water intake.

Stool softner (Dioctyl Sodium Sulfosuccinate, DOSS)

This anion detergent emulsifies colonic content by accumulation of water. Liquid paraffin should not be combined to it (Laxicon 100 mg tab, or 50 mg/5 mL). Hepatoxicity on prolong use. Nausea may occur because of its bitter taste. It may also be given as enema.

Lubricants (liquid paraffins)

Pharmacologically inactive, soften stool and lubricate hard scybali. Dose 15–30 mL/day, may produce:

- Foreign body granuloma
- Pneumonia
- Fat-soluble vitamin deficiency
- Leakage of oil at anal sphincter
- Healing of anorectal ulcer is delayed.

Irritant purgatives

These powerful purgatives irritate myoenteric plexus, accumulate water and electrolyte in gut lumen by inhibiting Na^+/K^+-ATPase in basolateral membrane of villous cells and increases secretion by PG synthesis. It may produce griping, fluid and electrolyte imbalance should not be used in pregnancy.

Phenolphthalein: This indicator is used as a purgative, now withdrawn from the US market.

Bisacodyl (Dulcolax 5 mg tablet): Irritates gut mucosa. Allergy, fixed drug reaction, Stevens-Johnson syndrome are important side effects. Suppository preparation evacuate bowel in 20–40 minutes. Mucosal damage may occur.

Sodium picosulfate (Laxicare 10 mg tablet): Diphenylmethane derivative bisacodyl hydrolyzed by colonic bacteria to active form, bowel movement occurs 6–12 hours of oral dose. Used for bowel preparation before coloscopic surgery.

Senna (Glaxenna 11.5 mg tablet): Obtained from leaves and pods of *Cassia* species. Passes to colon and acted upon by bacteria to produce anthrol. Taken at bedtime. Excreted with milk, so should not be used in lactating mother. Regular use for long time may cause pigmentation of colonic mucosa.

Castor oil: Obtained from seeds of *Ricinus communis* hydrolyzed by lipase in intestine to ricinoleic acid and glycerol. Ricinoleic acid is not absorbed and irritates mucosa. It is not used because of bad taste, severity of action, dehydration, after constipation and intestinal mucosal damage.

Tegaserod (Tegibis 2, 6 mg tablet): $5HT_4$ receptor's partial agonist, acts on intrinsic enteric afferent and enhances release of excitatory transmitter ACh and calcitonin gene-related protein (CGRP) to promote peristalsis. Used in IBS, chronic constipation. Only its small fraction is absorbed. Loose motion, flatulence, headache may occur. Should not be used in renal and hepatic diseases. It is withdrawn from market because of side effects of edema, heart attack and stroke.

Osmotic purgatives

All inorganic salts used as purgative, retain water osmotically and distend the bowel and enhance peristalsis. Magnesium salts contraindicated in renal disease whereas Na salt for CCF.

Magnesium sulfate (Epsom Salt): 5–15 gm bitter in taste.

Magnesium hydroxide (8% w/w suspension): 30 mL bland in taste (milk of magnesia).

Sodium sulfate (Glauber's salt): Bad in taste. Dose 10–15 gm.

Sodium phosphate: Dose 6–12 gm

Sodium potassium tartrate (Rochelle salts): 8–15 gm, relatively pleasant taste.

They are rarely used as purgatives because of after constipation, except in food and drug poisoning, colon preparation before surgery and worm infestations.

Lactulose (Duphalac 6.67 gm/10 mL) as semisynthetic disaccharide not absorbed in intestine. Broken down in colon by bacteria to retain more water. It reduces NH_3 to NH_4^+ salts which is not absorbed, therefore, effective in hepatic encephalopathy.

Other drugs which may be used to reduce blood ammonia are sodium benzoate and sodium phenyl acetate producing hippuric acid or phenyl acetic glutamine respectively which are excreted with urine.

Polyethylene glycol has replaced the use of oral sodium phosphate for colonic cleaning for surgical colonoscopy or endoscopic procedures.

Methylnaltrexone bromide and alvimopan are selective μ (mu) opioid receptor antagonist commercially available. Used for opioid induced constipation and postoperative ileus respectively. Dose methylnaltrexone 0.15 mg/kg every 2 days and alvimopan 12 mg cap 5 hours before surgery and twice daily after surgery till bowel becomes regular.

Prucalopride $5HT_4$ agonist without significant affinity for human ether-a-go-go-related gene channels like cisapride used to increase bowel movements.

Lubiprostone: A chloride channel activator is prostanoic acid derivative used in constipation of IBS. It can cause nausea.

Linaclotide is a guanylate cyclase C receptor agonist of luminal enterocyte and stimulates intestinal fluid secretion undergone clinical trial for use in chronic constipation.

Evasuant enema: Given gently to avoid bowel injury, causes liquifaction and fragmentation of faces.

Tap water, Soapsuds (natural), Isotonic NaCl (one level teaspon of common salt / half litre if water) vegetable oil, glycerine, docusate sodium, bisacodyl may be used. Do not use hot water, detergent, hypertonic salts

Tap water may cause water intoxication.

Enema is used for:
  i. Fecal impaction

  ii. For endoscopy, before radiography, before child birth

  iii. In patient of incontinance or colostomy

  iv. To reestablish reflex for rectum.

Drugs used to Treat Variceal Hemorrhage

Somatostatin   250 μg/hour
Octreotide   50 μg/hour

Given intravenously, reduces portal blood flow and variceal pressure by inhibition of gluca-gon and other peptide which alters mesenteric blood flow.

Vasopressin given IV causes splanchnic arterial vasoconstriction and lowers portal venous pressure.

Terlipressin: Vasopressin analog with less ADR.

β blocker: Decreases cardiac output and causes splanchnic vasoconstrictions caused by unop-posed α actions (propranolol and nadolol are used). It reduces recurrent bleeding.

56

Drugs of Inflammatory Bowel Disease (IBD)

Ulcerative colitis and **Crohn's diseases** are inflammatory bowel diseases with unknown etiologies. Drugs used are:

Sulfasalazine (5-ASA + Sulfapyridine)

Olsalazine (5-ASA + 5-ASA)

Balsalazide (5ASA + Amino benzoyl alanine)

(5-ASA= 5-Aminosalicylic acid)

- **Aminosalicylates** (sulfasalazine, olsalazine, balsalazide) and different forms of their time release are mesalamine and pentasa, when they reach terminal ileum or colon, colonal bacteria split them by azoreductase to release 5-ASA. Sulfapyridine is absorbed metabolised and excreted with urine but metabolized product of Balsalazide is not absorbed. Sulfasalazine is also used in RA.

- **Asacol** and apriso pH sensitive resin of masalamine dissolving in pH 7 of colon. **Rowsa** is enema formulation or canasa is suppository formultion of mesalamine. They release 5-aminosalicylic acid (5-ASA) topically in the areas of diseased mucosa of GIT. 5-ASA induces and maintains remission of ulcerative colitis, so first line drug to treat ulcerative colitis. The generic name of 5-ASA is mesalamine. 5-ASA inhibits local prostaglandin synthesis and nuclear factor kappaB.

ADR of sulfasalazine

More common with slow acetylators, nausea, GI upset, headache, arthralgia, myalgia, malaise, bone marrow depression, fever, exfoliative dermatitis, pancreatitis, pancarditis, pneumonia, hepatitis, hemolytic anemia, oligospermia (reverse on drug withdrawals). Impairs folate absorption.

Other aminosalicylate formulations are better tolerated. Olsalazine stimulates secretory diarrhea. Renal tubular damage, interstitial nephritis may occur.

- **Glucocorticoids (prednisolone (40–60 mg/ day):** Hydrocortisone enema, controlled release formulation of budenoside (9 mg/d). They inhibit inflammatory cytokines (TNFα IL-1) and chemokines (IL-δ), gene transcription of nitric oxide synthetase, phospholipase A2, cyclooxygenase 2, NF-κB.

Other corticosteroids used are prednisone, hydrocortisone and budesonide.

- **Purine analogues (Azathioprine and 6-mercaptopurine)**

- **Antitumor neurosis factor (*Infliximab, Adalimumab/Certolizumab*):** Dysregulation of T-helper cell type 1 (TH-1) response occurs in Crohn's disease. Infliximab is a antibody which binds to TNFα, a proinflammatory cytokines and blocks TNF receptors on inflammatory cell surface and suppresses downstream cytokines such as IL-1 and IL-6. Increased risk of lymphoma is there. Infliximab is approved for ulcerative colitis. Adalimumab (fully humanized IgG$_1$ antibody), certolizumab (polyethylene glycolated Fab fragment of humanized anti-TNF) both are given SC. They may produce reactivation of latent infection (tuberculosis, pneumonia), sepsis reactivation of hepatitis B, early mild reaction of fever, headache, urticaria, cardiopulmonary symptoms or delayed serum sickness symptoms like myalgia, arthralgia, jaw tightness, fever, rash, urticaria. The reactions are treated by paracetamol, diphenhydramine and corticosteroid. Multiple sclerosis, lymphoma and worsening of cardiac failure may occur with infliximab.

Anti-integrin therapy

Natalizumab is now approved for Crohn's disease targets α_4 subunits of integrin, not responding to other drugs. No other immunosuppressive should be co-administered because it can cause progressive multifocal leukoencephalopathy.

Purine analogue

Azathioprine and 6-MP given IV who experience frequent induction and remission of ulcerative colitis or Crohn's disease.

Cyclosporine: It induces remmision in ulcerative colitis not responding to corticosteroids.

Methotrexate: It controls relapsing Crohn's diseases not respnoding to corticosteroid.

Antibiotics: Metronidazole, Ciprofloxacin may help Crohn's disease so does some probiotics. These are lyophilized putative beneficial bacteria given orally.

Since ulcerative disease confined to colon whereas Crohn's disease affects both small and larges intestine. Sulfasalazine is ineffective in small bowels Crohn's disease because 5-ASA is liberated in colon.

Drugs used for Irritable Bowel Syndrome (IBS)

Irritable bowel syndrome is due to transient visceral hypersensitivity in genetically predisposed person producing long lasting sensitization of neuronal pain circuit. It is psychosomatic disease with multifactorial cause.

Drugs used for Irritable Bowel Syndrome (IBS)

The features of IBS is pain in abdomen, bloating, and altered bowel habits either constipation or diarrhea. If diarrhea is dominant, drugs used are: (i) **Loperamide** or **Diphenoxylate**, (ii) Kappa antagonist **Fedotozine**, (iii) Reserpine analog—Mebeverine, (iv) $5HT_3$ antagonist—alosterone also reduces pain and (v) Clonidine also reduces distension and increases visceral compliance.

If IBS is dominated by constipation then drugs used are $5HT_4$ agonist Tegaserod and prucalopride. Lubiprostone (it is a chloride channel activator opening in intestine to increase liquid secretion and decrease transit time. Nausea can occur). Antispasmodic anticholinergics like dicyclomine and hyoscyamine are also used for irritable bowel syndrome.

Trimebutine: It has mu agonistic and antimuscarinic effects.

Pinaverium: It is CCB with antimuscarinic effect and otilonium bromide is also CCB with antimuscarinic action. All these drugs are used to treat irritable bowel syndrome.

Linaclotide: This guanylyl cyclase-c agonist activates cystic fibrosis transmembrane conductance regulator (CFTR) increases chloride rich intestinal secretion, also used for IBS. It should not be used in pregnancy.

Other drugs which are used for IBS.

- Dietary restriction and fibre supplementation.
- Tricyclic antidepressant **(Nortriptylin)**.
- SSRI **(Citalopram)**
- Chlordiazepoxide
- Phosphodiesterase - 4 inhibitor as smooth muscle relaxant, *viz.* **droteverine**.

Antidiarrheal Drugs

Diarrhea: Diarrhea is a frequent passage of poorly-formed stool.

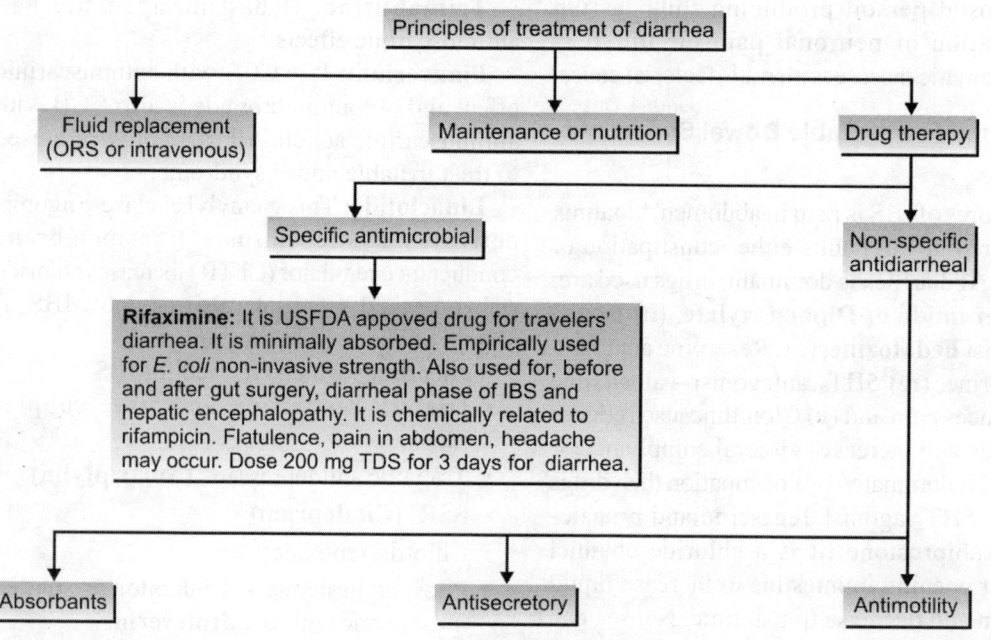

Principles of treatment of diarrhea

- Fluid replacement (ORS or intravenous)
- Maintenance or nutrition
- Drug therapy
  - Specific antimicrobial
  - Non-specific antidiarrheal

Rifaximine: It is USFDA appoved drug for travelers' diarrhea. It is minimally absorbed. Empirically used for *E. coli* non-invasive strength. Also used for, before and after gut surgery, diarrheal phase of IBS and hepatic encephalopathy. It is chemically related to rifampicin. Flatulence, pain in abdomen, headache may occur. Dose 200 mg TDS for 3 days for diarrhea.

Absorbants

Used for IBS and colostomy:
- Ispaghula
- Psyllium
- Methyl cellulose
- Bile salt binding resin (cholestyramine or colestipol) Dose 4–5 gm OD to TDS
- Kaolin (hydrated and aluminum silicate 1–1.5 gm after each loose motion
- Pecting is indigestible carbohydrate of apple pomace, adsorbs bacteria, toxins and fluids. Dose 1–1.5 gm after purge. May be used alone or with pectin.

Antisecretory

Used in ulcerative colitis:
- Sulfasalazine
- Mesalazine (mesacol 400 mg tab, 3 tab QDS)
- Bismuth subsalicylate in traveler's diarrhea
- Atropine

Antimotility

Used after anal surgery:
- Codeine
- Diphenoxylate
- Loperamide

Following antidiarrheal drugs are banned in india:
Kaolin, pectin, activated charcoal, attapulgite (absorbants), neomycin, streptomycin, sulfaguanidine, phthalylsulfathiazole, succinyl-sulfathiazole, diphenoxylate, loperamide, belladona hydroxyquinoline. Antidiarrheal with electrolyte.

A	B	C
Absorbants	**Antisecretory**	**Antimotility**

A — Absorbants

Antimicrobials have no roles in:
- Irritable bowel syndrome
- Coeliac disease
- Tropical Sprue
- Thyrotoxicosis
- Enzyme deficiency of pancreas

B — Antisecretory

- **Octreotide**
- **Somatostatin** analogue in refractory diarrhea of carcinoid tumor, AIDS–This 14aa peptide inhibits secretion of gastrin, glucagon, cholecystokinin, GH, insulin. VIP, 5HT; pancreatic secretion, gallbladder and intestinal motility, portal pressure and secretion of anterior pituitary hormones. **ADR**, flatulence, pain in abdomen, fat-soluble vitamin deficiency. Alters balance of insulin and glucagon, hypothyroidism. Other uses are diarrhea due to VIP-oma, carcinoid, vagotomy and dumping syndrome induced diarrhea, intestinal pseudo-obstruction secondary to scleroderma. Dose 50 μg SC; GI bleeding, pancreatic fistula, pituitary tumour (acromegaly).

Clonidine is indicated for diabetics with chronic diarrhea.

Bile salt binding resins (like cholestyramine, colestipol or colesevelam) decrease diarrhea due to excess bile acids in feces. Fecal impaction, bloating, flatulence, exacerbation of fat, malabsorption, constipation may occur. Colesevelam does not interfere much with drug absorption, but cholestyramine and colestipol do it.
- **Opioid** is used for short-term.
- **Racecadotril** (cadotril 100 mg, 1 cap TDS) converted to thiorphan, an enkephalinase inhibitor preventing degradation of endogenous enkephalin (μ agonist) lowering mucosal cAMP. Nausea, vomiting, drowsiness, flatulence may occur.

Probiotics in diarrheal disease: Gut flora is disturbed in diarrheal disease treated with antibiotics. Microbial cell preparation in live culture or lyophilized powder is used to restore it. Natural curd is a source of lactic acid producing organism. Commercial preparations contain *Lactobacillus* species, *Bifidobacterium*, *Enterococcus* sp; *Streptococcus faecalis, yeasts, Saccharomyces boulardii.* Routine use of probiotics is not justifiable. They rarely cause infection and acidosis.

Drugs for Peptic Ulcer

59

Peptic ulcer is defined as a sharply circumscribed loss of tissues in those parts of gastrointestinal tract, where acid pepsin digestion takes place. In gastric ulcer the acid secretion is generally low, but in duodenal ulcer it is either high or normal. The etiology of peptic ulcer, is multi-factorial, ranges from central versus peripheral causes or offensive versus defensive factors or *H. pylori* infection. The ulcer-prone areas are lower esophagus, stomach (lesser curvature) duodenum and Mickel's diverticulum.

Mechanism of HCl Secretion

The oxyntic cell's mitochondria, rich in zinc-containing enzymes carbonic anhydrase produce carbonic acid which in turn splits into bicarbonate HCO_3^- and hydrogen ion H^+ passes towards secretory surface and produce hydrochloric acid (HCl) combining with chloride Cl^-, HCO_3^- passes towards mucosal surface, since it is impervious to secretory surface. (Fig. 59.1)

Principles of Treatment

Decrease in offensive factors (acid, pepsin, NSAID, treat *H. pylori*) and increase in mucosal resistance.

When NSAIDs are administered by oral route the base of the ulcer lies generally on mucosal surface, but when administered by parenteral route the base of peptic ulcer lies on serosal surface (Figs 59.1 and 59.2).

Approaches for Treatment

a. Neutralization of gastric acid (antacids)

- **Local:** Magnesium hydroxide, magnesium carbonate, magnesium trisilicate, aluminium hydroxide, magaldrate, calcium carbonate.

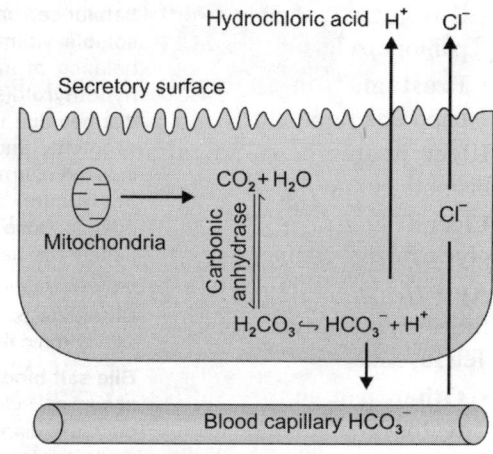

Fig. 59.1: Mechanism of secretion of hydrochloric acid

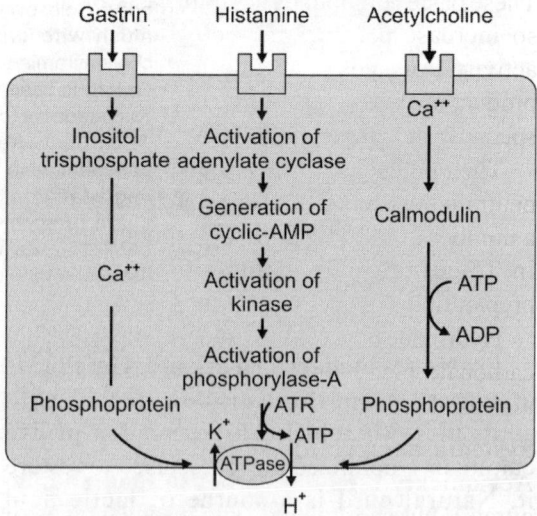

AMP=Adenosine monophosphate; ADP=Adenosine diphosphate; ATP=Adenosine triphosphate

Fig. 59.2: Cellular events of gastric acid

- **Systemic:** Sodium bicarbonate, sodium citrate.

b. Reduction of gastric acid secretion

- **Reducing gastrin secretion:** Antagonist by proglumide 800–1200 mg/day, but costly. Oxethazaine inhibits gastrin release.
- **H$_2$ antihistaminicis:** Cimetidine, ranitidine, famotidine, roxatidine, nizatidine, loxatidine.
- **Anticholinergic:** Propantheline, oxyphenonium, doxepin, pirenzapine.
- **Proton pump inhibitor:** Omeprazole, its S isomers (esomeprazole) lansoprazole, pantoprazole, rabeprazole, *etc.*
- **Prostaglandin analogue:** Misoprostol, enprostil, rioprostil.

c. Ulcer protectives: Sucralfate, colloidal bismuth citrate

d. Ulcer healing drugs: Carbenoxolone sodium, glycyrrhizinized liquorice

e. Anti-*H. pylori* drugs: Amoxycillin, clarithoromycin, Metronidazole, Tinidazole, Tetracycline

- **Other acid suppressants and cytoprotectors:** Rebamipide, ecabet.

Antacids or Acid Neutralizers

These basic compounds neutralize gastric acids, so increase pH and indirectly reduce peptic activity. Antacids *per se* do not decrease acid production, but by raising pH they release gastrin specially in patients of duodenal ulcer.

Their potencies are measured in terms of acid neutralizing capacity (ANC) which is defined as a number of mEq of 1N HCl is brought pH 3.5, in 15 minutes by a unit dose of antacid preparation.

Hydroxide bases are commonly employed, but carbonate, bicarbonate, citrate and trisilicates are also used.

Systemic antacids

Act quickly (sodium carbonate and sodium citrate), but short acting. The disadvantages of systemic antacids are:

- They produce alkalosis, particularly in renal diseases.
- Increase Na load which may be deleterious to hypertension and CCF patients.

- Stomach may distend to produce discomfort by CO_2 produced by it. Used to alkalise urine. Sodium citrate is similar to Na bicarbonate.

Non-systemic antacids

Poorly basic compounds react in stomach forming corresponding chloride salts which react with intestinal bicarbonate.

Magnesium salt

Hydroxide (milk of magnesia) efficious antacids with mild rebound acidity.

Magnesium carbonate

Reacts with HCl slowly, CO_2 evolved is gradual.

Magnesium trisilicate

Has low solubility, reactivity, silica produced by reaction with HCl is gelatinous and adsorbs pepsin to protect ulcer base. May produce problem in renal insufficient patient. Releases cholecystokinin and imbibes water and acts as a osmotic purgative.

Aluminum hydroxide gel (Aludrox tabs, suspension): Weak, slowly reacting antacid, slowly polymerize on keeping, so loses acid neutralizing capacity. Since Al relaxes smooth muscle and its astringent action causes constipation, may cause intestinal blockage, if given in large doses. It decreases peptic activity. Binds phosphate in intestine to prevent its absorptions, causing hypophosphatemia and osteomalacia, but may be used in kidney phosphate stones.

Magaldrate (PH$_4$, Ulgel): It is a hydrated complex of hydroxymagnesium aluminate. Initially reacts with acid to produce $Al(OH)_3$ which reacts slowly.

Calcium carbonate

Potent, rapidly acting causing distension of stomach, Ca^{2+} absorbed may produce hypercalcemia, hypercalciuria, alkalosis renal stone.

Milk alkali syndrome

Characterized by headache, anorexia, weakness, abdominal discomfort, renal stones, alkalosis due to large quantity of milk and $CaCO_3$ or $NaHCO_3$

used to treat peptic ulcer in the past. It is rarely seen nowadays.

Therapeutic Uses of Antacids

- Duodenal ulcer
- Reflux esophagitis
- Prophylaxis for aspiration pneumonia during endoscopic, emergency, comatose patient (stress ulcer), surgery.
- In pancreatitis
- $Al(OH)_3$ used at times as antidiarrheal agent.

Reduction of Gastric Acid Secretion

No drug available effective against hormone gastrin. (Proglumide is a gastrin antagonist, but not used because cheaper drugs are available.)

H_2 antagonist: Cimetidine, ranitidine, nizatidine and roxatidine are competitive. Competitive noncompetitive for famotitine, non-competitive with loxatidine are presently available in market.

H_2 blockers reduce gastric secretion in all phases (basal, psychoneurogenic, gastric) and to all stimuli (ACh, gastrin, insulins, alcohol, food) acid output, volume, pepsin and intrinsic factor secretion (though B_{12} deficiency does not occur). They do not alter esophageal sphincter tone or esophageal motility.

Cimetidine is orally absorbed, crosses placenta and milk, but penetration in brain is poor. Excreted in urine and bile unchanged or oxidized.

Adversed effects of cimetidine: Generally well-tolerated, occasionally produce headache, dizziness, dry mouth, confusion, hallucination, delirium. Bolus IV can release histamine. It causes bradycardia, arrhythmia and cardiac arrest. It has got antiandrogenic effect (by displacing dihydrotestosterone from cytoplasmic receptor), inhibits degradation of estradiol in liver and increases prolactin level, decreases sperm count temporarily and impotence. High dose may produce gynecomastia. Rise in aminotransferase, fever, neutropenia. Inhibits cytochrome P450 and metabolism of many drugs.

Use of H_2 antagonist

- Duodenal ulcer

- Gastric ulcer
- Stress induced ulcer
- Zollinger-Ellison syndrome
- Gastroesophageal reflux
- Prophylaxis to aspiration pneumonia
- To treat urticaria with H_1 blockers.

Ranitidine (zinetac 150, 300, rantec 150, 300 50 mg/2 mL): 5 times potent to cimetidine, longer acting, no antiandrogenic effect, does not inhibit hepatic metabolism of other drugs. Adverse effects are comparatively less.

Famotidine

8 times more potent to ranitidine and longer acting. Adverse effects are less because of higher potency and long acting, suitable for ZE syndrome (topcid, 20, 40; facid 20, 40 20 mg/2 mL).

Roxatidine (rotane 75 and 150 mg SR)

Long acting and two times potent to ranitidine. No antiandrogenic effect or enzyme inhibition property.

Nizatidine

Higher oral bioavailability, plasma half-life 1–1.5 hours. Dose 300 mg at bedtime.

Loxatidine

Powerful non-competitive H_2 antagonist.

Anticholinergics

Non-selective antimuscarinics (atropine, propantheline, oxyphenonium) produce side effects. The newer M1 receptor blockers pirenzepine and telenzepine (more potent than former) used in flatulent dyspepsia. Antiulcer dose 50 mg BD or TDS for pirenzepine.

Trimipramine and doxepin are tricyclic antidepressants with anticholinergic properties and weak proton pump inhibition action, reduce gastric acid secretion and promote ulcer healing.

Proton Pump Inhibitors—Omeprazole (Omez 20)

It is substituted by benzimidazole. Proton pump inhibitors after absorption accumulate in parietal cell of stomach. Substituted benzimidazole is a hit and run drug inhibits the final step of gastric acid secretion at pH less than 5. Charged cationic form (sulfenic acid and sulfenamide configuration) reacts covalently with the SH group of H^+/K^+-ATPase enzyme and inhibits it irreversibly. Acid secretion starts when new H^+/K^+-ATPase molecules are synthesized. It is orally absorbed, highly protein-bound, metabolized in liver and metabolites are excerted with urine. No dose adjustment required for elderly and renal disease. Secretion resumes gradually from 3–5 days after stopping of the drug. Long lasting suppression may produce compensatory hypergastrinemia and proliferation of parietal cells and gastric carcinoid tumors in rats. To prevent the degradation of PPI in acidic pH of stomach, it is supplied as:

- Enteric coated tablets with gelatin capsules
- Enteric coated granules or tablets
- Powdered drug with sodium bicarbonate.

Uses of Omeprazole or PPI

- Peptic ulcer (now an integral component of *H. pylori* therapy)
- Gastroesophageal refulx disease (GERD)
- Zollinger-Ellison syndrome
- Other hypersecretory states like mastocytosis endocrine adenoma.

Adverse effects are rare like nausea, loose motion, rash, leukopenia, atropic gastritis on prolong use.

It increases level of diazepam, phenytoin and warfarin by inhibiting their oxidation.

Lansoprazole (lan 30, lanzol 30): Faster, more potent, more bioavailable; but reversible blocker of H^+/K^+-ATPase. Other effects are similar to omeprazole.

Pantoprazole (Pantocid/Panotdac 40 mg): Risk of drug interactions is less, because it has lower affinity for cytochrome P450 compared to omerprazole and lansoprazole. Recently **rabeprazole** (Rezo) and **esomeprazole** have been marketed with some pharmacokinetic superiorities. S-enantiomer of omeprazole (esomeprazole) and S-pantoprazole are more potent. These are examples of me-too drugs, *i.e.* drugs with same function with very little structural difference produced by manufactures. Tenatoprazole is a new PPI.

Prostaglandin analogues

Promote mucus secretion, HCO_3 secretion, inhibit acid and gastric secretion and strengthen mucosa which is buffered by HCO_3, maintain circulation of gastric and duodenal region prone to ulcer. Since natural PGs have short t/2, stable PGs are developed. Misoprostol (800 µg/ day), enprostil (70–140 µg/day), rioprostil (600 µg/ day) are given in 2–4 divided doses, heals duodenal ulcer in 4–8 weeks. Major adverse effects are diarrhea, abdominal cramps, uterine bleeding, abortion and acceptability of patient is poor because they are poor reliever of ulcer pain.

Ulcer Protectives

a. **Sucralfate (ulcerfate 1 gm tab)**

Basic aluminum salt of sulfated sucrose, at pH < 4 produces gel-like consistency and strongly adheres to ulcer base and remains there for more than 6 hours. Precipitates surface protein and acts as physical barrier to acid, pepsin and bile. Dietary protein gets deposited producing another layer. It has no antacid property. It is minimally absorbed from GIT used to treat duodenal, gastric ulcer specially who continue with their smoking habits. Recently, it has been trialed to treat stomatitis ulcer with its suspension in glycerol. Dose 1 gm, one hour before 3 major meals for 4–8 weeks. Other uses are bile reflux, gastritis, phosphate stone of kidney. It interferes with the absorption of many drugs (*viz.* tetracycline fluoroquinolone, phenyotins, *etc.*)

b. **Colloidal bismuth subcitrate (trymo, pylocid, 120 mg)**

Precipitates at pH < 5. Heals ulcer at 8 weeks almost 80%. It increases secretion of mucus and bicarbonate probably through PGE_2 production, coats over ulcer (forms glycoprotein bicomplex) acting as diffusion barrier. Separate *H. pylori* from mucosa and kills them, reduces pepsin output by adsorption. Ulcer heals with lower relapse rate.

Not absorbed. **Side effects**—headache, dizziness, osteodystrophy, encephalopathy due to bismuth toxicity. Black stool, and black colored denture and tongue may occur. Milk and antacids should not be given simultaneously.

Ulcer Healers

Carbenoxolone sodium (Gastric ulcer 50 mg caps): 100 mg TDS for 4–6 weeks obtained from liquorice has been shown to enhance glycoprotein synthesis. Prolongs life span of gastric epithelium. Orally completely absorbed, highly protein-bound. It exerts mineralocorticoid action leading to Na^+ retention and K^+ excretion. GTT may be altered, edema and rise of BP may occur. Not used much because of side effects.

Glycyrrhizinate liquorice (Degliq 0.4 gm cap): 1–2 caps TDS. Less effective than carbenoxolone. It is free of Na and H_2O retaining effect.

Anti-*Helicobacter pylori* Drug

H. pylori attaches to the surface epithelium underneath the mucus, with high urease activity producing ammonia, maintaining neutral environment around bacteria and promotes back diffusion of H^+ ions causing chronic gastritis, dyspepsia, peptic ulcer, gastric carcinoma, lymphoma. Antibacterials found effective against *H. pylori* are Amoxycillin, Clarithromcyin, Tetracycline, Metronidazole and Tinidazole.

Some Anti-*Helicobacter pylori* Regimens

Two week regimes (mg)
- Amoxycillin 750 BD/Clarithromycin 500 BD + Omeprazole 40 mg OD.
- Amoxycillin 500 TDS/Tetracycline 500 QDS + Metronidazole 400 QDS/Tinidazole 500 BD + Bismuth 120 mg QDS.
- Amoxycillin 750 TDS + Metronidazole 500 TDS + Ranitidine 300 OD.

One week regimes (mg)
- Amoxycillin 500 TDS/Clarithromycin 250 BD + Metronidazole 400 TDS/Tinidazole 500 BD + Omeprazole 20 BD

- Amoxycillin 500 TDS + Clarithromycin 250 TDS + Omeprazole 20 BD

Miscellaneous acid suppressants and cytoprotectants

Rebamipide: Used in some parts of Asia, increases PG generation and by scavenging reactive oxygen.

Ecabet: Increases PGE_2 and PGI_2 formation used mostly in Japan.

Indications of operations in peptic ulcer disease

- Intractable recurrent pain with loss of work especially after previous hemorrhage.
- Complications of ulcers.
- Ulcer present for 5 years.

Nowadays incidence of peptic ulcer treated with operation has declined, but incidence of its complication has increased due to inadequate treatment by poor motivation to complete therapy.

Clinically antiulcer drugs can be evaulated by following criteria

- Accelerate healing
- Reduce pain of ulcer
- Prevent complication
- Prevent recurrence of ulcer
- Avoid side effects of ulcer

Criteria for ideal peptic ulcer drugs

- Accelerate healing of ulcer
- Reduce pain of ulcer
- Prevent complications of ulcer
- Result in low relapse rate when discontinued
- Produce no side effect
- Is based on good scientific program and its mechanism of action known
- Facilitate patient compliance and their mode and schedule of intake be simple
- Effective against both gastric and duodenal ulcers
- Inexpensive.

NB: New drug: Potassium competitive acid blocker, **Revaprazan** inhibits H^+/K^+-ATPase.

Barry J Marshall and J Robin Warren (2005) got Nobel Prize for discovering *H. pylori*.

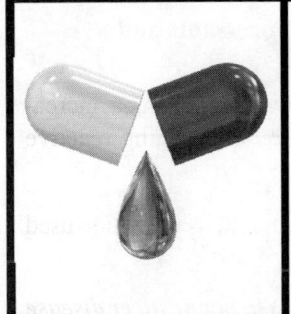
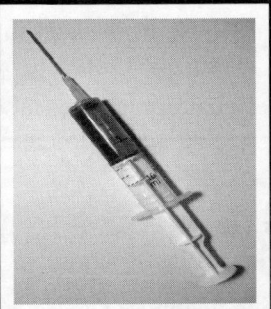
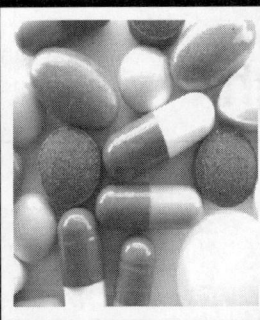
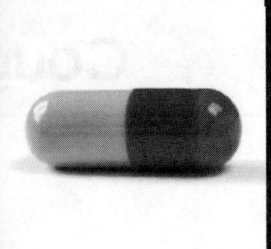

SECTION 7

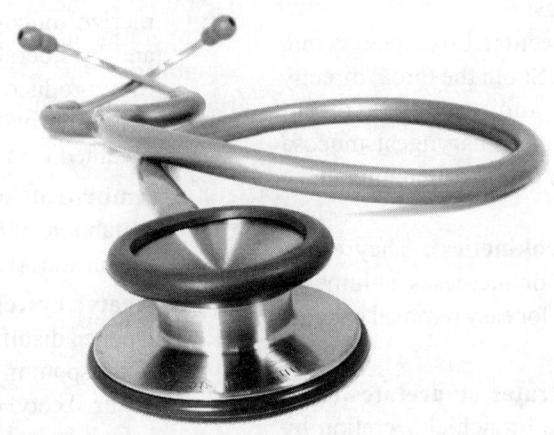

RESPIRATORY SYSTEM

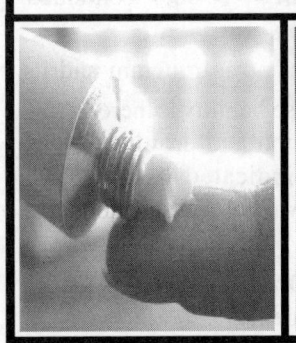
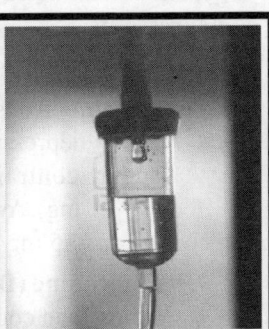
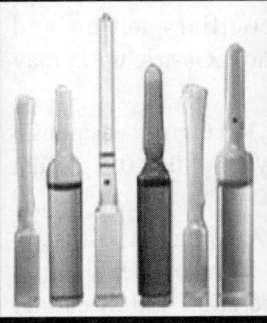
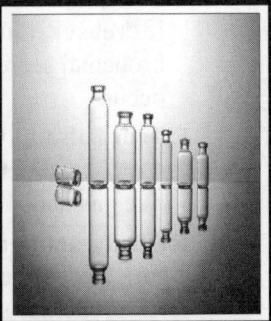

60

Cough

Cough is a protective reflex for expulsion of respiratory secretion and foreign particles from the air passage. Productive cough drains out the air passage, but unproductive cough should be suppressed. Cough may be treated as symptom with the following drugs:

1. **Pharyngeal demulcents:** Lozenges, syrup, glycerine, liquorice. Sooth the throat directly or by salivation and reduce afferent impulses from irritated pharyngeal mucosa and give relief of dry cough originating in the throat.

2. **Expectorants (mucokinetics):** They either decreases viscosity or increases volume of respiratory secretion for easy removal by cilia.

   A. **Directly acting**
   - **Na and K citrates or acetates** (0.3–1 gm) increase bronchial secretion by salt action.
   - **Potassium iodide** (0.2–0.3 gm) secreted by bronchial glands and irritate them to increase their secretion. Goiter may occur.
   - **Guaiphenesin** (Guaiacol 100–200 mg) increases mucociliary action and bronchial secretion. Gastric upset may occur.
   - **Tolu balsam** (0.3–0.6 gm); **Vasaka** 2–4 mL, **terpin hydrate** 0.1–0.3 gm act like guaiacol.

   B. **Reflexly acting:** Ammonium salt (0.3–1 gm); Ipecac (0.6–1.8 mL) reflexly stimulates bronchial secretion and sweating. Used in subemetic doses.

Mucolytic
- **Bromhexine** (8 mg TDS, 4 mg BD for children 1–5 years and 4 mg TDS for above 5 years).
- **Mucolytic and mucokinetic:** Depolymerize mucopolysaccharides directly and by liberating lysosomal enzymes. May produce rhinorrhea, lacrymation. It is a derivative of alkaloid vasicine obtained from *Adhatoda vasica*.
- **Ambroxol (ambril 30 mg tab)** is a metabolite of bromohexine with similar action and ADR. Dose 15–30 mg TDS.
- **Acetyl cysteine and carbocisteine:** Opened disulfide bonds in mucoprotein of the sputum. GI irritation and rash may occur. Acetyl cysteine is given directly into respiratory tract by aerosol in tracheostomy patient.
- **Carbocisteine:** Used orally 250–750 mg TDS with some benefits in chronic bronchitis patient.

3. **Antitussives acting on cough center as depressants**

   A. **Opioids**
   - **Codeine:** Abuse liability is there, respiratory depression and drowsiness can occur, contraindicated in asthmatic (10–30 mg). Available as codeine 15 mg tab and 15 mg/5 mL liquid.
   - **Pholcodine (Dose 10–15 mg)** is longer acting than codeine.
   - **Ethylmorphine (Dose 10–15 mg)**

- **Morphine** 2–4 mg IM rarely used as antitussive.

B. **Non-opioids**
- **Noscapine** useful for spasmodic cough, 15–30 mg (coscopin 7 mg/5 mL or coscotab 25 mg tab). No narcotic, analgesic and dependence potential, headache; nausea can occur. Releases histamine which can produce asthma.

- **Dextromethorphan (10–20 mg)** does not depress muociliary function. Nausea, dizziness and ataxia can occur.

- **Carbetapentane (30 mg TDS)** is an antitussive, anticholinergic, weak local anesthetic.

- **Oxeladin (Pectamol 10–30 mg)** is cough depressive, centrally acting.

- **Chlophedianol (detigon 20–40 mg)** with less effects, slow and longer acting.

- **Pipazethate (selvigon 40 mg/mL):** Phenothiazine with antitussive. Dose 40–80 mg.

C. **Antihistaminics** are promoted to treat allergic cough except in asthmatics.

Chlorpheniramine 2 mg TDS, diphenhydramine 15–25 mg TDS, promethazine 15–30 mg TDS.

Fixed drug combinations with antihistaminics, bronchodilator and antitussives are present in Indian market, but those are banned.

Aromatic chest rub has no benefit in pathological cough.

61

Therapeutic Gases

Oxygen, carbon dioxide and helium (an inert gas) have therapeutic utilities apart from anesthetic gases. Oxygen when inspired (air contains 21% oxygen) carried with hemoglobin mainly and with physical solution in plasma (can be increased by increase in ambient pressure). Oxygen delivery decreases globally when cardiac output falls or in local areas when regional blood flow is obstructed or compromised. Hypoxia occurs when oxygen transport from capillaries to tissues is decreased as in cyanide poisoning.

OXYGEN

Causes of Oxygen Deprivation

- Low inspired oxygen
- Increase in diffusion barrier
- Hypoventilation
- Ventilation perfusion mismatch
- Venous admixture or shunt

It is monitored physically by examining cyanosis, arterial oxygen saturation by transcutaneous pulse oximetry. It measures Hb saturation not PO_2.

Effects of Oxygen Administration

- **Ventilation:** Initially decreases then stimulates ventilation. Decreases sensitivity of respiratory center to carbon dioxide.
- **CVS:** Heart rate decreases, cardiac output decreases, dilates pulmonary vessels; but coronary and cerebral blood flow are reduced. Does not modify BP significantly.

- **Nitrogen concentration:** Reduces partial pressure of nitrogen in alveoli, subsequently it is eliminated from body cavities *via* alveoli. Inhaled oxygen does not produce detectable change in its consumption, CO_2 production or glucose utilization and respiratory quotient.

Methods of Administration of Oxygen

It may be delivered by: (i) Low flow or (ii) high flow system. It is delivered by inhalation except during extracorporeal ciruclation, it is dissolved in circulating blood.

Ventimask available in 3 models delivers 24%, 28% to 35% of oxygen. Actual delivered oxygen depends on rate, tidal volume, inspiratory flow, *i.e.* on ventilators pattern.

- Through cannula, catheter or ventimask operates thorugh Bernoulli's principle, achieves steady concentration. Less than 60% in inspired air. 1–6 L/minute ensures 24–44% of inspired oxygen. Larger flow is wastage.
- Aims to ensure highest concentration of oxygen in inspired air in high altitude pulmonary edema, bronchial asthma given by closely fitting aeronasal mask with a non-return valve and either a reservoir bag or a demand valve on oxygen supply. It should be humidified before administration because oxygen is a respiratory irritant.

Oxygen toxicity: Probably due to production of H_2O_2, reactive agents like superoxide anion, singlet oxygen, hydroxyl radical which attack and damage lipid and protein macromolecules of biological membrane. Superoxide dismutase, glutathione peroxidase and catalase to scavenge toxic oxygen by-products. First starts in lungs with increased capillary permeability and decreases lung function.

Adverse Effects of Oxygen Therapy

- **Respiratory tract:** Damages pulmonary epithelium, inactivates surfactants producing atelectasis and respiratory distress.
- **CNS:** Paresthesia, mental disturbances, loss of consciousness, convulsion, twitching.
- **Carbon dioxide narcosis:** Clinical manifestations are sweating, raised intracranial pressure, twitching, drowsiness, papilledema and convulsion. It occurs with COPD, status asthmaticus, *etc*. Group of patients where respiration maintained by hypoxemic drive and administration of oxygen will reduce ventilation.
- **Retrolental fibroplasia** (caused by hyperbaric oxygen) produces this occlusal proliferative retinal disease.
- Potential fire hazard.

Preparations

Oxygen IP dispensed in compressed state in cylinders painted black with white shoulders. Oxygen mixed with carbon dioxide cylinders, are black having gray and white quarterings on neck and shoulder.

Therapeutic Uses of Oxygen

- *Hypoxia* (which not only stops machinery but also wrecks the machine).

Bowel distension from ileus or obstruction
- Embolism
- Pneumothorax
- To reduce partial pressure of inert gas

Hyperbaric oxygen therapy has two components, i.e.
- Increased hydrostatic pressure and
- Increased oxygen pressure

As diluent of anesthetic gas
Hyperbaric oxygen is administered at higher than atmosphere pressure and is used for:

- Respiratory distress of newborn
- Carbon monoxide poisoning
- Decompression sickness
- Anerobic infection *(Cl. welchii)*
- Aerobic infection *(Pseudomonas* in burn or refractory chronic osteomyelitis)
- Circulatory disturbances (myocardial infarction, shock, *etc.*)
- Surgery (open heart, organ transplantation, *etc.*)
- Malignancies to render them sensitive to radiotherapy.

CARBON DIOXIDE

It is produced in body during tissue and food metabolism, has marked effects on CNS, respiration and circulation.

Effects of Carbon Dioxide Inhalation

It is rapid, potent stimulus of ventilation. Increases rate and tidal volume of respiration by its direct action, chemical drive and stimulation of peripheral arterial chemoreceptor.

Circulation: Decreases heart rate, force of contraction, relaxes vascular smooth muscle, causing vasodilatation. The direct circulatory effects are antagonized by sympathetic activation induced by it. Cerebral and coronary vessels, splanchnic and skeletal muscle's blood vessels dilate. It is most potent cerebral vasodilator.

CNS: Stimulates cerebral cortex and reduces seizure threshold, higher concentration depresses the cortex and stimulates subcortical areas with cortical projection.

Adverse effects: Headache, dizziness, confusion, palpitation, dyspnea, rise in BP, loss of consciousness (if gas exceeds 10%).

Preparation

- Carbon dioxide IP marketed in steel cylinders painted gray in liquid form at 58 to 72 atmospheric pressures.
- Carbogen has 5–10% carbon dioxide and rest is oxygen.

- Solid carbon dioxides
  - (a) Dry ice   (b) CO_2 snow

Therapeutic uses of carbon dioxide

1. Respiratory depression (5–10% CO_2 is used)
2. **CO poisoning:** CO_2 is used with oxygen to stimulate respiration and wash out CO.
3. **Hiccup:** 10–25% CO_2 in intractable hiccup
4. In anxiety neurosis and personality maladjustment (30% CO_2 with 70% oxygen)
5. CO_2 snow is used locally to destroy **warts, naevi** with minimal scaring and pain, the adjacent tissue should be covered with paraffin for protection.
6. Miscellaneous
   - Increases speed of induction and emergence of anesthesia.
   - To prevent postoperative atelectases
   - To terminate petit mal seizure
   - Supersaturated solution of CO_2 is used as mild rubefacient.
   - Carminatives
   - To mask unpleasant taste of saline purgative.
7. Insufflation during endoscopy because it is soluble and non-inflammable.
8. Open heart surgery
9. To do cardiopulmonary bypass. Extracorporeal membrane oxygenation (ECMO). To adjust pH when patient is cooled for bypass.

Helium

This inert gas has low density, low solubility and high thermal conductivity supplied in brown cylinder and used:

- As an intermittent inhalation to treat prolong asthma resistant to other drugs because it lowers density and minimizes breathing efforts.
- For pulmonary function testing
- As a level in imaging studies
- For Caisson's disease
- As a non-inflammable diluent to oxygen in open heart surgery anesthesia

- To treat laryngeal spasm and edema
- During laser surgery on the airway. (It takes away heat from the point of contact of laser because of its high thermal conductivity.)
- As a laser polarized helium and is used as a contrast agent for pulmonary magnetic resonance imaging. It is a costly gas.

NITRIC OXIDE

It is a free radical gas with endogenous signaling capacity. It is long-known as an air pollutant and potential toxicity. NO endogenously produced from L-arginine by enzyme, NO synthetase. In vessel, it causes vasodilatation in response to stress or vasodilator. It inhibits platelet aggregation, adhesion. Impaired NO production causes atherosclerosis, hypertension, spasm of coronary and cerebral vessels. It acts as a mediator in nerve. It is implicated to mediate control of nociceptive pathways, as mediator of inflammation, if overproduced. It causes macrophage-induced cytotoxicity.

Therapeutic uses

- To dilate pulmonary vasculature with minimal cardiovascular effect.

Diagnostic uses

- In cardiac catheterization.
- To determine diffusion capcacity across alveolar-capillary unit.
- To assess severity of asthma and RTI by measuring exhaled NO.
- It should be withdrawn gradually because sudden discontinuation may cause pulmonary artery hypertension.
- It is administered as 50 ppm or 50 parts per billion. Higher concentraion is toxic.

NO toxicity

Partly it is due to its oxidation product NO_2.
- Methemoglobinemia
- Impairs left ventricular performace by dilating pulmonary circulation.

Precautions

- Continuous NO and NO_2 measurements.

- Use certified cylinders of NO.
- Measure methemoglobin lebel.
- Give lowest NO for therapeutic effect.

Methods to administer: By close fitting mask, nasal prong administration for pulmonary hypertension, it should be withdrawn gradually to avoid rebound pulmonary artery hypertension.

Some toxic gases
- Carbon monoxide (CO)
- Sulfur dioxide (SO_2)
- Ozone (O_3), but nowadays it is used for low back pain due to disk prolapse.
- Nitrogen dioxide (NO_2)
- Cyanide.

62

Bronchial Asthma

The word asthma is derived from the Greek verb *aazein* meaning to pant, to exhale with the open mouth, clinically characterized by increased responsiveness of tracheobronchial tree to a variety of stimuli, resulting in variable airway obstruction. Pathologically, asthma is a disease of bronchial smooth muscle contraction, mucosal edema, inflammation and viscid mucous secretion and all leading to airflow obstruction.

Four groups of drugs are mainly used for asthma. They are: (a) Sympathomimetic amines,

(b) anticholinergics, (c) xanthine derivatives and (d) anti-inflammatory corticosteroids.

Sympathomimetic amines

β_2 receptors relax the bronchial smooth muscle by virtue of their stimulation of adenyl cyclase and increase cyclic-AMP within the smooth muscle of bronchus, which in turn sequesters Ca^{2+} of smooth muscle of bronchus and makes it relaxed. The indirectly acting sympathomimetic release of adrenaline from nerve terminals, runs

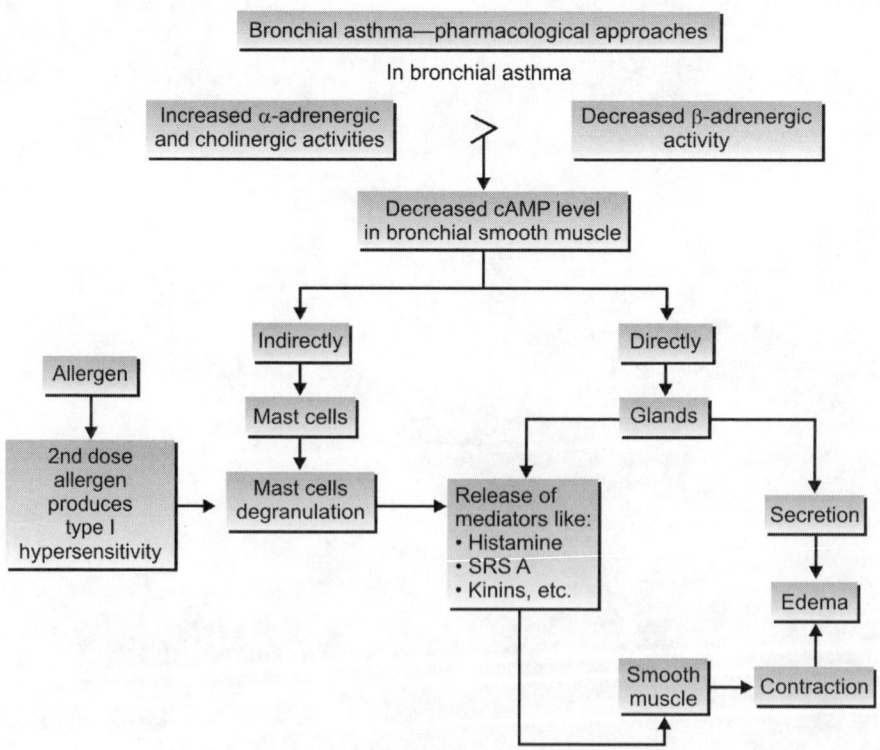

Table 62.1: Some sympathomimetics with doses and route or administration

Sl. no.	Drugs with dose	Routes	Acts on	Remarks
1.	Adrenaline 0.2 to 0.5 mL of 1:1000 solution	SC; IM (in oil)	α and β_1 and β_2	Needle should not be in vein. It should not be used if its color is changed.
2.	Ephedrine 30 mg at bedtime	Oral	α and β_1 and β_2	–
3.	Isoprenaline 0.4–0.8 mg inhalation, 10–20 mg SL or 1–2 mg IM	Sublingual; inhalation IM	–	Sudden death and cardiac arrhythmia may occur.
4.	Orciprenaline (Alupent) Oral; SC or IM inhalation. Dose 20 mg oral, 0.5–1 mg IM or SC, 0.65–1.3 mg by inhalation	β_2	–	Not a substrate for COMT so orally effective.
5.	Terbutaline (Bricarex) 5 mg oral 0.25 mg SC; 250 µg by inhalation	Oral; IV inhalation	β_2	–
6.	Salbutamol (Asthalin). Dose 2–4 mg oral, 0.25–0.05 mg IM or SC,100–200 µg by inhalation	Oral; IV inhalation	β_2	Palpitation, nervousness, restlessness, ankle edema may occur. Undergoes presystemic metabolism in gut wall.
7.	Isoetharine 1% soluble	Inhalation	β	(Not available in India)
8.	Feneletrol	Oral; inhalation	β	(Not available in India)
9.	Rimiterol	Inhalation	β_2	(Not available in India)
10.	Salmeterol (Serobid) 25 µg by metered dose 2 puff BD It is partial B_2 agonist	Inhalation; long acting used for nocturnal asthma	β_2	–
11.	Formoterol 12–24 µg BD, 12 µg/unit inhalant power 1% solution for inhalation. It is full agonist.	Inhalation	β_2	–
12.	Bambuterol 10–20 mg OD Not yet approved in USA	Orally	β_2	Prodrug of terbutaline. Hydrolyzed by pseudocholinesterase in lung and plasma.

the risk of tachyphylaxis and it should not be used with other directly acting sympathomimetic because it will potentiate the action of other sympathomimetics (like increasing pulse rate and BP). Sympathomimetics by increasing cAMP in mast cells, decrease antigen-antibody induced mediator release. Salmeterol and formoterol are called long acting Beta agonist (LABA). Ultralong acting Beta agonists are indacaterol. Olodaterol vilanterol. These drugs are approved for COPD and along with corticosteroid in bronchial asthma.

Anticholinergics

Atropine methonitrate, ipratropium bromide, tritropium bromide useful in refractory bronchial asthma, but cannot be used in glaucoma and prostate hypertrophy patients. New drug in this group is glycopyrolate used in inhalation for COPD. Glycopyrolate is discussed with anticholinergic drugs.

Xanthine Derivatives

- Inhibit phosphodiesterase enzymes leading to intracellular accumulation of cAMP, which sequesters intracellular calcium to relax bronchial smooth muscle.
- Inhibit catechol-orthomethyltransferase (COMT) responsible for destruction of intrinsically released adrenaline and increasing its titer at syno-effector junction.
- Releases catecholamine from adrenal medulla, may be mediated by cAMP.
- Antagonizes adenosine receptors.
- Enhances histone deacetylation. Histone acetylation is necessary for activation of inflammatory gene transcription.
- Low dose theophylline restores responsiveness of corticosteroids. Commonly used xanthines are theophylline and aminophylline.
- Doxophylin (Oxypur) 400 mg OD or BD for children 12 mg/kg.

Pentoxyphyllin is a PDE inhibitor used for intermittent claudication.

Reflumilast is PDE$_4$ inhibitor approved for COPD but not used for bronchial asthma.

Conditions increasing theophylline levels are: Age more than 50, obesity, liver disease, CCF, COPD, acute viral infection, high carbohydrate low protein diet, cimetidine, allopurinol, erythromycin, ciprofloxacin, influenza virus vaccines.

Conditions decreasing theophylline level: Young age, cigarette smoking, low carbohydrate high protein diet, phenytoin, phenobarbitone.

Pharmacokinetics: Theophylline is orally absorbed and distributed in all tissues, crosses placenta, secreted in milk, 50% protein-bound, metabolized by demethylation and oxidation, 10% unchanged excreted in urine.

Preparation: Theophylline (anhydrous) 100–300 mg TDS, 15 mg /kg/day; aminophylline 100–200 mg orally or, IV slowly.

Therapeutic use: Bronchial asthma, COPD and apnea in premature infant.

To reduce the toxicities of PDE4 keeping therapeutic efficiency in different isoforms of PDE4 are developed, *viz.* **roflumilast, cilomilast, tofimilast** which are used for COPD, but withdrawn after clinical trials because of toxicities except roflumilast.

Anti-inflammatory Corticosteroids

The mechanism of action of corticosteroids in bronchial asthma:
- It increases β-adrenergic receptors.
- It causes eosinopenia, basopenia and neutropenia.
- Reduces inflammation.
- Reduces IgE synthesis.
- Stabilizes mast cell.
- Inhibits histamine release.
- Releases adrenaline from adrenal medulla *via* portal system.
- Inhibits mucus secretion.
- Induces vasoconstriction.

Orally administered corticosteroids in order of increasing potency are as follows:

Cortisone > Hydrocortisone > Prednisone > Prednisolone > Methyl prednisolone > Triamcinolone > Dexamethasone > Betamethasone.

Systemic corticosteroid therapy is given in two situations: (1) Severe asthma, (2) status asthmaticus and acute exacerbation of asthma. They should be tapered gradually.

Side effects
- Peptic ulcer
- Hypertension
- Diabetes mellitus
- Latent tuberculosis may flare up.

Inhaled Steroids

These are steroids with topical action and low systemic activity due to poor absorption and marked first pass metabolism. Beclomethasone and budesonide are marketed in India. They should be prescribed when more than three β agonists puff and sodium cromoglycate are ineffective.

The inhaled steroid: (i) Decreases bronchial hyperactivity and increases peak expiratory flow rate; (ii) prevents episodic asthma and reduce need for β agonist inhalation. They are not useful in acute attack or status asthmaticus. Peak effects are seen after 4–7 days.

Horse voice, dysphonia, sore throat, **candidiasis** can occur as side effects. By use of spacer, gargle after every dose (wash off drug deposited) for prevention and treat with topical nystatin. Mucosal damage and chest infection are not increased by inhaled steroid on prolong use.

Preparations Available

Beclomethasone dipropionate 50, 100 and 200 μg per metered dose inhaler or 100–200 μg powder per rotacap. Intranasal spray 50 μg in each nostril BD or TDS to treat perennial rhinitis.

Budesonide: Non-halogenated steroid with high topical activity; dose 200–400 microgram BD-QD by inhalation in asthma, 200–400 μg/day by intranasal spray for allergic rhinitis (Pulmicort or Budecort 100 μg/metered dose inhalation and Rhinocort 50 μg/metered dose nasal spray).

Flunisolide, triamcinolone acetonide, fluticasone propionate are other inhalation steroids. Fluticasone propionate is devoid of systemic action. Flunisolide used for seasonal and perennial rhinitis. **Ciclesonide** 80–160 μg by inhalation. It is a prodrug released after cleaved by bronchial esterase. In plasma it is protein-bound. Dose 80–160 μg by inhalation.

SOME INHALED CORTICOSTEROIDS

- Fluticasone (Flovent) 44; 110; 220 μg/puff.
- Beclomethasone (QVAR) 40; 80 μg/puff.
- Budesonide (Pulmicort) 160 μg/activation
- Flunisolide (Aerospan) 80; 250 μg/puff
- Mometasone (Asmanex twisthaler) 110; 220 μg/actuation
- Triamcinolone (Azmacort) 75 μg/puff.
- Ciclesonide (ciclez) 80-160 μg OD.

Mast Cell Stabilizers (Sodium Chromoglycate)

Used for prevention of asthma by preventing degranulation of mast cells and release of mediators like histamine, leukotriene, interleukin, inflammatory TXA_2, *etc.* Long-term treatment decreases cellular inflammatory mediator of anaphylaxis, PAF, PG, superoxide and inflammatory response. Bronchial hyperactivity is reduced, bronchospasm to allergen irritantly cold air, exercise may be prevented. It is not bronchodilator and does not prevent Ag-Ab reaction, so not effective during attack.

It is not absorbed orally so given as aerosol 1 mg/dose, 2 puff QDS.

Uses

- Bronchial asthma (as inhaler)
- Allergic rhinitis (as nasal spray)
- Allergic conjunctivitis (as 2% eyedrop)

Adverse effects: Bronchospasm, throat irritation, cough, rarely nasal congestion, headache, dizziness, arthralgia, rash, dysuria have been reported.

Nedocromil

It differs structurally from cromolyn, but shares the common mechanism of action. It alters the function of delayed chloride channel in cell membrane and inhibits cell activation and so inhibits cough and in mast cells inhibits release of mediators by antigen. It is more potent. Does 4 mg (2 puff BD).

Ketotifen orally active, used prophylactically, has some phosphodiesterase inhibitor action, restricts Ca^{2+} entry into cell, and LTD4/C_4 antagonism. Not bronchodilator *per se*. Other uses are conjunctivitis, urticaria and food allergy, rhinitis. Orally absorbed, 50% bioavailability due to first pass metabolism. Sedation and dry mouth are common adverse effects (Ketovent 1 mg BD).

Mediator blockers: Azelastine blocks H_1 and leukotriene receptors, LT synthesis inhibitor; zileuton are trialed.

Hospitalization in bronchial asthma: When FEV1 is less than 30% or does not increase to 40% after vigorous therapy.

Sedation should be avoided but: Chloral hydrate, diazepam, chlorpromazine are less dangerous.

Other Drugs

Amitriptylline has an antihistaminic antagonist, inhibits uptake of NAd and inhibits phospho-diesterase.

Tetrahydrocannabinol increases FEV1 but has addiction liability.

Immunosuppressant and **immunomodulator** may be used when allergic substance is known.

Omalizumab: It is IgE monoclonal antibody, inhibits further binding of IgE to mast cells, and thus it inhibits its degranulation. It lowers IgE level significantly after 10 weeks of use. Given SC and reduces corticosteroid requirements and reduces frequency of attacks.

ADR: Injection site reaction and rarely anaphylaxis.

New drugs: Montelukast (ventair 10/5/4 mg tablets) is a leukotriene receptor antagonist effective in aspirin induced asthma, exercise induced asthma and for tapering the dose of corticosteroid. Given once daily. Metabolized in liver.

Other drug which blocks LTD4 receptor is zafirlucast. Zileuton inhibits 5-lipoxygenase and so prevents leukotriene synthesis available in 60 mg extended release tab. Seretra is Thromboxane inhibitors also promoted for asthma prevention.

Future trends

* Monoclonal antibodies directed against cytokines; interleukins 4, 5 and 13.
* Antagonist of cell adhesion molecules
* Protease inhibitors
* **Immunomodulator:** Etanercept, which is a TNFα antagonist also used for rheumatoid arthritis and ankylosing spondylitis has got potentialities in the treatment of bronchial asthma.

Treating chronic airway infection of *Chlamydia pneumoniae* and *Mycoplasma pneumoniae* with macrolide antibiotics to prevent aggravation of asthma by these organisms.

Inhaled drugs for bronchial asthma

Following group of drugs are prescribed by inhalation in bronchial asthma: (i) β_2 agonist, (ii) anticholinergics, (iii) cromoglycate and (iv) corticosteroid.

The efficacy of aerosolized drug depends upon particle size. Smaller particles are exhaled out, larger particles get deposited in oropharynx, but particle size of 1–5 millimicron diameter deposits on bronchi.

Treatments of status asthmaticus

i. Hydrocortisone hemisuccinate 100 mg IV stat followed by 100–200 mg; 4–8 hourly.
ii. Nebulized salbutamol (2.5–5 mg) + Ipratropium bromide.
iii. Humidified oxygen by inhalation
iv. Mechanical ventilation
v. Suitable antibiotics to treat infeciton of the chest.
vi. Correction of acidosis by sodium bicarbonate or lactate infusion. Correlation of dehydration.
vii. Subcutaneous terbutaline since in severe spasm drug may not reach the bronchi.

Controlling asthma below 12 yrs of age (Step wise)

Step 1: Short acting beta agonist. If no response.

Step 2: Low dose inhaled steroid or cromolyn or leukotriene receptor antagonist (LTRA) or theophyllines if no response.

Step 3: Low dose steroid inhalation + long acting beta agonist or low dose inhaled gluco steroid + Zileuton or leukotriene receptor antagonist and theophyllin. If no response.

Step 4: Then medium dose inhaled steroid + long acting beta agonist alternatively with glucosteroid inhalation LTRA theophylline or zileuton may be added If there is no respnose then.

Step 5: High dose inhaled steroids + LABA. Omalizumab may be added if there is allergies. Even if there is no response then.

Step 6: High dose inhaled steroid + LABA + oral glucocorticoids. Consider Omalizumab for allergies patient. Control environment, patient education, etc. of such step.

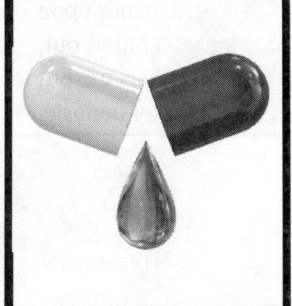
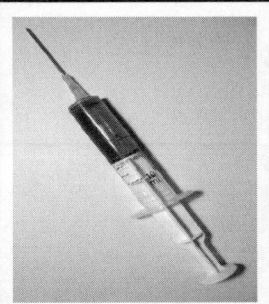
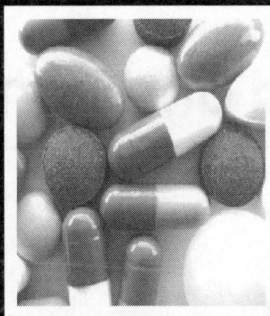
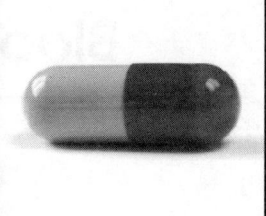

SECTION 8

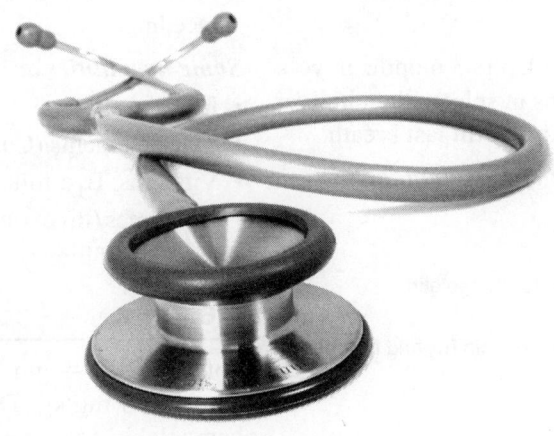

HEMOPOIETIC SYSTEM

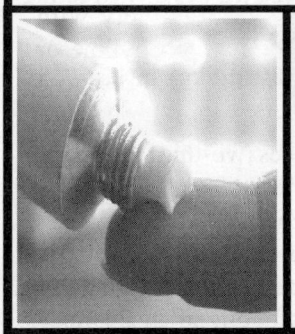
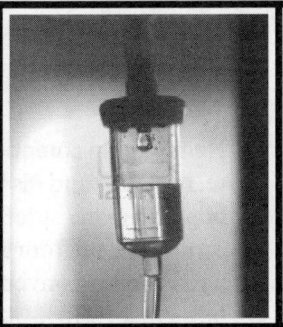
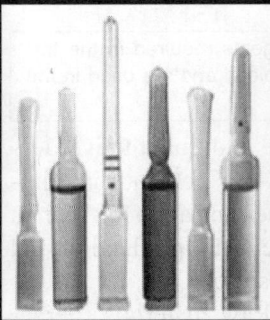
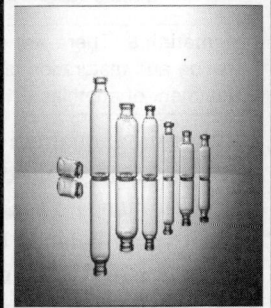

63

Blood and Iron

Blood is a liquid connective tissue comprising red blood cells (erythrocytes), white blood cells (leukocytes) and platelets (thrombocytes) suspended in fluid medium of plasma. Erythrocyte differs from majority of body cells that the mature functioning cells differ physically from their precursors.

Development of RBC: Up to 3 months in yolk sac, then up to 6 months in spleen, then in liver and in adult in bone marrow till last breath.

Stages of development of RBC and factors involved in it

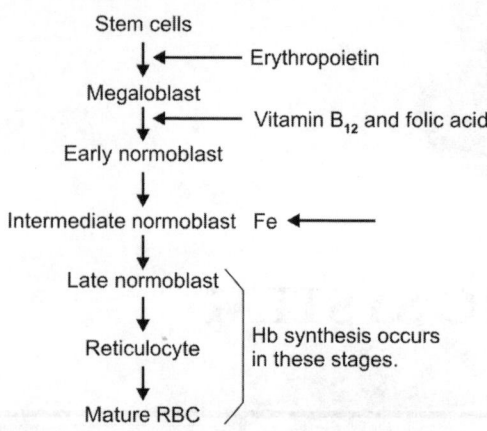

Hematinics: There are agents required in the formation and maturation of blood and are used in the treatment of anemias.

Anemia is qualitative and quantitative decrease in hemoglobin or RBC or both in comparison to standard age, sex and altitude. Anemia occurs when balance between production and destruction of RBC is disturbed, *viz.*

- **Premyeloid stages:** Raw materials (hematinics) for production of RBC are less.

- **Myeloid stage** (lock out in RBC factory)— aplastic anemia.

- **Postmyeloid stage**, *i.e.* production and formation is all right, but there is excessive destruction of RBC (intrinsic or extrinsic defect of RBC leading to hemolysis) or excessive bleeding.

Some hematinics are

- Iron
- Trace elements (Cu, Co, Mo)
- Vitamins: B_{12}, folic acid, pyridoxine, *etc.*
- Hormones (thyroxin, androgen, corticosteroid)
- Proteins of high biological value.

IRON

Total iron 2.5–5 gm. In man 50 mg/kg and in women 38 mg/kg. Distributed more on RBC hemoglobin 66%; myoglobin 3%; ferratin and hemosiderin as stores 25%; in parenchyma, as an enzyme 6%.

Daily requirement

Male	0.5–1 mg (13 µg/kg)
Female	1–2 mg (21 µg/kg) menstruating
Infants	60 µg/kg
Pregnancy	3–5 mg (80 µg/kg) in last 2 trimesters.

Hemoglobin comprises two-third of total iron store, rest one-third (as ferratin and hemosiderin) in bone marrow, spleen and muscles. Most of the iron released from 3×10^6 of RBC destroyed every second is converted to hemoglobin.

6.3 gm of Hb% is cyclized in 24 hours. Average western diet contains 10–15 mg of iron/day, normal man absorbs 10% of dietary iron (1–1.5 mg/day). Anemic patient absorbs more 30%. Iron loss/day by desquamation 0.5–1 mg, menstrual loss 13.5 mg/period. Pregnant woman needs 2–4 mg of iron/day for fetus.

WHO Criteria of RBC counts and Hb%		
	RBC (× 10^{12}/L)	Hb%
Men	$5.5 \pm 1.0 . 10^{12}$/L	15.5 ± 2.5 gm/dL
Women	$4.8 \pm 1.0 . 10^{12}$/L	14.0 ± 2.5 gm/dL
Infants	$5.0 \pm 1.0 . 10^{12}$/L	16.5 ± 3 gm/dL
Full term (cord blood)	$4.4 \pm 0.8 . 10^{12}$/L	12.0 ± 1 gm/dL
10–12 years	$4.7 \pm 7.0 . 10^{12}$/L	13.0 ± 1.5 gm/dL

Absorption of Iron

Iron is absorbed from whole GIT, but main site is duodenum. Absorption depends upon:

- Requirement of body and forms of iron (Fe^{2+} is better absorbed than Fe^{3+}).
- Organic heme is better absorbed than inorganic.
- Routes of administration (if large amount is given IV, whole is retained)
- Certain factors help iron absorption like hydrochloric acid, bile salts, chlorophyll, 1st class protein, vitamin C.
- Certain factors reduce iron absorption like food, phosphates, phytates, antacids and excessive mucus.

Iron is absorbed either by

1. **Passive transportation**—operating in supra hemostatic quantities of iron (when large amount of iron is ingested then it combines with certain amino acids, *i.e.* glycine, serine, *etc.* and absorbed by passive diffusion), when dose is slightly more than normal, it remains within epithelial cells or epithelial villi and after three days, if not taken by the body then cells are exfoliated and excreted through feces.

2. **Active transport (mucosal block theory):** This operates in hemostatic quantity. Ferrireductase duodenal cytochrome B present on luminal surface reduces iron to ferrous state. Ferrous iron is a substrate for divalent metal transporter 1 (DMT1) which transports iron to the base. It is oxidized to ferric by hephaestin (a transmembrane copper-dependent ferroxidase).

Hepcidin is a negative regulator of iron absorption, stimulated by inflammation or by iron overload. Its production is increased by anemia of chronic diseases. Apoferritin is continuously being produced by mucosal cells, combines colloidal hydroxide of ferric salt to form ferritin. The ferritin remains in mucosal cells (2–4 days) called ferritin curtain, when all the apoferritins present in the mucosal cells are saturated, further absorption of iron is stopped.

Transport: In blood, iron is transported in combination with β_1 globulin (glycoprotein) called transferrin. Total plasma content of iron is about 3 mg and it is recycled 10 times everyday.

Storage: It is stored in spleen, bone marrow, liver as ferritin and hemosiderin.

Excretion: It is tenaciously conserved by the body. Excretion in adult male 0.5–1 mg as exfoliated skin, GI mucosal cell, feces, urine, sweat, menstruating loss 0.5–1 mg/day (Figs 63.1A and B).

Indications for iron therapy

- In iron deficiency due to chronic blood loss.
- Pregnancy
- Various abnormalities of GIT
- Premature babies
- In pernicious anemia with cyanocobalamin as iron stores get exhausted by sudden increase in blood formation.

Preparation of Iron

Oral

- Ferrous gluconate (35 mg/5 mL)
- Ferrous sulfate (60 mg/5 mL)
- Colloidal Fe (IC) hydroxide (free from GI upset)
- Ferrous fumarate (65 mg)

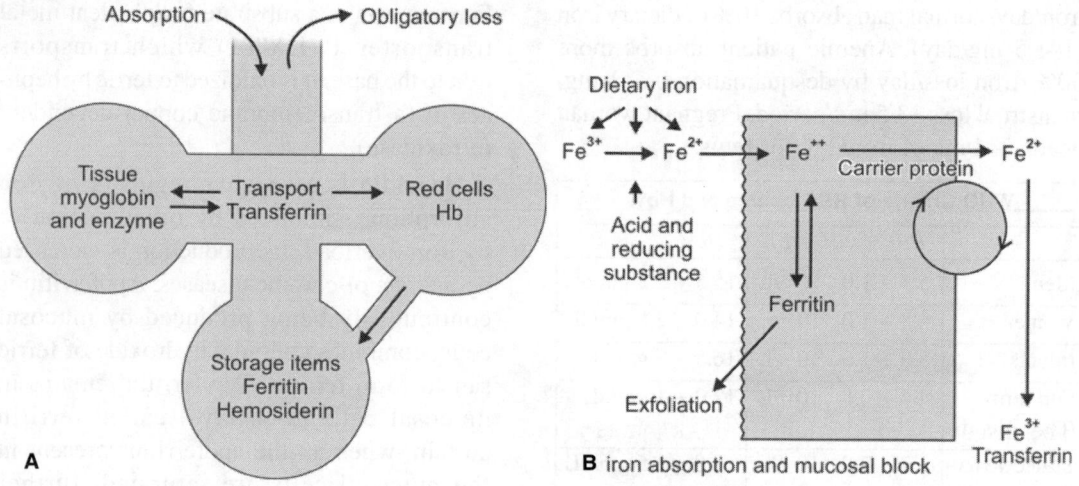

Figs 63.1A and B: Absorption of iron

- Ferric ammonium citrate mixture (scale iron)
- Hemoglobin 0.33% iron.

Parenteral

- Iron dextran (imferon) given IM or IV.
- Iron sorbitol citric acid given IM (Jectofer)
- **Iron sucrose (uniferon):** May be given IV. Less chance of anaphylactic reaction, but it may produce tubulointerstitial disease of kidney. Following IV injection taken up by RE system and dissociates iron.
- **Ferric carboxymaltose:** Ferric hydroxide core is stabilized by carbohydrate shell. It is given IV diluted with saline.

Adverse effects of iron therapy

- Epigastric pain
- Heart burn
- Nausea
- Metallic taste
- Staining of teeth
- Constipation or diarrhea.

Indication of parenteral iron therapy

- Failure to absorb iron as in bowel resection or malabsorption
- Inability to tolerate oral iron
- Where average daily loss equals or exceeds absorption
- Noncompliance

Calculation of iron dose

If body wt = W

Blood vol = 70 W

Hb : H gm%

1 gm Hb contains 3.4 mg of iron

$$\frac{70\,W\,(15-H)\times 3.4}{100} = 2.38\,W\,(15-H)$$

Adverse reaction to parenteral iron therapy

Local: Pain, skin discoloration, abscess formation, lymphadenopathy

Systemic: Headache, fever, arthralgia, hemolysis, tachycardia, anaphylactic shock, black urine with iron sorbitol complex.

Treatment of iron poisoning

- Stomach wash with 1% $NaHCO_3$
- DTPA (diethylene triamine pentaacetic acid) 35–40 mg/kg.
- Desferrioxamine 20 mg/kg in saline every 6 hours for 2 days. It may be given IM also.
- Supportive measures like IV fluid BP support and diazepam for convulsion. **BAL is contraindicated, as it forms toxic complex with iron.**
- Deferiprone and Deferasirox are given orally to treat iron poisoning.

Other uses of desferrioxamine

- Acute iron intoxication
- Hemochromatosis

64

Vitamin B$_{12}$ and Folic Acid

The discovery of vitamin B$_{12}$ is dramatic and started from 180 years and includes two Nobel Prize winning discoveries. Combe and Addison reported megaloblastic anemia. Whipple first said that liver is a potent source of hemopoietic substances. Hodgkin discribed crystalline structure of B$_{12}$ by X-ray diffraction. Austin Flint first said gastric atrophy causes pernicious anemia (incurable). Minot and Murphy demonstrated effectiveness of liver extracts in pernicious anemia.

Chemistry of vitamin B$_{12}$

It has three major portions.
- Planner group or corrin nucleus
- 5, 6-dimethylbenzimidazole nucleotide links to corrin nucleus at right angle.
- A variable group R.

When variable group is (–CN) = Cyanocobalamin; (–OH) = Hydroxycobalamin; (–CH$_3$) = Methylcobalamin (–5′ deoxyadenosyl) = 5′–Deoxyadenosyl cobalamin.

Source: Only animal. Commercial source is from *Streptomyces griseus,* a by-product of streptomycin plant.

Daily requirement 1–3 µg; in pregnancy and lactation 3–5 µg.

Deficiency of Vitamin B$_{12}$ (Fig. 64.1)

It occurs in:
1. Inadequate supply
2. Inadequate intrinsic factor
3. Ileal disease
4. Congenital absence of TC II

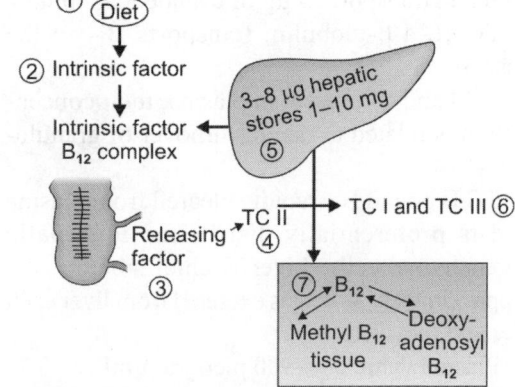

Fig. 64.1: Absorption and distribution of vitamin B$_{12}$

5. Rapid depletion of hepatic, enterohepatic circulation.
6. Abnormal appearance of TC I and III.
7. Normal supply to cell with inadequate folic acid.

Metabolic function: Vitamin B$_{12}$ is intricately linked with folate metabolism, the active coenzyme forms of B$_{12}$ deoxyadenosyl cobalamin and methyl cobalamin generated in the body.

1. It is essential for the conversion of homocysteine to methionine.
2. Essential for hemopoiesis (early normoblasts)
3. Essential for epithelial cells.
4. Production of myelin sheaths

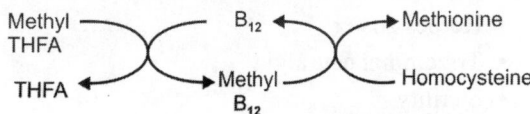

5. Malonic acid is converted to succinic acid and links carbohydrate and lipid metabolism. Inhibition causes accumulation of malonic acid and fatty acids with odd number of carbon atoms leading to neurological disorders.
6. Required for –SH group in reduced form.
7. Lipotropic function.

Intrinsic factors: It is glycoprotein in nature of molecular weight 60,000. The value fluctuates with HCl acid secretion. Deficiency occurs in gastrectomy. One oral unit of intrinsic factor will bind and transport 15 µg of cyanocobalamin.

TC II, a β-globulin, transports B_{12} to the tissues.

TC I and III present in plasma, their concentration is related to rate of turnover of granulocytes.

TC II bound B_{12} rapidly cleared from plasma and is preferentially distributed to hepatic parenchymal cells. Liver is chief storage site. Approximately 3–8 µg is excreted from liver each day and recycled.

Plasma value 200–900 picogram/mL.

Therapeutic indications of B_{12}: It should be given prophylactically only when there is reasonable ground. It should be specific, shotgun therapy may be dangerous.

Indications of B_{12}

a. **Megaloblastic anemia due to**
- Deficient intake
- Intrinsic factor deficiency
- Inadequate utilization

b. **Neuropathies**
- Subacute combined degeneration of spinal cord
- Tobacco or tropical amblyopia

c. **Empirical use**
- Infective hepatitis
- Psoriasis
- Multiple sclerosis
- Herpes zoster
- Trigeminal neuralgia
- Sterility

Contraindications of B_{12}: Undiagnosed anemia, single dose may interfere with diagnosis for a week.

Preparation of B_{12}

Cyanocobalamin:	Redisol, macrabin 35 µg/ 5 mL
Hydroxycobalamin:	Redisol-H, 500–1000 µg/mL
Methylcobalamin:	Diacobal 500 µg/mL

FOLIC ACID

Chemistry: Consists of three groups. Pteridine ring, para-aminobenzoic acid and glutamic acid (chemically pteroyl glutamic acid).

DIETARY SOURCES

Vegetable: Spinach, green leafy vegetables

Animals: Meat, liver, egg, milk, synthesized in gut flora, but not available for absorption.

Daily requirement: Adult 200 µg/day; 300–400 µg/day in pregnancy and lactation. Normal serum value 6–20 ng/mL.

Utilization: Folic acid is present in food as polyglutamates, additional glutamate residues are split off primarily before it is absorbed in upper intestine. Reduction and methylation also occur at this site. It is transported in blood mostly as methyl THFA partly bound to plasma proteins. It is also absorbed by carrier mediated active transport. Large dose may be absorbed by passive diffusion fractionally.

It is rapidly taken up by tissues and stored in cells as polyglutamates. Liver takes up large part and excretes methyl THFA which goes into enterohepatic circulation.

Metabolic function: Folic acid is activated to coenzyme forms DHFA and THFA by enzyme folate and dihydrofolate reductase. THFA mediates a number of one carbon transfer reactions by carrying a methyl group.

1. Purine and pyrimidine biosynthesis

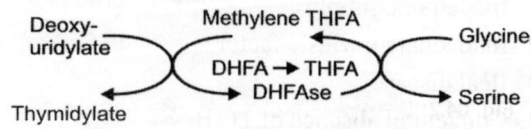

2. Amino acid metabolism
- Serine → Glycine (B$_6$ required)
- Histidine → Glutamic acid
- Homocysteine → Methionine (B$_{12}$ required)

3. Generation of fumarate

DISTRIBUTION OF FOLIC ACID AFTER ABSORPTION

Deficiency of folic acid (Fig. 64.2)

It occurs in:
1. Inadequate supply
2. Defective absorption
3. Defective folate binding protein (uremia, hepatitis, alcoholism)
4. Defective enterohepatic circulation
5. Folate trap

Manifestation of folic acid deficiency: Megaloblastic anemia, epithelial damage, glossitis, enteritis, diarrhea, steatorrhea, debility, weight loss.

Preparation: Folic acid (Folvite) 5 mg tab, 1 tab daily.

Folinic acid: Calcium leucovorin 3 mg/mL

Therapeutic indications of folic acid

1. Megaloblastic anemia
- Nutritional deficiency
- Increased demand (pregnancy, lactation)
- Impaired absorption (malabsorption)
- Helminth infestation (*D. latum*)
- Impaired utilization (liver disease)
- While treating with B$_{12}$

2. Methotrexate toxicity (folinic acid) is used.
3. Citrovorum rescue factor to rescue normal cells in methotrexate therapy.

Adverse effects: Orally completely safe, folinic acid injection rarely causes hypersensitivity.

Hematopoietic Growth Factors

Erythropoietin

(Carnot and Deflandre in 1906)

It is a sialoglycoprotein hormone (mol wt. 34000) produced by peritubular cells of kidneys, acts on bone marrow erythroid cells to proliferate it from G0 phase (Fig. 64.3). Its titer increases in Bartter syndrome, AV fistula; hypoxia. PGE2 and cAMP appear to be implicated in renal production of erythropoietin (EPO). It is not sole growth factor for erythropoiesis, but is important regulator for proliferation of **C**olony **F**orming **U**nit (CFU-E) and their immediate progeny. Kidney detects O$_2$ delivery to modulate erythropoietin secretion. Hypoxia-inducible factor 1 (HIF-1), a heterodimer (HIF-1α and -1β) transcription factor to stimulate multiple hypoxia inducible genes like vascular endothelial growth factor and erythropoietin which in turn stimulate rapid expansion of erythroid progenitor. After secretion, EPO binds to membrane receptor of erythroid progenitor in the marrow and internalized. Its feedback loop is disrupted by kidney disease, nerve damage, vitamin and iron deficiencies.

It is possible that hypothalamus senses tissue oxygen level and triggers erythropoiesis either through neurohypophyseal humoral mechanism or *via* sympathetic nervous system. Alternatively

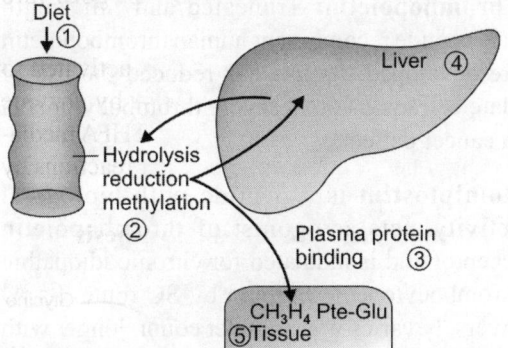

Diet

Liver

Hydrolysis reduction methylation

Plasma protein binding

CH$_3$H$_4$ Pte-Glu Tissue

Fig. 64.2: Distribution of folic acid after absorption

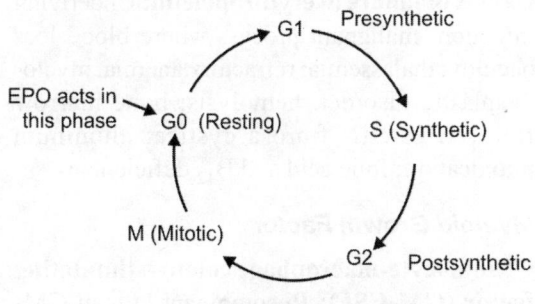

Presynthetic — G1

EPO acts in this phase → G0 (Resting)

S (Synthetic)

M (Mitotic)

G2 — Postsynthetic

Fig. 64.3

variation in vascular dynamics of blood oxygenation leads to its liberation.

EPO production is increased by CO_2, androgen, decreased oxygen and inhibited by oxygen.

Recombinant human erythropoietin (Epoetin) is commercially available. Plasma $t\frac{1}{2}$ 6–10 hours given IV or SC. It is an orphan drug.

EPO is used in anemia

- Chronic renal failure 25–100 U/kg bi- or tri-weekly reduces need for transfusion, SC administered epotin reduces dose requirement.
- Other uses are anemia of AIDS, cancer. Specially those on zudovudine therapy.
- Autologous transfusion during surgery. Athletes use it (blood doping).

Adverse effects of erythropoietin: Non-immunogenic. Sudden increase in hematocrit viscosity and vascular resistance, hypertension, seizures, flu-like symptoms (lasting 2–4 hours), clot formation in AV shunts in dialysis patient (Hemax 2000 U/mL; 4000 U/mL, Eprex 2000 U and 4000 U/mL in 0.1 mL prefilled syringe given IV or SC.

More recently novel erythropoiesis stimulating protein (NESP) or Darbepoetin alfa is approved for treatment with similar indication.

Darbepoetin: It is long acting erythropoietin with addition of the carbohydrate chain improving its biological activity and it has decreased clearance rate, so $t\frac{1}{2}$ is increased. It has no value in acute treatment for anemia.

Peginesatide is approved for treatment in CRF. It is peptide in nautre but postmarketing reports of anaphylaxis compelled a recall.

Causes of failure in erythropoietin: Underlying infection; malignant process where blood loss occultly; thalassemia; refractory anemia, myelodysplastic disorder, hemolysis; bone marrow fibrosis; osteitis fibrosa cystica; aluminum intoxication; folic acid and B_{12} deficiencies.

Myeloid Growth Factor

Granulocyte-macrophage colony-stimulating factor (GM-CSF): Recombinant human GM-CSF (sargramostim amino acid glycoprotein produced in yeast) is used subcutaneously after hematopoietic stem cell implantation or after intensive chemotherapy.

Side effects

- Bone pain
- Flu-like symptoms
- Flushing
- Nausea
- Vomiting
- Dyspnea
- Capillary leak syndrome
- Supraventricular arrhythmia. Raise creatinine
- Bilirubin may rise.
- Hepatic enzymes may rise.
- Frequent blood counts are essential.

Granulocyte-colony stimulating factor (G-CSF): Filgrastim recombinant G-CSF produced in *E. coli* (Neupogen) used in autologous hematopoietic stem cell transplantation and high dose cancer therapy, neutropenia of AIDS patient on zidovudine. It is given SC or IV over ½ hour at 1–20 µg/kg/day.

Thrombopoietic Growth Factors

Interleukin 11: Stimulates megakaryocyte maturation. Recombinant human interleukin, oprelvekin (Neumega) is obtained from bacteria. Used SC in non-myeloid malignancies with thrombocytopenia. It causes fluid retention, tachycardia, palpitation edema, shortness of breath, rash, paresthesia.

Thrombopoietin: Truncated and full length polypeptide recombinant human thrombopoietin are developed. Its use has reduced the use of platelet transfusion in severe thrombocytopenia in cancer patient.

Romiplostim is a peptide with biological activity, acts as agonist of thrombopoietin receptor and is indicated for chronic idiopathic thrombocytopenic purpura by SC route. Its $t\frac{1}{2}$ inversely varies with platelet count, longer with patient with thrombocytopenia and shortest with patient whose platelet count has recovered to normal. Eltrombopag is orally active agonist of thrombopoietin receptor used for idiopathic thrombocytopenia.

Trace Elements in RBC Formation

Cobalt: It is used successfully in primary red cell disease, chronic disease leading to anemia. Previously, it was thought that cobalt inhibits oxygen transporting enzyme leading to anoxia but in 1985 Gold Wasser *et al.*, showed it is due to rise of erythropoietin.

Copper: Helps in three ways:
- Helps in the absorption of iron
- Helps in the mobilization of iron from depot
- Stimulates heme synthesis.

Molybdenum: Decreases gastric upsets.

Agents used to treat sickle cell diseases: Hydroxyuria relieves painful clinical course of sickle cell disease.

ADR: Bone marrow suppression, cutaneous vasculitis. Other uses of hydroxyuria are CML; polycythemia.

Hormones

a.

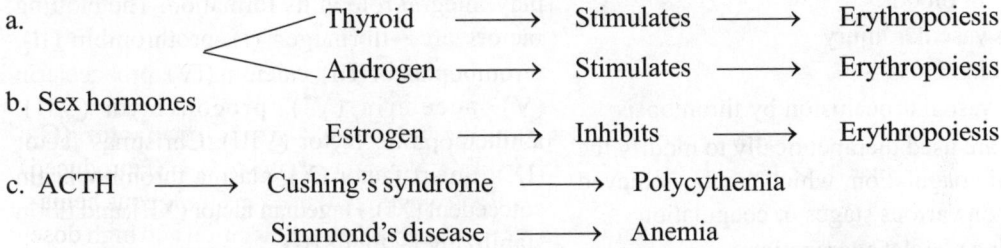

Thyroid $\longrightarrow$ Stimulates $\longrightarrow$ Erythropoiesis

Androgen $\longrightarrow$ Stimulates $\longrightarrow$ Erythropoiesis

b. Sex hormones

Estrogen $\longrightarrow$ Inhibits $\longrightarrow$ Erythropoiesis

c. ACTH $\longrightarrow$ Cushing's syndrome $\longrightarrow$ Polycythemia

Simmond's disease $\longrightarrow$ Anemia

d. Corticosteroid suppresses antigen-antibody reaction used with benefit in hemolytic anemia.

Shotgun antianemic preparation: Use of antianemic preparations containing multiple ingredients like liver extracts, iron, folic acid, B$_{12}$, copper, cobalt, manganese, *etc.* are called shotgun preparation. These should be avoided because some ingredients are not required at all or some may interfere with diagnosis. A commercial preparations containing multiple ingredients are present in subtherapeutic concentrations.

65

Drugs of Blood Coagulation

Hemostasis is a dynamic process which maintains:

- Fluidity of blood
- Repairs vascular injury
- Limits blood loss
- Avoids vascular occlusion by thrombosis

Drugs are used therapeutically to modify the process of coagulation, which can be achieved by acting on various stages or coagulation:

- Inhibiting platelet aggregation
- Clot or fibrin formation
- Fibrinolysis

Various clotting factors (13 factors) control the formation of clots, but platelets and fibrin play integral role in its formation. The clotting factors are—fibrinogen (I), prothrombin (II), thromboplastin (III), calcium (IV), proaccelerin (V), accelarin (VI), proconvertin (VII), antihemophilic factor (VIII), Christmas factor (IX), Stuart factor (X), plasma thromboplastin antecedent (XI), Hageman factor (XII), and fibrin stabilizing factor (XIII).

Clotting factors are proteins in plasma in inactive forms activated by partial proteolysis.

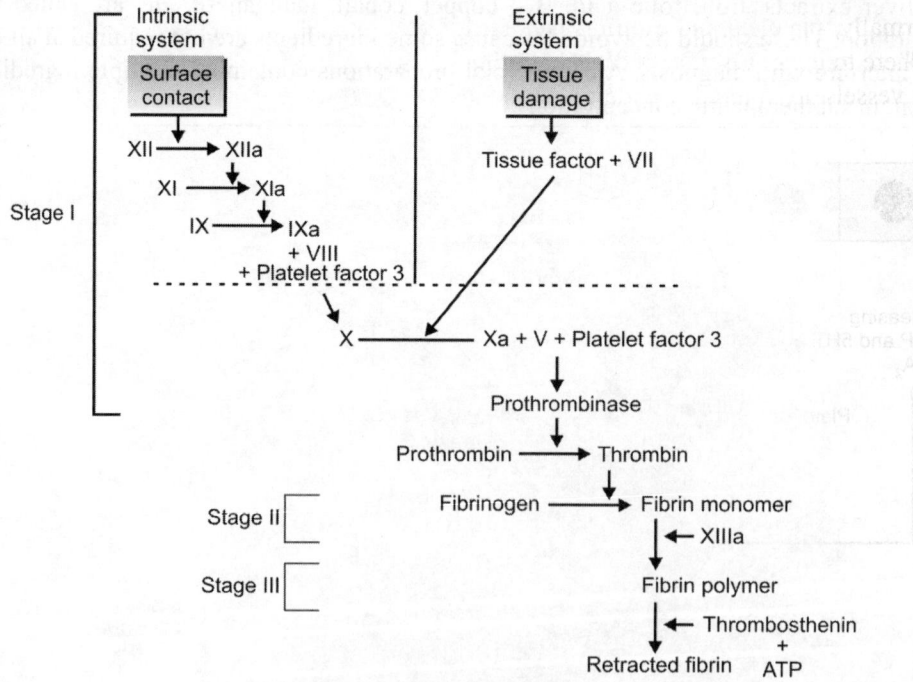

Fig. 65.1: Stages of clotting

The intrinsic pathways, extrinsic pathways and common pathway can be detected by following tests.

	Intrinsic pathway	Extrinsic pathway	Common pathway
Prothrombin time	Normal	Increased	Increased
Activated partial thromboplastin time	Increased	Normal	Increased

Thrombin activates many upstream factors and amplifies its own generation to produce clot formation. Antithrombin proteins C and S; antithromboplastin, fibrinolysis system oppose coagulation and help lysis of the clot. If these two systems are out of control then there will be generalized clotting and bleeding called disseminated intravascular coagulation (DIC).

Mechanism of Clotting

Mechanism of clotting can be divided into three stages:

Stage I : Formation of thromboplastin required for conversion of prothrombin to thrombin.

Stage II : Conversion of prothrombin to thrombin.

Stage III : Conversion of fibrinogen to fibrin.

Normally, platelets and clotting factors do not adhere to intact vascular endothelial lining. When vessels are injured it undergoes a series of changes towards procoagulant activities like exposing subendothelial matrix proteins (collagen von Willebrand factor) resulting platelet activation, synthesis and secretion of vasoconstrictors and molecules recruiting platelets. TXA2 is synthesized from arachidonic acid. Platelet granules secrete ADP and 5HT. Platelet activation causes conformation changes in α_{II} and β_{III} integrin (IIb/IIIa) receptors to bind fibrinogen which cross-links adjacent platelets causing their aggregation and formation of platelet plug (Fig. 65.2).

Coagulation system is also activated by producing thrombin generation and formation of fibrin plug which stabilizes platelet plug.

AGENTS USED TO CONTROL BLEEDING

Used locally

- Thrombin
- Tromboplastin
- Fibrin
- Gel foam
- Oxidized cellulose

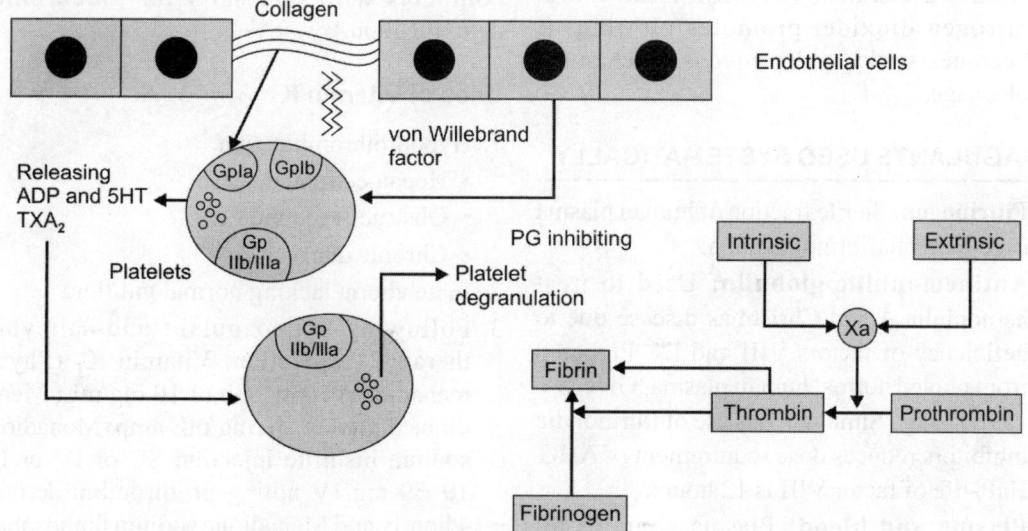

Fig. 65.2: Thrombin formation in damaged vascular site

Used systematically

- Fibrinogen
- Antihemophilic globulin
- Plasma or blood
- Calcium
- Vitamin C and rutin
- Snake venoms
- Vitamin K
- Epsilon-aminocaproic acid (EACA)
- Sclerosing agent
- Tranexamic acid

LOCALLY USED COAGULANTS

a. **Thrombin:** Obtained from bovine plasma, inactive below pH 5. Stored at 2–8 °C. Locally used to stop oozing and anchoring skin grafts.

b. **Thromboplastin:** Used to determine prothrombin time and local hemostatic, obtained from acetone extract of brain and lungs of rabbits.

c. **Fibrin:** Obtained from human plasma, dehydrated to form sheets, cut for use of desired size of bleeding surface.

d. **Gel foam:** Pressed form of gelatin sponge moistened with sterile isotonic solution, before using in suturing or operating wounds in conjunction with thrombin. Completely absorbed in 4–6 weeks.

e. **Oxidized cellulose (oxycel):** Treated with nitrogen dioxide, promotes clotting. It becomes sticky and provides mechanical blockage.

COAGULANTS USED SYSTEMATICALLY

a. **Fibrinogen:** Sterile fraction of human plasma used to treat afibrinogenemia.

b. **Antihemophilic globulin:** Used to treat hemophilia A and Christmas disease due to deficiency of factors VIII and IX. Prepared from pooled normal human plasma. Given IV 15–60 U/kg. Simultaneous use of fibrinolytic inhibitors reduces dose requirement of AHG. Half-life of factor VIII is 12 hours.

c. **Plasma and blood:** Plasma contains all clotting factors. Whole blood for replacement of clotting factors may increase cardiac load and risk or transfusion reaction is there.

d. **Calcium:** By parenteral route stops bleeding.

e. **Vitamin C and rutin:** Used in case of scurvy causing increased erythropermeability. Oral dose of rutin 20–30 mg and vitamin C 50–100 mg TDS.

f. **Snake venom:** Of Russel viper and Copper head snakes enhances coagulation by stimulating thrombokinase.

g. **Ethamsylate (Ethamsyl 250–500 mg TDS):** Reduces capillary bleeding, when platelets are adequate (*viz.* menorrhagia, epistaxis, hematuria, *etc.*)

VITAMIN K

Naphthoquinone derivative, fat-soluble vitamin occurs in two forms K_1 and K_2. It is essential for synthesis of prothrombin and factors II, VII, IX and X. It is also shown to be involved in electron transport (coenzyme) and oxidative phosphorylation.

Absorption: Produced by gut flora, this fat-soluble vitamin is absorbed by bile salts.

Adverse reactions are rare after oral administration. Intravenous use may be fatal. Large dose may produce hemolytic anemia, kernicterus in newborn, hyperbilirubinemia because it competes with bile salts for glucuronide detoxification.

Uses of Vitamin K

1. Hypoprothrombinemia
   - Hepatocellular disease
   - Obstructive jaundice
   - Chronic diarrhea

2. In newborn, lacking normal gut flora

3. Following anticoagulant and salicylate therapy. Preparation: Vitamin K_1 (Phytomenadione) 10 mg tab or 10 mg/mL; Menadione 5 mg/tab, 10 mg/mL amp; Menadione sodium bisulfite injection SC or IV or IM 10–50 mg IV noting prothrombin activity 4 hourly and Menadione sodium diphosphate (Synkavite 5 mg/tab, 10 mg/mL).

Epsilon-aminocaproic acid: Structurally related to lysine, may be given orally or parenterally, blocks plasminogen activity by competitive blockade, reducing fibrinolytic activity. Excreted by kidney unchanged. It may cause nasal stiffness, dyspepsia, hypertension, nausea, conjunctival erythema, skin rash.

Dose of epsilon-aminocaproic acid (Amicar) 5 gm. Orally or slow IV to reduce hypotension, 1 gm hourly. Use to control bleeding in abruptio placentae and prostatectomy, PPH and hemorrhage following surgery, adjunct therapy of hemophilia; bleeding from fibrinolytic therapy; intracranial aneurysm. It is not effective in thrombocytopenia. It is not used in DIC or upper genitourinary bleeding.

Other drugs of this group are tranexamic acid, AMCA, **p-aminomethyl benzoic acid (PAMBA)**.

Tranexamic acid: Dose of tranexamic acid is 15 mg/kg orally loading followed by 30 mg/kg every 6 hourly.

Serine Protease Inhibitors

Aprotinin: It inhibits fibrinolysis, plasmin-streptokinase complex (patient received thrombolytic agent). Previously used for open heart surgery or liver transplantation, but withdrawn due to its ADR.

ADR: Risk of myocardial infarction, stroke and renal damage.

Recombinant factor VIIa

This is approved for treatment of hemophilia A or B with inhibitors Glanzmann's thrombosthenia, congenital or acquired hemophilia, factor VII deficiency given as bolus injection.

Desmopressin: It increases factor VIII activity used for minor surgery like tooth extraction. Other preparations of plasma fractions are:
- Autoplex (factor VIII correctional activity)
- FEIBA (factor eight inhibitor bypassing activity)
- Recombinant activated factor VII (novo seven)

Sclerosing Agents

Irritates to obliterate varicose vein or to close hernia.

Preparations

- Phenol in almond oil or peanut oil.
- Quinine + Urethane
- Ethanolamine oleate 5% in 25% glycerine
- Sodium tetradecyl sulfate (anionic detergent)
- Sodium morrhuate ⎤ *These are salts of*
- Sodium linoleate ⎦ *fatty acids*

66

Anticoagulants

Anticoagulants are the drugs reducing blood's coagulability. Normally clot is controlled by— (i) prostacycline, (ii) antithrombin, (iii) protein C and (iv) heparan sulfate liberated by endothelial.

Anticoagulant drugs may be classified as:

Drugs Modifying Platelet Function

- Prostacyclin, PGI_2 inhibit platelet aggregation; these are at trial level.
- Dazoxiben blocks thromboxane A_2 production, orally active. Under investigational level.
- Dipyridamole (presantine) inhibits platelet aggregation, blocks platelet phosphodiesterase enzyme leading to increase in cAMP.
- Aspirin, sulfinpyrazone (uricosuric drug), dextran (plasma expander) inhibit platelet aggregation.

Fast Acting Anticoagulant

Heparin was first isolated by McLean in 1916. In 1918, Howel and Holt named it heparin due to its abundance in liver. It is a heterogenous straight chain anionic mucopolysaccharide called glycosaminoglycan of mol wt 15,000 dalton. Less than 1% of native glycosaminoglycans are obtained by alkaline hydrolysis from a covalently conjugated protein core of heparin. It consists of two repeating disaccharide units: (i) d-glucosamine and L-iduronic acid and (ii) d-glucosamine and d-glucuronic acid. Most samples of heparin sodium contains 8–15 sequences of each disaccharide unit, but not necessary in equal portion. It is prepared from bovine lung or intestinal mucosa of pork, sheep and whales. It is acidic because of its covalent linkage with sulfate and carbolic acid group. Incidence of thrombocytopenia is less with porcine heparin. It clears hyperlipemic plasma. Features of heparin-induced thrombocytopenia (HIT) start 5–10 days after heparin, common with unfractionated heparin, producing commonly venous thrombosis.

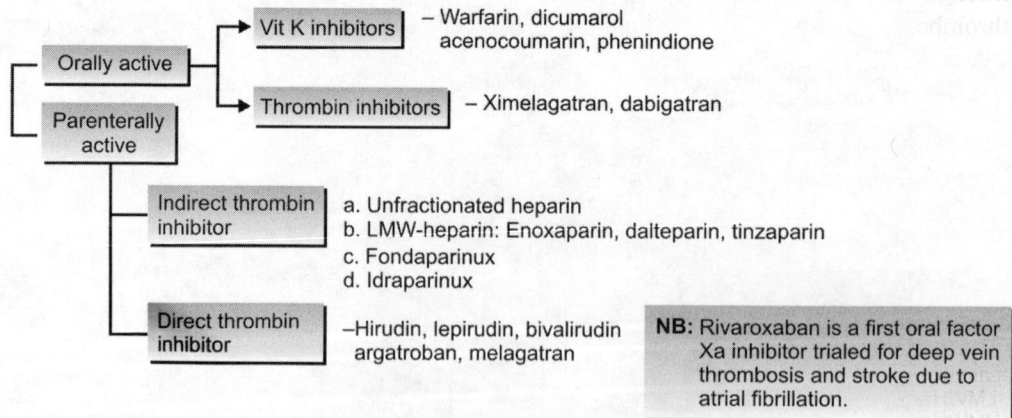

NB: Rivaroxaban is a first oral factor Xa inhibitor trialed for deep vein thrombosis and stroke due to atrial fibrillation.

HIT is a heparin-induced thrombocytopenia which is systemic hypercoagulable state generally treated by unfractionated heparin. It is less common in pediatric patient and rare with pregnant woman.

Heparin acts by accelerating the action of two naturally occurring plasma inhibitors, antithrombin III and heparin cofactor II and inhibits activated coagulation factors of intrinsic and common pathways including thrombins Xa and IXa. High doses of heparin interfere platelet aggregation. Close monitoring of activated partial thromboplastin time is necessary for inhibiting Xa. Low molecular heparin acts by binding antithrombin III with longer t½ and more bioavailability. Heparin is metabolized in liver and does not cross the blood placental barrier and is not secreted in milk.

The indirect thrombin inhibitors act on antithrombin. High molecular weight haparin or unfractionate heparin (UFH), low molecular weight haparin (LMWH) and synthetic pentasaccharide. Fondaparinux binds to antithrombin and enhances activation of factor Xa.

Direct thrombin inhibitors hirudin and bivalirudin bind to active and substrate recognition site of thrombin whereas argatroban and melagatran being small molecules bind to only thrombin active site.

Full dose heparin 5000 IU given in bolus followed by 1200–1600 IU/hour by infusion pump. aPTT should be monitored. SC heparin given for long-term management. Low dose heparin is given prophylactically to prevent deep vein thrombosis.

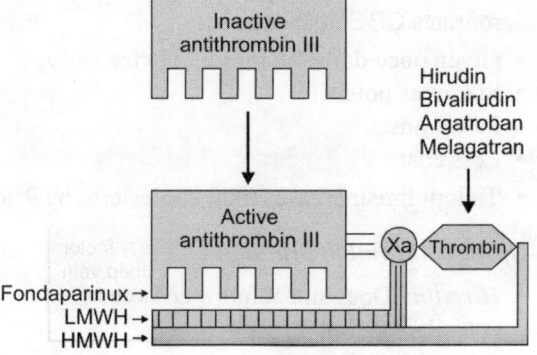

Inactive antithrombin III

Hirudin
Bivalirudin
Argatroban
Melagatran

Active antithrombin III — Xa — Thrombin

Fondaparinux →
LMWH →
HMWH →

Indications of low molecular weight heparins are

- Deep vein thrombosis
- Pulmonary embolism
- Unstable angina
- Myocardial infarction
- To maintain patency of cannula and shunt of dialysis patient.
- Defibrination syndrome (Heparin is used paradoxically)

Some LMW heparins are

- Enoxaparin
- Nadroparin
- Tinzaparin
- Reviparin
- Dalteparin
- Ardeparin

Heparinoids: They are mixture of low molecular weight sulfate glycosaminoglycans, *e.g.* danaparoid, lepirudin, bivalirudin, argatroban, ancrod, drotrecogin alfa causing less bleeding. Bioavailability 100% after SC. Argatroban can prolong INR, *i.e.* international normalized ratio. Bivalirudin has t½ of 25 minutes.

Advantages of LMW-Heparin: Better bioavailability; longer t½ so less injection prick (SC) required with predictable response and no need of monitoring, low risk of HIT syndrome and osteoporosis.

Contraindications of Heparin

- Bleeding disorder, thrombocytopenia
- Severe hypertension
- Threatened abortion, bleeding piles, peptic ulcer
- Neurosurgery
- Aspirin should be withheld before heparin therapy.
- Ocular surgery
- Lumbar puncture

Comparison between heparin and oral anticoagulant

- Heparin is given IV or SC but oral anticoagulants by oral routes.
- Heparin action starts quickly, puts oral anticoagulants which take 1–3 days to produce their action.

- Heparin is active *in vivo* and *in vitro,* but oral anticoagulants act *in vivo* only.
- Oral anticoagulants action can be antagonized by vitamin K, but heparin action is blocked by protamine sulfate.
- Warfarin produces fetal warfarin syndrome, but heparin does not cross placental barrier.
- Heparin therapy monitored by a PTT, but oral anticoagulant action is monitored by PT.
- Heparin is used for initiating therapy, but oral anticoagulants are used for maintenance.

Protamine sulfate: A strongly basic compound antagonizes action of heparin (1 mg neutralizes 100 units of heparin). Obtained from sperm of fish. In absence of heparin, it acts as an anticoagulant by acting on platelets.

Coumarin type anticoagulants: Warfarin Na inhibits vitamin K_2, epoxide in liver and decreases factors II, VII, IX and X and two natural endogenous inbibitor proteins C and S. It is slow acting, crosses placental barrier and may cause hemorrhages in fetus and also growth retardation, hypoplasia of nose and hand bones called contradi syndrome or fetal warfarin syndrome. Its dose is adjusted by prothombin time (PT).

International normalized ratio

$$(INR) = \left(\frac{PT\ of\ patient}{PT\ of\ reference} \right)^{ISI}$$

ISI stands for international sensitivity index depends on the sensitivity of WHO's reference of a thromboplastin which guides management of warfarin overdose. If INR <5, stop the drug or give lower dose; INR 5–9, give vitamin K, oral (1–2.5 mg) > 9, but no bleeding, give vitamin K_1 oral with 3–5 mg. More than 20 with bleeding treated with fresh frozen plasma. Reversal of excessive warfarin action can be achieved by oral or parenteral vitamin K_1; fresh frozen plasma, prothrombin complex concentrates (Bebulin; proplex T) recombinant factor VIIa (rFVIIa). Because of long t½ of warfarin single dose of vitamin K or rFVIIa may not reverse warfarin effect.

Warfarin sodium: Oral anticoagulants may be used parenterally (word warfarin is derived from **Wisconsin Alumni Research Foundation** with **Arin**).

Indandione derivative (phenindione, diphenindione, anisindione, chlorphenindione)
Similar to coumarin derivative.

Ximelagatran: Orally absorbed, metabolized to melagatran which inhibits thrombin.

Uses of anticoagulants

- Deep vein thrombosis
- Pulmonary embolism
- Myocardial infarction
- Unstable angima
- Rheumatic heart disease
- Atrial fibrillation
- Cerebrovascular accident
- Defibrination syndrome

Drug interaction of oral anticoagulants

- Chlofibrate, disulfiram, thyroxine, anabolic steroids, cimetidine intensify action of oral anticoagulants.
- Barbiturates, chloral hydrate, griseofulvin by stimulating microsomal enzymes decrease its action.
- Tolbutamide, phenytoin inhibit warfarin's metabolism.

Newer Drugs

Inhibition of ADP receptors, ticlopidine and clopidogrel. Combined thromboxane synthetase inhibitors, ridogrel and picotamide.

Prasugrel is similar to clopidogrel but should not be given in patient of TIA and more than 75 years of age.

Advantages of Clopidogrel Over Ticlopidine

- Drugs do not have neutropenic effect so routines CBC not required.
- Given once daily (ticlopidine twice daily)
- Six times potent
- Faster onset
- Less cost
- Ticlopidine increases total cholesterol by 9%

Specific thrombin inhibitors

- *Hirudin:* Does not require cofactor for anticoagulant activity.

- *Hirulog:* Interacts with catalytic site of thrombin.
- *Argatroban:* Competitively blocks fibrinogen cleavage and platelet activation of thrombin.
- *Melagatran:* Low mol wt, reversible, potent, selective, thrombin inhibitor.
- *Inogatran:* Selective inhibitor of thrombin and platelet aggregation.
- *Efegatran:* Tripeptide; direct thrombin inhibitors.
- Others are Ximelagatran, Dabigatran.

Thrombolytic Drugs

Activate plasminogen form plasmin and help lysis of thrombus.

- **Streptokinase**—activates plasminogen to plasmin obtained from beta-hemolytic streptococci. It is an antigenic and produces neutralizing antibodies. So less effective on repeated use.
- **Urokinase** (obtained from human urine). It is non-antigenic and non-pyrogenic. These are contraindicated in hypofibrinogenemia.
- **Prourokinse**—single chain urokinase.
- **Recombinant**—tissue plasminogen activator
- **Staphylokinase**
- **Alteplase, reteplase, tenecteplase** (reteplase and tenecteplase are long acting so also called bolus fibrinolytics mainly used for acute myocardial infarction and lifethreatening pulmonary embolism).

Therapeutic uses of antithrombotic therapy

- Cardiac chamber thromboembolism
- Non-valvular atrial fibrillation
- Cardioversion
- Ventricular thrombus
- Nonischemic dilated cardiomyopathy
- Coronary artery disease
- Cardiac valve replacement
- Prevention of IHD.

Contraindications of antithrombotic therapy

- Hypersensitive to drugs
- Bleeding tendencies (hemophilia and purpura)
- Bacterial endocarditis

- Active tuberculosis
- Ulcerative colitis
- GIT bleeding
- Lumbar puncture
- Intracranial tumor.

Antiplatelet Drugs

Aspirin: Blocks production of thromboxane A_2 and inactivates COX-1.

a. **Dipyridamole** is a vasodilator interferes platelet function by increasing intracellular cAMP. Used in postoperative primary prophylaxis of thromboembolism in prosthetic heart valve in combination with warfarin.

b. **Cilostazol:** Phosphodiesterase inhibitor causes vasodilatation and inhibits platelet aggregation. Used for intermittent claudication.

c. **Blocking platelet glycoprotein II B/III A receptors:** This group of drugs targets platelet II B/III A receptor complex of the final common pathway of platelet aggregation. Drugs are abciximab; eptifibatide and tirofiban. They are used parenterally for acute coronary syndrome.

Other anticoagulants

- *Danaparoid* used for deep vein thrombosis, mixture of 84% heparin sulfate, 12% dermatan sulfate and 4% chondriotin sulfate.
- Bromadiolone, brodifacoum, diphendione, chlorphenacinone and pindone are rodenticide with their poisoning and anticoagulant action. Treated by vitamin K.
- Drotrecogin alfa is a human-activated protein C (recombinant form), inactivates factors Va and VIIIa. It decreases mortality of severe sepsis patients. It has anti-inflammatory activity.

Some *in vitro* anticoagulants

- Physical method by cooling or by collecting in coated vessels.
- **Chemical agents:** (a) Oxalates, (b) citrates, (c) ethylenediaminetetraacetic acid (EDTA) and (d) heparin.

Drug-Induced Blood Dyscrasias

LEUKOPENIA, AGRANULOCYTOSIS

- Tranquilizers : Chlorpromazine, meprobamate
- Analgesics : Amidopyrin, phenylbutazone, indomethacin
- Antibacterials : Chloramphenicol, sulfonamide, septran, furazolidine
- Antithyroids : Thiouracil, methimazole, propyl thiouracil
- Miscellaneous : Gold salts, troxidone, imipramine, thiacetazone, procainamide.

Hemolytic Reaction

Antibacterials: Sulfonamide, furazolidine, nitrofurantoin, chloramphenicol, dapsone.

Antimalarials: Quinine, mepacrine, primaquin, pamaquine.

Miscellaneous: Phenacetin, naphthalene, vitamin K, salicylates.

Drugs causing thrombocytopenia

Quinidine, procainamide (antiarrhythmic); phenytoin valproic acid, carbamazepine (antiepileptic); ranitidine, cimetidine (H_2 blockers); thiazide, furosemide (diuretics); sulfonamide, penicillin, rifampicin (antimicrobials). Alpha-methyldopa, danazol quinine, gold compound (miscellaneous).

Plasma Expanders

These high molecular substances when infused (IV) exert oncotic pressure and retain fluid in the vascular compartments.

Desirable properties of plasma expanders

- Should be pharmacologically inert, non-antigenic and non-pyrogenic.
- Should remain in circulation for considerable time and exert oncotic pressure comparable to plasma.
- It should be cheap, stable and sterilizable.
- Should not interfere with blood grouping.

   Human plasma and reconstituted albumin are the best, but runs the risk of hepatitis and AIDS.

Contraindications of plasma expanders

- Severe anemia
- Cardiac failure
- Kidney failure
- Pulmonary edema

Uses of Plasma Expanders

As a substitute of plasma, viz. burn, hypovalemic shock, endotoxin shock, severe trauma with tissue damage, as temporary measure of whole blood loss. (It does not have oxygen-carrying capacity.)

Table 68.1: Commonly used plasma expanders

Plasma expanders	Remarks	Uses
Human albumin 20% (Albudac)	100 mL of solution is equivalent of about 400 mL of frozen plasma or 800 mL of blood.	Used in burns, hypovolemic shock, hypoproteinemia, cardiac bypass, liver failure and dialysis
Dextran 70 and 40 have mol wt. 70,000 and 40,000 (lomodex) respectively. It is polysaccharide obtained from sugar beat.	Does not interfere with blood grouping, non-antigenic anaphy-laxis may occur, dextran 40 is quick acting and prevents RBC sludging. Dose 20 mL/kg in 24 hours.	Commonly used plasma expander, can be stored for 10 years. It may interfere crossmatching; platelet and coagulation function and may be antigenic.
Degraded gelatin polymer (Hemaccel) 500 mL as 3.5% solution in isotonic electrolyte medium	Polypeptide, MW = 30,000, does not interfere with blood grouping. Plasma expansion lasts for 12 hours. Expensive than lomodex	Used for heart, lung and dialysis machine.
Hydroxyethyl starch (HES)	Colloidal oncotic property of 6% HES = Human albumin	Used to harvest granulocytes.
Polyvinylpyrrolidone as 3.5% solution buffered in normal saline (osmoplasma, sio-plasma).	MW = 40,000 interferes with blood grouping and histamine releasing.	Less used

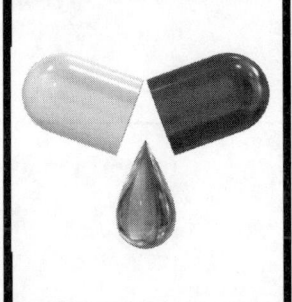
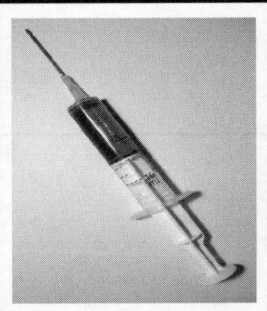
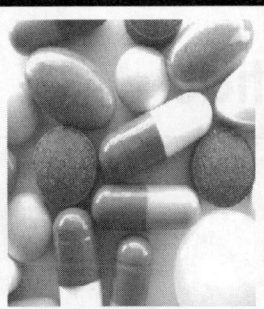
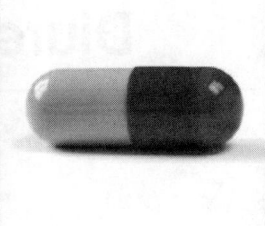

SECTION 9

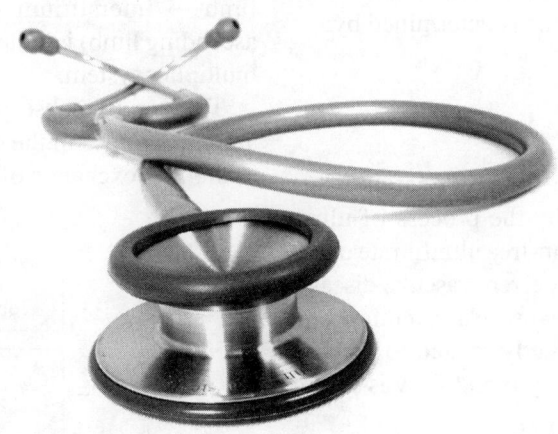

DRUGS ACTING ON KIDNEY, WATER AND ELECTROLYTE METABOLISM

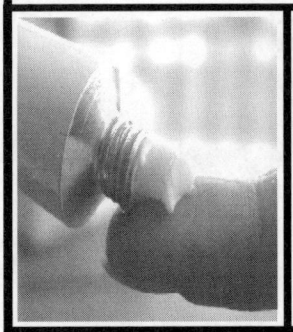
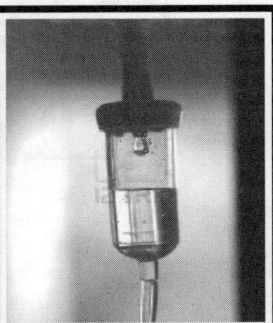
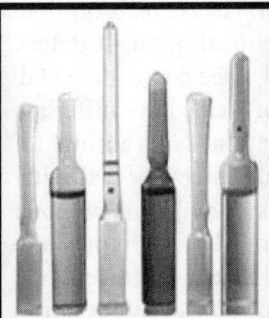
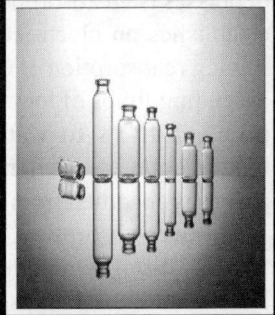

69

Diuretics

Kidneys are responsible for regulating volume and compositions of body fluids, apart from its main function of excretion. The functional unit of a kidney is called *nephron.*

Physiology of urine formation: The composition and volume of urine is determined by:

- Glomerular filtration
- Tubular reabsorption
- Tubular secretion.

Glomerular filtration: Urine formation starts in the glomerular tuft by the process of ultra-filtration, which is protein-free ultrafiltrate of the plasma. The cardiac failure, renovascular disease, vasoconstrictor, NAd cause Na retention and edema. The GFR is directly related to cortical blood flow, the medullary blood flow is not of much importance there.

The major portion of Na, K amino acids, glucose are reabsorbed actively, along with water, it is also absorbed (obligatory absorption), so fluids within the lumen remain isotonic with plasma. The expansion of extracellular fluid volume releases natriuretic hormone, which depresses Na reabsorption. The Na reabsorption establishes an electrochemical gradient determining reabsorption of Cl^-. The descending and ascending limbs of loop of Henle have different permeabilities to water and Na^+ acting as hairpin countercurrent multiplier. The Na^+ with anions is absorbed from ascending limb without free water absorption and deliver hypotonic fluids to distal convoluted tubule. In descending limb, water diffuses out into hypertonic surroundings and Na^+ enters tubular lumen from there, hence tubular fluids gradually becomes hypertonic from isotonic at beginning and gradually becomes hypotonic at ascending limb because of active extrusion of Cl^- with Na^+. This circular and repeatitive transfer of Na (ascending limb → interstitium → descending limb → ascending limb) is called hairpin countercurrent multiplier system.

The active reabsorption of Na^+ along with anion continues in the distal convoluted tubule, at this site exchange of Na^+ for K^+ and H^+ ions

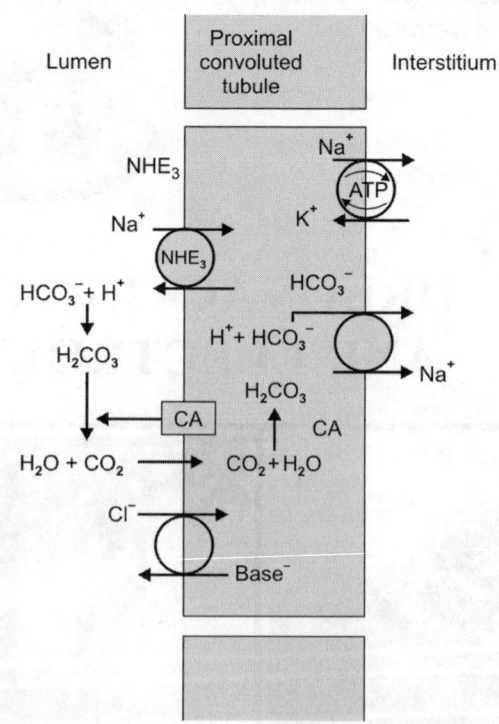

Fig. 69.1: Proximal convoluted tubular site

occurs which are influenced by aldosterone hormone which causes Na retention and K^+ depletion.

The proximal tubular cells contain carbonic anhydrase producing carbonic acid given as follows:

$$H_2O + CO_2 \rightleftharpoons H_2CO_3$$
$$H_2CO_3 = H^+ + CO_3$$

The H^+ derived from carbonic acid is exchanged for sodium with the help of Na^+/H^+ exchanger 3 (NHE3) located in the luminal membrane of proximal tubule epithelial cells (Fig. 69.2).

From tubular lumen which combines with HCO_3 of tubular cells and return to ECF as $NaHCO_3$. H^+ of tubular fluid makes the urine acidic. NH_3 is also produced by tubular cells which diffuse out of lumen reacting to H^+ producing NH_4 which is not absorbed.

Urine enters collecting tubule as isotonic to plasma. Here under the influence of ADH from posterior pituitary becomes permeable to water regulating the insertion of preformed water channel (Aquaporin AQP_2) into apical membrane *via* G-protein coupled cAMP-mediated process. Urea is transported by urea transporter UT_1 also stimulated by ADH which reinforces the medullary hypertonicity during water deprivation, which passes freely to hyperosmotic renal medulla.

Kidney produced autacoids and diuretic activity:

Adenosine: Acting through A_1, A_{2a}, A_{2b} A_3 Adenosine increases Na^+ resorption mainly via A1 receptor in preglomerular afferent arteriole and several segments.

Prostaglandins: PGE_2 blunts Na+ resorption and enhances diuretic activity and its blockade by NSAID blunts dinretic activity.

Natriuretic Peptides: ANP, BNP and CNP induce natriuresis.

Sodium-Glucose Cotransporter (SGLT-2)-inhibitors: Dapaglifozin, serglifozin, remoglifozin, canaglifozin, promoted as antidiabetic agent have diuretic action as it promotes Na^+ excretion operates in proximal convoluted tubule.

Site of Action of Diuretic (Fig. 69.2)

1. CA inhibitors (proximal convoluted tubule) (Fig. 69.1)
2. Osmotic agents (proximal tubule)

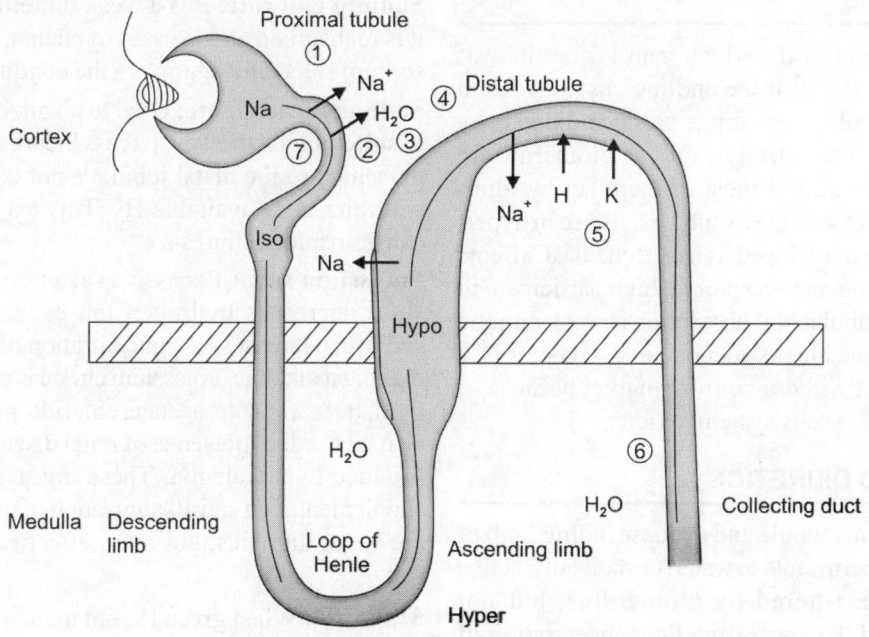

Fig. 69.2: Countercurrent hairpin multiplier and site of action of different diuretics

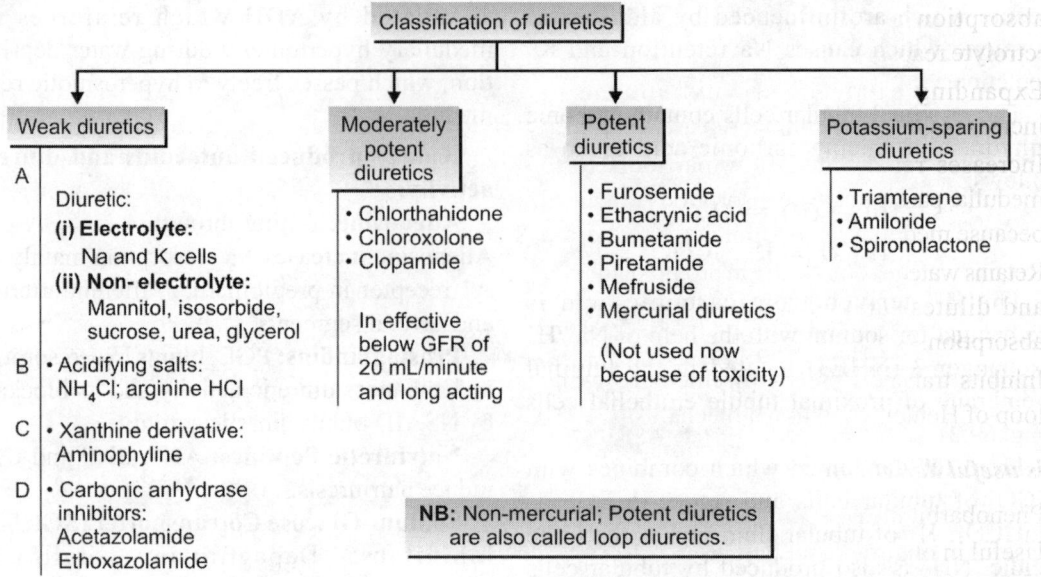

3. Loop diuretics (thick ascending limb)
4. Thiazides (distal convoluted tubule)
5. Aldosterone antagonist
6. ADH antagonist.
7. Through Adenosine (A_1) receptor.
8. Sodium-Glucose co-transporter inhibitors (SGLT-2 inhibitors)

DIURETICS

Diuretics are drugs which cause a net loss of Na^+ and water in urine and increase formation of urine. Only a few drugs produce diuresis by increasing the filtration rate at glomeruli are week diuretics, but most of them act by interfering Na^+ resorption by tubules. Its use in hypertension has outstripped its use in edema. Caffeine blocks adenosine receptors which participate in proximal tubular Na^+ absorption is weak diuretic Rolophylline blocks adenosine A_1 receptor is a diuretic but withdrawn from market because of its central nervous system toxicity..

OSMOTIC DIURETICS

The proximal tubule and the descending limb of Henle are permeable to water. Osmotically, active agents are filtered by glomerulus, but not reabsorbed. By increasing the concentration of osmotically active substances of plasma, the glomerular concentration of these substances can be raised. Increased solute of fluids passing the renal tubules opposes the reabsorption of water by its osmotic activity.

Ideal osmotic diuretics should not be metabolized or reabsorbed after being filtered out. It should be freely filtrable and pharmacologically inert.

Sodium chloride: It is a weak diuretic because it is reabsorbed and in cases of edema, excess of sodium salts only aggravate the condition.

Sodium bicarbonate: Used to alkalize the urine in sulfonamide therapy. Excess bicarbonate load presented to the distal tubule is not completely neutralized by available H^+. This excess anion causes osmotic diuresis.

Potassium salts: Excessive secretion of potassium decreases hydrogen ion exchange with sodium, decreases H^+ concentration of the urine making it alkaline. Potassium citrate is commonly used; but carbonate, acetate, chloride, nitrate may also be used. In presence of renal disease, it may produce hyperkalemia. These are used for K^+ supplementation and alkalinization of urine. They are weak diuretics, but more effective than Na salts.

Mannitol: When given IV, not metabolized and rapidly filtered by glomeruli with almost without reabsorption and limits tubular water and electrolyte reabsorption by:

- Expanding extracellular fluid volume → increases GFR and inhibits release of renin.
- Increases renal blood flow particularly to medulla, passive salts reabsorption is reduced because medullary hypertonicity is reduced.
- Retains water isosmotically in proximal tubules and dilutes luminal fluid opposing NaCl absorption.
- Inhibits transport process in thick ascending loop of Henle by unknown mechanism.

It is useful diuretic in

- Phenobarbitone poisoning
- Useful in oliguric renal failure
- Surgery in deeply jaundiced patient
- Aortic surgery
- Hemolytic transfusion reaction
- To reduce raised intracranial pressure
- Glaucoma

It is not absorbed orally, given IV as 10–20% solution (Mannitol 10%; 20% in 100–350 mL and 500 mL bottles).

Contraindications of Mannitol

- Acute tubular necrosis
- Pulmonary edema
- LVF

Headache is common, nausea and vomiting may occur in hypersensitive patient.

Isosorbide: Dihydric alcohol, produced by removal of water from sorbitol, used to treat cirrhotic edema. With thiazide it is synergistic in action as diuretic. It is effective orally. Dose 1–2 gm/kg as 50% solution.

Glucose and sucrose: Sucrose is not metabolized or reabsorbed, acts as diuretic. Temporary renal tubular nephrosis may occur with sucrose.

Glycerol: IV 10% glycerol in normal saline or 5% dextrose is used for reducing cerebral edema because it avoids rebound edema. May be used in CCF. Rapid infusion in 30% may produce hemolysis.

Urea (30%): No longer used as osmotic diuretic because of many disadvantages.

Xanthines: Theophylline and aminophylline increase renal blood flow by cardiac action, inhibits tubular reabsorption of Na and its diuretic action not affected by acid–base balance. Aminophylline given in dose 0.25–0.5 gm diluted with 20 mL of 5% glucose slowly IV.

Caffeine blocks adenosine receptors which participate in proximal tubular Na^+ absorption, is a weak diuretic.

CARBONIC ANHYDRASE INHIBITORS

The enzyme, carbonic anhydrase (CA) presents in renal cortex, gastric mucosa, pancreas, eye and CNS. It catalyzes the reaction $CO_2 + H_2O = H_2CO_3$, the enzyme plays an important role in reabsorption of Na^+ and HCO_3 ($H_2CO_3 = H^+ + HCO_3^-$) by providing carbonic acid which provides hydrogen ion for exchange with sodium. Acetazolamide is a sulfonamide derivative, inhibits CA at proximal tubule non-competitively, but reversibly slows the hydration of CO_2 leading to decreasing availability of H^+ to exchange with luminal Na^+. Lack of H^+ leading to excretion of Na, along with water is excreted. Continued action of acetazolamide depletes HCO_3^+ in the body and causes acidosis, little HCO_3^- is filtered by glomerular and acting as self-limiting diuretic.

Other extrarenal actions of acetazolamide

- The intraocular tension is decreased.
- Decreased gastric HCl and pancreatic $NaHCO_3$ secretion at very high doses.
- Increased CO_2 level of brain, this decreases pH of CSF which raises seizure threshold and sedation.
- Alters CO_2 transport in lung and tissues, but actions are masked by compensatory mechanism.
- Decreases thyroidal uptake of iodine.

Therapeutic uses of carbonic anhydrase inhibitors

- Glaucoma (decreases aqueous humour formation)—generally, topically active agents (dorzolamide and brinzolamide) are used to

avoid systemic metabolic effects.
- Alkalizes urine and promotes excretion of certain drugs like cystine or uric acid, but prolong use requires HCO_3^- administration.
- Mountain sickness because it decreases CSF formation.
- Periodic paralysis
- Epilepsy.

Adverse effects: Acidosis, hypokalemia, drowsiness, paresthesia, fatigue, fever, rash, bone marrow depression and renal stone formation (rare, but fatal). Contraindicated in liver disease because it may precipitate hepatic coma by interfering elimination of NH_3 due to alkaline urine. Acidosis in patient of COPD. It may cause renal potassium wasting, but this can be countered by simultaneous administration of potassium. Dose of acetazolamide is 250 mg OD or BD (diamox).

Dichlorphenamide: Greater duration of action and Cl^- depletion, used for glaucoma. Dose 50–200 mg.

Ethozolamide is twice potent than acetazolamide as CA-inhibitor.

Methazolamide is used in the dose of 50–100 mg BD. Used for glaucoma, more potent than acetazolamide.

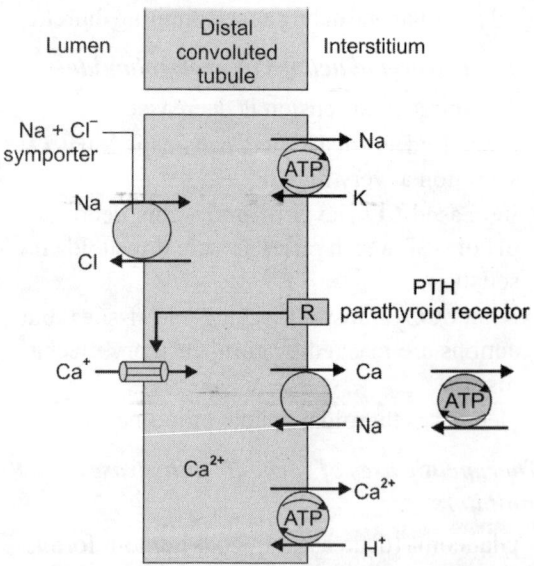

Fig. 69.3: Ionic exchange in distal convoluted tubule

BENZOTHIADIAZINES

Southworth (1937) observed that sulfanilamide is an antibacterial drug possesses diuretics action without inhibiting carbonic anhydrase significantly. Important pharmacological actions of benzothiadiazines are as follows.

Kidney and electrolytes: They act proximal to Na^+ and K^+ exchange region of distal tubule to prevent reabsorption of Na and Cl. The GFRs are not effected. Due to inhibition of carbonic anhydrase, it may cause some loss of HCO_3^-. It enhances Ca^{2+} reabsorption in contrast to loop diuretic which inhibits Ca^{2+} absorption. The calcium absorption in distal convoluted epithelial cell occurs *via* apical calcium channel and Na^+/Ca^{2+} exchanger which is regulated by PTH hormone acting on PTH receptor (Fig. 69.3).

Because of inhibition of Na reabsorption, large Na is available to distal segment where exchange of Na for K takes place in presence of aldosterone, causes excess K loss. Excess loss of Na, Cl and K leads to hyponatremia, hypochloremia, hypokalemia and alkalosis.

Blood vessels: They cause hypotension due to their actions on Na metabolism and on prolong action produces vasodilatation.

Metabolic actions: Hyperglycemia, glycosuria occur. Catecholamine is released secondary to volume depletion, inhibits insulin release and hypokalemia are possible mechanisms of hyperglycemia. Decreases excretion of uric acid and it decreases urine volume in diabetes insipidus (nephrogenic type).

Pharmacokinetics

- Orally absorbed
- Crosses placental barrier
- Secreted by tubules
- Excreted with urine
- The long acting benzothiadiazines are long acting because of plasma protein binding and lipid solubility.

Adverse effects

- Hypokalemia
- Hyponatremia

- Metabolic alkalosis
- Hyperuricemia
- Impaired GTT
- Hypochloremia
- Thrombocytopenic purpura
- Dermatitis
- Blood dyscrasia
- Hyperlipidemia
- Photosensitivity
- Weakness
- Paresthesia
- Impotence
- Kidney and liver failures may be precipitated.

Chlorthalidone (Hythalton)

(Dose 25–50 mg orally OD)

- Phthalimidine derivative
- Absorbed slowly
- Preferred for treatment of hypertension, also useful for treatment of hypoparathyroidism without causing hypercalcemia like vitamin D therapy.

Hydrochlorthiazide: Dose 25–100 mg orally OD.

Chorexolone (Nefrolan): Pthalimidine derivative more effective than chlorthiazide. Dose 25–100 mg.

Indapamide (dose 2.5–10 mg orally) and xipamide: Chemically related to chlorthalidone used as antihypertensive.

Clopamide: Diuretic action similar to bendroflumethiazide. Long acting, better tolerated. Dose 20–60 mg.

Quinazolinones [Quinethazone (50 mg) and Metolazone (5 mg tab)] belong to this group have diuretic properties similar to benzothiadiazines. Metolazone has additive action with frusemide. Inhibits PO_4 resorption. Other thiazides are: Bendroflumethiazide 2.5–10 mg orally OD; chlorthiazide 500 mg–2 g orally twice daily; metolazone 2.5–10 mg OD; polythiazide 1–4 mg orally and hydroflumethiazide 12.5–50 mg in two divided doses.

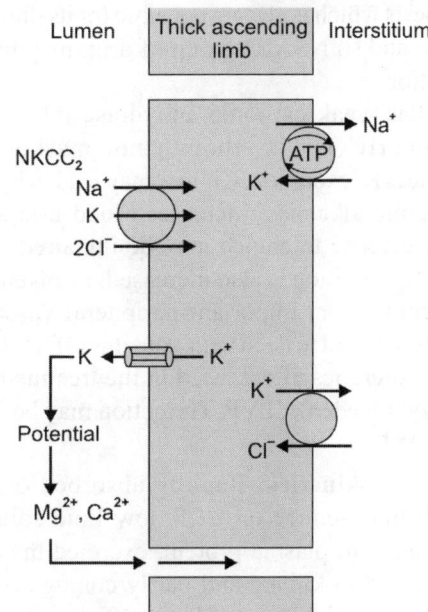

Fig. 69.4: Ascending loop of henle

Therapeutic Uses of Diuretics (Benzothiadiazine group)

- Edema
- Hypertension
- Diabetes insipidus
- Hypercalciuria (hydrochlorthiazide 50 mg BD)

Potent High Ceiling Diuretic (Frusemide, Bumetamide, etc.)

Frusemide (as a prototype of high ceiling, loop diuretic): Its natriuretic effect is greater than that of other classes. Diuretic effect increases with doses and it is active in relatively severe renal failure. It possesses halogenated sulfamoyl benzene ring. Its onset of action is prompt and short acting.

Pharmacological action: It acts on entire nephron except the distal site where Na^+ is exchanged for K^+ and H^+.

This group of drug inhibits the luminal Na^+-K^+-$2Cl^-$ transporter in this ascending loop of Henle and reduces resorption of NaCl. It also diminishes lumen positive potential which occurs due to K^+ recycling. As a result of this reduced potential loop diuretic increases Mg^{2+} and Ca^{2+} excretion. Loop diuretic also induces renal PG synthesis which is also responsible for its diuretic action and so NSAID group of drug may blunt its action.

It has weak carbonic anhydrase inhibition action, HCO_3^- loss though not marked, It enhances K^+ excretion, Cl^- loss may lead to hypochloremic alkalosis, increases blood uric acid level, glucose tolerance may be impaired, Ca^+ and Mg excretion is also increased. Intravenous frusemide is an important peripheral vascular pooler of blood in deep veins and this effect starts before diuretics effect, used in the treatment of pulmonary edema; LVF. The action may be PG-mediated.

Pharmacokinetics: Rapidly absorbed orally which may reduce on CCF, low lipid-soluble and bound to plasma protein, excreted mainly, unchanged in kidney and partly conjugated as glucuronic acid. Dose of Lasix 40 mg, sal inex 40 mg, 20 mg/2 mL injection; Lasix high dose 500 mg tab or 250 mg/25 mL injection (solution degrades spontaneously on exposure to light). 20–80 mg is injected at breakfast, for kidney insufficiency 200 mg 6 hourly IM or IV, in pulmonary edema 40–80 mg IV is given.

Torasemide (Dytor 10, 20, 100 mg tabs): Rapidly and completely absorbed orally. Used for hypertension, edema and renal failure.

Adverse effects: Na, K, Cl, and H_2O loss, patient complains for weakness, fatigue, cramps, postural hypotension, in elderly urinary retention, skin rash, diarrhea, pancreatitis, thrombocytopenia, neutropenia, diabetes mellitus, hyperuricemia, hearing loss may occur.

Not recommended as antihypertensive because of short duration, high diuretic potential and high dose requirement. Thiazides are preferred agents.

Mefruside: The pharmacological effect of this frusemide congener resembles more to benzothiadiazines, dose 12.5–50 mg orally and diuretic effect lasts for 20–24 hours. It is more potent than frusemide.

Bumetamide (Bumet 1 mg tab, 0.25 mg/mL injection) 40 times more potent than frusemide. Hyperuricemia, K^+ loss, glucose intolerance and ototoxicity are less than frusemide, but may cause myopathy. It is not effective in rats. Used in pulmonary edema. Lipid-soluble, plasma protein-bound and partly metabolized.

Piretanide (Dose 6–12 mg OD; 30–60 mg/ day in renal failure): Loop diuretic, 3–5 times potent than frusemide.

Ethacrynic acid (Edecrin): Synthesized as SH reactive agent, unsaturated ketone derivatives of phenoxyacetic acid. Sparingly soluble in water, but its Na salts are water-soluble, potent oral diuretics. Acts by inhibition of $Na^+/K^+/2Cl^-$ co-transport in ascending loop of Henle, without inhibiting carbonic anhydrase. Loss of K^+ is less, but chances of hypochloremic alkalosis are greater.

Orally rapidly absorbed, excreted through kidney, largely unchanged and as cysteine complex.

Side effects: Apart from electolyte changes may produce rashes, thrombocytopenia, agranulocytosis, vertigo, hepatotoxicity and hearing loss.

Ethacrynic acid tab 50 mg (dose 50–200), Na ethacrynate injection 0.5–1 mg/kg diluted with 50 mL of normal saline or 5% dextrose. Used in severe or resistant cases of pulmonary edema.

Uses of high ceiling diuretics

• Edema
• Pulmonary edema following MI or LVF
• Cerebral edema
• Forced diuretics in poisoning
• Useful in bromide, fluoride and iodide's toxic ingestion. Saline should be replaced for urinal loss.
• Hypertension
• With blood transfusion in anemia to prevent after load
• Since they increase calcium excretion in hypercalcemia used for renal stone.
• **Acute renal failure:** They increase the rate of urine flow; increase K^+ excretion.
• Hyperkalemia.

Organic mercurial diuretics: Accidentally discovered by a medical student. Strong diuretic, inhibit $Na^+/K^+/2Cl^-$ cotransport in ascending loop of Henle, probably acts with sulfhydryl enzymes of kidney tubules. It has to be given by parenteral route intermittently, because regular use causes alkalosis and refractoriness. These groups of diuretics are rarely used nowadays because of the availabilities of better drugs and the toxicities of these drugs.

Potassium sparing diuretics: They prevent K^+ secretion by antagonizing the effect of mineralo-corticoid hormone, aldosterone in collecting tubule (spironolactone and eplerenone). Amiloride and triamterone inhibit Na^+ influx through luminal membrane ion channels.

Spironolactone (Aldactone): Steroid with structural similarity with aldosterone, competitive inhibitor of aldosterone, prevents K^+ secretion and decreases Na reabsorption, weak diuretic. It enters epithelial cell from basolateral membrane and binds to mineralocorticoid receptor (MR) which translocates to nucleus to regulate multiple gene product called aldosterone-induced protein (AIP) which increases Na^+ conductance in luminal membrane and sodium pump activity.

The action of aldosterone antagonists depends on renal prostaglandin secretion so its action is bluned by NSAID.

Orally 75% bioavailable, metabolized in liver to active metabolite canrenone. Dose 25–50 mg BD. It is cumulative.

Uses of spironolactone

- Edema (cirrhotic or nephrotic)
- To counteract K^+ loss with thiazide or loop diuretics
- Hypertension
- Conn's syndrome.

Side effects

- Hirsutism
- Gynecomastia
- Menstural irregularities
- Impotence
- Drowsiness
- Hyperkalemia
- Acidosis in renal patient

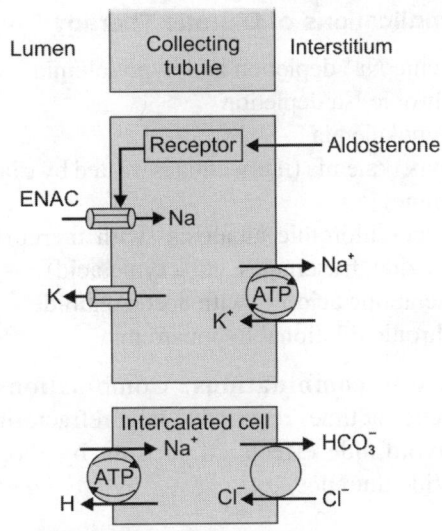

Fig. 69.5: Collecting duct of nephron

Drug interaction: Carbonexolene's action in peptic ulcer is reduced. Aspirin inhibits spirono-lactone by inhibiting its tubular secretion. It increases plasma digoxin lebel.

Eplerenone: More selective aldosterone anta-gonist. Less likely to produce gynecomastia; impotence and menstrual irregularities. It is available as 25, 50 and 100 mg tabs.

Triamterene: Dytac 100–200 mg orally. Incompletely absorbed orally, partly protein-bound.

Triamterene and amiloride interfere Na^+ entry through epithelial sodium ion channel in ENaC collecting tubule. Since K^+ secretion is coupled with Na^+ entry in this collecting tubule they are able K^+ sparing diuretics not aldosterone antagonists, induce hyperkalemia, may produce diarrhea. Used in:

- Pseudoaldosteronism characterized by hypertension, hypokalemia. Not associated with increased aldosterone secretion.
- With other diuretics in nephrotic syndrome and liver cirrhosis.

Amiloride: A guanidine derivative, in higher doses inhibits Na reabsorption. Orally absorbed, not bound to plasma protein, and its duration of action is also longer than triamterene.

Complications of Diuretic Therapy

- Acute Na^+ depletion and hypovolemia
- Chronic Na depletion
- Hypokalemia
- Hyperkalemia (if uricemia is treated by triamaterene)
- Hyperchloremic alkalosis (with mercurials, thiazide, frusemides, ethacrynic acid)
- Metabolic acidosis with acetazolamide
- Chronic dilutional hyponatremia.

Diuretic combinations: Combinations of diuretics at times required to treat refractoriness or avoid side effects (K loosing by loop or thiazide diuretics).

- Loop and thiazide may be given together.
- Potassium sparing may be combined with loop and thiazide diuretics to avoid potassium loss.

Non-oedematous states where diuretics are used

i. Hypertension: Loop or thiazides

ii. Nephrolithiasis: Thiazides

iii. Hypercalcemia: Loop diuretic

iv. Diabetes insipidus: Thiazide

Sodium-Glucose Cotransporter-2 in ($SGLT_2$) inhibitors *viz.* (discussed with diabetes mellitus) **Dapagliflozin canaglifozin** inhibit sodium-glucose reabsorption.

70

Antidiuretic Agents

ANTIDIURETIC HORMONES (ADH)

It is produced in supraoptic and paraventricular nuclei of hypothalamus travels along the hypothalamohypophyseal tract to posterior pituitary. It is a nonapeptide. In supraoptic and paraventricular nerve cell bodies, it is synthesized as a large precursor peptide along with binding protein "neurophysin". Rate of secretion is determined by hydration and contraction of ECF volume. Its secretion is enhanced by angiotensin II, PGs, histamine, ACh, neuropeptide and inhibited by GABA; atrial natriuretic peptide. Impulse from baroreceptor and higher centers also influence synthesis of ADH and its release. It acts through ADH receptors, which are of two types V_1 and V_2. The ADH receptors are G-protein coupled cell membrane receptor.

V_1 receptor = All vasopressin receptors except those of CD cells and some of blood vessels. The V_1 receptor is further divided into V_1a (present in smooth muscle, vasculature platelet, liver) and V_1b (present in anterior pituitary).

V_2 receptors present in collecting ducts of kidney, regulate water permeability, activating cAMP and through aquaporin in CD. Lithium and demeclocycline partially antagonize ADH action. Carbamazepine and chlorpropamide also potentiate its action.

Functions of ADH

- Blood vessels contract
- BP raises
- Smooth muscle contracts, so gut peristalsis increases
- Uterus contracts.

- In CNS, it is involved in temperature regulation, circulation, ACTH release.
- Induces platelet aggregation and hepatic glucogenolysis.
- It releases factor VIII and von Willebrand's factor from vascular endothelium *via* V_2 receptor.
- Orally inactive given as nasal puff or parenteral route.

Vasopressin Analogues

Lypressin: Terlipressin and desmopressin are vasopressin analogues.

Lypressin (Petresin 20 IU/mL): It is a 8-lysine-vasopressin acts both on V_1 and V_2 receptors. Given IM, SC or IV diluted with dextrose, over 10–20 minutes

Terlipressin (Glypressin 1 mg freeze dried powder with 5 mL of diluant): Used for esophageal varices. It is a produrg of vasopressin.

Desmopressin: Given intranasal 10–40 µg/day; 0.1–0.2 mg/TDS, SC or IV 2–4 µg/day in 2–3 divided doses

Uses of ADH

1. Diabetes insipidus (neurogenic)
2. Bed-wetting in children and adults
3. Renal concentration test
4. Hemophillia and von Willebrand's disease (desmopressin is preferred). It checks bleeding 0.3 mg/kg in 50 mL saline given IV for 30 minutes. It releases factor VIII and von Willebrand's factor.

5. Bleeding in esophageal varices

6. Abdominal radiography to drive out intestinal gas.

• 1 to 4 actions are mediated *via* V$_2$, 5 and 6 *via* V$_1$ receptors.

Preparation and Dosage

• Vasopressin IP inj. (Pitressin) 20 IU/mL. Dose 0.25–0.75 mL by SC or IM.

• Vasopressin tannate NF in oily suspension 5 U/mL; dose 0.5 mL in 24–72 hours. The ampules should be warmed and shaken before use, as drugs settle on standing.

• Desiccated posterior pituitary powder as snuff by insufflation 10–50 mg every time bladder is emptied.

• Synthetic vasopressin DDAVP (I deamino 8-D arginine vasopressin; desmopressin) 15 µg BD intranasaly, has got greater anti-diuretic and less pressor activity.

• 8-lysine-vasopressin (syntopressin) used as intranasal spray and is more stable.

Benzothiadiazines: Used to treat pituitary and nephrogenic diabetes insipidus, they probably act by reducing GFR and causing negative Na balance. Long acting drug like polythiazide is preferred, because of convenience and cheap. K$^+$ supplementation required.

Amiloride is used to treat lithium-induced diabetes insipidus.

Indomethacian reduces polyuria of diabetes insipidus (renal).

Chilorpropramide: Oral hypoglycemic, effective in diabetes insipidus of pituitary origin, probably increases sensitivity of renal tubules to low and ineffective concentration of vasopressin. Action is blunted by ethanol.

Carbamazepine: This antiepileptic agents probably releases vasopressin and sensitizes kidney to ADH. The action is blunted by ethanol.

Clorfibrate: Hypolipidemic drug effective in neurogenic diabetes insipidus in the dose of 1–2 gm/day. The side effects restrict its use.

Vasopressin antagonists: Conivaptan and tolvaptan are vasopressin antagonists. Elevated vasopressin concentrations are found in hyponatremia and heart failure. Conivaptan has high affinity for V$_1$a and V$_2$ receptors whereas tolvaptan has high affinity for V$_2$ receptor and conivaptan is approved by IV route for hyponatremia, but not for heart failure.

71

Nephrotoxic Drugs

Since kidneys are major organ for excretion, it is vulnerable to toxic action of drug which may be acute or chronic. Certain conditions correct after cessation of therapy. Serum creatinine is useful to guide and assess the severity of renal impairment.

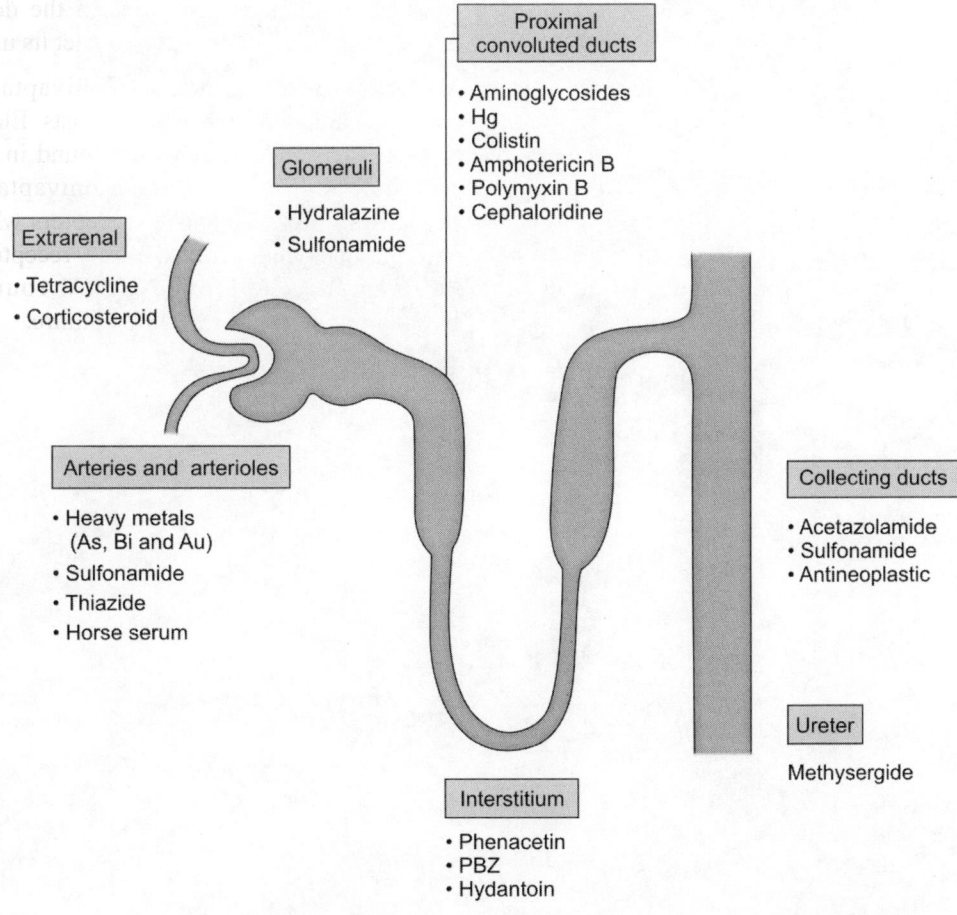

Fig. 71.1: Site of action of some nephrotoxic drugs

Table 71.1: Drugs causing nephrotoxicity

Site of action	Drugs	Nature of toxicities
Extrarenal	Tetracycline, corticosteroids	Azotemia by increasing protein breakdown
Arteries and arterioles	Heavy metals (As, Bi and Au), sulfonamide, horse serum, iodide	Vasculitis
Glomeruli	Hydralazine, sulfonamide	Vasculitis, glomerulopathy
Convoluted tubules	Aminoglycosides, mercury, colistin, amphotericin B, polymyxin B	Necrosis of proximal and distal tubular epithellium
Intrestitium	Phenacetin, PBZ, hydantoin	Papillary necrosis, interstitial nephritis
Collecting ducts	Acetazolamide, sulfonamide, antineoplastic	Crystaluria hyperuricemia
Ureter	Methysergide	Retroperitoneal fibrosis

72

Water, Sodium, Potassium and Hydrion Metabolism

The average water content in human body is 60, 51 and 77% of body mass in male, female and one month infant respectively. The body fluid is divided into:

- Intracellular fluid [ICF] (fluid inside cell) like dispersed phase of emulsion. 27% of total 60% of water.
- Extracellular fluid [ECF] 60% (outside the cell wall fluids) like continuous phase of emulsion acts as transport medium for various substances, which are moving into and from cell. It is further divided into extra- and intravascular. The main difference of these two are that intravascular protein is high. Otherwise they are continuous. The CSF, aqueous humor, GI tract fluid, tracheobronchial tree fluids constitute 2.5% of total body fluids known as transcellular fluids. ECF water is 33% of total 60% of water.

The ionized particles carrying positive and negative charges are called electrolytes. The electrolyte contents of ICF and ECF differ. The Na, Cl, and HCO_3 are extracellular, while K, Mg, and PO_4, SO_4 are generally intracellular. The electrolyte content of both extra- and intracellular fluids is not very different, the existing difference is essential to carry out specialized function by them.

FUNCTIONS OF ELECTROLYTES

- Maintenance of osmotic pressure
- Maintenance of electroneutrality
- For impulse conduction
- Production of energy

- Intracellular K and Mg are essential for various enzymes, P is required for ATP synthesis.
- **Miscellaneous:** Blood clotting and bone formation require calcium.

Water metabolism: Water content of healthy body is maintained in normal limits. Approximately 300 mL of water is produced daily during oxidation of food. The output is 100 mL with feces. 1000 mL in expired air and sweating and mainly through urine. Under basal conditions water balance can be calculated as follows: (24 hours intake + 300 mL from oxidation of food) – (24 hours urinary volume + 1000 mL of skin and lungs loss). The insensible water loss is high in hot–dry climatic condition. Water balance is maintained by intake (regulated by thirst) and output (regulated by ADH). Thirst and ADH activities are very sensitive to small changes in the osmolality.

Water depletion: Selective water deficiency is not common. It is usually associated with electrolyte metabolism. Relative water deficiency occurs in:

- Reduced intake of water in extreme lethargy and coma.
- Defective water absorption (diarrhea)
- Excessive sweating in fever
- Chronic renal failure (some cases)
- Diabetes insipidus.

Infant's ability to concentrate urine is less so they are more prone to water depletion than adults. Unrestricted administration of fluid produces excess water, if there is insufficient urinary output.

Sodium metabolism: Sodium is present mainly in ECF. Besides ECF, it is present in bone and cartilages. Body content of Na depends upon intake and output. Na craving for salt is observed in sodium depletion as thirst in water depletion excessive sweating in tropics (Heat exhaustion). Diarrhea and cholera may produce excess Na loss. Na is absorbed from jejunum by passive absorption mainly by:

- Concurrent glucose and fructose absorption (solvent drag).
- Glucose stimulates active sodium absorption.
- Intraluminal jejunal sodium concentration increases Na absorption.
- Na absorption of ileum occurs by active transport process. About 1000 mEq of Na is secreted daily in alimentary tract which is totally reabsorbed. Aldosterone promotes absorption of Na from intestine and colon.

Urinary excretion of sodium: 98% of filtered Na (13–20 mEq per minute) is reabsorbed. Sodium retention occurs in CCF due to decreased sodium filtration and in Addison's disease due to reabsorption failure causing sodium depletion. Sodium excretion is regulated by renal blood flow (depends upon cardiac output, local condition of kidney vessels) and by hormone aldosterone. Sodium depletion causes decrease in ECF and plasma volume resulting in rise in the hematocrit and serum protein concentration.

Natriuretic peptide is a vasoactive peptide released from atrium and brain plays role in sodium hemostasis. Apart from this hydrocortisone, estrogen and testosterone cause Na^+ retention. ADH indirectly affects sodium hemostasis.

Causes of sodium loss
- Gastrointestinal loss—diarrhea, discharge from fistula.
- Renal loss—diuretics therapy, diabetic coma, starvation, acute tubular necrosis, Addison's disease, polyuria with normal sodium (excretion occurs in diabetes insipidus).

- In hot–dry environment.
- In draining ascitic fluid.

Symptoms of Na loss: Loss of appetite, lethargy, muscle cramps (100–200 mEq depletion). Massive sodium depletion (1000–1500 mEq) will produce shock—BP will fall. Vasoconstriction of skin and kidney will take place, eyeball shrunken, skin turgor is lost.

Hyponatremic syndrome: Here toal body sodium is normal or high, but plasma sodium level is low. Hyponatremia may be due to sodium loss, potassium loss, excess water or their combinations. At times it is due to inappropriate ADH secretion.

Excess sodium: Always associated with water retention may be due to:
- Intrinsic kidney disease (nephritis)
- Excessive resorption of sodium (aldosteronism)
- Decreased renal blood flow as in congestive heart failure or shock.

Treatment of hypernatremia
- Restricting sodium intake
- Increasing sodium output by diuretics
- Improving renal perfusion by digitalis in CHF or intravenous infusion in oligemic shock.

Hypernatremia may be due to
a. Primary sodium excess
b. Primary potassium excess
c. Water depletion
d. Combination of (a + b + c)

The treatment is reducing Na level by 5% dextrose in water till serum sodium level declines to normal. Then ½ of normal saline is administered till salt deficit is rectified.

POTASSIUM METABOLISM

The distribution of potassium is related to the cell mass 70% in muscle, 20% in brain and large viscera and 10% in skin subcutaneous tissues.

The total body potassium content can be estimated by:

- Analysis of Cadavers
- Isotope dilution technique
- Measuring whole body radiation from naturally occurring isotope of K^{40}.

Potassium intake and excretion: Daily intake varies from 50–150 mEq, more in vegetarians. It is secreted by kidney tubules. Increased Na intake increases the potassium loss. 5–10 mEq of K is excreted in stools. The potassium concentration of sweat in infant is 3.9 mEq/L. Potassium loss is significant in sweating in fever and dry heat.

Potassium Depletion and Hypokalemia

- Occurs in dietic deficiency
- Gastrointestinal loss—vomiting, pyloric obstruction, fistula, steatorrhea, purgative use chronically
- **Renal loss:** Sodium overload, starvation, acidosis, protein catabolism, excessive aldosterone, hydrocortisone and diuretics, nephrotic syndrome, Fanconi's syndrome, diabetic acidosis, if treated with insulin.
- Excessive sweating.

Clinical features: Lethargy, malaise, weakness of muscular activity, anorexia, thirst, paralysis, conduction defect in heart, paralytic ileus, skeletal muscle fiber shows Zenker's degeneration, ST depression, prolong QT, T inversion and prominent U wave.

Treatment: Potassium by mouth, coconut water, orange, banana. By oral route as KCl. K citrate. It should not be given directly into vein, which may cause sudden death.

Potassium excess: Hyperkalemia is fairly common and fatal complication occurs in chronic renal insufficiency, diabetes, respiratory acidosis and some drugs like ACE-inhibitors, trimethoprim, pentamidine, spironolactone, amiloride, heparin, succinylcholine, cyclosporine, and in Addison's disease. Manifestations are arrhythmia, cardiac arrest in diastole, ECG shows ST depression, wide QRS, T tentative, PR prolongation.

Treatment of potassium excess

- Dietary restriction of K, calorie should be given as carbohydrate and fat, not as protein.
- Preventing tissue breakdown by anabolic steroids
- Promoting entry of potassium into cells by 5–10 units of insulin with 5% glucose and corrective acidosis
- Promoting K excretion by cortisone in Addison's disease
- Ion exchange resins
- Peritoneal or hemodialysis
- Controlling infection and acidosis
- Toxic effect of K^+ on heart can temporarily conrtrolled by 10% calcium gluconate 5–10 mL, may be repeated. Dialysis is life-saving.

ACIDOSIS AND ALKALOSIS

According to present concept, an acid is a proton donor; molecule or ion which provides a proton [a hydrion H^+] is a positively charged particle and lowers the pH of a solution into which it is placed. Water can act as acid or base depending on circumstances. The pH of body fluid is constant by three mechanisms as:

- Buffer systems
- Renal mechanisms
- Respiratory mechanism.

Metabolically hydrions are produced in body in two forms

a. *Potential hydrion*

 As CO_2 produced by combustion of foods like carbohydrates, fats, proteins.

b. *Non-volatile hydrion*

- Incomplete oxidation of carbohydrate, fat producing organic acid.
- Sulfuric acid produced following oxidation of sulfur-containing amino acids.
- Phosphoric acid produced during oxidation of phosphoproteins.

 A fall in carbonic acid or rise in bicarbonate will produce alkalosis and rise in carbonic acid and fall in bicarbonate will produce acidosis.

ACIDOSIS

Acidosis is the increase of potential and/or non-volatile hydrion content of the body. Hydrion concentration in plasma is termed acidemia. Acidosis without acidemia is compensated acidosis.

Acidosis can occur in

a. Metabolic acidosis

b. Renal acidosis

c. Respiratory acidosis

   a. *Metabolic acidosis* due to retention of carbon dioxide.

   • Fever, starvation, dehydration, diabetic ketoacidosis.

   • Administration of drugs: Salicylates, NH_4Cl, methanol.

   • Excessive loss of alkaline fluids: Diarrhea.

   • Lactic acidosis by oral hypoglycemic biguanides.

   • Administration of large quantities of normal saline.

   • Accumulation of lactic acid.

   b. *Renal acidosis:* Body hydrion is increased due to defective renal excretion (renal tubular acidosis, glomerulonephritis, diabetic nephropathy, Addison's disease) with carbonic anhydrase inhibitors.

   c. *Respiratory acidosis:* Increase in potential hydrion occurs in chronic lung disease, cor pulmonale, respiratory muscle paralysis. Plasma bicarbonate and PCO_2 are raised, urine is acidic.

Clinical features: Hyperpnea, muscle twitching, mental confusion, Kussmaul respiration, bone pain due to demineralization of bones, alkaline phosphatase raised with chronic renal failure.

Treatement of acidosis: Correct electrolyte disturbance in Na and K along with treatment of 7.5% $NaHCO_3$, quantifies sufficient rise in plasma bicarbonate concentration. Use of sodium lactate to correct acidosis is not justified, because it depends upon oxidative mechanism for conversion of bicarbonate and it causes lactic acidosis. Excess alkali administration in presence of kidney damage may cause tetany, pulmonary edema. Acidosis with renal failure is better managed with dialysis. Respiratory acidosis is difficult to treat and is terminal event. IV or oral sodium bicarbonate is given in emergency, intermittent oxygen, bronchodilator and respiratory infection should be treated.

ALKALOSIS

Alkalosis is defined as reduction of hydrion of body and alkalemia is reduction in hydrion concentration of the plasma manifested as increase in pH of blood. Alkalosis without alkalemia is called compensated alkalosis.

Types of Alkalosis

• Metabolic

• Hypokalemia

• Contraction

• Respiratory

   a. **Metabolic:** Alkali ingestion in presence of renal damage, excessive vomiting, excessive ingestion of milk (milk alkali syndrome).

   b. **Contraction alkalosis:** With mercurial diuretics. Ratio of PCO_2/HCO_3 decreases. Administration of NH_4Cl corrects chloride loss.

   c. **Hypokalemic alkalosis:** Occurs with thiazide diuretics.

   d. **Respiratory alkalosis:** Hyperventilation in anxiety, fever, high altitude climbing, salicylates, analeptic, hot bath, hypothalamic tumor. Excess washing out of hydrion raises pH of blood.

Clinical features: Feeling of tingling and muscle cramps. Tetany in alkalosis due to lowering of plasma ionized calcium, chronic alkalosis causes anorexia, apathy, mental disturbances.

Treatment: Aims at removal of cause, correction of body fluids, *viz.* vomiting causing chloride loss is treated by IV normal saline, 5% arginine hydrochloride is better than IV NH_4Cl because it may cause acidosis and ammonia poisoning.

MANAGEMENT OF WATER AND ELECTROLYTE DISTURBANCES IN CHOLERA AND ACUTE DIARRHEA

- Correction of water electrolyte and acidosis.
- Administration of suitable antibiotics.
- Treatment of complications.
- Supportive therapy with IV glucose (for nutrition); antidiarrheal (doubtful role). Specific gravity of plasma measured by $CuSO_4$ solution (normal is 1.025). For increase of 0.001 of plasma specific gravity, adult patient requires 4 mL/kg body weight of fluids. IV fluids are given rapidly, initially at the rate of 100 mL per minute. In an emergency, isotonic saline and sodium bicarbonate in 2 : 1 ratio is given which will rectify Na loss and acidosis. Coma and convulsion indicating hypoglycemia requires IV glucose.

WHO's recommended oral rehydration therapy

1. Sodium chloride   – 2.6 gm/L
2. Potassium chloride   – 1.5 gm/L
3. Trisodium citrate dihydrate – 2.9 gm/L
4. Glucose   – 13.5 gm/L

                Total   **– 20.5 gm/L**

All are mixed in 1 liter of boiled cooled water.

Home-made ORS

- Sodium chloride ¾ teaspoon full
- Potassium citrate ½ teaspoon full
- Trisodium dihydrate citrate ¾ teaspoon full
- Glucose 1½ tablespoon full in 1 liter of boiled cooled water.

Cereal-based oral rehydration solution (CORS)

Here glucose is replaced by rice or other starchy foods. It reduces vomiting and severity of diarrhea along with replacing body fluids. It needs digestive enzymes for its success which is not a problem for adults except in infants below 4 months where intestinal glycoamylase is not fully developed.

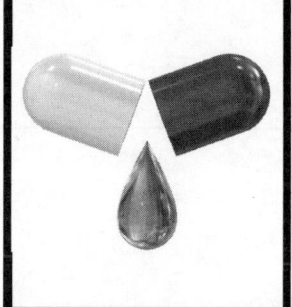
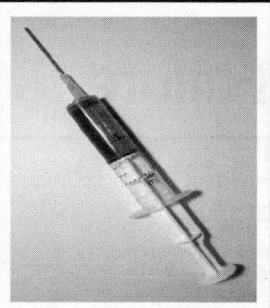
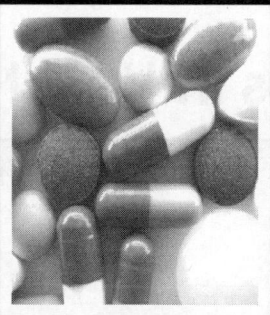
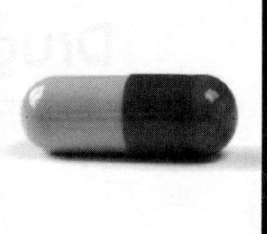

SECTION 10

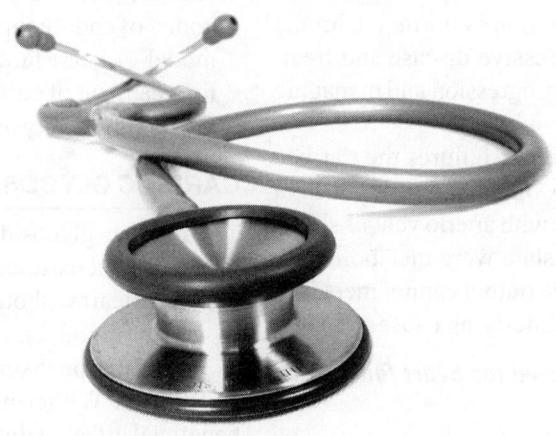

CARDIOVASCULAR SYSTEM

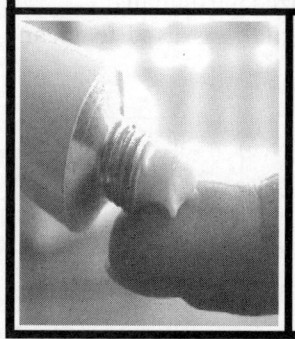
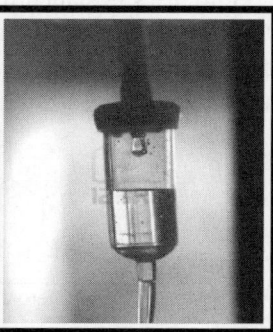
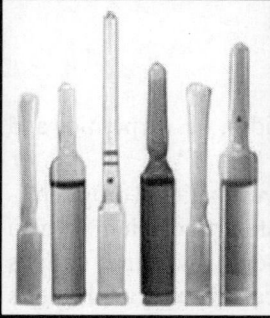
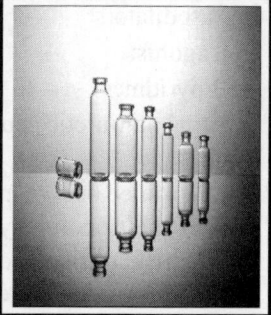

73

Drugs in Heart Failure

Heart failure is a syndrome of multiple causes occur when cardiac output of the heart is inadequate to provide oxygen demand of the body. In systolic failure, mechanical pumping and ejection fraction is reduced and in diastolic failure loss of relaxation of cardiac muscle reducing cardiac output but ejection fraction is normal. Chronic heart failure is a progressive discase and treatment aims at reducing progression and managing decompensation.

Commonly in all heart failure, the cardiac output is low called low output failure but in high output failure as occurs with arterio venous shunt, anemia, hyperthyroid state were metabolic rate is increased and cardiac output cannot meet it. It is treated by treating underlying cause.

Drugs which can be used for heart failure are

- Cardiac glycosides
- Diuretics
- Aldosterone receptor antagonist
- Angiotensin receptor antagonist
- Angiotensin converting enzyme inhibitors
- Renin inhibitor: Aliskiren
- β blockers
- Vasodilators
- β agonist
- Bipyridines
- Atrial natriuretic peptides, *viz.* carperitide and ularitide
- Levosimedan is an investigational drug sensitizes the troponin system to calcium. It also inhibits phosphodiesterase and causes vasodilatation. **Omecamtiv mecarbil** alters binding of myosin to strongly binding actin

without increasing energy consumption. Istaroxime inhibits Na^+ / K^+ ATPase and sequesters $Ca2^+$ by SR, so less arrhythmogenic.

- **Bosentan** and **tezosentan** are orally and intravenously active nonselective competitive antagonist of endothelin, effective in experimental model of heart failure. Bosentan is approved for treatment of pulmonary hypertension. ADR are teratogenicity and hepatoxicity.

CARDIAC GLYCOSIDES

The cardiac glycosides have cardiac inotropic properties, increase cardiac contractility of hypodynamic heart without proportionate increase in O_2 consumption (*cf.* cardiac stimulants increase O_2 consumption disproportionately).

William Withering in 1785, described the beneficial effect of digitalis obtained from decoction of foxglove, used by old lady to treat dropsy, mentioned in his famous book *An Account of Foxglove and Some of its Medicinal Uses.* Mackenzie and Cushney in 1911, demonstrated digitalis block atrioventricular conduction. Henry Gold in 1938 standardized the digitalis.

By convention, digitalis is used to mean cardiac glycosides.

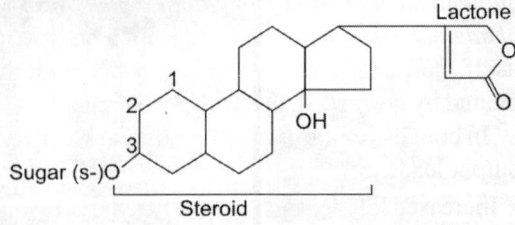

Fig. 73.1: Structure of glycoside

Table 73.1: Some cardiac glycosides and their sources

Sl. no.	Source	Glycosides
1.	*Digitalis purpurea* (Leaf)	Digitoxin, gitoxin, gitalin
2.	*Digitalis lanata* (Leaf)	Digitoxin, gitoxin, digoxin
3.	*Strophanthus kombe* (Seed)	Strophanthin K
4.	*Strophanthus gratus* (Seed)	Strophanthin G (Ouabain)
5.	*Urginea maritima* (Bulb)	Proscillaridin A
6.	*Thevetia nerltifolia* (Nut)	Thevetin
7.	*Convallaria majalis*	Convallotoxin
8.	*Bufo vulgaris*	Bufotoxin
9.	*Semisynthetic*	Acetyl digoxin, acetyl-strophanthidin, desacetyl-lantoside

Structure of Glycoside (Fig. 73.1)

The active constituents of glycosides represent a combination of an aglycone or genin with one or more sugars. Aglycone is a cyclopentano-perhydrophenanthrene is a steroid nucleus, with a lactone attached to it. The pharmacological action lies on aglycone which is less potent and transient in action. The sugars in glycoside increase potency of:

- Aglycone
- Increase water solubility and
- Increase cell permeability. The hydroxyl present in aglycone determines polarity. Acid hydrolysis of glycosides separate sugar and aglycone.

PHARMACODYNAMICS

Digitalis increases force of myocardial contraction in CCF patient and slows the ventricular rate in presence of atrial fibrillation and flutter.

The failure of heart may be defined as *"Inability of the heart to maintain an output adequate to meet the body's metabolic need in spite of adequate venous return"*. It is not a disease in itself, but a syndrome, which can be properly treated by correcting the underlying cause.

In congestive cardiac failure, the low cardiac output leads to:

- Increased left ventricular volume and pressure
- Ventricular hypertrophy
- Increased circulating catecholamine

- Increased systemic vascular resistance
- Activation of renin-angiotensin aldosterone system
- Increased vasopressin secretion

Mechanism of Action of Digitalis

The extracellular concentration of $[Na^+]$ and intracellular $[K^+]i$ is maintained by Na^+/K^+-ATPase pump [said to be receptor of digitalis]. It binds to α-subunit of sarcolemmal Na^+/K^+-ATPase. The intracellular concentration of Ca^{2+} is regulated by exchange for Na^+ (exchange site). The active extrusion of Na^+ is decreased by digitalis leads to increase in $[Na^+]i$ which in turn causes increase in $[Ca^{2+}]i$. The Ca^{2+} also enters the cell by L-type Ca^{2+} channel during depolarization, triggers release of stored intracellular calcium from sarcoplasmic reticulum *via* ryanodine receptor (RyR) which is available for activation of actin-troponin-tropomycin complex [plant alkaloid ryanodine interferes with the release of calcium from SR]. During the repolarization Ca^{2+} is sequestered in SR by Ca^{2+}-ATPase mostly $SERCA_2$ and remainder by high capacity Na^+/Ca^{2+} exchanger which exchanges $3Na^+$ for $1Ca^{2+}$. β agonist and PDE inhibitors increase cAMP and probabilities of opening L-type Ca^{2+} channel and RyR Ca^{2+} channel.

Mechanism of Action of Digitalis in Heart Failure (Figs 73.2 and 73.3)

- Inhibits Na^+/K^+-ATPase pump and increases

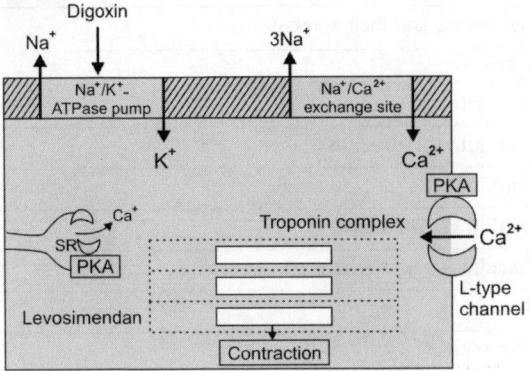

Fig. 73.2: Mechanism of action of digitalis

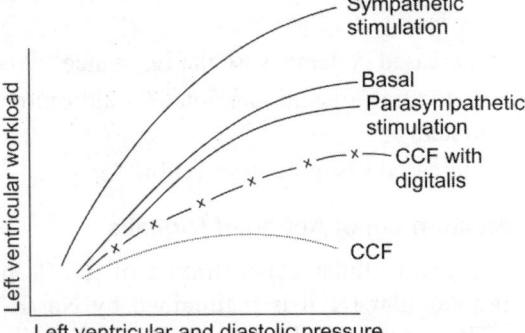

Fig. 73.3: Left ventricular workload in digitalis treated patient

intracellular calcium in patient of heart failure for efficient cardiac contraction.

- Resets baroreceptors
- Decreases sympathetic nervous system activity
- Slows down ventricular rate in patient of atrial fibrillation
- By efficient cardiac contraction increases renal blood flow and acts as diuretics.

Istaroxime is an investigational steroid which also inhibits Na^+/K^+-ATPase and apart from that, it increases entry of Ca^{2+} in sarcoplasmic reticulum. It seems, it will be less arrhythmogenic than digoxin. It is in phase II clinical trials.

Levosimendan inhibits PDE and sensitizes myocardium to Ca^{2+}.

Pharmacological Actions of Digitalis

A. Heart rate: Heart rate is decreased by digitalis, more marked in CCF due to improved circulation, positive inotrophic action restoring vagal tone and abolishing sympathetic activity. It slows heart rate by vagal [reflexly through].

  i. Nodose ganglion sensitization and amplifying parasympathetic discharge to the heart.

 ii. Direct stimulation of vagal center.

iii. Sensitization of SA mode to ACh. Extravagal direct action on SA and AV nodes. The anti-adrenergic action is increased. The vagal action of digitalis can be blocked by atropine.

B. Electrophysiological activity: Differs in different fibers qualitatively and quantitatively, the Purkinje fibers and automatic conducting tissues and atria are more sensitive.

a. At Purkinje fibers: There is decrease in maximal diastolic potential, increase in slope of phase 4 depolarization and decrease in action potential duration, because of increase in slope of phase 4 depolarization, the fiber becomes automatic.

b. In SA and AV nodes, automaticity is reduced at therapeutic concentration by vagal action, which hyperpolarizes these cells and reduces their phase 4 slope. In toxic doses, reduce resting membrane potential of SA cells by direct action and cease impulse generation.

Action potential duration and amplitude of atrium is decreased. The effective refractory period of atrium is decreased by vagal action and that of AV node is increased by direct action.

c. ECG: May produce arrhythmia.

- Decreases amplitude or T inversion
- Slowing AV conduction (increased PR interval) and AV block at toxic doses
- QT shortening
- Depressed ST segment (at high doses due to interference with depolarization)

Abnormal QRS of WPW syndrome is

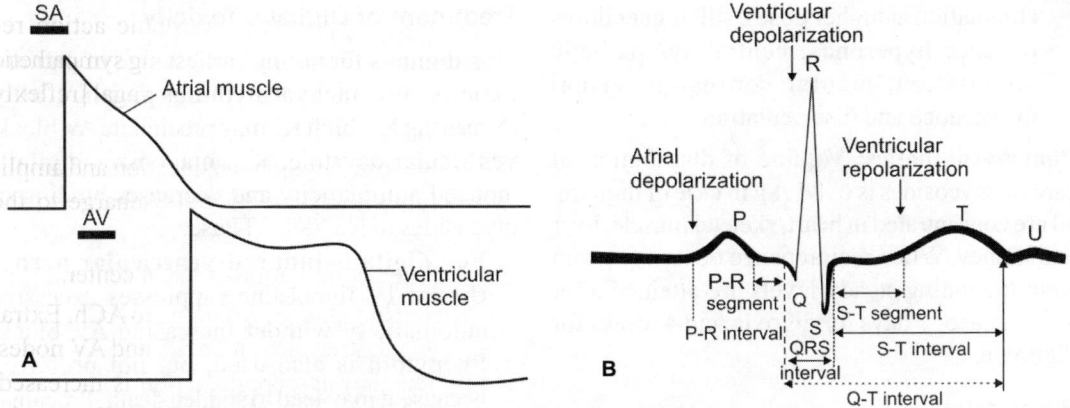

Figs 73.4A and B: Normal action potential of cardiac muscle and normal ECG.

widened because conduction through normal AV bundle is slowed, but not by abbarant Kent's bundle.

C. **Blood vessels:** Mild vasoconstriction effect, but in CCF patient improvement of circulation occurs indirectly because reflex sympathetic overactivity is withdrawn and peripheral resistance is decreased. No prominent effect on BP, though it directly constricts coronary artery, but coronary insufficiency is no contraindication of its use.

D. **Kidney:** Improves circulation in CCF, increases renal perfusion and causes diuresis. No effect in normal person.

E. **CNS:** Nausea and vomiting due to CTZ

Table 73.2: Pharmacokinetics of different digitalis preparations			
Properties	*Digitoxin*	*Digoxin*	*Ouabain*
Number of –OH groups	One	Two	Five
Polarity	Least	More	Most
Oral absorption	Very good (90–100%)	Good (60–80%)	Erratic and little
Protein binding	95–97%	25%	Very little
Time course onset	½–2 hours	15–30 min	10–15 min
Action	6–12 hours	2–5 hours	1–2 hours
Peak duration	2–3 weeks	2–6 days	1–2 days
Plasma t/2	5–7 days	40 hours	20 hours
Plasma concentration	15–30 ng/mL	0.8–2 ng/mL	–
Potency	Least	Intermediate	Highest
Daily maintenance dose	0.05–0.2 mg	0.125–0.5 mg	–
Dose elimination	10–15%	35%	60–70%
Route of elimination (mainly)	Hepatic metabolism	Renal excretion	Renal excretion
Administration	Oral	Oral/IV	IV
Duration of action	Prolong about 2–3 weeks	3–6 days	1–3 days
Daily loss first order kinetics	Cumulative in nature (10%)	37% less cumulative	No need
Generally used for	Maintenance	**Routine treatment and emergency**	Emergency

stimulation at higher doses, still higher doses produce hyperpnea, central sympathetic stimulation, mental confusion, visual disturbance and disorientation.

Pharmacokinetics: Volume of distribution of cardiac glycosides is 6–8 L/kg in case of digoxin, all are concentrated in heart, skeletal muscle, liver and kidney. When maintenance doses are given from beginning steady levels are attained after $4 \times t^{1/2}$, *i.e.* 6–7 days for digoxin and 4 weeks for digitoxin.

Preparation

Digoxin: Lanoxin 0.25 mg tab. 0.05 mg/mL or 0.5 mg/2 mL injection.

Digitoxin: Digitalin 0.1 mg

Lantoside C: 0.25 mg tab (Cadilanid)

Deslanoside: Deslanoside 0.25 mg/mL injection

Strophanthin K: Strophosid 0.25 mg/mL injection. (similar to ouabain)

Acetyldigoxin: Acylanid 0.2 mg tab, 0.5 mg/2 mL injection.

IM route recommended for deslanoside because other preparations produce irritation and muscle necrosis. Parenteral route is preferred in emergency, vomiting and unconscious patient.

Therapeutic Uses of Digitalis

• Congestive cardiac failure
• Atrial flutter and fibrillation
• Paroxysmal supraventricular tachycardia

The dose of digitalis has to be adjusted according to the type of preparation, age, weight, renal function and concomitant use of other drugs. The range of therapeutic and toxic doses of digitalis is very narrow, therefore, toxicity is very common. **The extracardiac manifestations** like anorexia, vomiting, headache, agitation, mental confusion, hyperapnea, visual disturbance, diarrhea, skin rash, gynecomastia are rare. **Cardiac toxicity** includes pulsus bigeminus, ventricular extrasystole, tachycardia, partial to complete heart block.

Treatment of Digitalis Toxicity

Stop digitalis for noting earliest sign of digitalis toxicity. For tachyarrhythmia give K^+, after measuring K^+, high K^+ may precipitate AV block, ventricular asystole. K^+ antagonizes digitalis induced automaticity and decreases binding of glycosides to Na^+/K^+-ATPase.

a. **For digitalis-induced ventricular arrhythmia:** IV lignocaine suppresses excessive automaticity without increasing AV block. Phenytoin is also used, but not preferred because it may lead to sudden death. Procainamide and quinidine are contraindicated.

b. **Supraventricular arrhythmia:** Propranolol

c. **AV block and bradycardia:** Atropine. Cardioversion by DC shock is contraindicated. Because of high Vd it is not suitable for dialysis and elimination by diuretic.

Antibodies Fab fragment is marketed in Europe digibind (38 mg vial) given IV, improves survival of digitalis intoxication. It is an orphan drug and costly.

Important Drug Interaction of Digitalis

• Diuretic may precipitate arrhythmia due to K loss.
• Calcium: Precipitates toxicity, synergises digitalis.
• Quinidine: Plasma concentration increases due to reduction of tissue binding.
• Verapamil, diltiazem, captopril, amiodarone, increase plasma concentration of digoxin.
• Potassium sparing diuretics reduce renal excretion of digoxin.
• Adrenergic drugs and succinylcholine produce arrhythmia.
• Absorption is decreased by sucralfate, metoclopramide and increased by tricyclic antidepressant atropine, erythromycin, omeprazole and tetracycline so increases bioavailability. Phenobarbitone induces enzymes and decreases $t^{1/2}$ of digitoxin.

Contraindications and precautions of digitalis

- Digitalis toxicity
- Hypokalemia—enhance toxicity
- Myocardial infarction
- Thyrotoxicosis—more prone to arrhythmia
- Partial AV block converted to complete block
- Acute myocarditis—prone to arrhythmia
- Wolf-Parkinson-white syndrome because decreases the refractory period in bypass tract causing VF.

Other Drugs of CCF Diuretics

The diuretics increase the rate of urine formation. Three groups of diuretics are commonly used.

- Thiazide group
- High ceiling or loop diuretics
- Potassium sparing diuretics

The thiazide diuretics (hydrochlorthiazide/chlorthalidone) are mild diuretics, which may be used as first line drug in heart failure patients. When they are used with loop diuretics in patient of resistant cases they cause sequential blocking of nephron. Metalozone is a potent thiazide diuretic which exerts action on proximal and distal nephrons. Use of diuretics may be complicated with hypercalcemia, hyperuricemia, hyperlipidemia, hypophosphatemia, rash pancreatitis and ototoxicity.

The loop diuretics (drugs of this group are frusemide, bumetamide, ethacrynic acid): Ethacrynic acid is better choice in sulfur sensitive patient, but it is more ototoxic. The action of above-mentioned diuretics is blunted by NSAID group of drugs except sulindac.

Spironolactone, eplerenone, amiloride, triamterine are potassium-sparing diuretics. Spironolactone and eplerenone are competitive inhibitors of aldosterone. Amiloride and triamterine act to inhibit Na and K exchange in distal nephron. In combination with thiazide or loop diuretic, they mutually potentiate their action and hypopotassiumic effect is less. Action of spironolactone is blunted by carbenoxolone sodium, an antipeptic ulcer drug.

Some causes of apparent diuretic resistance

- Incorrect use of diuretic
- Electrolyte volume imbalance
- Poor renal perfusion, diuretic-induced hypovolemia
- Excess circulating catecholamine
- Activation of renin angiotensin aldosterone system
- Interfering drugs.

Sympathomimetic agents

Dopamine: Endogenous catecholamine with positive inotropic properties due to β_1 adrenostimulation. It improves renal perfusion in doses 2.5 µg/kg/min. In higher doses it increases systemic vascular resistance. **Fenoldopam,** a dopamine agonist has also been trialed in treatment of heart failure. Dose 0.1 µg/kg/min and increases gradually up to 1.6 µg/kg/min.

Dobutamine: It is a synthetic β_1 adrenoceptor stimulant with positive inotropic properties. Dose 2–8 µg/kg/min IV.

Levodopa: Antiparkinsonian drug converted peripherally to dopamine trialed for heart failure.

Ibupamine: Dopaminergic drug has got inotropic, vasodilator and natriuretic effects with beneficial effects in heart failure. It acts by releasing in the blood epinine with properties similar to dopamine. It increases renal blood flow.

Prenaterol: β_1 agonist, increases cardiac output in patient of heart failure in cardiac shock, cardiac surgery and treating side effects of β blockers.

Xamoterol: It is a partial β_1 blocker with intrinsic sympathomimetic effect, has moderate ino- and chronotropic effects, has got antianginal properties. Dose 200 mg twice daily.

PHOSPHODIESTERASE III INHIBITORS (BIPYRIDINES)

This group of drugs increases myocardial contraction. They inhibit breakdown of cyclic adenosyl monophosphate by inhibiting phosphodiesterase isoenzyme-3. They are effective orally and parenterally. Prototypes of this group of drugs are amrinone, milrinone, enoximone, vesnarinone which are inodilators (inotropic + vasodilator). Amrinone is given in the dose 0.75 mg/kg bolus followed by 5 µg/kg/IV min. Now it is called inamrinone. In amrinone now withdrawn from USA. Does not mix it with glucose and keep it away from sunlight. Inamrinone is marketed as inocor 5 mg/mL as lactate 20 mL amp. Platelet count should be done periodically to check thrombocytopenia. Other ADRs are nausea, vomiting, and arrhythmia. Milrinone 10 times more potent than amrinone and dose 50 µg/kg followed by 375–750 ng/kg/min.

They decrease preload and afterload in patient of heart failure. Commonly used vasodilators are:

Levosimendan: Apart from inhibiting phosphodiesterase, it also sensitizes myocardium to Ca^{2+}. It also causes some vasodilatation.

VASODILATORS

- **Nitrate:** Relaxes vascular smooth muscle by increasing 3', 5'-cGMP. Recommended when digoxin and ACE inhibitor fail to give adequate control.
- **Hydrazine:** Arterial dilator due to 3.5' GMP accumulation.
- **Prazosin:** Alpha receptor antagonist, trialed for CCF. Other drugs of this group are doxazosin, terazosin, *etc.*
- **Sodium nitroprusside:** Has to be given IV. Vasodilatation starts within 1 minute and dissipates when stopped. May lead to cyanide toxicity.

- **Angiotensin-converting enzyme inhibitors (ACI):** This group of drugs inhibits the production of potent vasoconstrictor angiotensin II. The other actions of angiotensin I are antinatriuretic effect and facilitator of sympathetic neurotransmission. Stimulant of aldosterone and arginine vasopressin (AVP). All are antagonized by ACI so it is a balanced vasodilator. A big list or ACE inhibitors is available in the market which are broadly classified into:

Class I: Captopril like

Class II: These are prodrugs converted into active drugs by metabolism. The drugs of class II ACE inhibitors are benzepril, cilazepril, enalapril, fosinopril, perindopril, quinapril, ramipril, *etc.*

Class III: These are water-soluble drugs. The example of class III drugs is lisinopril which is a water-soluble molecule. Nowadays angiotensin II receptor antagonists are also available in the market and effective for CHF. The following side effects are encountered with ACE inhibitors:

- Cough
- Hypotension
- Renal side effects like low pressure precipitating reversible renal failure
- Angioedema, a rare life-threatening condition due to formation of kinins. Treatment is SC adrenaline
- All ACE inhibitors are embryopathic.

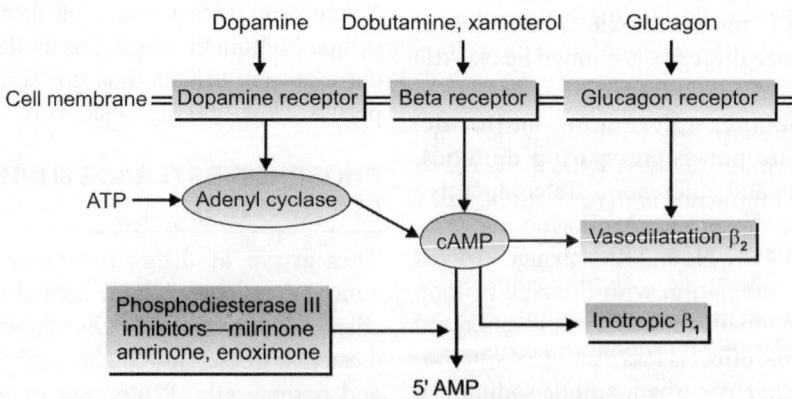

Fig. 73.5: Site of action of different inotropic drugs

Individual ACE Inhibitors

Captopril (acetan 25 mg tab, 1 tab BD to TDS): It is sulfhydryl dipeptide surrogate of proteins having property to abolish pressor action of angiotensin I. It increases plasma kinin level which also potentiates hypotensive action. Its action on BP also depends on Na^+ states (as with dietary restriction or diuretic therapy). Reflex sympathetic stimulation does not occur. It does not affect coronary, cerebral and renal blood flows. Plasma angiotensin and renin are increased. 70% absorbed, partly metabolized and excreted. It retards diabetic retinopathy.

ADR: Hypotension, hyperkalemia (specially if used with K^+-sparing diuretics, NSAID, impaired kidney function patient), cough, rash, urticaria, dysgeusia (loss of taste), embryopathy, headache, nausea, dizziness, precipitation of acute renal failure, proteinuria and granulo-cytopenia.

Enalapril (Enias 5, 10 and 20 mg tabs): Converted to tripeptide analogue enalaprilat (available as injection in some countries). It is more potent, single dose or BD therapy and long acting. ADR as rash or taste problem is less.

Perindopril (Coversyl 2, 4 mg tabs): Prodrug and long acting.

Lisinopril (Lispril 25, 5, 10 mg tabs): Lysine derivative of enalapril, does not require hydrolysis, long acting. May cause reduction of venous return, cardiac contractility and output.

Fosinopril (Fovas 10, 20 mg): Phosphinate derivative, eliminated by liver and kidney both. First dose hypotension may occur.

Trandolapril (Zetpril I, 2 mg tab): Carboxyl prodrug; absorption delayed with food. Meta-bolized partly. Eliminated both in urine and feces.

Ramipril (Cardace 1.25, 2.5, 5 mg caps): Long acting. Inhibits local renin angiotensin system. Prodrug, converted to active ramiprilat. Slow release of tissue-bound drug increases its $t\frac{1}{2}$.

Imidapril (Tanatril 5, 10 mg tabs): Prodrug and long acting OD dose.

Benazepril (Benace 5, 10, 20 mg tabs): Non-sulfhydryl prodrug; excreted *via* kidney. Dose 10 to 40 mg OD.

Uses of ACE inhibitors

- Hypertension
- CCF
- Myocardial infarction
- As a prophylaxis in high cardiovascular risk patient
- Diabetic and non-diabetic nephropathies prevention
- Sclerodema crisis
- Captopril test to diagnose renovascular hypertension.

ACE inhibitors can also be classified chemically as follows

Sulfhydryl containing ACE-I

- Captopril
- Pivolopril
- Fentiapril
- Zofenopril
- Alacepril
- Dose   12.5–50 mg/day

Dicarboxyl containing ACE-I

- Enalopril   2.5–40 mg/day
- Lisinopril   5–40 mg/day
- Benazepril   10–40 mg/day
- Quinapril   5–80 mg/day
- Moexipril   7.5–30 mg/day
- Ramipril   1.25–20 mg/day
- Spiapril   12.5–50 mg/day
- Perindopril   1–16 mg/day
- Indolapril
- Pentopril
- Cilazepril   2.5–5 mg/day

Phosphorus containing ACE-I

- Fosinopril   10–40 mg/day.
- **Angiotensin receptor blockers (ARBs):** Losartan, candesartan, valsartan, telmisartan, irbesartan and olmesartan are AT_1 receptor blockers.

- **Renin inhibitor:** Aliskiren is a renin inhibitor approved for hypertension and is undergoing as trial for heart failure.

Individual ARBs

Losartan (Giftan 25, 50 mg tabs): Competitive AT_1 antagonist, orally absorbed 33% due to first pass metabolism. Partly carboxylated in liver to active metabolite (E3174). Both are plasma protein-bound. Dose reduction required for liver dysfunction patients.

ADR: Hypertension, hyperkalemia, angio-edema, headache and dizziness may occur.

Candesartan (Candesar 4, 8 and 16 mg tabs): Produces long unsurmountable antagonist. Eliminated by liver metabolism and renal excretion. Dose 4–8 mg OD or BD. 4 mg OD doses in liver and kidney diseases.

Irbesartan (IRBEST 150–300 mg): Oral bio-availability is high, excreted by bile. Dose 150–300 mg OD.

Valsartan (Valzaar 40, 80, 160 mg): Food interferes absorption. Elimination occurs *via* liver.

Telmisartan (Telvas 20, 40, 80 mg tabs): Does not produce active metabolites like losartan. Mainly excreted unchanged *via* bile. Dose reduction requires in liver disease.

Olmesartan (Olmesar 20 mg tab)

Therapeutic uses of ARBs

- Hypertension
- CCF
- Myocardial infarction
- Diabetic nephropathy.

Flosequinan is a vasodilator, used for mild, moderate and severe CCF, seems to be alternative to ACE-I.

Phentolamine: Given IV, causes vasodilatation and has got adrenoceptor blocking properties.

Nesiritide: It is a recombinant product of endogenous peptide, brain natriuretic peptide (BNP), which increases cGMP in smooth muscle cells, reduces venous and arteriolar tones and causes diuresis too. It is given IV bolus because of short $t/\frac{1}{2}$. Hypotension may occur.

Carperitide and ularitide are synthetic analogs of atrial natriuretic peptide and urodilantin are in investigational label for drugs of heart failure.

Bosentan and Tezosentan: These are affective in experimental model of heart failure, but not on clinical trial. These are competitive inhibitor of endothelin and orally active. Bosentan is teratogenic and hepatotoxic. It is approved for pulmonary hypertension petients.

β Blockers

Bisoprolol, carvedilol and metoprolol; if used cautiously at low dose after several months of treatment, raise ejection fraction, slower heart rate and reduce symptoms of heart failure.

Bradycardiac Drug: Ivabradine is relative selective. I_f sodium channel blocker inhibits hyperpolarization activated sodium channel in the SA node causing bradycardia may be of benefit heart failure.

Vasopeptidase Inhibitors

This group of drugs simultaneously inhibits ACE; neutral endopeptidases (NEPs) and antihypertensive agent. NEP degrades atrial and brain natriuretic peptides. So their inhibitors **omapatrilat** improves exercise capacity, symptoms of heart failure. It also reduces death risk and frequent hospitalization in chronic heart failure. Other drugs of this group are sampatrilat, fasidotrilat.

Cardiac Resynchronization

Patients who have normal sinus rhythm and wide QRS will have impaired ventricular contraction. Particularly left ventricular contraction dimination will decrease cardiac output. Biventricular pacing will reduce the risk of mortality who is already on drugs of heart failure.

VAPTANS

Heart failure with hyponatremia presumably due to increased vasopressin activity, V1A and V2 receptor antagonist, conivaptan or V2 antagonist, **tolvaptan, conivaptan** may be used.

74

Pharmacotherapy of Hypertension

In cardiovascular disease vascular component is as important as cardiac part. Hypertension reflects the vascular component.

Hypertension affects over one billion adults and 25% of all population world wide. The hypertension is a state in which systolic blood pressure is more than 140 mmHg and diastolic pressure is more than 90 mmHg. It is characterized by elevation of blood pressure, normal cardiac output, increased peripheral vascular resistance with pathological changes in arterioles of kidney, heart, brain.

Two major types of hypertension

- **Primary or essential** where no cause is known.
- **Secondary** to kidney diseases (chronic glomerulonephritis, pyelonephritis, polycystic kidney, *etc.*); endocrinal (Cushing syndrome, primary hyperaldosteronism, pheochromocytoma, *etc.*); vascular (coarctation of aorta, renal artery disease, *etc.*).

Blood pressure is the product of cardiac output (CO) x peripheral vascular resistance (PVR). Peripheral vascular resistance is exerted by

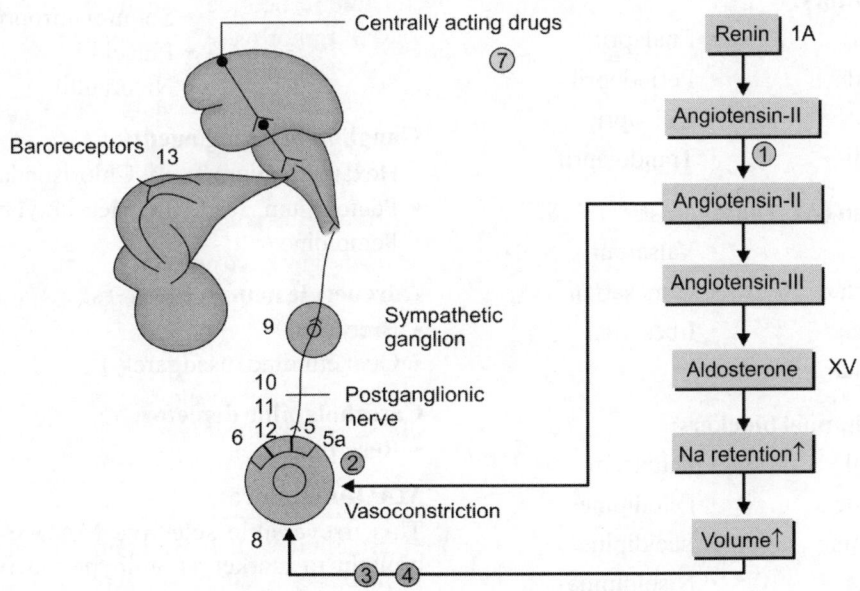

Fig. 74.1: Site of action of antihypertensive drugs

arterioles and post capillar venules. Other control site of systemic BP are baroreflex controlled by autonomic nerves, along with humoral mechanism viz. Renin-angiotensin system, and local vasoactive substance like nitric oxide, endothelin-1 which are vasodilator and vasoconstrictor respectively.

Stages of hypertension (Joint National Committee VIII)

	SBP (mm of Hg)	DBP (mm of Hg)
Normal	< 120	80
Prehypertension	120–139	80–89
Stage I HTN	140–159	90–99
Stage II	≥160	≥100

Drugs of hypertension can be classified according to the site of action as shown in Fig. 74.1.

Drugs Classification

Renin inhibitors:
- Aliskiren
- Remikiren
- Enalkiren

ACE inhibitors:
- Captopril
- Lisinopril
- Ramipril
- Moexipril
- Enalapril
- Perindopril
- Quinapril
- Trandolapril

Angiotensin (AT₁) antagonists:
- Losartan
- Candesartan
- Eprosartan
- Telmisartan
- Valsartan
- Olmesartan
- Irbesartan

Calcium channel blockers:
- Verapamil
- Nefedipine
- Nitrendipine
- Isradipine
- Clevidipine
- Diltiazem
- Felodipine
- Lacidipine
- Nisoldipine

Diuretics:
- Mild diuretic : Indapamide
- Thiazides : Chlorthalidone Hydrochlorthiazide
- High ceiling : Furosemide
- K⁺ sparing : ◆ Spironolactone,
  ◆ Eplerenone,
  ◆ Triamterine,
  ◆ Amiloride

β blockers:
- Propranolol, Atenolol
- Metoprolol
- Labetalol (α + β blocker), etc.

α-adrenergic blockers:
- Prazosin
- Phentolamine
- Indoramin
- Terazosin
- Phenoxybenzmine

Central sympatholytics:
- Clonidine
- Methyldopa

Vasodilators:
- **Arteriolar**
  ◆ Hydralazine
  ◆ Minoxidil
  ◆ Diazoxide
- **Arteriolar + venous dilators:**
  ◆ Sodium nitroprusside,
  ◆ Pinacidil,
  ◆ Nicorandil

Ganglion blocking agents:
- Hexamethonium,
- Pentolinium,
- Pempidine
- Chlorisondamine,
- Meacamylamine,

Adrenergic neuron blockers:
- Bretylium
- Guanethidine (used rarely)

Catecholamine depletor:
- Reserpine

MAO-inhibitor:
This irreversible selective MAO-B-inhibitor brought to market as antihypertensive but no longer used.
- Pargyline

Miscellaneous:

- α-methyl-p-tyrosine, Veratrum alkaloid.

Veratrum alkaloid:

I. Renin inhibitor (Aliskiren)

It inhibits enzymatic activity of renin. Reduces angiotensin I, II and aldosterone. Used for hypertension and also trialed for heart failure. Used orally.

ADR: Hyperkalemia, kidney impairment, teratogenic (dose 150–300 mg).

II. Angiotensin-converting enzyme (ACE) inhibitors

It is a preferred drug in all grades of essential hypertension and renovascular hypertension except bilateral renal artery stenosis. Diuretics or β-blockers may be added to it. It retards diabetic nephropathy, vascular hypertrophy, LVH. Appropriate antihypertensive in patient with diabetic nephropathy, LVF, CCF, angina and post-MI patient.

III. Angiotensin antagonist

Losartan acts on AT1 receptor antagonist, losartan K (50 mg tab OD dose) marketed as replace with losacar.

Irbesartan: Orally absorbed, metabolized in liver to inactive metabolite, 90% bound to plasma protein, excreted with urine. Not recommended for pregnancy (because it may cause neonatal skull hypoplasia), anuria, oligohydramnios leading to fetal limbs contraction, hypoplastic lung. It is better to avoid in lactating mother.

Adverse effects are headache, cough, anaphylaxis, rash, nervousness, anxiety. Dose 150 mg daily to 300 mg daily (irovel 150 mg).

Other AT receptor antagonists are discussed elsewhere with drugs of heart failure.

IV. Calcium channel blockers

All calcium channel blockers (dihydropyridines, *e.g.* nifedipine); phenylalkylamines, *e.g.* veraparnil and benzothiazepines, *e.g.* diltiazem) are equally potent antihypertensives, decrease peripheral resistance without lowering cardiac output, and fluid retention. Ankle edema is due to increased hydrostatic pressure across capillaries as a result to reflex postcapillary vasoconstriction.

Advantages of calcium channel blockers (CCBs): Can be given to asthma, angina and gout patients. Do not impair renal perfusion or alter lipid profile or electrolyte balance, no sedation and sexual function impairment. Can be used in pregnancy.

The concerns of CCB as antihypertensives are its negative ino- and chronotropic effects, may worsen CCF, nifedipine decreases insulin release, may accentuate bladder voiding difficulties in elderly male, and gastroesophageal reflux.

Mechanisms of action of CCB

The common property to inhibit entry of Ca^{2+} into the cell *via* slow calcium channels. Diltiazem was launched in 1975 from Japan. Three types of Ca^{2+} channels are described in smooth muscles and excitable tissues identified in Germany.

- Voltage sensitive channel
- Receptor operated channel
- Leak channel.

The voltage sensitive calcium channel in heart and smooth muscle consists of 4 units α_1, α_2, β, γ, δ of which α subunit is more important, as it contains calcium channel pores and binding sites for calcium antagonist.

Voltage sensitive calcium channels are divided into L type (long lasting) and T type (transient current). Transient channel does not interact with standard antagonist. L channel works at less negative potential and linked to muscular excitation, contraction coupling and blocked by standard calcium antagonist. The CCB binds to α_1 subunit and restricts Ca^{2+} entry. The different CCBs may have different affinities for various site specific isoforms of the L channel responsible for different actions exhibited by different CCBs.

Classification

Phenylalkylamine

- Verapamil
- Gallopamil

Dihydropyridines

- Nifedipine
- Nicardipine
- Felodipine
- Nisoldipine
- Nimodipine (cerebroselective vasodilator used for reversing compensatory vasoconstricton after subarachnoid haemorrhage)
- Clevidipine (ultrashort acting used for hypertensive emergencies (given IV)

- Nitrendipine
- Isradipine
- Amlodipine

Benzothiazepines

- Diltiazem

Others

- Bepridil

Cardiovascular Indications of Calcium Channel Blockers (CCBs)

1. **Ischemic heart diseases**
   - Stable angina
   - Unstable
   - Non-Q infarction
   - Myocardial revascularization.
   - Variant
   - Prinzmetal's angina
   - Silent ischemia

2. **Hypertension**
   - Systemic hypertension
   - Hypertensive emergencies
   - Preoperative hypertension
   - Regression of LVH

3. **Cardiomyopathy**
   - Hypertrophic dilated

4. **In CCF**, it is contraindicated as such, but verapamil reduces sudden death

5. **Cardiac arrhythmia**
   - Atrial flutter and fibrillation
   - Supraventricular tachycardia
   - Ventricular arrhythmia

6. **Prevention of cardiomyopathy**

7. **Postcardiac transplantation**

8. **Primary pulmonary hypertension**

9. **Peripheral vascular disease**
   - Raynaud's disease
   - Intermittent claudication
   - Mesenteric artery insufficiency.

V. Diuretics

Thiazide, high ceiling and K-sparing diuretics are used.

Mechanism of action

- Initially diuresis reduces plasma and extra-cellular fluid volume reducing cardiac output.
- Decreases intracellular Na which leads to decreased stiffness of vascular wall and dampens responsiveness to noradrenaline and angiotensin II.

Indapamide (Natrilix 2.5 mg tab): Mild diuretic, reduces BP at doses which cause little diuresis, electrolyte imbalance and K^+ loss. Possesses additional vasodilator effect exerted through alteration of ionic fluxes across vascular smooth muscle cell. Orally absorbed single dose 2.5 mg is sufficient (Lorvas 2.5 mg tab). It is indole derivative of chlorosulfonamide.

Xipamid: This drug has diuretic and hypotensive effects and adverse effects like thiazide given in a single 20–40 mg daily (available as 20 mg tab). Other diuretics used as antihypertensives discussed in appropriate chapter.

VI. β blockers

Discussed ealier in autonomic nervous system.

Labetatol (Normadate 50, 100, 200 mg tabs): α + β blockers given IV for rapid reduction of BP in cheese reaction or clonidine withdrawal. Available as oral tablets also. Dose 20 to 40 mg every 10 minutes till response is achieved. Orally start with 50 mg BD up to 100–200 mg TDS.

VII. α-adrenergic blockers

Non-selective α blockers (phentotamine, phenoxybenzamine) block α_1 and α_2 receptors. Used in hypertension. Disappointing because fall in BP reflexly increases HR and CO. Reserved for special conditions like pheochromocytoma and clonidine withdrawal, cheese reaction where circulating catecholamine is high.

Prazosin (Minipress XL 2.5 mg and 5 mg tabs): Selective competitive α blockers dilate vessel. Renal blood flow is maintained.

Postural hypertension called **first dose effect** disappears gradually. Suitable for diabetics, favorable effect on lipid profile, uric acid metabolism, helpful in CCF patients, improves benign prostatic hypertrophy. Adverse effects are postural hypotension, dry mouth, palpitation, nasal blocked, impaired ejaculation, blurred vision. Not used as first drug.

Terazosin and doxazosin are long acting congeners of prazosin. Indoramin, urapidil are selective α_1 blockers used as antihypertensives in some countries.

VIII. Central Sympatholytics

Clonidine

Imidazoline derivative, having an adrenergic agonistic activity to α_2 receptor, decreases sympathetic outflow and NAd release. It exhibits therapeutic window phenomenon, i.e. higher doses do not alter therapeutic effect. Orally absorbed, excreted through kidney.

Arkamin 100 µg tab starts with 100 µg and increases gradually up to 300 µg TDS. It is useful for migraine also. Transdermal therapeutic system is available in the USA.

New drugs **moxonidine** and **rilmenidine** are congeners of clonidine which are selective for imidazole receptors (IR_1) and modulate central α_2 receptor. They are having longer t½. They have less adverse drug effects and have beneficial effects on carbohydrate and lipid metabolism.

Adverse effects: Sedation, mental depression, dry mouth, nose and eyes, impotence, bradycardia, postural hypotension, sudden removal causes sudden release of catecholamine and syndrome similar to pheochromocytoma.

Other uses of clonidine

- Opioid alcohol and smoking cessation
- Analgesics
- Loose motion of diabetic neuropathy
- Attenuate vasomotor symptoms of menopausal syndrome.
- Clonidine suppression test for pheochromocytoma. It reduces plasma NAd to < 5 ng/mL in essential hypertension, but not in pheochromocytoma.
- In diagnosis of growth hormone deficiency as it stimulants GH release.

Methyldopa

The isomers of α-methyl analogue of dihydroxyphenylalanine (DOPA), the precursor of dopamine and noradrenaline, was introduced to treat hypertension in 1960. The mechanism of action of methyldopa is not established yet with certainty as originally postulated to inhibit the enzyme dopa decarboxylase enzyme concerned with synthesis of noradrenaline.

α-methyl noradrenaline is a metobolite of methyldopa acts as a false neurotransmitter fails to explain many actions of methyldopa.

The α-methyl NA formed in the brain from methyldopa (α_2 agonist) decreases sympathetic activity. It decreases total peripheral resistance more than heart rate and cardiac output, may be acting on different population of neurons in vasomotor center than clonidine. It decreases renin release and increases prolactin level. It is orally absorbed, transported by amino acid carrier, partly metabolized and partly excreted unchanged. Antihypertensive effect starts 4–6 hours after and lasts 12–24 hours. It may accumulate in system in cronic administration and in renal insufficiency.

Adverse effects: Sedation, lethargy, reduced mental capacity, can be minimized by giving at bedtime, dry mouth, nasal stuffiness, weight gain, postural hypotension, positive Coombs' test with hemolytic anemia, fever, rash rebound hypertension on withdrawn. It should not be prescribed with tricyclic antidepressant (reverses its action) or reserpine and halloperidol accentuate mental symptoms (alphadopa 250 mg tab. Dose 1 tab BD to QD).

IX. Vasodilators

Hydralazine: Causes arterial vasodilation. Angina may be precipitated by hyperdynamic circulatory state induced by it. The vascular smooth muscle relaxation is partly due to stimulation of cGMP and partly endothelial derived generation of NO (nitric oxide). Direct effect on membrane potential and on Ca^{2+} fluxes also been proposed. Diuretic or β blockers should be given to avoid tolerance. Orally absorbed **acetylated may produce** LE syndrome; available as 25, 50 mg OD or TDS (nepresol) and can be given IV or IM in hypertensive emergencies.

Minoxidil: It is a prodrug, K^+ channel opener, orally absorbed, metabolized in the liver and exerted in urine. Used with β blockers in hypertensive emergencies, associated with renal disease. It increases cutaneous blood flow to produce excess of hairs (used in alopecia, mintop 2% scalp lotion). Pericardial effusion may occur.

Diazoxide: A thiazide derivative on IV injection promptly decreases the tone of resistance vessels, K^+ channel opening causes smooth muscle hyperpolarization, insulin serection is inhibited, gout may be precipitated.

Highly protein-bound. Also used as uterine relaxant to arrest premature labor and in insulinoma.

Pinacidil and cromakalim are K^+ channel activators initiated for hypertension discussed with antianginal drugs.

Sodium nitroprusside: Quick acting, dilates both arteriole and venules, decreases venous return, so myocardial work is reduced, ischemia not accentuated.

Endothelial cells, RBC splits nitroprusside to generate NO which relaxes smooth muscle.

Nitroprusside is used in hypertensive emergencies 50 mg in 500 mL 5% dextrose bottle. Infusin started 0.02 mg/min. Nitroprusside is converted to thiocyanate in liver which is exerted slowly.

Adverse effects

- Fatigue anorexia
- Vomiting
- Cyanide toxicity
- Nausea
- Prespiration

Therapeutic uses

- Hypertension (refractory), CHF
- Mitral regurgitation to improve ventricular performance by reducing preload and afterload.
- Sonide: Pruside 50 mg in 5 mL injection.

X. Ganglion Blockers

- **Pentolinium** used SC
- **Trimethaphan** (Arfonad) IV short acting used to produce hypotension during surgery.

Oral preparations are (chlorisondamine, mecamylamine, pempidine) rarely used because of adverse effects.

Adverse effects of ganglion blockers

Parasympathetic blockade: Mydriasis, cyclopegia, blurred vision, dry mouth, paralytic ileus, urine retention.

Sympathetic blockade: Hypotension, sexual function disturbance, syncope, pulmonary edema, with hexamethonium therapy.

Central action by secondary and tertiary amines crossing blood-brain barrier causing mental confusion and tremor (seizure mecamylamine; pempidine).

Tolerance is common except with mecamylamine.

Trimethapan produces anuria, vascular thrombosis.

XI. Acting on postganglionic sympathetic nerve ending

Adrenergic neuron blocking agents inhibit nerve impulse to release NAd. Drugs are:

- *Bretylium:* Initial results are good, but tolerance develops very soon.
- *Guanethidine (ismelin):* Taken up by adrenergic nerve ending by active amine transport to produce following functions.
  - ◆ Displace NAd from storage granules stoichiometrically
  - ◆ Inhibits nerve impulse release of NAd (guanethidine sulfate 10 and 25 mg tabs)

ADR

Postural hypertension, failure to ejaculate, diarrhea.

Contraindicated in pheochromocytoma. Polyarteritis nodosa on prolong therapy may occur.

Bethanidine (Esbatal)

- Quickly absorbed
- Rapid hypotensive action
- Adverse effects same as guanethidine.

Dose 5 mg TD or QD orally.

Debrisoquine sulfate (Declinax): Dose 10 mg 2–3 times a day till satisfactory control is achieved. Tolerance develops, adverse effects are like guanethidine.

Gaunoxan (envacar): Blocks adrenergic neurons and α-adrenergic blocker. Initial dose is 20 mg increased gradually. Liver damage may occur.

Gaunochlor (vatensol): Similar to guanoxon.

XII. Catecholamine Depletors

Reserpine: Alkaloid obtained from roots of *Rauwolfia serpentina* (Sarpagandha), an indigenous to India, acts at the membrane intraneuronal granules which store NAd, 5HT and DA. Irreversively inhibits active amine transport, and monoamines are gradually depleted and degraded by MAO. The effects last longer after the drug is eliminated, because CA stores are restored gradually and the phenomenon is called hit and run drugs (Serpasil 0.25 mg tab or 1 mg/mL inj, Adahlphane 0.1 mg + 10 mg dihydralazine tab).

Adverse effects: Sedation, depression, parkinsonism, overactivity of parasympathetic activity, acid secretion, diarrhea, bradycardia, other effects are suicidal tendencies, postural hypotension, weight gain and impotence.

XIII. MAO-inhibitors pargyline

Rarely used nowadays as antihypertensive because of adverse effects and drug interactions.

XIV. α-Methyl-p-tyrosine

It blocks synthesis of CA by inhibiting tyrosine hydroxylase useful in the pretreatment of surgery in pheochromocytoma.

XV. Drug Acting Reflexly

Veratrum alkaloid: The primary site of action of this drug is on afferent receptors, predominantly present in the heart and in the carotid sinus area where the afferent receptors are sensitized, peripheral sympathetic tone is reduced, producing fall in BP; vagal tone is increased simultaneously inducing bradycardia. The thera-

peutic index of this drug is low, with frequent adverse effects so rarely used.

Antihypertensive of some special situations

Migraine: Propranolol; **Depression:** Vasodilator ACE-I; CCB; α-blockers but reserpine, clonidine, beta blocker should be avoided. **In bradycardia** CCB and beta blockers should not be used. **In angina pectoris** hydrallazine should be avoided preferred drug is beta blocker and CCB. **In fluid retention** diuretics are given. **In prostratic hyperplasia** α-blockers are preferred. Thiazide is preferred in **osteoporosis** and **renal calculi.** In thyrotoxicosis beta blockers are given but without intrinsic sympathomimetic activity. In **diabetes mellitus** CCB; ACE-I; ARB is prescribed, K^+ sparing diuretic should be avoided. **Hypertension with hyperlipidemia** is treated with low dose thiazide; ACE-I; α-blocker. Beta blockers should be avoided here. **Hypertension** with **mitral valve prolapse** is treated with beta blocker. **Left ventricular hypertrophy** is treated with ACE-I, ARB. **Hypertension** with **bronchial** asthma treated with vasodilators, CCB. **Congestive heart failure** is treated with ACE-I, ARB, diuretics, vasodilator, CCB is contraindicated. **Hypertension with TIA** is treated with CCB, ACE-I, ARB. It should be treated with ACE-I; ARB; vasodilators. Vasodilators should not be prescribed in palpitation patients **Raynauds phenomenon** patient should be treated with CCB not beta blockers.

Orthostatic hypotension: When BP decreases by 20 mm Hg systolic and 10 mm of diastolic within 3 minutes of standing from supine is called orthostatic hypotension generally occurs with diuretics, nitrates, phenothiazines. TCA; antihypertensives, antiparkinsonian drugs, with autonomic failure in diabetes. Drugs prescribed are: **Midodrine** a agonist, (10 mg TDS) **pseudoephedrine** (30–60 mg TDS); **Phenylephrine** 10 mg every four hourly. **Fludrocortisone** in severe cases.

Requirements of an Ideal Antihypertensive

- It should produce predictable reduction in both systolic and diastolic BPs in supine and errect positions.

- Should have rapid action with sufficient duration of action.
- Should not produce tolerance.
- It should not reduce circulation to vital organs like brain, kidney, heart, and should be free from toxic effect.
- It should be cheap and synergic with other anti-hypertensive.

  Only thiazide diuretics come nearest to ideal antihypertensive.

Safe antihypertensive drugs for pregnancy

Beta blockers, Atenolol is safe in third trimester, but may cause IUGR and fetal bradycardia, labetalol (may be hepatotoxic) Methyldopa, Clonidine, Nifedipine, Hydralazine, Prozosin. But ACE inhibitors and ARB are contraindicated.

Some newer antihypertensives

- Endopeptidase inhibitors: Candoxatril
- Dopamine (D_1) agonist: Fenoldopam
- Serotonin (5HT2A) antagonist: Kentanserin
- α_1 and Ca^{2+} antagonists: Monetepil
- ACE and endopeptidase inhibitor: Alatriopril

Pulmonary Hypertension

Classical systemic antihypertensive are not useful in pulmonary hypertension. Drugs which can be used for idopathic pulmonary hypertension are:

- **Bosentan: Ambrisantan** both endothelin receptor antagonist. Newer drug of this group is **Macitentan.**
- **Phosphodiesterase-5 inhibitors:** Sildenafil, **Tadalafil.**
- **Prostaglandins: Epoprostenil, Treprostinil Iloprost.**
- **Riociguat** it increases cGMP level. Headache gastritis; diarrhea, hypotension, hemorrage may occur should not be given with PDE-I and nitrate.
- **Nitric oxide** inhalation
- **Diuretics:** Furesomide

Warfarin to counter tendency of hemorrhage

- **Perfenidone** suppresses pulmonary fibrosis. It is pyridine immunosuppressants with marginal benefits.

75

Antianginal Drugs

Angina is a syndrome of chest pain due to adverse demand supply disparity to a portion of the myocardium provoked by exercise, emotion, eating, coitus and subsides when increased demand is withdrawn (classical angina). Variant angina (Prinzmetal's angina) is due to localized coronary vasospasm where attacks occur at rest or during sleep. Unstable angina is caused due to increased epicardial coronary artery tone or small platelets clots nearer to atheromatous plaque.

Antianginal drugs relieve cardiac ischemia, but without any effect on coronary artery pathology.

Pharmacological approach to modify oxygen demand in IHD.

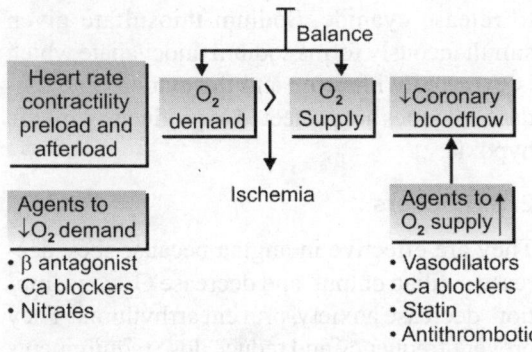

Drugs may relax the vascular smooth muscle as follows

- Increasing cGMP which facilitates dephosphorylation of myosin light chains
- Decreasing intracellular Ca^{2+}
- Stabilizing vascular smooth muscle cells
- Increasing cAMP in vascular smooth muscle.

CLASSIFICATION OF ANTIANGINAL DRUGS

1. **Nitrates**
   - *Short acting:* Glyceryl trinitrate
   - *Long acting:* Isosorbide dinitrate (short acting by sublingual route), isosorbide mononitrate, erythrityl tetranitrate, pentaerythritol tetranitrate.
2. **β blockers:** Proparanolol, metoprolol, atenolol etc.
3. **Calcium channel blockers:** Nifedipine felodipine, nicardipine, amlodipine, nitrendipine, nimodipine, lacidipine.
4. **Potassium channel openers:** Nicroandil, pinacidil, cromakalim.
5. **Miscellaneous:** Dipyridamole, lidoflazine, ivabradine, oxyphedrine.

1. Nitrates

Organic nitrates are polyol esters of nitric acid, but inorganic nitrites are esters of nitrous acid. Nitrate esters ($-C-O-NO_2$) and nitrite esters ($-C-O-NO$) are characterized by sequence of carbon–oxygen–nitrogen, but nitrocompounds which are not vasodilators possess carbon–nitrogen bond $-C-NO_2$. Thus glyceryl trinitrate is erroneously called nitroglycerin. Amylnitrate is highly volatile, organic nitrates are of low molecular weights are moderately volatile. High molecular weight nitrate esters erythrityl tetranitrate, isosorbide dinitrate are solid in the pure form, nitroglycerine is explosive.

All nitrates are smooth muscle relaxants, vary in the time course.

Mechanism of actions of Nitrates

- Organic nitrates are quickly denitrated in smooth muscle cell to release NO as reactive free radical which activates guanylyl cyclase, leading to increased cGMP which dephosphorylates myosin light chain kinase (MLCK). Reduced availability of MLCK interferes with activation of myosin, fails to act with actin-causing relaxation.
- The production of PGE or PGI_2 and membrane hyperpolarization is also involved to cause muscle relaxation.
- Raised cGMP reduces Ca^{2+} entry causing relaxation.
- Raised cGMP decreases platelet aggregation.
- Nitrates dilate vein and arteries, but more the former, which decreases venous return and preload as a consequence end diastolic pressure and volume. The decreased ventricular wall tension decreases O_2 consumption.
- Nitrates by virtue of arterial dilatation decrease the afterload and blood pressure, with higher doses reduction of BP may produce reflex sympathetic stimulation of heart and angina may be precipitated.

Beneficial and deleterious effects of nitrate in IHD.

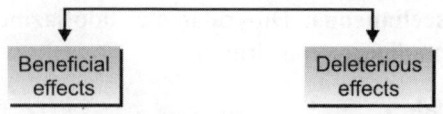

Beneficial effects	Deleterious effects
• Decreased ejection time	• Tachycardia
• Arterial pressure	• Decreased diastolic
• Ventricular volume	perfusion time
• Epicardial coronary	due to tachycardia
artery dilation	
• Increased collateral	

It redistributes blood in bigger conducting vessels. It is effective in angina because: (i) It dilates vessel's spasm and (ii) decreases cardiac output. It does not have any effect on heart *per se*. It causes flushing of face; and headache (because of meningeal vessel's dilation). It decongests lung and decreases renal and splanchnic blood flow.

Pharmacokinetics: All nitrates are absorbed from buccal mucosa, intestine and skin. All nitrates except isosorbide mononitrate undergo extensive first pass metabolism in liver, rapidly denitrated by glutathione reductase.

Adverse effects: Tolerance and cross-tolerance with other nitrates, throbbing headache, flushing, weakness, sweating, palpitation, methemoglobinemia and decreased oxygen carrying capacity in blood with severe anemia. Pentaerythritol tetranitrate may cause rash.

The tolerance may be due to reduced ability to generate NO due to depletion of –SH radicals. Volume expansion, sympathetic stimulation or humoral pathways may contribute to nitrate tolerance. It is advisable to withdraw nitrates gradually because sudden withdrawal may precipitate spasm of coronary arteries.

Therapeutic uses of nitrates

- Angina pectoris
- CCF and LVF
- Myocardial infarction
- Interventional cardiac procedure
- Biliary colic and esophageal spasm
- Cyanide poisoning
- In anal fissure.

Nitrates in cyanide poisoning (mechanism of action): Nitrates produce methemoglobin, which has high affinity for cyanide radicals to produce cyanomethemoglobin which dissociates to release cyanide. Sodium thiosulfate given simultaneously forms sodium thiocyanate which is excreted with urine and the cytochrome oxidase enzymes are protected to produce cytotoxic hypoxia.

2. β Blockers

They are effective in angina because they decrease cardiac output, and decrease O_2 consumption, decrease anxiety, prevent arrhythmia. They prevent frequency and reduce dose requirements of NTG in angina. It is not effective in variant angina.

β blockers are described in details earlier in autonomic nervous system.

3. Calcium Channel Blockers (CCBs)

CCBs are effective in reducing frequency and severity of classical and variant angina act due to reduction of cardiac work due to afterload reduction, increase exercise tolerance and increase coronary flow in normal individual. It is not the firstline drug in unstable angina. Calcium channel blockers are dealt in details with antihypertensives.

4. Potassium Channel Openers

It is a new class of drugs that modulate potassium channel (K^+) in cell membrane (nicorandil, cromakalim, pinacidil). Nicorandil was first synthesized in 1975 at Central Research Laboratories of Chugai, Japan, under the name of Sigmart. It is a niacinamide derivative with a nitrate group in its chemical structure. It hyperpolarizes the vascular smooth muscle membrane, increases intracellular synthesis of cGMP and increases the release of prostacycline from microsomes. Nicorandil is a nicotinamide and nitrate with its ability to increase. K^+ conductance through cardiac and vascular smooth muscles. This property possessed neither by nicotinamide nor by conventional nitrates.

Potassium channel openers hyperpolarizes vascular cell membranes causing voltage operated Ca^{2+} channel to close as a consequence reduction in free intracellular Ca^{2+} concentration which results in decreased vasomotor tone, particularly in coronary resistance vessels (their actions are antagonized by sulfonylurea).

Potential therapeutic uses of potassium channel opener

- Angina pectoris
- Hypertension
- CCF
- Myocardial salvage in MI
- Insulinoma
- Alopecia
- Bronchial asthma
- Urinary incontinence
- Raynaud's and cerebrovascular diseases
- Premature labor
- Penile erection disorders.

Table 75.1: Individual organic nitrates

Drugs	Preparations	Dose route	Duration	Remarks
Nitroglycerine	Angised (0.5 mg tab, Nitro-mack), angispan TR 2.5 mg, Angispan SR 6.5 mg, Nitrocontin 2.6; 6.4 mg, Nitromack 5 mg/5 mL, Millisrol 5 mg/10 mg, Nitrodern TTS 5 or 10 mg/24 hours patch	0.5 mg S/L 5–15 mg orally 5–10 mg/min IV	10–30 min 4–8 hours Till used	Volatile liquid absorbed in inert matrix in tightly closed glass container. Transdermal patch is incorporated in polymer-bonded adhesive patch IV used in unstable angina LVF. MI cardiac surgery 5 µg/min.
Isosorbide dinitrate	Sorbitrate 5/10 mg, Isodril 5 mg, Isomack-retard 20–40 SR cap	5–10 ng SL 10–20 mg oral 6–10 hours	20–40 min 2–3 hours	Solid can be taken SL or orally
Isosorbide 5-mono-nitrate	Monotrate 10; 20	20–40 mg oral	6–12 hours	Active metabolite of iso-sorbide dinitrate
Erythrityl tetra-nitrate	Cardilate 5 mg, 15 mg tabs	30–60 mg oral	4–6 hours	Long acting nitrate for prophylaxis use
Pentaerythritol-tetranitrate	Peritrate SA 80 mg	50–80 mg orally	3–5 hours 8–12 hours	—do—
Mannitol hexa-nitrate	15–30 mg tab	30–60 mg orally	4–6 hours	Used for prophylaxis

Miscellaneous Antianginal Drugs

- **Dipyridamole:** Dilates coronary vessels by preventing uptake and degradation of adenosine, a local mediator involved in auto-regulation of coronary flow. Cardiac work is not decreased. It causes coronary steal pheno-menon so it is a therapeutic failure. Dose 25–100 mg TDS (persantin 25, 75, 100 mg tabs). It inhibits platelet aggregation so used as prophylaxis for angina.

- **Adenosine** causes marked vasodilatation acting on A_{2A} receptor but its action is brief also, slows AV conduction. **Regadenoson** is selective A_{2A} agonist used for coronary circulation imaging.

- **Lidoflazine:** 60–120 mg OD-TDS (clinium 60 mg tab) decreases frequency of angina probably blocking Ca^{2+} channel.

- **Oxyphedrine:** Improves myocardial meta-bolism so they sustain hypoxia better. It alters taste sensation (Ildamen 8, 24 mg tabs, 4 mg/2 mL inj)

Table 75.2: Anti-ischemic drugs used for peripheral vascular disease	
Cyclandelate 200–400 mg TDS (Cyclospasmol)	Like papaverine relaxes smooth muscle and increases cutaneous, skeletal and cranial bloodflow.
Xanitol nicotinate (Complamina) 300–600 mg TDS	Vasodilator used to treat cere-brovascular disorder and PVD.
Pentoxiphylline 300 mg/2 mL given IV slowly (Trental	Reduce viscosity by (400 mg BD) improving RBC flexibility and rheological property, *i.e.* property of flow. No chance of steal syndrome. Reduces some cytokines and reduces portal pressure.

Therapeutic uses of peripheral vasodilators (Pentoxiphylline)

- Non-hemorrhagic stroke
- Cerebrovascular insufficiency (low drive, vertigo, tinnitus, memory defect)
- Tropic ulcer
- Intermittent claudication

- Retinal and cochlear disturbances
- Improve sperm motility
- Hepatorenal syndrome

Drugs for peripheral vascular disorders

β-agonist-Nylidrin, CCB nifidipine and α blockers: Phenoxybenzamine, prazosin, tolazoline but they can produce steal syndrome. Antioxidants are another approach.

New Drug: Cilostazol (Pletoz 50–100 mg tablets) used for pain-free walking in intermittent claudication. It is phosphodies terase-3 inhibitor. It has vasodilating and selective antiplatelet effects.

Ideal antianginal agent

- Selectively dilates coronary arteries, without producing significant alteration of other vessels.
- CO, BP and HR, oxygen consumption should remain unchanged.
- Should protect heart from stress-induced adrenergic effects.
- Should act promptly for sufficient duration without producing tolerance.

None fulfills those requirements.

Treatment of angina (Principles)

i. Relief and prevention of individual attack
ii. Chornic prophylaxis
   - Nitrates
   - β blockers
   - Calcium channel blocker
   - Digitalis in nocturnal angina (an expression of LVF)
   - Advice of way of life, to avoid smoking, alcohol, overeating
   - Treatment of associate conditions.

Principles of conservative treatment of myocardial infarction

- For pain, anxiety and apprehension opioid, diazepam
- Oxygenation
- Maintenance of blood volume, tissue perfusion and microcirculation

Flowchart 75.1: Treatment of myocardial infarction

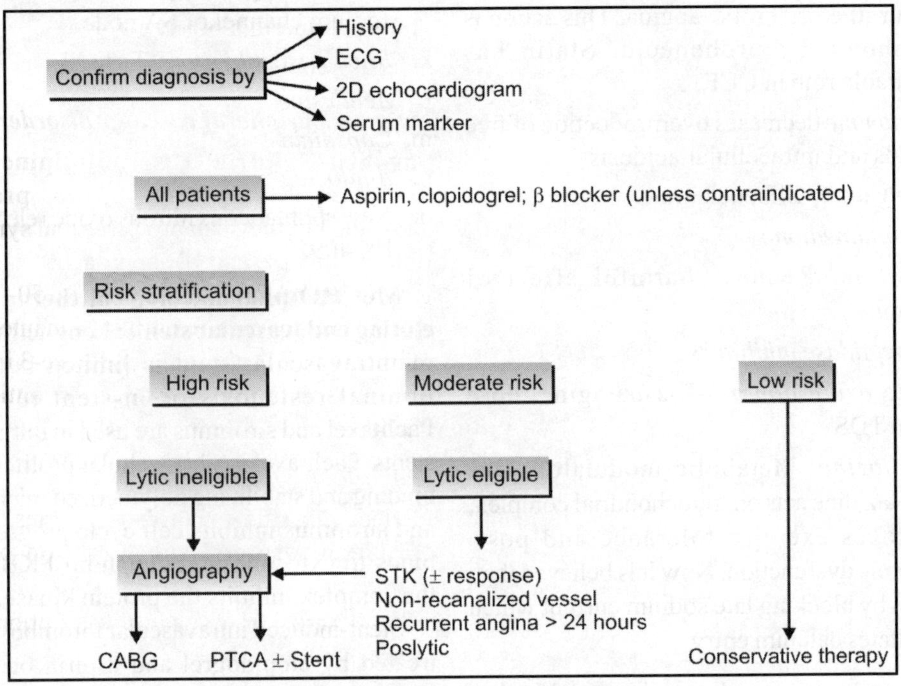

Confirm diagnosis by → History / ECG / 2D echocardiogram / Serum marker

All patients → Aspirin, clopidogrel; β blocker (unless contraindicated)

Risk stratification

High risk — Moderate risk — Low risk

Lytic ineligible — Lytic eligible

Angiography ← STK (± response) / Non-recanalized vessel / Recurrent angina > 24 hours / Poslytic

CABG   PTCA ± Stent   Conservative therapy

- Correction of acidosis by IV sodium bicarbonate.
- Prevention of arrhythmia
- Pump failure ┬ Frusemide
              ├ Vasodilator
              └ Inotropic agent
  (dopamine, dobutamine, rarely digitalis)
- Prevention of thrombus extension and embolism by heparin followed by oral anticoagulant.
- Thrombolytics, streptokinase/urokinase/alteplase
- Prevention of remodeling and subsequent CHF by ACE inhibitors
- Prevention of future attacks by aspirin and treatment of hyperlipidemia.

Newer Antianginal Drugs

A. Hemodynamically Active

a. *Newer nitrates*
  - Molisidomine (does not develop tolerance)
  - Pirisidomine
  - Linsidomine

b. *Newer β blockers*
  - Bisoprolol
  - Mepindolol
  - Carteolol
  - Celiprolol
  - Betaxolol
  - Penbutolol

c. *Newer CCBs*
  - Miberfradil
  - Elgodipine
  - Felodipine
  - Bepridil
  - Isradipine
  - Nislodipine
  - Nicardipine
  - Nimodipine

B. Acting at cellular Level (Metabolically Active)

a. *Trimethazidine* improves ATP production in ischemic tissues. It inhibits long chain 3-keto acyl CoA-thiolase (LC_3KAT), the enzyme which oxidizes fatty acid and increases glucose metabolism. Since ischemic myocardium shifts to fatty acid as a substrate which requires more O_2 and its shifting back to substrate reduces oxygen demand. It protects against O^+ free radicals.

b. *Allopurinol:* High dose of this xanthine oxidase inhibitor inhibits oxidative stress and endothelial dysfunction and prolong exercise time in atherosclerotic angina. This action is not shown by probenecid. Statin has favourable role in CCF.

c. *Linsidomine* decreases overproduction of free radicals and intracellular acidosis.

d. *Sulfonylurea:* Glibenclamide

e. *Thiazolidinedione*

f. *Carnitine:* Reduces harmful effect of ischemia.

g. *Vasopeptidase inhibitors*

h. *Nitric oxide donor*—L-asparagine, dose 1 gm TDS.

i. *Ranolazine:* Metabolic modulators like trimetazidine acts on mitochondrial complex, improves exercise tolerance and post-ischemic dysfunction. Now it is believed that, it acts by blocking late sodium current which facilitates calcium entry.

j. *Ivabradine* is a sodium channel blocker (If = funny current) which reduces heart rate by inhibiting the hyperpolarization activated sodium channel of SA node.

k. *Rhokinase inhibitors:* Fasudil

l. *Acadesine*

m. *Capsaicin*

n. *Amiloride*

o. New spontaneous nitrous oxide releasers like FK 409.

MeCHO pharmacological therapy: Drug eluting endovascular stents: Long-term efficacy of intravascular stent is limited because of luminal restenosis or in-stent restenosis. Paclitaxel and sirolimus are used in intravascular stents. Paclitaxel inhibits cellular proliferation by binding and stabilizing polymerized microtubules and sirolimus inhibits cell cycle progression. It binds to cytosolic immunophilin FKBP12 and the complex inhibits the protein kinase.

Stent-induced intravascular thrombosis can be treated by clopidogrel and aspirin or heparin, intravenously administered GP IIb/IIIa inhibitors (abciximab, tirofiban and eftifibatide).

76

Cardiac Arrhythmia and its Treatment

The transmembrane potential of cardiac muscle is determined by water-soluble Na^+, K^+, Ca^+ and Cl^- ions which can diffuse only through aqueous channels which are specific pore-forming proteins for diffusion. Fluxes of ions through channels are thought to be controlled by gates which are probably flexible peptide chains or energy barrier.

The equilibrium or reversal potential for ions is determined by Nernst equation,

$$E_{ion} = 61 \times \log \left(\frac{C_{extracellular}}{C_{intracellular}} \right)$$

The interior of cardiac muslces is (–80 to –90 mv) negative to exterior due to Na^+/K^+-ATPase and fixed anionic charges within the cell. The normal cardiac cells can permeate K^+ which determines resting potential because of inward rectifier channels are open. The cardiac muscle cells undergo depolarization and repolarization 60 times/minute, the shape and duration of it is determined by the ion channel protein complexes in the cardiac cell membrane. Ischemia, scarring, sympathetic stimulations all disturb cardiac cells to produce arrhythmia.

When atrial or ventricular cell at rest is depolarized, Na^+ channel's conformation changes from closed (resting) to open (conducting) state which allows Na^+ to enter the cardiac cells lasting few milliseconds after which Na^+ channel's protein rapidly goes to inactivated no conducting state. Inward Na^+ current produces series of activation and inactivation of other channels. (Fig. 76.1)

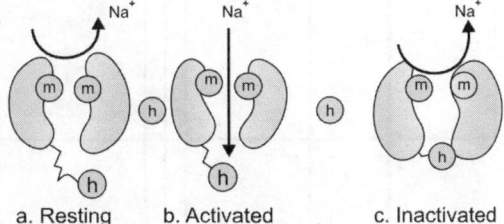

a. Resting b. Activated c. Inactivated

Fig. 76.1: Resting, activated and inactivated Na^+ channels

Cardiac sodium channel has been cloned.

Depolarization to threshold voltage results in opening of activation of (m) gates which subsequently opens (h) gates to activate the channel to increase sodium permeability (Fig. 76.1).

Transient outward K^+ causes outward repolarizing K^+ current called (I_{Ko}) causing phase I notch seen in action potential which is also inactivated rapidly. Phase II platue due to Ca^{2+} inward depolarizing current (Fig 76.2) which is balanced by repolarizing current of K^+ channel (delayed rectifier current is also called I_K).

Subsequently, Ca^{2+} current is inactivated to repolarize the cardiac cell (phase III). Delayed rectifier current generated by the expression of human ether-a-go-go-related genes (HERG) and it has become a new path for research for antiarrhythmic drugs.

Calcium channels are also activated and inactivated like sodium channel.

Two types of action potentials in cardiac muscles are possible:

• Slow channel

• Fast channel which differs from slow channel as given in Table 76.1.

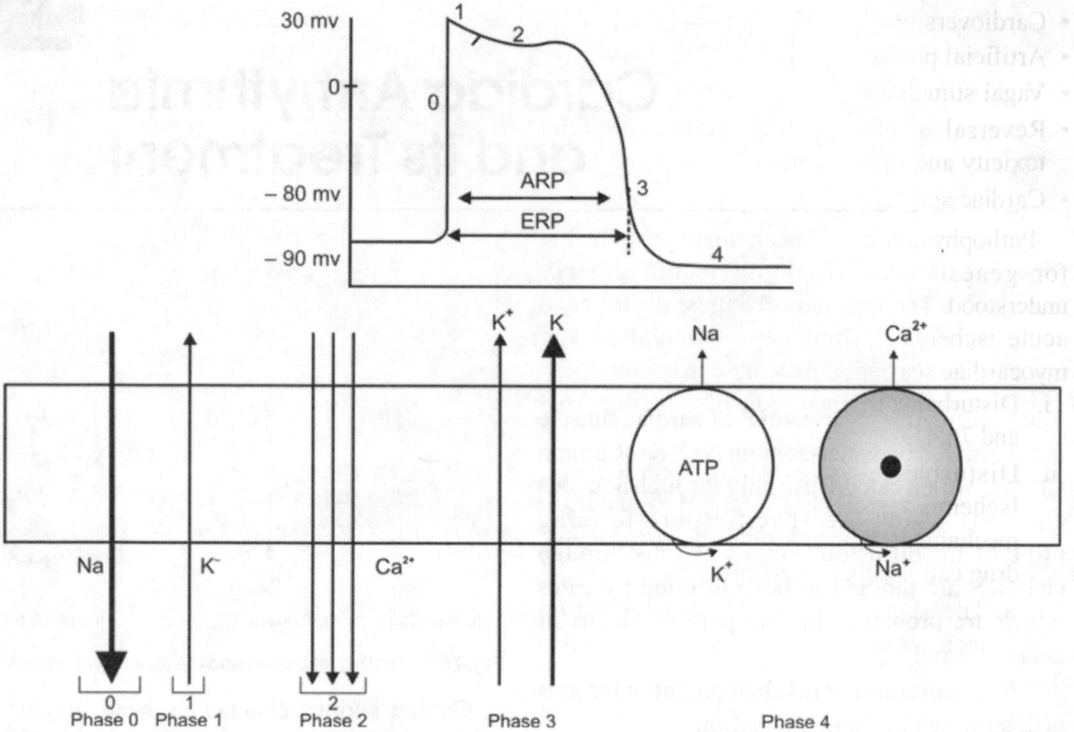

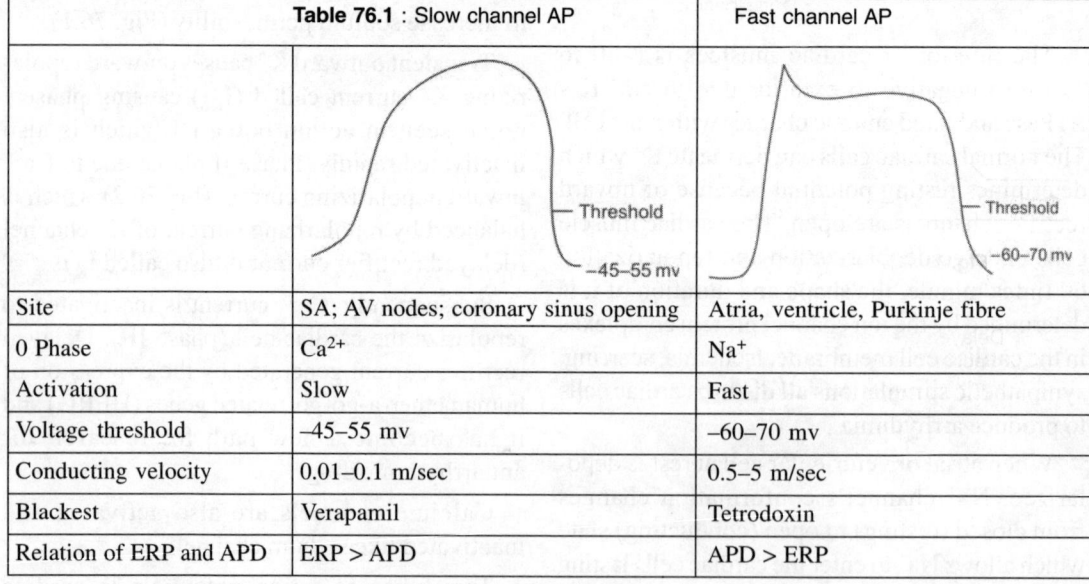

Fig. 76.2: Action potential of Purkinje fiber

Table 76.1 : Slow channel AP	Fast channel AP

	Slow channel AP	Fast channel AP
Site	SA; AV nodes; coronary sinus opening	Atria, ventricle, Purkinje fibre
0 Phase	Ca^{2+}	Na^+
Activation	Slow	Fast
Voltage threshold	–45–55 mv	–60–70 mv
Conducting velocity	0.01–0.1 m/sec	0.5–5 m/sec
Blackest	Verapamil	Tetrodoxin
Relation of ERP and APD	ERP > APD	APD > ERP

Heartbeat is the rhythm of life, therefore, any arrhythmic condition of the heart should not be taken lightly and considered for treatment accordingly. It is common with digitalis and anesthetic treatments and after myocardial infarction. Various types of treatments for cardiac arrhythmias are:

• Antiarrhythmic drugs

- Cardioversion
- Artificial pacing
- Vagal stimulation
- Reversal of precipitating factors (digitalis toxicity and hypokalemia)
- Cardiac surgery.

Pathophysiological mechanism responsible for genesis of arrhythmia is not clearly understood. The ion channel can be disturbed in acute ischemia, sympathetic stimulation and myocardiac scaring. It may arise in condition of:

i. Disturbance in impulse formation (Figs 76.3 and 76.4).

ii. Disturbance in impulse conduction. Ischemia, electrolyte and pH imbalance, mechanical injury, stretching, neurogenic drug can produce arrhythmia by:

a. The slope of phase IV depolarization increased pathologically in the autonomic or ordinary fibers resulting tachycardia or extrasystole, *i.e.* enhanced or ectopic pacemaker.

b. **After depolarization** is a secondary depolarization in normal or premature action potential and of two types:

- **Early after depolarization:** Repolarization during phase III is interrupted and membrane potential oscillates neighboring tissues are activated and impulse may be propagated (Fig. 76.3).

- **Delayed after depolarization:** Generally, results from Ca^{2+} overload (digitalis toxicity or ischemia) after attaining RMP secondary deflection occurs, may reach threshold potential to initiate premature AP (Fig. 76.4).

c. **Re-entry** (Fig. 76.5)

- **Circus movement:** Premature impulse passes around one way obstacle by temporarily blocked in one direction

Early premature action potential

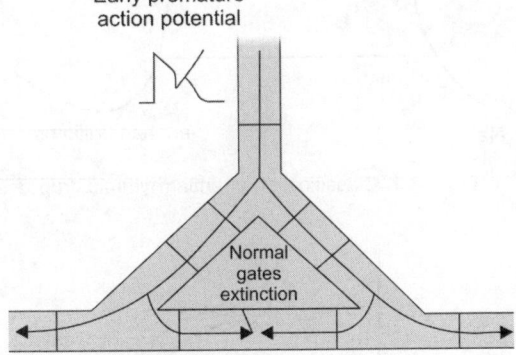

Fig. 76.3: Early afterdepolarization

Delayed premature action potential

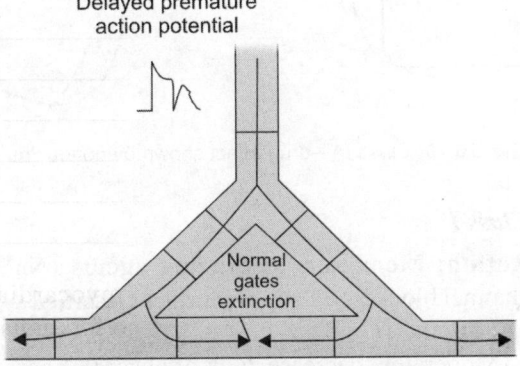

Fig. 76.4: Delayed afterdepolarization

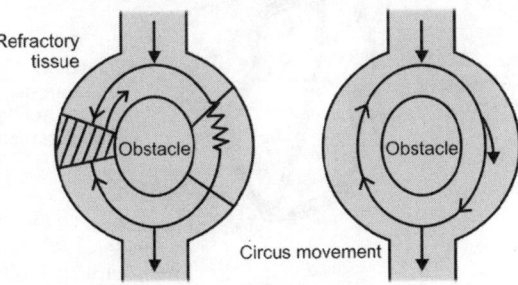

Fig. 76.5: Re-entry

goes to original spot in advance state of recovery and excites it, *e.g.* WPW syndrome.

- **Microentry circuits:** One of the branches of Purkinje fiber is depolarized to produce unidirectional block (Fig. 76.5).

d. *Torsades de pointes:* When QT interval is long, may produce ventricular tachycardia. Drugs which can prolong QTc interval: Terfenadine, Cisapride, Astemizole, Amiodarone, Disopyramide, Quinidine, Bretylium, Sotalol, Procainamide, Gatifloxacin, Sparfloxacin,

Thioridazone, Mefloquine, Halofantrine, Ziprasidone.

e. Fractionation of impulse: Under vagal over activity when atrial effective refractory period is brief, asynchronous activity of atrial fiber occurs leading to atrial fibrillation.

f. Conduction block: Prolong PR, signifying AV conduction block.

Classification of Antiarrhythmic Drugs

i. Clinical classification (as shown in the Fig. 76.6)

ii. Vaughan-Williams and Singh

Vaughan-Williams and Singh (1969) proposed a 4 class system taking into account important electrophysiological property of a drug. The system is arbitrary because many drugs exert multiple effects.

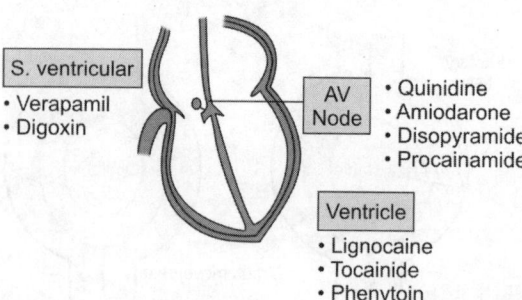

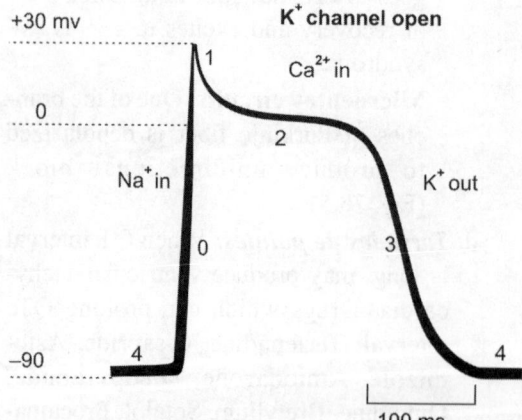

Fig. 76.6: Clinical classification of antiarrhythmic drugs

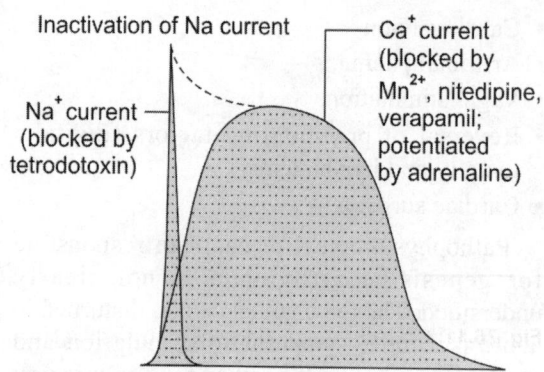

Fig. 76.8: Drugs interfering ionic flow of cardiac muscle action potential

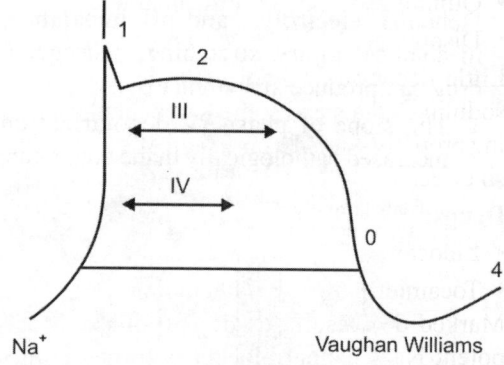

Fig. 76.9: Classification of antiarrhythmic drug

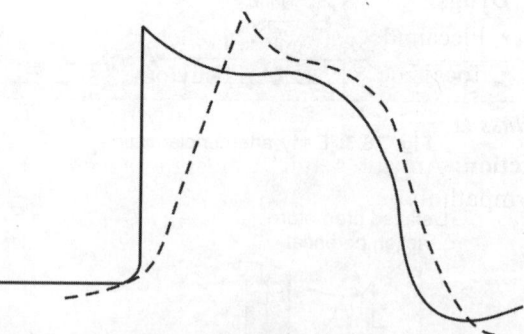

Fig. 76.10: Class IA—drug effect shown by dotted line

Class I

Action: Membrane stabilizing agents (Na$^+$ channel blockers). They are further classified as 1A, 1B and 1C.

a. Moderately decrease dv/dt of phase 0. These drugs block open Na$^+$ channel and block

Fig. 76.7: Ionic flow in cardiac action potential

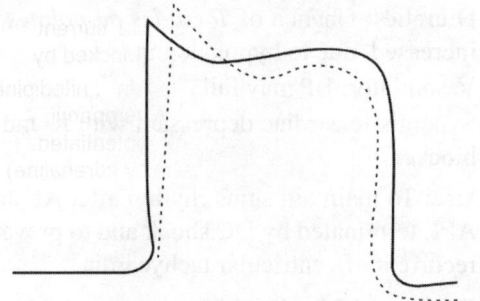

Fig. 76.11: Class IB—drug effect shown by dotted line

cardiac K^+ channel so delays repolarization and prolongs APD (Fig. 76.10).

Drugs:

- Quinidine
- Procainamide
- Disopyramide
- Moricizine

b. Little decrease in dv/dt of 0 phase. Blocks sodium channel and some K^+ channels opening properly with fast onset and offset kinetics so effective on faster heart rate (Fig. 76.10).

Drugs:

- Lidocaine
- Mexiletine
- Tocainide
- Phenytoin

c. Marked decrease in dv/dt of 0 phase. Most potent Na^+ channel blocker with negligible effect on K^+ channel so there is no effect on APD (Fig. 76.10).

Drugs:

- Flecainide
- Mexiletine
- Tocainide
- Phenytoin

Class II

Action: Antiadrenergic β-blocking agents, *i.e.* sympatholytics. Useful for supraventricular

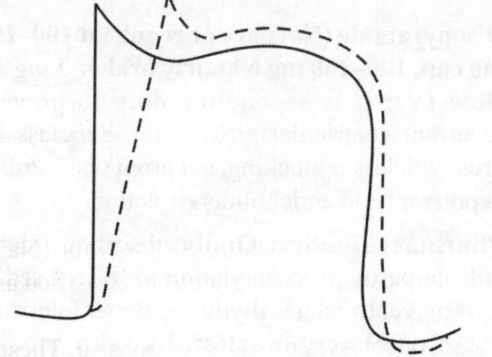

Fig. 76.12: Class IC—drug effect shown by dotted line

tachycardia. Decreases slope 4 which is responsible for automaticity.

Drugs:

- Propranolol
- Esmolol
- Sotalol (also class III)

Class III

Action: Agents widen AP (prolong repolarization and ERP). Blocks K^+ channel. Increases QT interval so may precipitate *torsades de pointes*.

Drugs:

- Amiodarone
- Bretylium (also class II)
- Defetilide
- Ibutilide

Class IV

Action: Calcium channel blocker (L-type voltage gated)

Drugs:

- Verapamil
- Diltiazem

In addition for PSVT: Adenosine, digitalis

For AV block: Sympathomimetic—isoprenaline. Anticholinergies—atropine

Digitalis is used in AF and AFL to control ventricular rate.

Mechanism of Action of Antiarrhythmic Drugs

- Delaying spontaneous depolarization to decrease rate.
- Increasing excitation threshold (procainamide)
- Increasing diastolic intracellular negativity.
- Increasing effective refractory period.

Individual Drugs

1. Quinidine: Obtained from *Cinchona* barks is a dextro-isomer of quinine.

Class I

Limits the conductance of Na^+ across cell membranes with local anesthetic action.

Subclass IA

- Na channel blocker
- Suppresses AV conduction and prolongs PR, QRS and QT.
- Prolong action potential duration.

Pharmacological action on heart: Antivagal + class IA + class III. Decreases automaticity of Purkinje fibers and other ectopic foci. It has little effect on afterdepolarization. SA node automaticity is little affected, but sick sinus aggravated. Refractory period is prolonged. Its antivagal action serves to terminate PSVT; atrial flutter and fibrillation. It depresses myocardial contractility so failure may be precipitated.

BP: Decreases by α blocking action and in higher doses by direct vasodilatation.

Quinidine blocks CYP2D6 and increases t½ of propafenone and conversion of codeine to morphine.

Skeletal muscle, GIT and uterus: Decreases contractility. Bitter and irritant taste may produce vomiting. Uterus may be stimulated to contract, but not useful as oxytocics and antimalarial action poorer to quinine.

Pharmacokinetics: Orally absorbed, about 90% protein-bound to albumin acid and α_1 acid glycoprotein, metabolized in liver by hydroxylation and excreted in urine. Therapeutic plasma concentration 2.5 µg/mL. Given orally or by slow IV not IM (may lead to necrosis). Quinidine sulfate 200 mg tab as gluconate 800 mg/10 mL inj. Dose 200–400 mg TDS.

Adverse effects: Not well-tolerated, sudden death due to cardiac arrest or VF may occur. Nausea, vomiting, ringing of ear, vertigo, visual disturbance, mental changes, idiosyncracy, fever, asthma, vascular collapse may be precipitated, arrhythmia *(Torsades de pointes)* paradoxical tachycardia.

Contraindications of quinidine

- Heart block
- Intolerance (thrombocytopenia)
- CCF and low BP
- History of embolism.

Important drug interactions of quinidine

1. Increase plasma digoxin concentration by:
   - Displacing it from tissue binding.
   - Decrease its biliary and renal clearance.

2. Diuretics: Chance of *Torsades de pointes* is increased, due to hypokalemia.
3. Vasodilator: BP may fall.
4. Synergistic cardiac depressant with K and β blockers.

Use: To maintain sinus rhythm after AF and AFL terminated by DC shock and to prevent recurrent of ventricular tachycardia.

2. Procainamide: Amide derivative of local anesthetic procaine possesses antiarrhythmic property like quinidine, but dose per dose less potent, less depressant to cardiac contractions and AV block. Antivagal action less and not a blocker so fall of BP is less.

Pharmacokinetics: Orally absorbed, well-distributed, less binding to protein, metabolized in liver by acetylation to N-acetyl procainamide which blocks K^+ channels and prolongs APD. There is pharmacogenetic differences as slow and fast acetylators like INH.

(Pronestyl—0.25 gm/tab or 1 gm/10 mL. Dose 0.5–1 gm oral or IM followed by 0.25–0.5 mg every 2 hours)

Therapeutic use of procainamide: Same as quinidine, but not a preferred drug for prolong oral therapy and it needs frequent dose adjustments. Used for ventricular extrasystole and ventricular tachycardia in lignocaine resistant cases.

Adverse effects of procainamide: Nausea, vomiting, weakness, mental confusion, cardiac paradoxical tachycardia, SLE in slow acetylators, fever, rash and agranulocytosis. It interferes with antimicrobial effect of sulfonamide by producing PABA.

Disopyramide (Norpace or regubeat 100–150 mg cap, 100–200 mg 6 hourly oral or 2 mg/kg slow IV): It is secondline drug to prevent recurrent ventricular arrhythmia. Subclass IA drug with less α blocking, but prominent cardiac depressant and anticholinergic action.

Pharmacokinetics: Orally absorbed, metabolized partly by dealkylation in liver. Used to prevent ventricular arrhythmia. Better tolerated.

Anticholinergic action like dry mouth, constipation, blurred vision may occur.

3. Moricizine: Subclass IA drug with less marked cardiac depressant and CNS effect used to suppress ventricular extrasystole and WPW syndrome. It delays Na$^+$ channel recovery. It is given orally in the dose of 200–300 mg TID. It is a phenothiazine derivative.

Subclass IB

- They block Na channels, but do not delay channel recovery.
- Do not depress AV conduction or prolong APD, ERP and QT interval.

4. Lignocaine: Commonly used as local anesthetic, is a blocker of inactivated Na channel more than that of open state. It is used to ventricular tachyarrhythmia, in emergency setting like cardiac surgery or MI, but not in atrial arrhythmia. Useful in digitalis toxicity because it does not depress AV block.

Xylocard 20 mg/mL; it does not contain any preservative like that present in local anesthetic.

Dose: 50–100 mg IV bolus action lasts only for 10–20 minutes because of rapid distribution. It is hydrolized, de-ethylated and conjugated before excretion. Metabolism is hepatic blood flow dependant (propranolol decreases hepatic blood flow and prolongs its t½).

Adverse effects: Drowsiness, nausea, nystagmus, twitching, fits, paresthesia.

5. Mexiletine (Maxitil): Local anesthetic, pharmacologically similar to lignocaine, orally effective antiarrhythmic. It increases threshold voltage, reduces phase 0 depolarization, decreases slope of phase 4, converts one-way block of Purkinje fiber into two-way block. Orally absorbed, metabolized in liver, excerted in urine. Morphine reduces its absorption, phenytoin and rifampicin induce its metabolism.

ADR: Bradycardia, hypotension and AV block, tremor, nausea, vomiting, blurred vision, ataxia are common.

Mexitil 50–100 mg cap, 250 mg/10 mL inj orally or IV

Dose 100–200 mg TDS. Used for post MI arrhythmia, ventricular extrasystole and VT.

IV Dose: 100–200 mg IV over 10 min then 1 mg/min.

6. Tocainide: Orally active, lignocaine analogue, effective in ventricular arrhythmia rarely used for side effects of thrombocytopenia and pulmonary fibrosis. Dose 400–800 mg TDS.

7. Phenytoin: Blocks Na$^+$ channel (inactivated), depresses automaticity of ventricular and Purkinjee fiber, without effecting SA node. Promotes AV conduction and suppresses digitalis induced afterdepolarization. Narrow spectrum antiarrhythmic used for digitalis toxicity, ventricular arrhythmia.

Available as dilantin and Epsolin 100 mg/ 2 mL or 100–200 mg oral 2–6 hourly. Extravasation should not be there.

Subclass IC

- Most potent Na$^+$ blockers
- Delays conduction
- Prolongs PR and QRS with variable effect on APD.

8. Flecainide (Tambocor): Reserved for resistant cases of AF, supraventricular arrhythmia, WPW syndrome without CHF. It is fluorinated analogue of procainamide.

9. Propafenone: It depresses conduction and has β-adrenergic blocking property, so failure and bronchospasm may be precipitated. Has proarrhythmic potential, not marketed in India. (propafenone marketed as rhythmonorm 150 mg tabs BD used for ventricular arrhythmias, re-

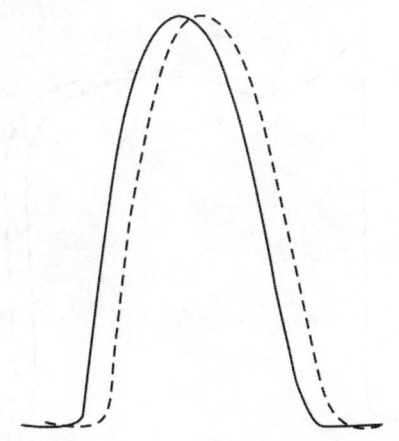

Fig. 76.13: Class II—drugs effect shown by dotted line (Decreasing phase 4 depolarization of pacemaker)

entrant tachycardia involving AV node and accessory pathways.)

Encainide is withdrawn from the USA market.

Class II

- Suppresses adrenergically mediated ectopics
- Decreases the slope of phase IV depolarization, and automaticity in SA node and Purkinje fibers and ectopic foci.
- Prolongs ERP of AV node.

10. Propranolol: Dose IV 1 mg/min, orally 40–80 mg TDS. Used for sinus tachycardia, atrial and nodal extrasystole, less effective than adenosine and verapamil in PSVT, used to treat WPW syndrome, but bradycardia may occur.

11. Sotalol (Betacardone): Prominent Class III action with prolonging repolarization, blocks K^+ channels, delays AV conduction. Used for VT, AF and AFL. May produce *torsades de pointes.*

12. Esmolol: Short acting β blocker (marketed as mini block 100 mg/10 mL. Dose 0.5 mg /kg/min) used to treat AF/AFL, supraventricular tachycardia and arrhythmia associated with anesthesia.

Class III (Fig. 76.14)

- Prolongs repolarization
- AP widened
- Increase ERP
- Re-entrant arrhythmia terminated.

13. Amiodarone (Cardarone, eurythmic 100–200 mg tab and 150 mg/3 mL inj): Used for ventricular and supraventricular arrhythmia and WPW syndrome. Incompletely and slowly absorbed. Action on oral route takes weeks to start. Accumulates in muscle and fats so close monitoring required.

Adverse effects: Hypotension, nausea, photo-sensitization, corneal microdeposit, pulmonary alveolitis and fibrosis, peripheral neuropathy, liver damage and hypothyroidism.

Interaction: Digoxin and warfarin levels are increased by reducing clearance through kidney and AV block in patient receiving Ca^+ channel blocker.

14. Dronedarone: Structurally similar to amiodarone without iodine atom, so no effect on thyroid metabolism. Used twice daily for atrial fibrillation.

15. Dofetilide: Used for maintenance of sinus rhythm in patient of atrial fibrillation.

16. Ibutilide: IV used to convert atrial flutter and fibrillation to normal sinus rhythm. QT prolongation occurs, leading to *torsade de pointes.*

17. Bretyllium: Adrenergic neuron blockers. Polar compound so oral absorption erratic. Introduced as antihypertensive agent, blocks

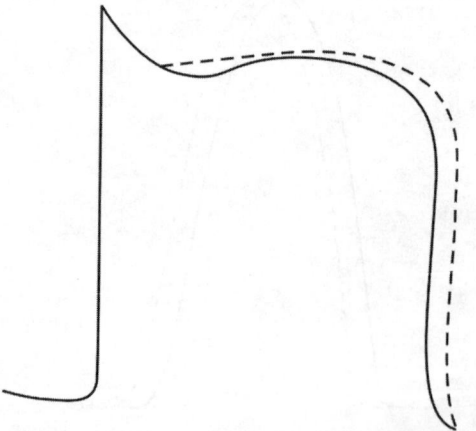

Fig. 76.14: Class III—drugs effect shown by dotted lines (blocking K⁺ channel during phase 3 of action potential)

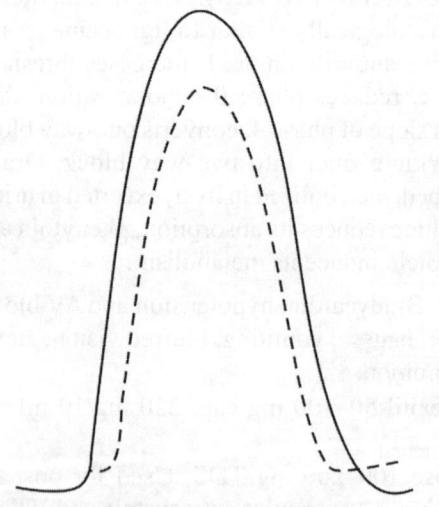

Fig. 76.15: Class IV—drugs effect shown by dotted lines which block L-type Ca²⁺ channel producing decreased phase 4 depolarization in SA and AV nodes

noradrenaline release, prolongs APD and ERP. Used to treat ventricular fibrillation, refractory to electrical defibrillation, short-term use recommended. Dose 5–10 mg/kg IV over 10 minutes.

Class IV

• Inhibits Ca^{2+} mediated slow channel inward current.

18. Verapamil is used to treat PSVT, to control ventricular rate in AFL as an alternative to digitalis. Diltiazem seldom used as antiarrhythmic.

OTHER ANTIARRHYTHMICS

19. Adenosine: Administered by rapid IV (1–3 sec) as free base 6–12 mg or as ATP (10–20 mg). Adenosine terminates PSVT within 30 sec. Activates ACh sensitive K^+ channel causing membrane hyperpolarization though A_1 type receptor on SA node causes pacemaker depression and bradycardia. In AV node, it prolongs ERP slowing conduction and in atrium shortens action potential and reduces excitability. Indirectly reduces Ca^{2+} current in AV node and depresses re-entrant circuits responsible for PSVT. It dilates coronary artery. Available as

Table 76.2: Pharmacological treatment of cardiac arrhythmia

Arrhythmia	Emergency treatment		Prophylaxis
	Preferred	Alternative	
SA node, sinus arrhythmia, sinus tachycardia, β blocker, sinus bradycardia, Atropine			
Atrial premature beats	Sedative, β blocker Procainamide Disopyramide	Quinidine	Qunindine, Procainamide Disopyramide
PAT	Vagal stimulation, IV verapamil	Digitalis IV β blockers	Quinidine, Procainamide Disopyramide Digitalis
PAT with homodynamic compromise	DC cardioversion	Quinidine	
AF	Digitalis Propranolol IV verapamil	Digitalis Quinidine DC cardioversion	
Atrial fibrillation	Same as flutter	—do—	
Ventricular premature beat	Lignocaine IV Procainamide	Quinidine, Procainamide, Disopyramide	Quinidine Procainamide
PVT	Same as ventricular premature beat		
PVT with hemodynamic compromise	DC cardioversion		Quinidine
Ventricular fibrillation	Difibrillation; IV Bretyllium	Lignocaine Procainamide	Quinidine Disopyramide
Digitalis induced tachyarrhythmia	Lignocaine	IV phenytoin	
Complete heart block	Atropine	Isoprenaline	Pacemaker

adenoject 3 mg adenosene base per mL in 2 mL and 10 mL amp. It has short t½ of 10 sec because it is taken up by RBC and endothilial cells, where it is converted to 5 AMP. ATP injected is converted to adenosine.

Drug interactions of adenosine: Dypyridamole blocks uptake so potentiate action, but theophylline and caffeine blocks receptors so antagonize action.

Uses of adenosine

• To diagnose tachycardia dependent on AV node
• Controlled hypotension during surgery
• Brief coronary dilatation during surgery for intervention procedure.

20. Magnesium: It is used for congenital acquired long QT syndrome. Also used in digitalis induced arrhythmia of Mg level is low. 1gm $MgSO_4$ is infused slowly over 20 minutes.

21. Vernakalant: It is multi-ion channel blocker. It is recommended for converting recent onset atrial fibrillation to normal sinus rhythm.

22. Ivabradine: Discussed earlier with drugs of heart failure. It is trialed for in appropriate sinus tachycardia.

23. Ranolazine: This drug originally developed as antianginal drug has shown anti arrhythmic activity for atrial fibrillation. It also suppresses ventricular tachycardia.

24. Potassium: Used in digitalis induced arrhythmia.

DRUGS FOR AV BLOCK

25. Atropine: Used for AV block due to vagal over- activity, *e.g.* digitalis toxicity, some cases

of MI. It shortens ERP in AV node and increases conduction velocity in bundle of His.

Dose: 0–6 to 1.2 mg/IV.

Sympathomimetic (adrenaline and isoprenaline): Shortens ERP in conducting tissues, used to overcome partial heart block till external pacemaker is implanted.

Some author places cardiac glycosides on class V and miscellaneous agents like phenylephrine, methoxamine, edrophonium in class VI antiarrhythmic drugs.

Ideal antiarrhythmic drug

• Effective against specific group of arrhythmia.
• Should not have adverse effect particularly cardiac
• Should be effective orally and intravenously
• Long acting
• Produce stable plasma levels, so that monitoring of drug is not necessary.
• Cheap and easily available

In fact all antiarrhythmic drugs are potentially arrhythmogenic.

Drug which can increase QT interval

• Antiarrhythmics: Amiodarone, disopyramide, procainamide, propaferone, qunidine
• Antimicrobials: Artimisinin, halofantrine, mefloquine, quinine, gatifloxacin
• Antihistamines: Terfenadine, astemizole
• Antidepressants: Tricyclics
• Antipsychotics: Thioridazine, resperidone
• Prokinetics: Cisapride

77

Drugs Used in the Treatment of Hyperlipoproteinemia

When the concentration of the ·cholesterol or tryglyceride carrying lipoprotein arbitrarily exceeds 95th percentile of random population, the condition is known as hyperlipoproteinemia, which is responsible for development of atherosclerosis with its sequela like thrombosis and infarction especially in the end arteries supplied organs (heart, brain).

Lipid Transport

Lipids are transported in association with apoprotein which is a coat of phospholipid, free cholesterol and apoprotein, inside core of which consisting of cholesterol esters and tryglyceride.

There are six classes of lipoproteins which differ in their shapes, sizes, density, proportion of tryglyceride and cholesterol esters. Each class of lipoprotein has a specific tissue of origin, and catabolism and has defined role in the transport of lipids.

Dietary lipids obsorbed from intestine with the help of bile salts and form chylomicrons, passed into lacteals to reach bloodstream *via* thoracic duct. Intestinal cholesterol absorption is mediated by Niemann-Pick C_1 like protein which is the target of ezitimibe. During its passage through capillaries, the endothelial lipoprotein lipase hydrolyzes triglyceride into

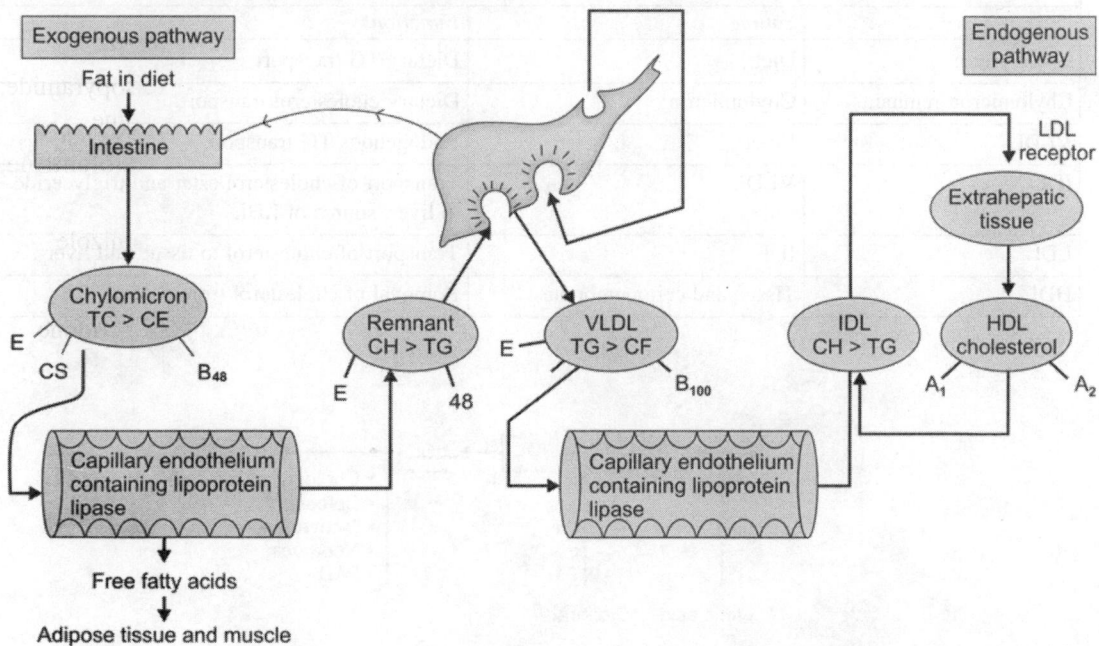

Fig. 77.1: Metabolism of lipoproteins (exogenous and endogenous)

fatty acids which cross endothelium and enter adipocyte or muscle cells are either oxidized to give energy or esterified and stored as triglyceride. Its size is reduced, content of triglyceride is diminished, but its cholesterol ester remain intact called chylomicron remnant, which is cleared by receptor mediated endocytosis in the liver cells, where the chylomicron remnant is digested, and the free cholesterol performs the functions of:

• Synthesis of cell membrane
• Excreted *via* bile
• Stored in liver.

Liver under stimulation of high calorie intake or carbohydrate intake secretes triglyceride and cholesterol in plasma in VLDL (very low density lipoprotein). The lipoprotein lipase of capillary endothelium acts on VLDL and fatty acids pass into adipose tissue. The remnant is called IDL (intermediate density lipoprotein) which contains more cholesterol esters than triglyceride. Half of IDL is taken by LDL receptors in liver and the rest becomes low density lipoprotein containing

only cholesterol esters (losing triglycerides). LDL remains in plasma for long time and is the major reservoir of cholesterol in human plasma. Rate of LDL uptake is regulated by LDL receptor synthesis. When liver or extrahepatic tissues require cholesterol for synthesis of steroid hormone, new cell membranes or bile acids synthesize LDL receptors. Thyroxine and estrogen enhances LDL receptor gene expression and has got LDL lowering effects.

When the cells of the body die, the cell membrane undergoes turnover, the free cholesterol is continuously replaced in plasma and high density lipoprotein (HDL) immediately takes it up, esterifies it with the help of enzyme of plasma called lecithin cholesterol acetyl transferase (LCAT) and transfer it back to LDL, IDL, chylomicron for completing cycle with the help of cholesterol ester transfer protein.

Lipoproteins are also disposed off by less specific pathways operating in macrophages and scavenger cells.

VLDL, IDL and LDL are atherogenic, while HDL is protective.

Table 77.1: Functions and sources of lipoproteins

	Source	*Functions*
Chylomicron	Diet	Dietary TG transport
Chylomicron remnants	Chylomicron	Dietary cholesterol transport
VLDL	Liver	Endogenous TG transport
IDL	VLDL	Transport of cholesterol ester and triglyceride to liver; source of LDL
LDL	IDL	Transport of cholesterol to tissue and liver
HDL	Tissue and cell membrane	Removal of cholesterol from tissues

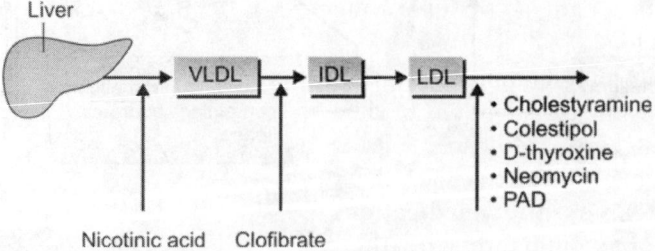

Fig. 77.2: Site of action of hypolipidemic drugs

Disease Causing Hyperlipoproteinemia

Primary

- Single gene defect
- Summation of multiple subtle gene.

Secondary

- Nephrotic syndrome
- Diabetes mellitus
- Hypothyroidism
- Alcoholism
- Oral contraceptive pills
- Biliary cirrhosis
- Uremia.

Strategies to Treat Hyperlipoproteinemia

- Diet: It should be low cholesterol, unsaturated animal fats or vegetable fats, but should provide normal calorie.
- There should be elimination of aggravating factors (OCP, alcohol, etc.)
- Drugs.

Drugs used for hyperlipoproteinemia are of two types

- Those which effect production of lipoprotein.
- Drugs effecting lipoprotein removal.

I. Cholesterol lowering drugs

- **Cholestyramine and colestipol:** Cholestyramine and colestipol are unabsorbed after oral administration, binds to bile acids in intestinal lumen, interfere with enterohepatic circulation and increase fecal loss of cholesterol. It decreases LDL cholesterol. Maximum effect observed in two weeks and returns to baseline in 3–4 weeks of discontinuation. Cholestyramine 4 gm or colestipol 5 gm sprinkled on food.

  ADR: Patient may complain of gritty texture of resins, constipation, bloated feeling, heart burn, flatulence, nausea; other drugs should be taken either 1 hour before or 4 hours after medications because it may interfere with their absorption.

- **Probucil:** Strong antioxidant, well-tolerated, reduces cholesterol, LDL cholesterol.

  ADR: Pain in abdomen, flatulence, nausea can occur, should be avoided in ventricular arrhythmia because it prolongs QT interval, fetal abnormality may occur, stored in body fats. Dose 250–500 mg BD for type IIa and type IIb hyperlipoproteinemia.

- **Fish oils (Maxepa 10 gm/day):** Reduce triglycerides by reducing hepatic VLDL synthesis, generally used with fibrates.

II. Drugs lowering cholesterol and triglycerides

- **Nicotinic acid:** This vitamin reduces plasma lipids, but its amide derivatives are ineffective. Reduces TG and VLDL rapidly, followed by modest LDL and cholesterol. It raises HDL. It decreases lipolysis in adipose tissue with reduction of FFA flux to the liver. Dose 100 mg TDS increased up to 2–6 gm/day, but in that dose produces vasodilatation, flushing, heat, itching. These effects may be reduced by starting with lower dose, or if given with aspirin. It is useful in types III, IV, V hyperlipidemia, should not be used in diabetes and cardiac arrhythmia.

- **Fibric acid derivative (clofibrate)** reduces plasma triglycerides, may be secondary effect to reduce lipolysis in adipose tissue, and increased activity of enzyme lipoprotein lipase. These are also activators of peroxisome proliferator activated receptor α which stimulates fatty acid oxidation. Enhances release of ADH. It is orally absorbed, metabolized and excreted with urine as glucuronide conjugation.

  Atromid 0.5 gm cap, dose 0.5–1 gm OD potentiates oral anticoagulants, displaces frusemide and phenytoin, from plasma proteins.

  Weight gain, increased appetite, myalgia, gallstone formation, hyperuricemia, reversible alopecia, decreased libido, cardiac arrhythmia may occur. It should not be used in kidney and liver diseases patient and to pregnant and lactating mother. It is not used now.

a. **Gemfibrozil (Iopid 300 mg):** Fibric acid derivative, useful in type III hyperlipoproteinemia.

Decrease clotting factor VII, epigastric distress, loose motion, eosinophilia, blurred vision, impotence, gallstone formation (not that common). Dose 300–600 mg BD before meal in type III, IV, and V diseases.

b. **Bezafibrate (bezalip 200 mg 1 tab TDS):** Fibric acid derivative used in types III, IV and V hyperlipoproteinemia.

GI upset, rash, myalgia may occur.

c. **Fenofibrate (Fenolip):** Fibric derivative, prodrug and greater action on LDL.

III. **3-hydroxy-3-methylglutaryl coenzyme-A reductase inhibitors (statin and vastatin)**

Acts by competitively inhibiting the enzyme HMG-CoA reductase, catalyzing rate limiting step in cholesterol synthesis.

HMG-CoA reductase inhibitors lower LDL cholesterol, in 4–6 weeks, raise HDL cholesterol. Since HMG-CoA activities are higher at night,

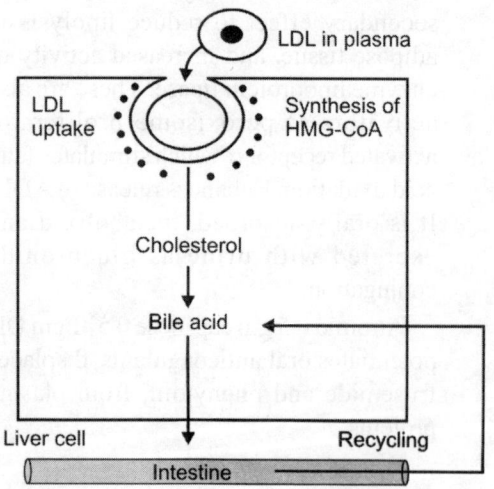

Fig. 77.3

so statins are better administered at night except atorvastatin and rosuvastatin which may be administered at any time because of their long t½.

Simvastatin (simcard 5–20 mg/day): It is a prodrug hydrolyzed in GI tract to active form.

Atorvastatin (aztor, atorva) 10–80 mg also has antioxidant properties (10, 20, 40 and 80 mg tabs).

Pravastatin also decreases plasma fibrinogen level. Other statins are fluvastatin, lovastatin, rosuvastatin. Lovastatin is available as 10, 20 and 40 mg tabs.

Statins are used for types IIa, IIb, V and for secondary hypercholesteremia (diabetes, nephrotic syndrome).

Headache, nausea, GI upset, rash, sleep disturbances, rise of serum transaminase, but liver damage is rare, increases CPK and causes muscle tenderness which is common, if given concurrently with gemfibrozil, erythromycin, cyclosporin. Statins are not advised to nursing mother and women wishing to conceive. Some statins are approved for children, *viz.* atorvastatin, simvastatin, lovastatin for children up to 11 years. Pravastatin is approved for children above 8 years.

Whom to treat with statin?

It is a firstline drug to lower lipid in postmenopausal women, men over 45 and female over 55 if lipid profile is high, cerebrovascular disease patient with high cholesterol, in peripheral vascular disease, type II diabetes mellitus patient, in postmyocardial infarction or revascularization patient.

• **Neomycin:** This aminoglycoside lowers LDL cholesterol by complexing with bile acids preventing their absorption. Decreases intestinal absorption, may produce steatorrhea, malabsorption, diarrhea. May be used as alternative to bile salt binding resins.

• **Gugulipids** of gum guggul moderately lowers CH and TG, well-tolerated and dose 25 mg TDS.

• **α-thyroxine:** Decreases LDL concentration.

- **PAS-C** may be used for type IIa and type IIb. Excessive alcohol offset of this effect.
- **β-sitosterol:** Plant sterol similar to cholesterol except for a substitution of ethyl group at C24 or its side chain. Not absorbed orally, decreases cholesterol absorption, generally taken t½ hour before meal at bedtime. Dose 30 mL.

Radical Therapy for Refractory Hyperlipidemia

- Ileal bypass: Ileum anastomosed with cecum to disrupt enterohepatic circulation.
- Portacaval shunts
- Liver transplantation will provide LDL receptors.

Extracorporeal Lipoprotein Removal

- LDL plasmapheresis.
- **HELP (Heparin extracorporeal LDL precipitation) system:** LDL is precipitated by lowering pH and removed by filters. The process also removes fibrinogen.
- **Gene therapy:** A retrovirus carrying DNA for LDL receptor and subsequent injection into portal vein in partial hepatectomy patient. It is a crude method. Better result expected in future.

Newer Drugs

Ezetimibe (Ezedoc 10 mg): Reduces exogenous cholesterol, decreases LDL and increases HDL. It does not affect intestinal triglyceride absorption. It is complementary therapy to statin, so combination tablets are available. It is water-insoluble, absorbed after glucuronidation in intestine and enters enterohepatic circulation 70% excreted with feces and 10% with urine. Its absorption is inhibited by bile acid sequestrants. May cause allergy and myopathy. Ezetimibe is contraindicated in pregnancy. It is not given with bile sequestrants.

Rosuvastatin (Rosuvas 5, 10, 20 mg): Newer, once a day statin, reduces LDL and increases HDL.

Pitavastin (Pitava 1–2 mg): Metabolized by CYP2C9, so chances of drug interaction are less. Should not be given to patient of cyclosporine therapy.

Avasimibe inhibits enzyme acyl coenzyme A. Cholesterol acyl transferase (ACAT-1) which forms cholesterol ester from cholesterol.

Torcetrapib: It inhibits enzyme cholesterol ester, triglyceride transport protein (CETP) and thereby increases HDL cholesterol. Another drug of this group is anacetrapib.

Recent drugs approved for adjunct therapy:

- **Icosapent ethyl:** An omega-3 fatty acids
- **Lomitapide:** Inhibits formation of VLDL
- **Mipomersen sodium:** An antisense oligo-nucleotide which inhibits synthesis of apo B-100.

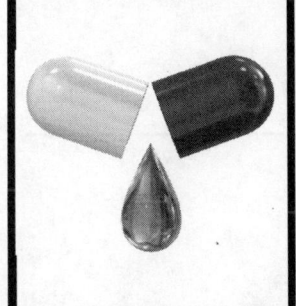
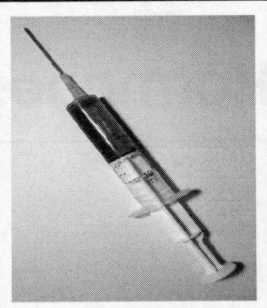
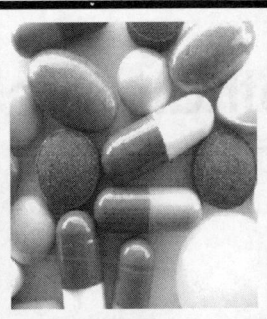
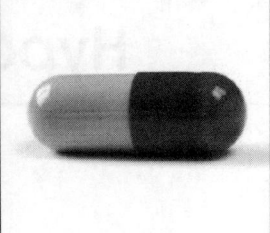

SECTION 11

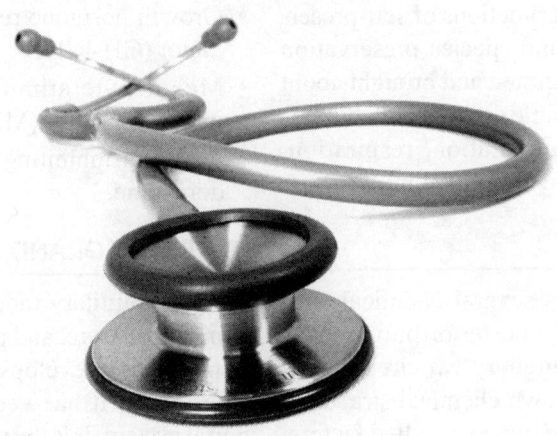

DRUGS OF ENDOCRINAL DISEASES

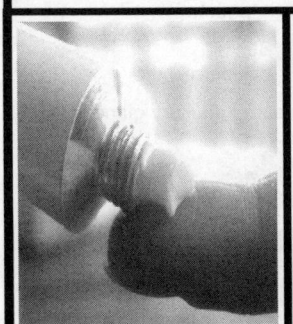
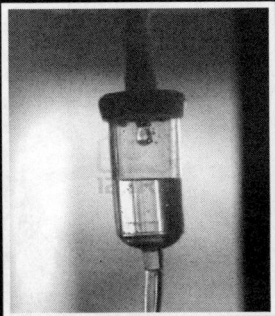
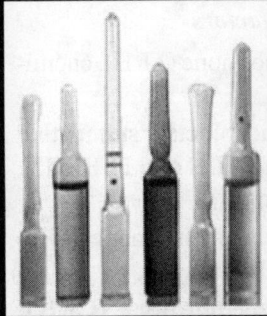
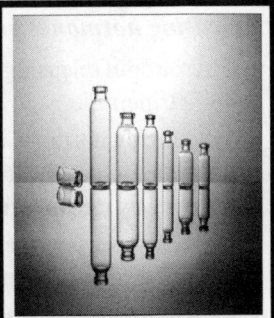

78

Hypothalamic Hormones

The Greek word *hormaein* means to stir up or to impel is defined as "a substance of intense biological activity, secreted by specialized specific cells in the body and transported through circulation to a distance where it exerts its effects on target cells". Important functions of self-preservation (homeostasis) and species preservation (reproduction) are integrated and brought about by neuroendocrine complex which collaborates various functions as circulation, respiration, digestion, excretion and reproduction.

HYPOTHALAMUS

Hypothalamus releases several chemical substances which reach the posterior pituitary *via* neurons and anterior pituitary *via* circulations. Those which are of known chemical structures are called hormones and other are called factors. Six releasing and three inhibiting factors till known, acting on anterior pituitary produced by hypothalamus.

Different Hormones and Factors Released by Hypothalamus

Releasing hormones or factors

- Thyrotropin releasing hormone (TRH), chemically tripeptide.
- Luteinizing hormone and follicular stimulating hormone releasing factor (LH and FSH-RH), chemically decapeptide.
- Growth hormone-releasing hormone (GH-RH), chemically peptide hormone.
- Corticotropin-releasing hormone (CRH), chemically peptide.

- Melanocyte stimulating hormone releasing factors (MSH-RF)
- Prolactin releasing factors (PRF)

Release inhibiting factors

- Growth hormone release inhibiting hormone factor (GH-RIH)
- Melanocyte stimulating hormone release inhibiting factor (MSH-RIF)
- Prolactin inhibiting factor (PIF), chemically dopamine.

PITUITARY GLAND

Anterior pituitary (adenohypophysis) develops from oropharynx and posterior pituitary (neurohypophysis) develops from floor of the brain (Fig. 78.1). It has very rich blood supply and portal system. It is the master of endocrine glands and elaborate number of peptide hormones. Their secretion is under control of hypothalamus

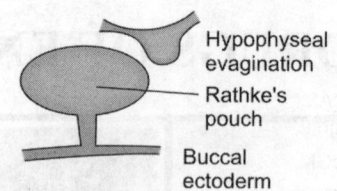

Fig. 78.1: Development of pituitary gland

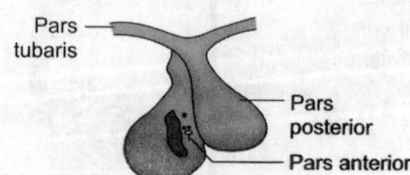

Fig. 78.2: Pituitary gland

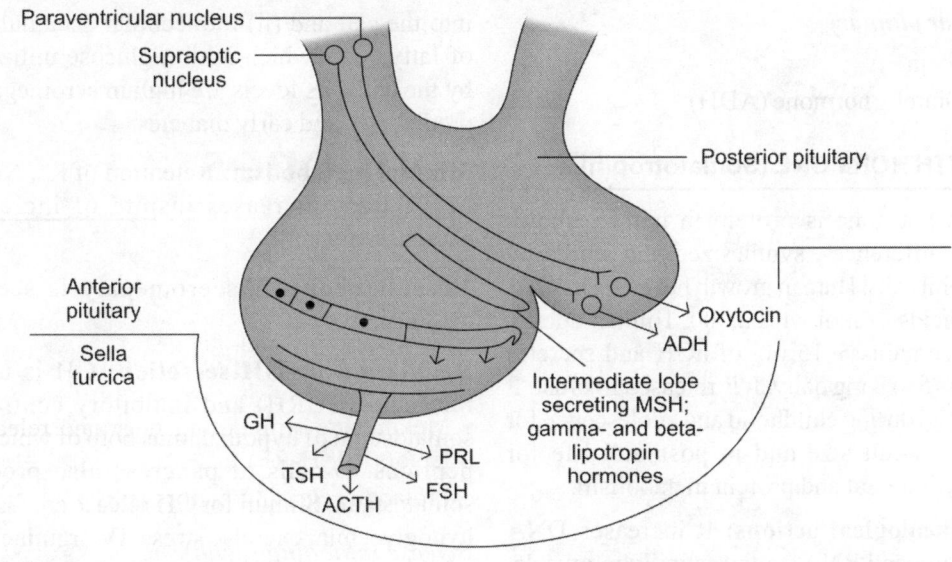

Fig. 78.3: Parts of pituitary and different hormones liberated by it

through releasing and inhibiting hormones. Histologically, anterior pituitary is either acidophilic or basophilic according to staining character and releases separate hormones.

HORMONES SECRETED BY PITUITARY

Anterior pituitary

• Growth hormone (GH) released by acidophil somatotroph.

• Adrenocorticotropic hormone (ACTH) released by corticotroph.*

• Thyroid stimulating hormone (TSH) released by thyrotroph.*

• Gonadotropins: FSH and LH released by gonadotroph.*

• Prolactin released by acidophilic lactotroph

• Melanocyte stimulating hormone (MSH) by intermediate lobe.

All are released by basophils

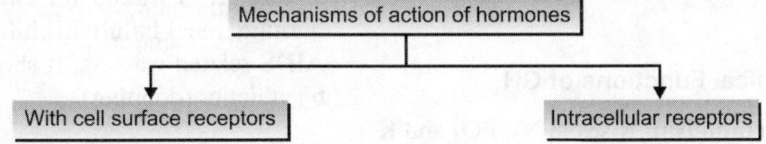

i. With cAMP as second messenger: ACTH, FSH, LH, MSH, PTH, glucagon, catecholamine, ADH, HSG, CRH, TSH and calcitonin

ii. With cGMP as second messenger: Atrial natriuretic factor (ANF)

iii. With Ca or phosphatidyl as second messenger: TRH, GnRH, catecholamine, gastrin, vasopressin, oxytocin, acetylcholine

iv. Mediated by tyrosine kinase: Insulin.

v. Cell surface receptor with unknown intracellular messenger: Growth hormone, prolactin and erythropoietin

Intracellular receptors

• Glucocorticoids
• Mineralocorticoids
• Estrogen
• Progesterone
• Androgen
• Calcitriol
• Thyroxine

*released by basophils

Posterior pituitary

- Oxytocin
- Antidiuretic hormone (ADH)

GROWTH HORMONE (Somatotropin)

Growth hormone is protein in nature, shows species differences, synthesized and stored by eosinophil cells. Human growth hormone has 191 amino acids of mol wt. 22,000. Human adenophysis contains 5–15 mg of hGH and secretes about 0.75 to 3 mg daily. It is released in brust. It is required during childhood and adolescence for attaining adult size and in postnatal life for carbohydrate, fat and protein metabolism.

Pharmacological actions: It increases DNA replication and RNA synthesis in liver, muscle, adipose tissue and cartilage. Production of glycosaminoglycans are increased, collagen synthesis and turnover is increased. Thyroid hormones are required for full effect of GH on DNA replications. GH has many effects on intermediary metabolism. It acts on cell surface JAK-STAT protein kinase receptor. Some of its effects are indirectly through elaboration of somatomedin or insulin-like growth factors IGF_1 and IGF_2 which are extracellular mediators of GH response, which acts as paracrine. Liver is a major source of IGF_1 and like insulin it promotes glucose uptake by muscle and lipogenesis. IGF_1 acts through its own receptor and through insulin receptor.

Physiological Functions of GH

Protein metabolism: Rises in N_2, PO_4 and K^+; blood urea falls, urinary excretion of hydroxyproline increases, increases transport of amino acids into the cells and accelerates intracellular protein synthesis.

Fat metabolism: Fasting FFA rises due to lipolytic action. It inhibits lipogenesis from glucose and acetate. GH released during sleep, has little effect on plasma fatty acids.

Carbohydrate metabolism: Produces carbohydrate intolerance probably due to: (i) Inhibition of phosphorylation of glucose after its entry into the cell and (ii) intracellular accumulation of fatty acids which inhibit glucose utilization by the cells. Its levels are high in acromegalies, prediabetes and early diabetes.

Mineral metabolism: Retention of K^+, Na^+, P, Mg^{2+}, Ca^{2+} increases inspite of increased excretion of Ca^{2+}.

Miscellaneous: Visceromegaly is seen in acromegaly.

Regulation or GH secretion: GH is under releasing (GHRH) and inhibitory control of somatostatin of hypothalamus both of which are peptides. D-cells of pancreas also produce somatostatin. Stimuli for GH release are fasting, hypoglycemia, exercise stress, IV arginine. It is inhibited by high dose corticosteroid, IGF_1; increased plasma free fatty acid levels.

Pathological involvement: Excess GH production causes acromegaly, hyposecretion causes pituitary dwarfism.

Preparation: Human growth hormone (Crescormon). 41U vial in lyophilized form, dissolved in 2 mL normal saline before use. Dose 0.06–16 IU/kg IM or SC three times a week. Two varieties of recombination DNA technique rhGH somatropin and somatrem are available. It is also used for Turner's syndrome and in children with renal failure. rhGH is used for constitutional short stature. It is trialed for catabolic states like burning, renal failure in children, osteoporosis; AIDS related wasting. It should not be abused by athletics (dopping).

Therapeutic uses

- Pituitary dwarfism
- Turner's syndrome
- Patient with total parenteral nutrition
- Antiaging

Adverse effects: Allergy or resistance to treatment, pain at injection site, lipodystrophy, hypothyroidism, glucose intolerance, salt and water retaintion are rare. Somatrem is more immunogenic, other toxicities are peripheral edema; carpal tunnel syndrome, increased level of cytochrome P450, proliferative retinopathy. Sermorelin and Hexarelin are recombinant GH-RH analogs used for pituitary dwarfism.

Sermorelin is a synthetic GH-RH used to diagnose GH secretion.

Mecasermin: Children with IGF_1 deficiency may not respond to exogenous GH, may be due to mutation of GH receptors and neutralizing antibodies to GH. Mecasermin is used to IGF_1 deficiency patient not responding to GH. It is a recombinant human IGF_1 given SC 0.04–0.08 mg/kg. Hypoglycemia may occur, so taken after snacks. Other ADRs are intracranial hypertension and raised liver enzymes.

Somatostatin: This 14 amino acid peptides, inhibit GH, TSH, PRL, secretion of pituitary, insulin and glucagon of pancreas, and gastrointestinal hormones including gastrin and HCl. Constricts splanchnic, hepatic and renal blood vessels, somatostatin decreases mucosal blood flow, useful for upper GI bleeding. Antisecretory action is beneficial in pancreatic, biliary or intestinal fistulae, but it is short acting, lacks specificity of action and rebounds after discontinuation. *Ocetreotide* overcomes these disadvantages. It is long acting synthetic surrogate of somatostatin. Its ADRs are abdominal pains, nausea, steatorrhea, gallstone due to bile stasis, diarrhea. It is preferred over somatostatin.

Somatostatin (stilmen 250 μg and 3 mg amp) 250 μg slow IV over 3 minutes followed by 3 mg infusion over 12 hours. Octreotide (Sandostatin) 50–100 μg in 1 mL amp. Initially 50–100 μg SC. 100 μg IV used for stopping esophageal bleeding.

Lanreotide: Analogue of somatostatin, long acting (acts for 10–15 days), used for acromegaly, acts like octreotide.

Pegvisomant: It is a GH antagonist used for acromegalic due to pituitary adenoma. It is a polyethylene glycol complexed mutant GH, binds to GH receptor, but does not produce signal transduction.

Prolactin (Single chain of 199 amino acids of MW = 23000): It is in conjuction with estrogen, progesterone and several other hormones; causes development of breast after parturition. When estrogen and progesterone secretion falls prolactin level rises. It inhibits hypothalamo-pituitary gonadal axis, therefore, breastfeeding causes lactational amenorrhea and inhibition of ovulation. It affects immune response through T lymphocyte. There is no clinical indication of prolactin. It is predominantly under inhibitory control of pituitary through PH-IH. Chemically, dopamine acts through D_2 receptor. Bromocriptine and cabergoline decrease plasma prolactin level whereas dopamine antagonist halloperidol and dopamine depletor, reserpine increase plasma prolactin level.

Bromocriptine (Proctinal Bromogen 2.5 mg tab): Ergot derivative acts on $D_2 > D_1$ dopamine receptor as agonist and α-adrenergic blocker. It is not uterine stimulant (oxytocic).

Action: Decreases prolactin, antigalactopoietic. Increases GH release in normal, but decreases the same in acromegaly patient. It has levodopa like action.

Decreases BP due to central action and due to α blockade. Decreases GI motility and causes vomiting and nausea.

Pharmacokinetics: Orally partially absorbed, high first pass metabolism, metabolized in liver and excerted by bile.

Therapeutic uses of bromocriptine

It is started in low dose and increased gradually to avoid side effects of vomiting.

• Hyperprolactinemia (2.5–10 mg/day)
• Suppression of lactation and breast engorgement in case of neonatal death, but risk is there.
• Acromegaly, relatively high dose 5–20 mg/day is required.
• Parkinsonism, dose 20–80 mg/day.
• Hepatic coma, it causes arousal.
• Diabetes mellitus.

Cabergoline (Caberlin 0.5 mg tab; dose starts with 0.25 mg twice weekly, if requried increased every 4–8 weeks up to 1 mg biweekly). It is D_2 agonist, long acting used to those patients not tolerating or responding bromocriptine. It is preferred for hyperprolactinemia and acromegaly.

Pergolide and **quinagolide** are other D_2 agonists used for hyperprolactinemia.

Side effects of bromocriptine: Nausea, vomiting, nasal blockage, hypotension, syncope, mental confusion, hallucination, psychosis, livedo reticularis, abnormal movements.

Gonadotropins (GNS): Two gonadotropins from anterior pituitary FSH and LH are glycoproteins with two peptide chains total of 207 amino acid residues and 23–28% sugar. FSH mol wt = 32,000, LH mol wt = 30,000, both act to promote gametogenesis and secretion of gonadal hormones. Disturbances in gonadotropin release from anterior pituitary are responsible for delayed puberty or precocious puberty. Inadequate secretion produces amenorrhea, sterility in female, oligospermia and impotence in men. All gonadotropins are given IM. They are partly metabolized and partly excreted unchanged in urine.

Menotropin obtained from urine of menopaused women contains FSH and LH. Chorionic gonadotropin is a placental hormone, urofollitropin is a FSH obtained from menopausal women is devoid of LH, **Follitropin alfa and beta** are human FSHs produced by recombinant DNA technology. Lutropin is a recombinant human LH.

FOLLICULAR STIMULATING HORMONE (FSH)

FSH in female induces follicular growth, helps to develop ovum to secrete estrogen. In male, it supports spermatogenesis and has trophic influence in seminiferous tubules.

Luteinizing hormone (LH) helps in ripening and triggering of ovulation followed by luteinization. It influences progesterone secretion. In male, it stimulates testosterone secretion by interstitial cells and called interstitial cell-stimulating hormone (ICSH). FSH and LH act through their distinct receptors; both of them are G-protein coupled receptors.

FSH and LH release are stimulated by single decapeptide hormone called GnRH released by hypothalamus. GnRH is released in pulses. The frequency and amplitude of pulses determine whether FSH, LH or both will be released. Estrogen and progesterone inhibit FSH and LH secretion, but preovulatory use of estrogen increases LH and FSH secretion. Inhibin inhibits FSH release and DA inhibits LH release. Gonadotropin increases in puberty. Gn level in menopausal women is high due to loss of feedback inhibition. Inappropriate secretion causes the following:

In childhood

- Excess causes precocious puberty
- Less causes delayed puberty.

In adult

- Excess causes polycystic ovaries
- Less causes amenorrhea, sterility, impotence, oligospermia.

Preparations

- Metrodin 75 and 150 IU/amp (FSH pure) [Pregnorm 75 IU FSH + 75 IU LH/amp.]
- Human chorionic gonadotropins (HCG). (Corion, Profasi 1000; 2000; 5000; 10000 IU) As dry powder with separate solvent.
- Recombinant human FSH (rhFSH): Follitropin α, follitropin β
- Recombinant human LH (rhLH): Lutropin
- Recombinant hCG (rhCG): Choriogonadotropin α

Therapeutic uses of gonadotropins

- Amenorrhea, infertility, menotropin (*i.e.* FSH and LH) 1M OD × 10 days, followed next day by 1000 IU of hCG.
- Hypogonadotropic hypogonadism in males, 1000–2000 IU of hCG IM bi-or triweekly and the FSH and LH after 3–4 months which will stimulate testosterone secretion and stimulate spermatogenesis.
- Cryptorchidism HCG or androgen is used.
- To aid *in vitro* fertilization (menotropin FSH + LH or pure FSH is used).

Adverse effects: Polycystic ovary, ovarian bleeding, precocious puberty in children, allergic reactions (skin testing should be advised), hormone dependent prostrate and breast malignancies, headache, edema, mood changes.

Two important adverse effect of women treated with gonadotropin and LCG are ovarian hyperstimulation syndrome and multiple pregnancy.

Gonadotropin-releasing hormone (GnRH): Gonadorelin-pulstile administration of gonadorelin is tried for infertility, delayed puberty or cryptorchidism is because of few weeks continuous use desensitizes pituitary gonadotropes and there is fall in gonadotropin level. This synthetic GnRH is injected IV 100 μg. It induces prompt release of LH and FSH and rise of gonadal steroids (GnRH analogues).

Superactive GnRH agonists: Buserelin, deslorelin, goserelin, leuprolide, nafarelin, histrelin, triptorelin used as pharmacological gonadectomy for precocious puberty, prostate cancer, endometriosis, premenopausal breast cancer, uterine fibroid, polycystic ovarian disease and to assist induced ovulation, as contraceptive for both male and female. These drugs stimulate gonadotropin secretion, if given in pulsatile manner and inhibit the release on continued administration. These drugs are generally used SC route; nafarelin and buserelin used by nasal route, goserelin used by SC implant. These drugs are more potent than natural GnRH and long acting with high affinity for GnRH receptor. Flare up reaction, *i.e.* initial gonadotropin release occur which may be dangerous for Ca prostate and endometriosis patient.

These are used in pulsatile manner for anovulatory infertility, hypogonadotropic hypogonadism, delayed puberty and cryptorchism whereas used continuously for precocious puberty, endometriosis, Ca-prostate, polycystic ovarian disease and uterine fibroid because reduction of gonadotropin is seen which is beneficial for those conditions.

Nafarelin (nasarel 2 mg/mL nasal solution). Therapeutic use in precocious puberty (800 μg/BD); and for endometriosis (200 μg BD × 6 months); assisted reproduction 400 μg BD intranasally; uterine fibroid 200 μg intranasally BD.

Triptorelin (Tryplog 2.5 mg/5 mL vial. Dose 2.5–3.5 mg IM every 3–4 weeks). It is long acting, used for cancer prostate, endometriosis, precocious puberty, uterine fibroid.

Adverse effects: Hot flush, loss of libido, vaginal dryness, osteoporosis, emotional lability.

Gonadotropin-releasing hormone antagonist: Abarelix, degarelix, ganirelix and cetrorelix have least histamine-releasing action compared to other gonadotropin RH antagonists. They inhibit LH surge in controlled ovarian stimulation undergoing *in vitro* fertilization. Loss of libido, osteoporosis, hot flushes are ADR of GnRH antagonists. Abarelix and degarelix are approved for use in prostate cancer and LH suppression in controlled ovarian stimulation. They are also used for uterine fibroid, endometriosis, as an adjunct during *in vitro* fertilization.

In vitro fertilization hMG is used to activate follicular development which may cause premature ovulation. GnRH antagonists are used to prevent this.

THYROID-STIMULATING HORMONE (TSH) (THYROTROPIN)

Thyrotropin: TSH has mol wt. 30,000 with 210 amino acids containing glycoprotein, stimulates thyroid to synthesize and release T_3 and T_4.

Produces hyperplasia and hypertrophy of thyroid follicles, increases their blood supply, promotes iodide trapping and its incorporation, proteolysis of thyroglobulin to release more T_3 and T_4. Its regulation is controlled by hypothalamus (thyroid-releasing hormone, TRH). Therapeutically used only to differentiate myxoedema due to pituitary dysfunction from primary thyroid disease. Recombinant thyrotropin is likely to be available soon.

Protirelin is a synthetic analogue of TRH.

Somatostatin and its longer acting analogues suppress TSH release.

Adrenocorticotropic hormones (ACTH; corticotropin) have been discussed with corticosteroids.

79

Thyroid and Antithyroid Drugs

The thyroid gland was discovered by Wharton in 1656. Gull (1874) described hypofunction of thyroid. Kendal in 1915 isolated and crystalized T_4 thyroxine. Harrington and Berger (1926) detected its chemical structure.

The thyroid gland synthesizes, stores and secretes iodinated amino acid hormones—L-thyroxine and L-triiodothyronine, which are incorporated with glycoprotein thyroglobulin enclosed within cavities surrounded by thyroid epithelial follicular cells which synthesize the hormones. It also secretes peptide hormones (calcitonin) responsible for calcium metabolism secreted by parafollicular C-cells (discussed with calcium metabolism).

Production and secretion of thyroid hormones, involves the following steps

- Uptake of iodide by thyroid follicular cells.
- Oxidation of iodide to iodine and iodination of tyrosine residual of thyroglobulin.
- Coupling of iodotyrosine residues to form thyroxine and triiodothyronine.
- Breakdown of thyroglobulin to release active hormones.

Uptake of iodine: The trapping of iodine in the thyroid gland is stimulated by TSH against electrical and concentration gradient by active transport process Na^+/I^- symporter or NIS which is also influenced by iodine content of thyroid gland, *viz.* less store activates and large store inhibits it. Skin, salivary gland, gastric mucosa, intestine, placenta also concentrate iodine, but not influenced by TSH.

Oxidation of ioidine and iodination of tyrosine: Trapped iodine is carried to the apical membrane by another transporter called pendrin and oxidized and with the help of H_2O_2 to iodinium I^+ or hypoiodous acid (HOI) or enzyme-linked hypoiodate which combines to tyrosil residues of thyroglobulin to form mono- and di-iodotyrosine, still attached to thyro-globulin.

Coupling of iodotyrosines: Iodinated tyrosine couple to form triiodothyronine (T_3) and thyroxine (T_4) catalyzed by thyroid peroxidase. Oxidation and coupling both are stimulated by TSH. Thyroglobulin is the most efficient protein with special configuration to support this coupling.

Storage release: Thyroglobulin containing iodinated T_3 and T_4 are transported to the interior of the follicle and remained stored as thyroid colloid, taken back into cells by endocytosis and broken by lysosomal proteases releasing T_3 and T_4. Monoiodotyrosine (MIT) and Diiodotyrosine (DIT) are deiodinated and iodine is reutilized while T_3 and T_4 go to circulation. The uptake of colloid and proteolysis is stimulated by TSH.

T_4 is converted to T_3 in liver and kidney by 5'-deiodinase which takes up T_4 and converts it to T_3. Here there is removal of one iodine from outer ring B by 5'-deiodinase type I (DID-I) present in liver and kidney and DID type II present in brain, pituitary, skeletal and cardiac muscles. Removal of iodine from inner ring produces inactive metabolite, reverse T_3 (rT_3), by DID type III present in placenta, skin and brain

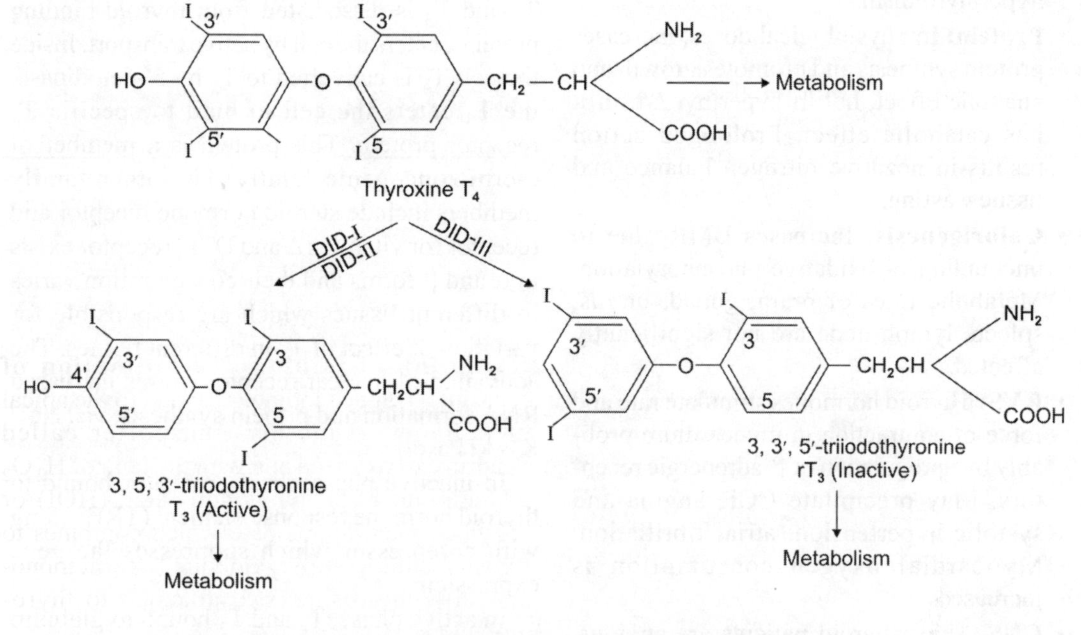

Fig. 79.1 Metabolism of Thyroxine DID =5' deiodinase enzyme

(Fig. 79.1). Presence of rT_3 in amniotic fluid indicates normal thyroid function of the foetus. Peripheral tissues take up T_3 except brain and pituitary. Propyluracil, propranolol (high dose), amiodarone and glucocorticoids inhibit this peripheral conversion of T_4 to T_3 (except in brain and pituitary).

Normal thyroid secretes 70–90 µg T_4 and 10–30 µg T_3/day. Thyroid hormone binds to plasma proteins thyroxine binding globulin, thyroxine binding prealbumin (transthyretin) and albumin. Only free hormones produce action. During pregnancy, protein-bound iodine (PBI) increases, but concentration of free hormone remains unaltered. The hormones are inactivated by deiodination and glucuronide/sulfate conjugation which are excreted in bile and some reabsorbed (enterohepatic circulation) and excreted in urine. Plasma $t\frac{1}{2}$ of T_4 = 6–7 days and T_3 = 1–2 days which is shortened in hyperthyroidism and prolonged in hypothyroidism due to faster and slower metabolisms.

Pituitary thyroid relationship: Thyrotropin hormone TSH is glycoprotein. Mol wt: 30,000, synthesized and released by basophil cells of anterior pituitary, under stimulation of TRH from hypothalamus. Circulating T_3 level modulates the response of pituitary to TRH. In additions to TSH, synthetic TRH stimulates release of prolactin, FSH (in man), LH (in woman) and GH. The TRH and TSH actions are mediated by enhanced synthesis of cAMP. TSH (high concentration) also act *via* IP_3 DAG which increases intracellular Ca^{2+} pathway in thyroid cells.

Function of Thyroid Hormones

Qualitatively T_4 and T_3 are similar.

1. **Growth and development:** Cretin, myxoedema, delayed milestone of development occur in hypothyroidism.

2. **Metabolism**
   - **Lipid:** Hyperthyroidism is characterized by hypocholesterolemia. All phases of cholesterol metabolism accelerated. It enhances lipolysis by potentiating action of catecholamine. LDL level of blood is reduced.
   - **Carbohydrate:** Absorption of glucose is increased, metabolism is stimulated, sugar utilization stimulated, glycogenolysis, gluconeogenesis in liver occur. All leads to

hyperglycemia with insulin resistance in hyperthyroidism.

- **Protein:** In physiological doses, increases protein synthesis and promotes growth and anabolic effect, but in hyperthyroidism it has catabolic effect. Prolonged action results in negative nitrogen balance and tissue wasting.
- **Calorigenesis:** Increases BMR, due to uncoupling of oxidative phosphorylation. Metabolic rates of brain, gonad, uterus, spleen, lymph node are not significantly affected.
- **CVS:** Thyroid hormones stimulate rate and force of contraction in myocardium probably by upregulation of β-adrenergic receptors. May precipitate CCF, angina and systolic hypertension, atrial fibrillation. Myocardial oxygen consumption is increased.
- **CNS:** Hyperthyroid patients are anxious, nervous with tremors and hyperreflexia. Hypothyroidism produces mental retardation.
- **Skeletal muscles** are flabby and weak in myxoedema, but in hyperthyroidism there is tremor; increased muscle tone and weakness due to myopathy.
- **GIT:** Peristalsis increases with T_3 and T_4 producing diarrhea.
- **Hemopoiesis:** T_4 helps in erythropoiesis.
- **Skin:** Thyroid deficiency causes deposition of complex mucopolysaccharides in connective tissue responsible for rough skin in myxoedema.
- **Reproduction:** Oligomenorrhea occurs and fertility is impaired in hypothyroidism. Normal thyroid function is essential for pregnancy and lactation.
- **Miscellaneous**
  i. Excess thyroxine impairs conversion of creatine to creatinine and phosphocreatinine leading to creatinuria.
  ii. Conversion of carotene to vitamin A is defective in hypothyroidism. Requirement of fat- and water-soluble vitamins increases with thyrotoxicosis.

Mechanism of Action of Thyroid

T_4 and T_3 is dissociated from thyroid-binding proteins, enters the cell by active transport. Inside the cell T_4 is converted to T_3 by 5'-deiodinase, the T_3 enters the cell to bind to specific T_3 receptor protein. This protein is a member of c-erbB oncogenic family. The other family members include steroid hormone receptor and receptor for vitamins A and D. T_3 receptor exists in α and β forms and their concentration varies in different tissues which are responsible for variation of effect of T_3 in different tissues. The activation of nuclear receptor causes increased RNA formation and prtoein synthesis, *viz.* Na^+/K^+-ATPase.

In inactive phase, the T_3 receptor bound to thyroid hormone response element (TRE) along with corepressor which suppresses the gene expression.

In active phase, T_4 and T_3 bound to globulin are released and free T_4 and T_3 enter to cells by active transport system, T_4 is converted to T_3 by 5'-deiodinase, T_3 goes towards nucleus and binds to ligand binding domain of thyroid receptor, promoting heterodimerization with retinoid X receptor (RXR) on thyroid hormone response element (TRE) displaces the corepressor and binds to coactivator. This thyroid receptor (TR) coactivator complex activates gene expression and protein synthesis (Fig. 79.2).

Difference between T_3 and T_4

- Thyroid secretes more T_4 than T_3.
- T_3 is five times potent to T_4 and T_3 is avidly bound to nuclear receptor. It has quicker onset of action.
- T_4 is convertible into T_3 in peripheral tissues, therefore, it may be said that T_4 is a prohormone of T_3.

Preparations: L-thyroxine Na (eltroxin, Thyrox 100 μg tab), triiodothyronine (liothyronine) 5, 25 μg tabs (used for myxoedema coma for quick response).

Pharmacokinetics: Absorption of L-thyroxine is incomplete for clinical purposes. L-thyroxine

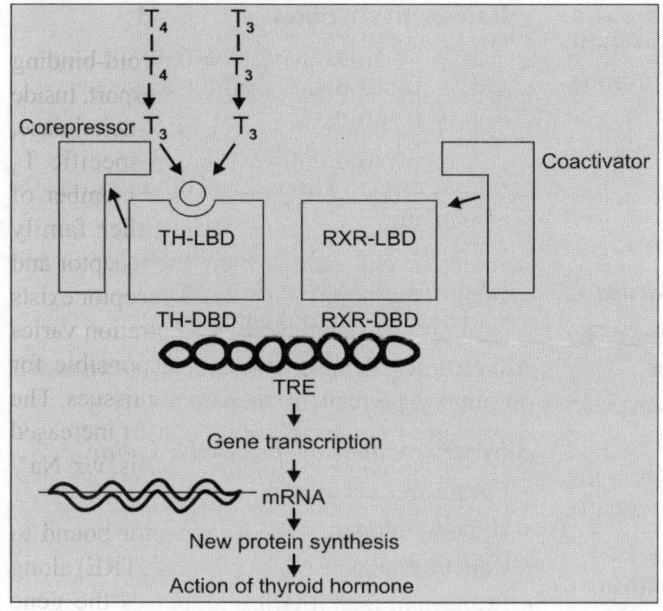

- **TH-DBD** : Thyroid hormone DNA binding domain
- **TH-LBD** : Thyroid hormone ligand binding domain
- **RXR-LBD** : Retinoid X receptor ligand binding domain
- **RXR-DBD** : Retinoid X receptor DNA binding domain
- **TRE** : Thyroid hormone response element

Fig. 79.2: Mechanism of action of thyroid hormone

is superior to triiodothyronine except for myxoedema coma.

Therapeutic uses of thyroid preparations

1. Cretinism
2. Adult hypothyroidism
3. Myxoedema coma (L-triiodothyronine is preferred)
4. Non-toxic goiter
5. Papillary carcinoma of thyroid: Suppresses TSH and produces temporary regression.
6. Empirical uses:
   - Refractory anemia
   - Obstinate constipation
   - Chronic non-healing ulcer
   - Menstrual disorder and infertility

THYROID INHIBITORS

Thyroid inhibitors lower functional capacity of hyperactive thyroid gland.

Thyrotoxicosis (hyperthyroid state)

Graves' disease is an autoimmune disorder due to IgG class of antibodies. Long acting thyroid stimulator (LATS) producing effects like TSH.

Toxic nodular goiter: Independent of TSH.

Classification of antithyroid drugs

1. **Goitrogens**
   a. **Thioamides** inhibit hormone synthesis: Propylthiouracil, methimazole, carbimazole (in the UK, carbimazole is used which is converted to methemazole *in vivo*, methimazole is about 10 times more potent to propyl thiouracil).
   b. **Inhibit ioidide trapping:** Thiocyanates, perchlorates, nitrates.
2. **Inhibit hormone release:** Iodine and iodides of Na and K; organic iodide.
3. **Destroying thyroid tissue:** Radioactive iodine ^{131}I, ^{125}I and ^{123}I.

Miscellaneous: Lithium (inhibits hormone release), amiodarone (inhibits conversion of T_4 to T_3), PAS and sulfonamide (inhibit thyroglobulins iodination).

ANTITHYROID DRUGS

They bind to thyroid peroxidase preventing oxidation of ioidide thereby inhibit:
- Iodination of tyrosine in thyroglobulin.
- Coupling of iodotyrosine to form T_3 and T_4. Propylthiouracil also inhibits peripheral conversion of T_3 and T_4.

Pharmacokinetics: Antithyroid drugs are absorbed orally and distributed widely, enter milk, placenta, metabolized in liver and excreted in urine.

Adverse effects of antithyroid drugs

- Hypothyroidism
- GI intolerance
- Joint pain
- Loss of hair
- Skin rash
- Agranulocytosis

Preparation and doses of antithyroid drugs

- Propylthiouracil 50–100 mg TDS followed by 25–50 mg BD or TDS as maintenance.
- Methimazole 5–10 mg TDS followed by 5–15 mg daily in 2 divided doses.
- Carbimazole (neomarcazole, thyrozole 5 mg tab) 1 tab TDS followed by 2.5–10 mg daily as maintenance.

Uses of antithyroid drug: Hyperthyroidism.

Iodine and iodides: They shrink enlarged glands which become less vascular and firm and make thyroid function euthyroid. Peak effect observed in 10–15 days after which due to thyroid escape thyrotoxicosis may occur. Hormone synthesis and release (thyroid constipation) are affected.

Preparation: Lugol's solution [5% iodine in 10% potassium iodide (KI) solution]. Lugol's solution; colloid iodine 10%, dose 5–10 drops/day, collosol iodine 8 mg iodine/5 mL liq (prophylactic dose 5–10 mg/day and therapeutic dose 100–300 mg/day for iodide).

Chronic iodine toxicity called *iodism* characterized by salivation, rhinorrhea, sneezing, inflammation of mucous membrane, all subsides on withdrawal of the drug.

Acute reaction produces swelling of lips, eyelids, angioedema, fever, joint pain, patechial hemorrhages, lymphadenopathy, thrombocytopenia.

Therapeutic uses of iodine preparation

- Preoperative prepration for thyroidectomy.
- Thyroid storm (Lugol's iodine 6–10 drops)
- Prophylactic in endemic goiter (Iodized salts are used)
- Antiseptic and expectorant
- Iodine containing contrast media (iopanoic acid; ipodate)

Radioactive iodines

^{131}I = t½ 8 days (commonly used)
^{123}I = t½ 13 hours used for diagnosis.
^{125}I = t½ 60 days
^{131}I = taken orally for:

- Diagnosis: Dose 25–100 μ curie for scanning.
- Therapeutic in toxic nodular goiter and Graves' disease. 3–6 m curie.
- Metastatic thyroid carcinoma.

Advantages: Simple, convenient, inexpensive, no surgery, permanent out patient therapy.

Adverse reactions of radioactive iodine

- Focal soreness in neck
- Hypothyroidism
- Genetic damage
- Damage of fetal thyroid
- Thyroid carcinoma

β blockers (Without sympathomimetic activity): Like **metoprolol, atenolol, propranolol** alleviate the manifestations of thyrotoxicity due to sympathetic overactivity. It is used till the effect of carbimazole or ^{131}I starts. Propranolol greater than 160 mg/day dose also reduces T_3 level by inhibiting conversion of T_4 to T_3.

Drugs for thyroid storm

Vigorous treatment required with:
- β blockers
- Propylthiouracil 200–300 mg QDS
- Iopanoic acid (0.5–1 mg)
- Corticosteroid (hydrocortisone 100 mg TDS given IV)
- Diltiazem to control tachycardia (60–120 mg), if not controlled by β blocker.
- Rehydration
- Anxiolytic
- External cooling
- Antibiotics, *etc.*

Antithyroid drug in pregnancy : 0.2% of pregnant women suffer thyrotoxicosis. They are treated with antithyroid drug. Propylthiouracil is better choice but methimazole can also be used.

80

Adrenocorticotropin and Corticosteroids

Adrenal glands are essential for life. It has two parts outer cortex and inner medulla, which are structurally and functionally different. The adrenal cortex structurally and functionally has three identifiable zones which are zona glomerulosa, zona fasciculata and zona reticularis without inwards. Hench first noticed therapeutic potential of corticosteroid in rheumatoid arthritis patient in 1949. Kendall, Reichstein and Hench got Nobel Prize in 1950. Now broad spectrum of actions of adrenocorticosteroids are well-known.

Pituitary-adrenal relationship: Basophil cells of adenohypophysis secrete ACTH regulating functions of adrenal cortex which is a polypeptide containing 39 amino acids of mol. wt. 4,500. The first 24 amino acids are common to hormone obtained from cattle, pig, sheep, and man while remaining 15 amino acids responsible for antigenicity of ACTH. Melanocyte stimulating hormone secreted from intermediate lobe of pituitary has sequence of amino acids identical to first 13 amino acids of ACTH.

ADRENOCORTICOTROPIN

Regulation of ACTH release: Hypothalamus releases corticotropin-releasing hormone (CRH) which reaches anterior pituitary *via* portal vein and stimulates ACTH release; CRH acts on CRH receptor on corticotropes which is G-protein coupled receptor. Rate of secretion of ACTH is maximum in early hours of morning, declining during day and minimum at midnight. Which appears to be related with sleep pattern. Metyrapone administration and in Addison's

disease, ACTH secretion is stimulated. A variety of stressful stimuli, trauma, surgery, pain, hemorrhage, *etc.* cause CRH release.

Pharmacological Actions of ACTH

On adrenal cortex

- Stimulates adrenal cortex to synthesize corticosterone, aldosterone and weakly androgenic hormones.
- Prolong ACTH administration produces hyperplasia of adrenal cortex.
- Hypophysectomy causes decrease in corticosterone secretion. Aldosterone secretion is not much affected.
- ACTH reduces cholesterol and ascorbic acid content of adrenal cortex.

Extra-adrenal action

- Lipolysis in adipose tissue
- Ketosis
- Cutaneous pigmentation
- Insulin resistance.

Pharmacokinetics: Protein in nature so should be given parenterally to avoid enzymatic digestion. Well-absorbed on IM administration, produces greater response, if given in morning.

Preparation of ACTH: Available as lyophilized powder becomes 40 IU/mL after reconstitution ACTHAR 5 mL vial, ACTHAR retard repository preparation in gelatinous solution. Cosyntropin is synthetic preparation containing 1–24 amino acids of human ACTH (0.25 mg IV in 24 hours) preferred over natural ACTH. Cosyntropin zinc-phosphate suspension 1.0 mg IM.

Therapeutic Uses of ACTH

Diagnostic

- When ACTH is administered urinary excretion of 17 ketosteroids are increased in normal adrenal cortex person, but not in suppressed adrenal function (Addison's diseases).

Therapeutic

- More or less same of carticosteroid hormones

- Patient receiving long-standing corticosteroid may require ACTH therapy to stimulate adrenal cortex or during steroid withdrawal.

Adverse reactions: *Allergy* (cosyntropin is less allergic) and other adverse reactions are due to hypersecretion of adrenocorticosteroid hormones like:

- Acne
- Na retention
- Hypokalemic alkalosis
- Thinning of skin may occur.

81

Adrenal Cortical Hormones

The zones of adrenal cortex elaborate three distinct groups of steroid hormones. Zona glomerulosa secretes aldosterone and desoxy-corticosterone (mineralocorticosteroids), zona fasciculata secretes cortisone, hydrocortisone (glucocorticoids), zona recticularis secretes dihydroepiandrosterone, androstenedione (androgens) trace of estrogen, progesterone produced as intermediary of other steriods, but probably not secreted. Corticosteroid hormones affect carbohydrate, protein and fat metabolism and also affect Na, K and fluid balance.

Biosynthesis: Gluco- and mineralocorticoids are cyclopentanoperhydrophenanthrene steroid nucleus containing 21 carbon atom molecules. With various functional groups (–H, –OH, –CH$_3$), atoms attached to it. Slightest structural changes produce marked differences in their biological activities (Fig. 81.1).

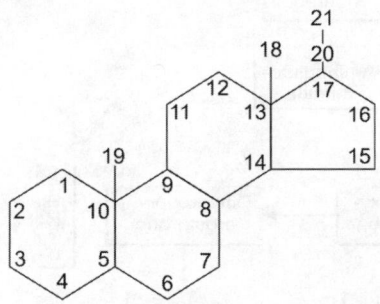

Fig. 81.1: Cyclopentanophenanthrene nucleus

Under the influence of ACTH, adrenal steroidogenesis takes place, more cholesterol are converted to pregnenolone, which is either converted to aldosterone, hydrocortisone or testo-sterone, but mainly hydrocortisone. Steroidal synthesis can be interfered by:

- Triparanol, blocks synthesis of cholesterol.
- Aminoglutethimide, inhibits conversion of cholesterol to pregnenolone.
- Metyrapone, specifically inhibits 11-β-hydroxylase which converts desoxycortisol to hydrocortisone used to test adrenal fucntion.
- Mifepristone is basically antiprogestine, in large doses blocks glucocorticoid receptor used in cushing syndrome due to adrenal carcinoma
- Ketoconazole, an antifungal drug nonselectively blocks adrenal and gonadal steroid syntheses at times used to treat cushing syndrome.
- Mitotane, causes adrenal cortical necrosis. It is an anticancer drug.
- **Etomidate** an general anesthetic inducer and sedative inhibits steroidogenesis, so does cyproheptadine.

ACTIONS OF GLUCOCORTICOIDS

A. Metabolic effects

- *Carbohydrate and protein metabolism*: Antianabolic (inhibits incorporation of amino acid into protein in peripheral tissues) and stimulates neoglucogenesis, hyperglycemia on chronic administration; peripheral glucose utilization is decreased.
- *Fat metabolism*: Mobilizes fat from peripheral fat depot by adrenaline and growth hormones, glucagon and thyroxine (permissive role). Excessive administration may produce buffalo hump, moon facies, fish

mouth, cAMP-induced breakdown of triglycerides are enhanced.

- Electrolyte and water metabolism: It is weak Na retainer and K excretor, essential to excrete water load in intoxication.
- Calcium metabolism: Intestinal absorption of calcium is decreased, renal excretion of calcium increases, produces spongy bone.

B. CVS: Permissive effect of adrenaline to pressure amine, restricts capillary permeability, maintains tone of arterioles and myocardial contractility. Hypertension may be observed.

C. Muscle: Weakness observed in both hypo- and hypercorticisms. Hypocorticism state produces weakness due to hypodynamic muscular circulation. Hypercorticism produces muscle wasting, myopathy whereas mineralocorticoids excrete K to produce weakness in muscles.

D. GIT: May aggravate peptic ulcer due to increased acid pepsin secretion.

E. CNS: Mood elevation, euphoria, restlessness.

F. Hemopoietic system: Increases RBC, platelet and neutrophil in circulation. Decreases lymphocyte, eosinophil and basophils by sequestering it and destruction of T and B lymphocytes.

G. Inflammation: Inflammation response is suppressed, reduces capillary permeability, local exudation, phagocytic activity, capillary proliferation, collagen deposition, fibroblastic activity. Equally effective on topical application.

H. Antiallergic responses: Suppress all varieties of hypersensitivity, prevents influx of calcium ion in mast cells, preventing its degranulation and liberation of different mediators. Has antipyretic and antigout effects.

I. Inhibits hypothalamohypophyseal axis: Small dose glucocorticoid or high dose intermediate acting on alternate days therapy are less likely to suppress hypothalamic-pituitary-adrenal axis. Prolonged use suppresses hypothalamopituitary adrenal axis.

Mechanism of Action of Corticosteroids (Cellular Level) (Fig. 81.2)

Glucocorticoid binds to glucocorticoid receptor (protein in nature of superfamily of molecular receptor including steroid; sterol; vitamin D; thyroid; retinoic acid and many other unknown ligands called orphan receptors). The polypeptide glucocorticoid receptor has three distinct domains, ligand binding domain; transcription activating domain and DNA binding domain.

Flowchart 81.1: Biosynthesis of steroid hormones

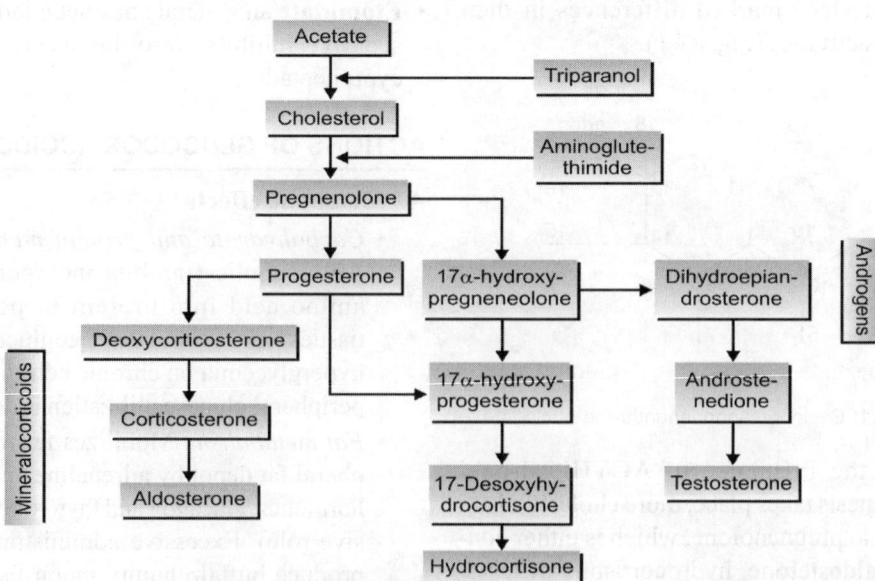

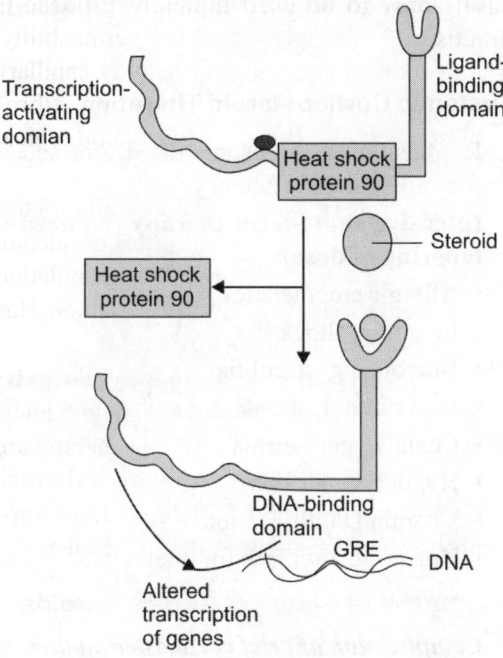

Fig. 81.2: Mechanism of action of corticosteroid

Heat shock protein (hsp90) binds to receptor when hormone is absent to prevent it for active conformation change in the receptor.

When hormone binds to receptor it dissociates hsp90 stabilizer and converts it to active configuration.

The interaction of glucocorticoid with glucocorticoid receptor element (GRE) may be activated by coactivator and inhibited by co-repressor collectively called coregulators. Some of its effects are due to its binding to aldosterone receptor (AR).

Absorption rate distribution: All natural and synthetic corticosteroids are effective by oral route, except DOCA. Hemisuccinates of hydro-cortisone are rapidly absorbed from IM site. Hydrocortisone undergoes high first pass metabolism, and 90% protein-bound to transcortin a globulin and albumin. They are metabolized in liver by hepatic microsomal enzymes. The metabolites are conjugated to glucuronic acid or sulfate and excreted in urine. Urinary excreted metabolized can be estimated as 17 ketosteroid and 17 ketogenic steroid.

Complication of corticosteroid therapy (systemic)

A. **Gastrointestinal**
   - Peptic ulcer (due to suppression of immunity and increase of growth of *H. pylori*) and increase in hydrochloric acid secretion.
   - Pancreatitis

B. **Musculoskeletal**
   - Myopathy
   - Osteoporosis
   - Aseptic necrosis of bone

C. **CNS:** Psychiatric disorder, pseudocerebral tumor, ophthalmoplegia, posterior subcapsular cataract, glaucoma.

D. **CVS:** Hypertension, Na and water retention, hypokalemia, alkalosis.

E. **Metabolic:** Precipitation of diabetes, hyperlipidemia, general obesity.

F. **Endocrine:** Growth failure, iatrogenic Cushing syndrome, secondary ameonorrhea, suppression of hypothalamic-pituitary-adrenal system, impaired wound healing, subcutaneous tissue atrophy, suppression of immune response and superimposition of bacterial, viral, fungal infections and parasitic infestation.

Preparation and dosage of glucocorticoids for systemic use

- **Hydrocortisone (efcorlin 100 mg/2 mL IV):** Acts rapid, but short acting. Used for shock, status asthmaticus, acute adrenal insufficiency. It has mainly glucocorticoids but also significant mineralocorticoids activity.

- **Cortisone (Corlin 5 mg tab; 25 mg/mL):** Oral or IM, less potent than hydrocortisone.

- **Prednisolone (wysolone, deltacortil 5 mg, 10 mg tab; 20 mg/mL):** Orally, IM or intra-articular used for allergy, autoimmune disease, or inflammatory or malignancies.

- **Methyl prednisolone** [Solumedrol 0.5 gm (8 mL) and 1.0 gm (16 mL) inj]: For IM or slow IV or 4–32 mg/day orally. More effective than prednisolone. Pulse therapy tried for rheumatoid arthritis, renal transplant, pemphigus with minimal suppression of pituitary-adrenal axis. Also given as retention enema in ulcerative colitis.

- **Triamcinolone** (Kenacort 1, 4, 8 mg tabs; 10 mg/mL or 40 mg/mL as acetonide for IM or intra-articular injections also used topically)
- **Betamethasone** (Betnesol 0.5 mg tab, 4 mg/mL IM, IV or 0.5 mg/mL oral drops).
- **Dexamethasone** (Dexona 0.5 mg tab, 4 mg/mL for IM or IV used for shock, cerebral edema, anti-inflammatory or antiallergic actions.)
- **Paramethasone:** Dose 2–20 mg/day orally.
- **Desoxycorticosterone acetate** (DOCA), only mineralocorticoid activity 2–5 mg sublingual or 10–20 mg IM biweekly or weekly for replacement therapy in Addison's disease.
- **Deflazacort (Defglu 6 mg tab):** It lacks mineralocorticoid potency and its glucocorticoid action is also lesser than glucocorticoids used for inflammatory and immunological disorders. Dose for adult 60–120 mg then 6–18 mg as maintenance per day.
- **Aldosterone:** Most potent mineralocorticoids, oral bioavailability is low so not used clinically.

Fludrocortisone: Potent mineralocorticoid, orally active and used for Addison's disease 50–200 µg/day. It is also used for idiopathic postural hypotension.

Topical steroids used for skin diseases described with skin and mucous membrane chapter.

Hydrocortisone eye ointment (NF 2.5% w/v) hydrocortisone acetate; hydrocortisone eyedrops (NF 1%).

Special Dosage Forms

For local therapy, topical ointment, cream, lotion are available for skin disease; ophthalmic solutions for eye diseases, for joint intra-articular injections, for asthma inhaled steroids, for ulcerative colitis hydrocortisone enema is used for local high concentration with low systemic effects.

Beclomethasone dipropionate; triamcinolone acetate, budesonide, flunisolide are available for nasal spray to be used topically for allargic rhinitis.

Systemic Corticosteroid Therapy

1. **Replacement:** Addison's disease or secondary adrenal insufficiency.
2. **Intensive short-term therapy (no need of tapering of dose):**
   - Allergic emergencies
   - Infection, shock
   - Necrotising vasculitis
   - Water intoxications
   - Cental hyperthermia
   - Hypoglycemic coma
   - Vitamin D intoxication
   - Hormone therapy for metastatic breast cancer.

Complication of brief corticosteroid therapy
   - Burning or itching at mucocutaneous junctions
   - Multifocal ventricular contractions
   - Precipitation of diabetic ketoacidosis
   - Ulceration of stomach.

3. **Prolonged high doses suppressive therapy (tapering required)**
   - Bronchial asthma
   - Ulcerative colitis
   - Subacute hepatic necrosis
   - Gluten sensitive enteropathy
   - Alcoholic hepatitis
   - Idiopathic thrombocytopenic purpura
   - Acute lymphatic leukemia
   - Hodgkin's disease
   - Nephrotic syndrome
   - Graft transplantation
   - Polymyositis
   - Dematocytosis
   - Giant cell temporal arteritis

4. **Low dose chronic palliative therapy**
   - Rheumatoid arthritis
   - Systemic lupus erythematosus

(erratic steroid doses or withdrawal may lead to pseudorheumatism).

5. **In tuberculosis:** Indicated in:
   - Pleural effusion
   - Pericardial effusion
   - Peritoneal effusion
   - Meningeal or Military tuberculosis
   - Allergic drug reaction with ATD drug

6. **Chronic inhibition of pituitary ACTH** in idiopathic hirsutism.

7. **Alternate days steroid therapy**
   - Bronchial asthma
   - Ulcerative colitis
   - Subacute hepatic necrosis
   - Chronic active hepatitis
   - Hemolytic anemia
   - Acute lymphatic leukemia
   - Hodgkin's disease
   - Sarcoidosis
   - Subacute thyroiditis.

Mineralocorticoids (Aldosterone)

It has main effect on Na retention and K excretion. Increases BP. Preparation available as DOCA, fludocortisone is used therapeutically in Addison's disease. Other uses are salt losing congenital adrenal hyperplasia, hyporeninemic hypoaldosteronism, severe postural hypotension from autonomic neuropathy of any etiology.

Contraindications of corticosteroids
- Peptic ulcer
- Diabetes mellitus
- Hypertension
- Pregnancy (risk of fetal defect)
- Tuberculosis and varicella infection
- Osteoporosis
- Herpes simplex keratitis
- Psychosis, epilepsy
- CCF
- Renal failure

Antagonist of Adrenocortical Agents

Synthesis inhibitor or antagonist of glucocorticoids:

Glucocorticoid antagonist (antiprogestin mifepristone) is evaluated for the treatment of Cushing's syndrome. It blocks glucocorticoid receptor in high doses by stabilizing hsp glucocorticoid receptor complex and alters its interaction with other coregulators.

Aminoglutethimide, **metyrapone**, **trilostane** and high dose of **antifungal ketoconazole** inhibit steroidogenic enzymes at livers, tried for Cushing's syndrome.

Metyrapone is used to test adrenal function. **Mitotane** has adrenolytic property in dog and to a some extent in human used for adrenal tumor (dose 12 gm/day). Diarrhea, nausea, vomiting, depression, somnolence, skin rash may occur. This prodrug used orally, studied for refractory cancer of prostate patient. It inhibits steroid.

Abiraterone: This prodrug used orally, studied for refractory cancer prostate patient. It inhibits steroid synthesis with compensatory increase in ACTH and aldosterone syntheses but this effect can be prevented by concomittent use of dexamethasone.

Etomidate used as inducing general anesthesia inhibits adrenal steroidogenesis.

Mifepristone: It is antagonist of steroid receptor used to treat ectopic ACTH or cushing patient. It is mainly used for post coital contraception.

Mineralocorticoid Antagonist

These steroid drugs csompete with aldosterone and decrease its action peripherally, *viz.*

a. **Spironolactone** (a potassium sparing diuretic) used in primary aldosteronism in the dose of 50–100 mg/day. It is slow acting and effect lasts for 2–3 days after its discontinuation.

b. **Eplerenone** is used in hypertension (dose 50–100 mg/day) with no reported action on androgen receptor. It is an aldosterone receptor antagonist. It may cause hyperkalemia.

c. **Drospirenone:** This oral contraceptive (progestin) also antagonizes aldosterone effect.

82

Insulin, Oral Hypoglycemic and Glucagon

ENDOCRINE FUNCTION OF PANCREAS

Pancreas contains scattered clump of cells throughout, particularly towards tail end called islet of Langerhans (about 1–2 million islets are weighing about 1 gm). Islet contains alcohol-soluble and water-soluble granules which stains bluish purple (β-cells) and pink (α-cells) with Mallory's triple stain containing insulin and glucagons respectively. The α-cells are of two types, $α_1$ or D cells secrete somatostatin (also secreted by hypothalamus) and $α_2$ cells secreting glucagons. The other hormones secreted by islets are islet amyloid polypeptide (IAPP) or amylin modulating gastric emptying, appetite and pancreatic peptide facilitating digestive processes.

INSULIN

deMeyer (1909) coined the name insuline (related to islets) later the 'e' was dropped. Banting and Best demonstrated the hypoglycemic activity in 1921. Abel prepared highly purified insulin in 1926. Structure of insulin was elucidated by Sanger in 1944–45. Leonard Thompson was the first patient to receive insulin in 12 Jan 1922.

Insulin contains two polypeptide chains A and B which contain 21 and 30 amino acids respectively. Insulin produced in β-cells as a single chain polypeptide precursor proinsulin consisting of 84 amino acids (Fig. 82.1). In Golgi apparatus, proinsulin is cleaved by trypsin like enzymes. During the cleavage, a large (with 33 amino acids) peptides called c-peptides are split off, leaving two chains connected by disulfide bonds. Thus Golgi apparatus is involved in

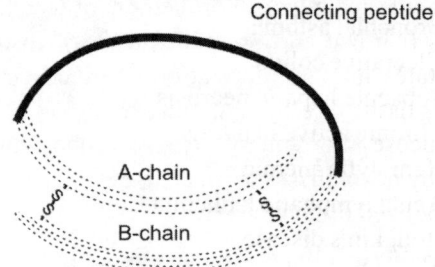

Fig. 82.1: Structure of human proinsulin

loading and storage of granules. Zinc in the granules of β-cells produces insoluble complex with insulin. Two atoms of zinc are attached to six molecules of insulin to produce crystals. The entire human pancreas contains 8 mg or 200 units of insulin, 20 units/1 mg used as assay purposes. Proinsulin is 10% as active as insulin, but C protein is inactive.

Half-life of insulin is few minutes, but their biological effects reach at maximum after 2–4 hours because it is taken up and bound to the tissues where it exerts its action (liver, kidney). Brain and RBC do not bind it.

It is destroyed by liver (first pass metabolism), pancreas, kidney, placenta by separation of two chains. Average insulin content in pancreas is 200 IU. Daily secretion rate 50 units, circulating concentration 20 microunits/mL; raised up to 50–150 microunits on stimulus. There are little differences between human, pork and beef insulins. Pig's insulin is less antigenic to human beings than beef.

> 1 IU of insulin decreases fasting blood sugar in rabbits to 45 mg/dL. 1 mg standard insulin = 24 IU.

Physiology of Carbohydrate Metabolism

The consumed carbohydrates in the form of starch, (polysaccharides) or sugar (disaccharides) are split of by salivary amylase, pancreatic amylase, lactase, maltase and invertase of intestinal juices into monosaccharides like glucose, galactose, fuctose and are absorbed in small intestine by diffusion and active transport.

Different tissues differ for their glucose requirements, *viz.* brain utilizes only glucose for its energy requirement, while other tissues utilize fatty acids and glucose for their energy requirements (cardiac and skeletal muscles). Insulin facilitates intracellularization of glucose and lowers tissue threshold of glucose.

Glucose after entering cells are phosphorylated by hexokinases to glucose-6PO$_4$, which is metabolized in several ways.

- **Glycolysis:** Glucose by anaerobic process is converted to pyruvate and lactate with efficiently producing ATP.

- **Pentose monophosphate shunt:** Aerobic process, is a source of TPNH, required for lipogenesis, deficiency leads to ketoacidosis.

- **Glucuronic acid pathway:** Produces uridine diphosphate, glucose utilized for synthesis of glycogen and produces glucuronic acid for conjugation of many substances.

- **Glycogenesis:** Derived largely from UDPG by action of glycogen synthetase.

- **Conversion of glucose:** Liver and kidney with the help of enzyme, glucose-6-phosphatase converts glucose-6PO$_4$ to glucose.

Insulin Release (Fig. 82.2)

Activity of β-cells (insulin secretion) is regulated by level of glucose in the interstitial fluid. Insulin is released from β-cells at low basal rate and is stimulated by glucose; due to hyperglycemia, glucose enters β-cells by GLUT$_2$ transporter causing raised intracellular ATP level which close the ATP dependent K$^+$ channel causing decreased K$^+$ efflux, resulting in depolarization of β-cells

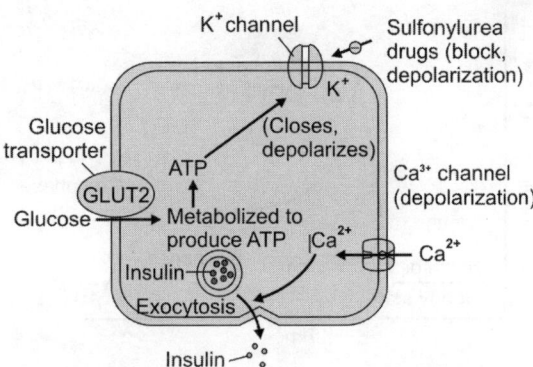

Fig. 82.2: Mechanism of insulin release

which opens up voltage gated calcium channels. The increased intracellular calcium triggers insulin release (Fig. 82.2). Drugs like sulfonylurea, meglitinide, D-phenylalanine act through this mechanism.

Glucose Transporters

GLUT$_1$: Present in RBC, brain and all tissues, transports glucose across blood-brain barrier.

GLUT$_2$: Present in β-cells of pancreas, liver and kidney and regulates insulin release and glucose homeostasis.

GLUT$_3$: Present in brain, kidney and placenta and uptakes glucose into neurons.

GLUT$_4$: Present in muscle and fat cells and helps insulin mediated uptake of glucose.

GLUT$_5$: It is present in gut and kidney and helps absorption of fructose.

There are 9–10 folds rise in insulin secretion in response to increase in plasma glucose from 70 to 150 mg/dL with simultaneous decrease in glucagon release from α-cells. Insulin release occurs in two phases—rapid phase of preformed insulin is released, starts within seconds, lasts for 10–15 minutes followed by slow rise, which remains high until blood glucose falls to base value (Fig. 82.3).

Other substances effecting insulin release: Amino acids (arginine), free fatty acids, non-glucose sugars, gastrin secretion, pancreozymin,

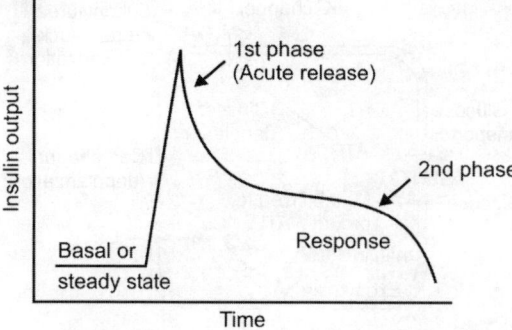

Fig. 82.3: Insulin release after rise in blood glucose

glucagon. Growth hormone, thyroxin, ACTH, glucocorticoids, xanthine, sulfonylureas stimulate insulin release.

Its release is inhibited by somatostatin, adrenaline, exogenous insulin, thiazides, phenytoin. Its release is enhanced by parasympathetic and selective β-stimulation and inhibited by vagotomy and α-adrenergic stimulation.

Actions of Insulin

- Facilitates glucose transport across cell membrane, fat cells. Skeletal muscles are sensitive. Its entry into liver, brain, RBC, WBC and renal medullary cells is independent to insulin. Ketoacidosis interferes with glucose utilization of brain leading to diabetic coma. Muscular exercises spare insulin and induce glucose entry.

- Glucose after entering cell is phosphorylated to glucose-6PO_4 enhanced by insulin through increased production of glucokinase. In liver, glycogen synthesis is enhanced by insulin and glycogenolysis is inhibited by inhibiting phosphorylase.

- It inhibits gluconeogenesis (production of glucose from non-carbohydrate source, *viz.* amino acids.

- Inhibits lipolysis and favors triglyceride synthesis.

- Insulin increases VLDL and chylomicron clearance by stimulating transcription of vascular endothelial lipoprotein lipase.

- Facilitates entry of amino acids and proteins in muscle and possibly other cells.

Insulin Receptors

Insulin initiates action by binding with glycoprotein receptors. Practically present in all cells; but liver, fat and muscle cells are rich. On cell surface which consists of α-subunits of mol wt 135000 binds with insulin and β-subunits of mol wt 95000 (which is insulin sensitive tyrosine specific protein kinase generates signal for insulin action on glucose, lipid and protein metabolism). Both subunits are linked by disulfide linkage. Commonly depicted model is $\alpha_2\beta_2$ (Fig. 82.4). The different events occurring with insulin receptor action are as follows:

A. Events in seconds
- Binding of receptor
- Confirmation change in receptor
- Receptor aggregation
- Change of receptor kinase
- Change in ion flux

B. Events in minutes
- Receptor internalization
- Generation of possible mediator substances
- Stimulation of glucose transports
- Stimulation of phospholipid turnover
- Activation of intracellular enzymes.

C. Events in hours
- Activation of amino acid transports
- Stimulation of protein and lipid syntheses
- Stimulation of RNA and DNA syntheses.

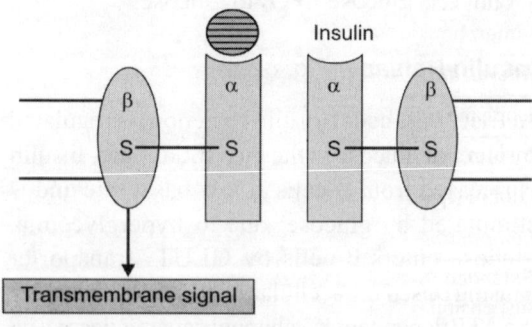

Fig. 82.4

D. Long-term effect of insulin: It regulates gene transcription and differentiation and governs protein synthesis, DNA-mediated synthesis of $GLUT_1$ to $GLUT_5$.

Transmembrane signal producing following functions

- Glucose transport
- Protein phosphorylation
- DNA synthesis and cell growth
- Activation of enzymes
- Protein synthesis

Physiological and Pharmacological Actions of Insulin

Insulin needs intact cells to produce its action and does not act on subcellular fraction.

Liver: Increases glucokinases and glycogen synthetase, results in glucose uptake and glycogen deposition. It stimulates fatty acid synthesis and inhibits protein breakdown.

Adipose tissue: Increases permeability and promotes utilization of glucose leading to increased synthesis of glycerol, a glycerophosphate and fatty acids, the last two combine to form triglycerides (lipogenesis). Glycerophosphate binds free fatty acids (antilipolytic action). It stimulates lipoprotein lipase of the adipose tissue cells and hydrolyzes the chylomicron in circulation.

Skeletal muscle: Increases glucose transport in muscle which is utilized by glycolytic pathways and partly for glycogen synthesis. Stimulates transfer of amino acids into cells and their incorporation into protein (protein anabolic action). Inhibits proteolysis and lipolysis of muscle.

Effects on carbohydrate, fat and protein metabolism: Discussed earlier.

Factors modifying insulin action

- **Muscular exercise:** Lowers blood sugar by enhancing entry of glucose in muscle cells and releasing bound insulin from muscles and vasculatures.
- **Hormones:** Discussed earlier.
- **Insulin antibodies:** Produce insulin resistance (requiring more than 200 IU/day) in patient on insulin therapy.

Table 82.1: Common insulin in use							
Type	*Appearance*	*pH*	*Protein*	*Onset action (hours)*	*Peak action (hours)*	*Duration of action (hours)*	*Can be mixed with*
Short acting							
Regular (soluble) insulin	Clear	3.2	–	1	2–4	6–9	All regular and lente preparation
Insulin zinc suspension (amorphous) semilente	Cloudy	7.2	–	1	3–6	12–18	
Intermediate acting							
Isophane (NPH)	Cloudy	7.2	Protamine	2	12	20	Regular
Insulin zinc suspension	Cloudy	7.2	–	2	6–8	24	Semilente
Globin (lente)	Clear	3.4	Globin	4	6–10	18	Regular
Long acting							
Extended insulin zinc suspension (ultralente)	Cloudy	7.2	–	7	16	36	Regular semilente
Protamine zinc insulin	Cloudy	7.2	Protamine	7	16	36	Regular

- **Synalbumin fraction of Valence-Owen:** Albumin related antagonist present in low concentration in non-diabetic and in high concentration in diabetic, pre-diabetic and myocardial infarction patients.

Preparations of Insulin

Conventional insulin is derived from beef or pork pancreas. Requires 2–3 injections daily, modified by adding zinc and proteins (protamine) to make it long acting modified retard preparations. Long acting are given SC but regular may be given IM or IV.

Insulin analogues: Insulin analogues have greater stability, consistency produced by using recombinant DNA technology. Following insulin analogues are present in market.

- **Insulin lispro (Humalog 100 U/mL):** It is first monomeric insulin marketed where B-chain proline at B28 is moved to B29 and lysine of B29 is moved to B28 which does not interfere its affinity to insulin receptor, but produces quick and short action of insulin. It is stabilized in hexamer form, given SC where it dissociates quickly to monomer.

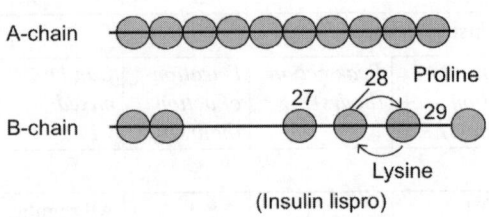

(Insulin lispro)

- **Insulin aspart (novalog 100 U/mL):** Here B28 proline is substituted by aspartic acid. Time of action is same as lispro.

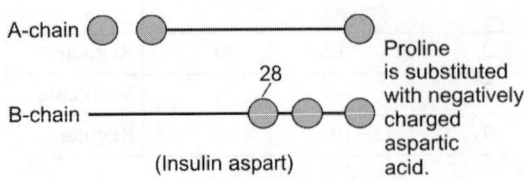

(Insulin aspart)

- **Insulin glulisine:** Here substitution of asparagine for lysine at B23 and glutamic acid is substituted for lysine at B29.

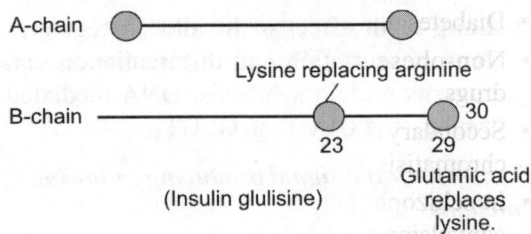

(Insulin glulisine)

- **Inhaled human insulin:** It causes pulmonary fibrosis. The preparations are **E**xubera and **A**frezza.
- **Insulin glargine:** It is long acting insulin analogue where 2 additional arginine in B-chain of carboxy terminal and glycine replaces aspergine in A21. It is soluble in acidic pH, but precipitates in neutral pH. It maintains a low insulin throughout the day (Lantus optiset 100 U/mL, 5 mL vial or 3 mL preloaded pen injector).
- **Insulin detemir:** Long acting insulin analogue. Here terminal threonine of B30 is dropped and myristic acid is attached to B29. Myristic acid is c-14 fatty acid chain.

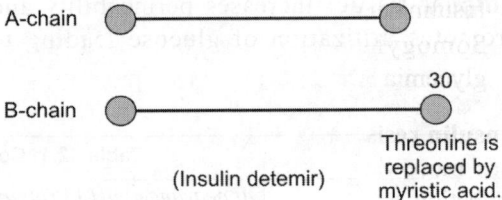

(Insulin detemir)

Types of diabetes mellitus

Type 1: Selective β-cells destruction with severe or absolute insulin deficiency.

Type 2: Tissues resistance to action of insulin with relative deficiency.

Type 3: Raised blood glucose to pancreatic diseases or drug therapy.

Type 4: First time detected during pregnancy, *i.e.* gestational diabetes.

Indications for Insulin Therapy

- Insulin dependent diabetes mellitus (IDDM) or type 1 diabetes mellitus.
- Diabetic ketoacidosis
- Non-ketotic hyperglycemic state
- Stress of surgery, infection, injury

- Diabetes during pregnancy (type 4)
- Non-obese NIDDM unresponsive to oral drugs.
- Secondary diabetes due to pancreatitis, hemochromatisis, *etc*.
- In schizophrenia insulin is given to produce convulsion.
- In the past it was used to improve appetite and body weight.
- Insulin tolerance test to determine the plasma HGH to test hypopituitarism.

Reaction to Insulin

- Hypoglycemia: Treatments—Glucose (orally or IV or glucagon 0.5 mg to 1 mg IV) or adrenaline 0.2 mg SC (less preferable)
- Local reaction: Swelling, erythema, stinging, lipodystrophy at injection site on prolong use.
- Allergy, urticaria, anaphylaxis, angioedema specially with protein contamination
- Insulin presbyopia
- Obesity
- Insulin neuropathy
- Somogyi phenomenon: Robound hyperglycemia following hypoglycemia.

Insulin resistance: Insulin requirement increases more than 200 IU/day may be acute (in infection, trauma, surgery, hyperglycemic agents, stress, corticosteroid therapy and ketoacidosis) or chronic with prolonged use of porcine or beef insulin producing antibodies. Pregnancy and oral contraceptive preparation produce low grade insulin resistance.

Purified insulin: Conventional insulin contains 10,000 ppm impurities in the form of proinsulin, pancreatic protein, insulin derivatives which are purified to make it non-antigenic. Preparations are:

Single peak: Contains 50–200 ppm proinsulin prepared by filtration, and crystallization. Available in 10 mL vial 40 IU/mL.

- Actrapid rapidica—purified pork (duration 8 hours) regular insulin.
- Lentard (duration 22 hours) pork lente insulin.

- Actraphane, rapimix—purified regular pork insulin 30% and isophane 70% (duration 24 hours).

Monocomponents: Monocomponents are further purified by gel exchange chromatography after gel filtration reducing impurities to 20 ppm.

- Actrapid MC—monocomponent regular insulin (duration 8 hours) 40 and 100 IU/mL.
- Monotard MC—monocomponent pork lente insulin, duration 22 hours available as 40 IU/mL.

Human insulins are produced by recombinant technologies in

- *E. coli* [proinsulin recombinant bacterial (prb)]
- Yeast [precursor yeast recombinant (pyr)]
- Enzymatic modification of porcine insulin (emp.) Cost of human insulin is coming down to same of pork MC.

Complication of Insulin therapy:

1. Hypoglycemia
2. Insulin allergy
3. Insulin resistance by circulating 1g G anti-insulin antibody.
4. Lipodystrophy with animal insulin.
5. Risk of cancer in insulin resistance cases.

Indications for pure/human insulin

- Insulin resistance
- Surgery
- Allergy
- Infection
- Lipodystrophy
- Ketoacidosis
- Pregnancy

Newer insulin delivery devices

- Insulin syringe these are prefilled syringe
- Pen devices use insulin cartridges
- Jet injectors
- Insulin pumps (continuous SC insulin infusion (CSII)
- Implantable pumps (electromechanical devices regulating insulin release).
- External artificial pancreas. Microprocessor controlled device.

- Intraperitoneal, oral (complexing insulin into liposomes), rectal, intranasal are also tried.

ORAL HYPOGLYCEMIC AGENTS (OHA)

Chief disadvantage of insulin is, it has to be given by injections.

History of Oral Hypoglycemic Drugs

- Herbal and minerals for ages
- Watanbe (1918) experimental proof of guanidine's hypoglycemic properties.
- Frank (1926) modified guanidine-synthalin A.
- Decrease use of synthalin A due to hepatoxicity.
- Ruiz (1932) noted the hypoglycemic effect of sulfonamide.
- 1956–60 Era of 1st generation sulfonylurea
- 1961–70 Controversial UGDP study
- 1970 second generation sulfonylureas
- 1977 Acarbose introduced
- 1957 Biguanide (phenformin) developed parallel to sulfonylureas.

Indication of oral hypoglycemic agent (OHA)

NIDDM of middle and elderly age group of recent origin diabetes (< 5 years) without end organ damage and other medical problem and failed on diet or exercise.

Contraindication of oral hypoglycemic agents (OHA)

- Insulin dependent diabatic, ketotic prone
- Inpaired renal and hepatic function
- Allergic to OHA
- Side effects of OHA: Skin rash, jaundice, hyponatremia
- Severe stress, infection, surgery
- Malnourished
- Chronic debilitating disease and severe diabetic and underweight
- Pregnancy
- Associated endocrinopathy.

A. Advantages of OHA

- Patients acceptability and independence
- Easy administration

- No need of exogenous insulin so less chance of insulin resistance
- Insulin being endogenous, it is more physiological in action in liver than to periphery
- No local reaction

B. Disadvantages of OHA

- Less medical supervision and disclination towards potential dangers of diabetes
- Chances of drug interaction and toxicities of drugs
- Increased therapeutic failure and limitation of dosage.

Classification of OHA

Sulfonyl urea

1st generation

- Tolbutamide
- Acetohexamide
- Chloropropamide
- Tolazamide

2nd generation

- Glibenclamide
- Gliclazide
- Glipizide
- Glimepiride

Biguanides

- Phenformin
- Metformin

Miscellaneous

- Alpha glycosidase inhibitor (acarbose, miglitol, voglitbose)
- Guargum; glucomannan
- Insulin secretagogues (repaglinide, nateglinide)
- Thiazolidinediones (ciglitazone, troglitazone, pioglitazone, rosiglitazone)

MECHANISM OF ACTION OF OHA (SULFONYLUREA)

- Releases insulin from pancreas acting on so called sulfonyl receptor on β-cells causing depolarization by reducing conductance of ATP sensitive K^+ channel leading to Ca^{2+} influx and degranulation and insulin release. 30% functional β-cells are essential for their action.
- Hepatic degradation of insulin is slowed. Reduces glucagon and increases somatostatin release.

- Sensitizes target tissue to insulin by increasing insulin receptor.
- Improves glucose tolerance.

Adverse Effects of Sulfonylurea

Nausea, vomiting, flatulence, diarrhea, hypoglycemia, hypersensitivity (rash, photosensitivity, purpura), leukopenia, jaundice by chlorpropamide, dilutional hyponatremia, antabuse reaction. Tolbutamide interferes iodide uptake and hypothyroidism, so should not be given to pregnant and lactating mother.

Biguanides

Mechanism of action of biguanide

Does not release insulin, but presence of some insulin is required. Metformin apart from type II diabetes mellitus also useful in polycystic ovarian disease

- Inhibits intestinal absorption of glucose hexose and vitamin B_{12}
- Suppresses hepatic gluconeogenesis
- Enhances insulin binding to receptors
- Promotes peripheral glucose utilization by interfering mitochondrial respiratory chain.
- Anaerobic glycolysis
- Increased glucose uptake and disposal in skeletal muscles and fat.
- Metformin is the only OHG which has been demonstrated to reduce macrovasculor events of DM type II

Adverse effects: Anorexia, nausea, metalic, diarrhea, tiredness, lactic acidosis (phenformin taking alcohol), vitamin B_{12} deficiency.

Pharmacokinetics: Orally absorbed, excreted with kidney.

Mechanism of action of alpha-glycosidase inhibitors acarbose (Glucobay 50 and 100 mg TDS): This oligosaccharides taken at beginning of meals reversibly inhibit a glucosidase enzymes in brush border of small intestinal mucosa, involved in digestion of carbohydrate. It decreases postprandial glycemia without increasing insulin level, decreasing digestion and absorption of polysaccharides. Regular use decreases HbA 1c, body weight and triglyceride.

Flatulence, diarrhea may occur. This group of drugs reduces the cardiovascular complications in patient with diabetes.

Miglitol: This is more potent than acarbose in inhibiting postprandial digestion; absorption of starch and disaccharides. It is six times potent to inhibit sucrose absorption.

Mechanism of guar gum (diataid 5 gm sachet): This polysaccharide fiber obtained from Indian cluster beans administrated before meal, slows gastric emptying and carbohydrate intolerance. Also reduces serum triglycerides. Flatulence, loss of appetite, feeling of stomach fullness, nausea may occur.

Glucomannan (dietmann 0.5 gm cap 1 gm sachet): This powder extract of tubers of konjar swells up in stomach absorbing water to reduce appetite, blood sugar, lipids. It also relieves constipation.

Repaglinide is insulin secretagogues, meglitinides derivative modulates insulin release by regulating potassium efflux through potassium channel. It is quick acting (within one hour of digestion) which lasts for 5–8 hours. Used for postprandial rise of blood glucose. Dose 0.25–4 mg just before meal. Its molecules are free from sulfur so can be given to sulfa-sensitive patient (where sulfonurea reacts). It is metabolized by CYP3A4. Should be used with caution in hepatic and renal impaired patients.

Nateglinide: D-phenylalanine derivative, insulin secretagogue. Given just before meal. Used for postprandial hyperglycemia. Metabolized in liver by CYP2C9 and CYP3A4. Safe in patient reduced kidney function. It restores insulin release in response to IV glucose which suppresses glucagon release. Useful for isolated postprandial hyperglycemia.

Other uses of hypoglycemics

- When tolbutamide 1 gm IV given to insulinoma patient, hypoglycemia occurs

Table 82.2: Differences between first and second generation sulfonyl urea	
First generation	*Second generation*
Hydrophilic	More lipophitic
Less affinity for β cells	Affinity for β cells high
Less potent, more toxic	More potent, less toxic
Absorbed partially	Absorbed completely
Easily displaced by other drugs	No easily displaced
Active metabolite	Inactive metabolite
Disulfiram action	Antabuse less common

- Diabetes insipidus

When not to take a particular OHA?

- Tolbutamide useful, if blood sugar level is around 200 mg or more.

- Chlorpropamide not preferred in elderly patient, renal insufficiency—Water logging disease (CCF, cirrhosis), alcoholics. Glibenclamide causes dangerous hypoglycemia, if fasting blood sugar is not very high.

Mechanism of action of thiazolidinediones (Tzd)

Reverses insulin resistance in liver, skeletal muscle, adipose tissue by raising number of glucose transporters ($GLUT_4$). Tzd is a ligand for peroxisome proliferator activated 'receptor, PPAR-γ part of steroid and thyroid superfamily, of nuclear receptor. Found in muscle, fat, liver and expresses gene involved in lipid and glucose metabolism, insulin signal transduction. Apart from its effects on fat, liver and muscle cells, it has effects on vascular endothelium, immune system and ovaries. These are hepatotoxic and some have hematological toxicities.

Difference between Primary and Secondary OHA Failures

Primary OHA failure

Definition: No response with OHA's maximum dose.

Causes

- Improper selection of patients
- Defective dietary compliance

- Occult infection or stress
- Idiopathic true failure

Secondary OHA Failure

Definition: Initial adequate response followed by a failure.

Causes

- Improper OHA selection
- Improper compliance (omission, reduction)
- Drug interaction
- Dietary non-compliance
- Pregnancy
- Over/occult aggravating concominent disorder
- Islet cell antibodies, antibodies, HLA-B_8, Pseudo-NIDDM.

New Approaches in Diabetes

Exenatide: Glucagon-like peptide-1 (GLP-1) is released from gut in response to oral glucose. It is difficult to use clinically because of rapid degradation by dipeptidyl dipeptidase-4 (DPP-4). Exenatide is recombinant chemically analogue of GLP-1, but resistant to DPP-4. It suppresses postprandial glucagon release and potentiates insulin release. It is given SC 1 hour before meal, 5 μg BD. It is the first incretin therapy available.

Other glycagon like peptide-1 are:

i. **Liraglutide** which is long acting (nausea, vomiting may occur)

ii. **Albiglutide** is GLP-1 fused with human albumin its t/2 is 5 days.

iii. **Dulaglutide:** Here two GLP-1 moelcule is linked to Fc fragment of human 1g G.

All of them increases the risk of pancreatitis.

Sitagliptin vildaglipti Linagliptin and saxagliptin: It inhibits DPP-4 enzyme to prevent degradation of endogenous GLP-1 (Glucogen, like peptide I). Given orally. Sitagliptin, vildagliptin and saxagliptins are chemically and pharmacokinetically different.

Islet amyloid polypeptide (IAPP; amylin): It is 37 amino acid peptide packaged with pancreatic β cells granules, co-secreted with insulin (1 molecule of amylin per 10 molecules of insulin), circulated on glycated active and nonglucated non-active form. It is a member of super family of neuroregulatory peptide. It produces negative feedback on insulin secretion. In pharmacological doses via vagus mediated mechanism, reduces glucagon secretion and gastric emptying, **Pramlintide** is amylin analog with proline substitution in 25, 28, 29 position, which makes it soluble and non-self aggregating.

Pramlintide: It is given SC before meal to reduce glucagon secretion and gastric emptying. It is synthetic amylin chemically. used as adjuvant therapy in types I and II diabetes mellitus. It suppresses glucagon release and delays gastric emptying. It has CNS mediated anorectic action also.

Bromocriptine as mesylate is used as adjunct to diet and exercise for glycemic control in type II DM because it targets D_2 receptor in the hypothalamus which alters insulin resistance.

Sodium-Glucose cotransporter-2 (SGLT-2):

Dapaglifozin, serglifozin, remoglifozin are undergoing clinical trial which inhibits glucose reabsorption from proximal tubule by sodium-glucose cotransporter-2 and increases glucose excretion. Its advantages are:

(i) There is weight loss.

(ii) Beneficial in hypertension patient

Table 82.3: Some OHAs with special features

Sl. no.	Sulfonylurea	Plasma $t\frac{1}{2}$ (hours)	Duration of action (hours)	Clearance action	Remarks
1.	Tolbutamide (restinon) 0.5 gm; Dose 0.5–3 gm/2–3 divided doses	6–8	6–8	Liver	Short action
2.	Chlorpropamide (diabenese) 0.25; 0.1–0.5 gm in 1–2 doses	30–36	36–48	Kidney, liver	Long action
3.	Acetohexamide, 0.5–1.5 gm in 1–2 doses	6–8	12–18	Liver	Produces active metabolite
4.	Tolazamide 0.125–1 gm; 1–2 divided doses	8	18–24	Liver absorption	Slow absorption
5.	Glibenclamide (daonil) 5 gm; tab 5–15 mg in 1–2 doses	4–6	18–24	Liver	Potent, slow acting
6.	Glipazide (glynase 5 mg) 5–20 mg in 1–2 doses	3–5	12–18	Liver	Fast acting
7.	Gliclazide (diamocron 80 mg) 40–240 mg in 1–2 divided doses	8–20	12–24	Liver	Antiplatelets action, delay retinopathy, decreases free radicals
8.	Glimapride (amarlyl) 1–4 mg once	5–8	Longer	–	Low insulin release, but stronger extrapancreatic action
9.	Phenformin (DBI, 25 mg) 25–150 mg in 1–3 doses	3–10	8–12	Liver, kidney	Lactic acidosis may occur.
10.	Metformin (Glyciphase 0.5 gm) 0.5 gm in 2–4 doses	1.5–3	6–8	Kidney	Less chance to produce lactic acidosis
11.	Glyburide 2.5 mg/day single morning	–	–	Metabolized in liver with low hypogly-cemic action.	Contraindicated in liver and renal disease patients

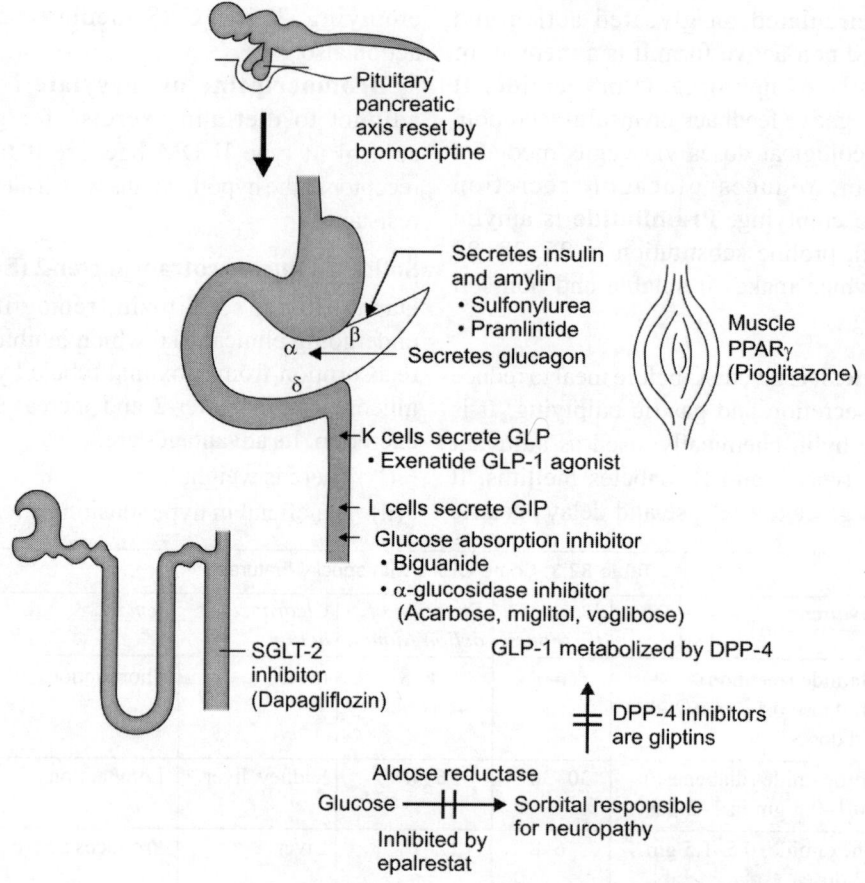

Fig. 82.5: Mechanism of actions of different antidiabetic drugs

(iii) Decreases insulin resistance

(iv) No hypoglycemic, but disadvantages are polyuria, increased incidence of UTI and sodium loss.

Epalrestat (Alrista 50 mg tab): Sorbitol is a metabolite of glucose metabolism produced by enzyme aldose reductase produced in diabetes responsible for complications like neuropathy where those are deposited. Aldose reductase inhibitor delays this deposition and delays the complications. Dose is 50 mg TDS.

Colesevelam is bile sequestrant acting by interrupting enterohepatic circulation and inhibiting Farnesoid X receptor (FXR) activation, used along with other antidiabetic drug in type-II DM.

GLUCAGON

This hyperglycemic hormone liberated from α-cells of pancreas of mol wt. 3,500 with 29 amino acids, in single chain. Glucose has opposite effect on insulin and glucagon release acts on receptor to activate adenylyl cyclase and increases cAMP in liver, fat cells and heart. Orally inactive, degraded in liver, kidney and plasma. Available as glucagon 1 mg inj.

Therapeutic uses of glucagon

- Hypoglycemia
- Cardiogenic shock
- Diagnosis of pheochromocytoma
- Relaxing gut, also tried for biliary colic, diverticulitis and in MRI imaging of gut as it releaxes it.

- β blocker poisoning because of ability to increase cAMP production.

Other hyperglycemics

- Diazoxide: Inhibits β cells to release insulin and oppose sulfonylurea.
- Somatostatin
- Thiazide
- Phenytoin
- Streptozocin: Damages β-cells of pancreas.

Sweetening Agents

These are non-carbohydrate substances with low calorie value used for sweetening of diet and beverages, *viz.*

- Saccharine
- Sodium cyclamate
- Aspartame: 200 times sweeter than sucrose
- Neotame: 30–60 times sweeter than aspartame
- Sucralose: 600 times sweeter than sucrose marketed as splenda.

83

Drugs Affecting Calcium and Magnesium Metabolisms

Calcium is the fifth most abundant element after C, O, H, and N in the body. Derangement of calcium metabolism is associated with various cellular functions and homeostasis. Milk and milk products, greenleafy vegetables, cereals are good sources of calcium. Milk and milk products calcium are better assimilable. Adult body weight's 1–1.5 kg is contributed by calcium mostly stored in bones and teeth, rest distributed in plasma and cells. Daily intake about 500–600 mg in infants, 600–700 mg in growing children. Mother needs 1 gm of calcium supplementation during pregnancy because from this source fetus gets about 30 gm of calcium. Normal plasma Ca level is 9–11 mg% of which 40% bound to plasma albumin, 10% complexed with citrate, phosphate and carbonate, remaining 50% unionized is physiologically important. Acidosis enhances ionization of calcium whereas alkalosis decreases calcium ionization.

Physiological roles of calcium
- Regulates excitability of nerves and muscles.
- Integrity of cell membrane and cell adhesion.
- Engaged in secretion of exocrine, endocrine and release of neurotransmitters.
- Acts as intracellular messenger for autacoids, hormones and neurotransmitters.
- Structural integrity of bones and teeth.
- Coagulation of blood.
- Automaticity and AV conduction in heart.

Absorption and excretion
Absorption takes place in small intestine. Intestinal absorption involves soluble ionized form of calcium in two separate steps:

- Calcium uptake at the mucosal pole
- Efflux at the serosal pole. Mucosal uptake of Ca^{2+} is carrier mediated, but mechanism is not understood. It is likely to involve Ca^{2+}-ATPase at serosal membrane.

Enhancer of calcium absorption: Vitamin D; parathormone.

Depressor of calcium absorption: Glucocorticoids, phytate, oxalates, phosphate, tetracycline, phenytoin, calcitonin. Urinary excretion depends upon filtration and resorption. There is a corelation between urinary Na and calcium. Calcium deficiency and low dietary calcium increase calcium absorption. Thiazide diuretics facilitate calcium resorption and impede calcium excretion.

Fibroblast growth factor 23, a newly discovered hormone, enhances phosphate excretion and inhibits production of vitamin D. Calcitonin, prolactin, growth hormone, thyroid hormone, corticosteroid and sex steroid all have their influence in calcium and phosphate hemostasis in some physiological conditions. Estrogen prevents bone loss in postmenopausal women, but has long-term side effects.

Selective estrogen receptor modulator (SERM), *Raloxifene* is used for bone loss in postmenopausal women without increasing risk of breast cancer or endometrial cancer.

Adverse effects of calcium: Constipation, intestinal obstruction, hypercalcemia (generally not by oral route), milk alkali syndrome, cardiac arrhythmia in digitalized patient. $CaCl_2$ is irritating by all routes. Extravasation of calcium salts may produce sloughing of skin.

Preparations

- CaCl$_2$ (irritant by all routes) 27% Ca
- Calcium gluconate (9% calcium preferred) for IV route, 0.5 and 1 gm tabs, 10% injection.
- Calcium lactate (13% Ca) given orally.
- Dibasic calcium phosphate (23% Ca) used oral as antacid and supplement Ca.
- Calcium carbonate used as antacid and calcium supplementation.

Dietary calcium as per recommendation of National Institute of Health (1994).

- Children 0.8–1.2 gm
- Young adult (11–24 years); pregnancy and lactation 1.2–1.5 gm
- Men 25–65 years 1.0 gm
- Women 51–65 years not on HRT 1.5 gm

Therapeutic uses of calcium

- Tetany: Start with IV calcium gluconate and switch over to oral calcium with vitamin D.
- Dietary supplement in children, pregnant and lactating mother, postmenopausal women and osteoporosis due to Cushing's syndrome, patient on corticosteroid therapy, rickets, osteomalacia, after removal of parathyroid tumor.
- Lead colic
- To counter the systemic effects of magnesium salts.
- Placebo
- As antacids
- Empirical uses: IV calcium gluconate is used for dermatosis, paresthesia, weakness and for vague symptoms. The benefit is probably psychological due to subjective effects by injection.
- Osteoporosis: It is used with hormone replacement therapy HRT/raloxifene, SERM/alendronate to prevent calcium deficiency.
- Components of Darrow's solution.
- Hyperkalemia and hypermagnesemia

Treatment of hypercalcemia

- Sodium phytate to inhibit absorption of calcium
- Correction of dehydration and solute diuresis by NaCl

- High dose corticosteroid (prednisolone 20–30 mg BD)
- K to counter the action of Ca on heart
- Mithramycin 25 mg/kg IV once or twice a week for hypercalcemia due to malignancy.
- IV phosphorous
- Gallium nitrate IV inhibits bone resorption
- Bisphosphonate: Zolendronate 4 mg IV to treat hypercalcemia of malignancy. Etidronate is used now.

Phosphorus

Abundantly present in all foods, deficiency rarely encountered in India. Daily requirement 0.9 mg, higher in growing children, pregnant and lactating mother.

Physiological functions of phosphorus

- Phosphorylation of endogenous metabolic reaction
- In storage of energy as ATP, structure of muscle and cytoplasm
- Regulation of hydrogen ion concentration.
- Formation of bone and teeth

Hypophosphatemia: Occurs in hyperparathyroid, vitamin D deficiency; dietary deficiency, Fanconi syndrome due to disorder in tubular resorption.

Hyperphosphatemia: Occurs in hypoparathyroidism, acromegaly and renal failure. Sevelamer is a cationic polymer binds to phosphate and lower phosphate level in patient of chronic renal failure. Lanthanum carbonate and calcium supplement is also used.

Therapeutic uses of phosphate: Neutral phosphate mixture used in hypercalcemia, vitamin D resistant rickets—prepared as follows, disodium hydrogen phosphate 3.66 gm and sodium dihydrogen phosphate 1 gm. Orange syrup 16 mL and make it 60 mL.

Magnesium Metabolism

Magnesium, an important constituent of human body, mostly present in bones and ECF intracellularly. Plasma level vary from 1.5–2 mEq/L. Cardiac and skeletal muscles, liver, brain, kidney contain appreciable amounts of magnesium. It is depressant to CNS, local anesthetic and depresses myoneural transmission. The action of Mg is antagonized by Ca^{2+}. Causes peripheral vasodilatation, cofactor for membrane ATPase, involved in uptake of catecholamine, activation of ribosomes by mRNA.

Calcium and magnesium have common transport mechanism across gut and renal tubules. Parathormone is essential for its absorption from gut and kidney. Renal tubular kidney disease produces magnesium toxicity even when used as antacid and purgatives.

Magnesium deficiency occurs in diarrhea, fistula discharge, malabsorption, hyperparathyroidism, diuretic therapy, renal tubular acidosis, hyperaldosteronism. Magnesium deficiency presents with weakness, restlessness, convulsion, tetany, involuntary movements.

Therapeutic uses of magnesium salts

- Magnesium deficiency
- CNS depressants and toxemia of pregnancy
- Antacids and purgatives
- As anticardioarrhythmia in postmyocardial infarct period.

Topical use

- $MgSO_4$ in 25–50% in glycerin topically used to alleviate inflammation.
- MgO as universal antidote
- Perrectally to reduce intracranial tension.

Parathormone (PTH)

In 1900, Vassale and Generali first performed selective parathyroidectomy and found it causing tetany and death. MacCallum and Voegtlin in 1909 showed parathyroidectomy decreases serum calcium. It was isolated in 1925. Parathormone secreted by chief cells of parathyroid gland. It is a single chain 84-amino acid polypeptide, cleaved in plasma into small fraction. It is synthesized as prepro-PTH, the excess amino acids are spit off in two steps and stored in intracellular vesicles. There is no tropic hormone for it and its secretion is regulated by Ca^{2+} level through a calcium-sensing receptor (CSR) which

is G-protein coupled receptor on parathyroid cells increasing cAMP level of the cell. Agents increasing cAMP can increase PTH release. Prolonged hypocalcemia causes hypertrophy of parathyroid. Vitamin D decreases PTH secretion. It is rapidly degraded in liver and kidney. Not available for therapeutic purpose. Only used therapeutically as diagnostically to differentiate pseudo- and true-hypoparathyroidism.

Physiological Action

- Bone: Increases resorption of calcium from bone.
- Kidney: Increases calcium reabsorption in the distal tubule and phosphate excretion.
- Intestine: Enhances formation of vitamin D in the kidney and thereby increases calcium absorption.
- PTH decreases Ca level in milk, saliva and ocular lens, may be reason of cataract formation in hypoparathyroidism.

Mechanism: Acts through PTH receptor. PTH receptors are not found in osteoclast. PTH acting on osteoblast induces "receptor for activation of nuclear factor KB ligand (RANKL)", which diffuses and combines with RANKL on osteoclast precursor to transfer it to osteoclast to develop bone-lysing ruffled surface. Another protein osteoprotegerin (OPG) produced by osteoblast and binds to RANKL and prevents it to bind osteoclast.

Denosumab a monoclonal antibody inhibits action of RANKL used to treat excess bone osteoporosis due to bone resorption.

Hypoparathyroidism: Presents with low calcium level, tetany, convulsions, laryngospasm, cataract, psychiatric problem. Pseudohypoparathyroidism occurs due to reduced sensitivity of target organs.

Hyperparathyroidism: Presents with hypercalcemia, decalcification, fractures, osteitis fibrosa generalisata, renal stones, constipation, anorexia and muscle weakness.

Cinacalcet: It activates Ca^{2+} sensing receptor in parathyroid gland to block PTH secretion. It is used in hyperparathyroidism due to renal disease and parathyroid tumor.

Teriparatide: It is a recombinant PTH (1–34 amino acid residues), given SC for osteoporosis. It stimulates bone formation. It is also used to diagnose pseudo- and true-hypoparathyroidism. In pseudohypoparathyroidism, it fails to increase calcium level, if given IV.

Calcitonin

A polypeptide (32 amino acids, mol wt. 3,600) produced by ultimobronchial bodies of para-follicular C cells of thyroid, first discovered by Copp in 1962. Its synthesis and secretion is regulated by plasma Ca^{2+} level. High Ca^{2+} level stimulates it. It inhibits bone resorption by osteoclast, tubular Ca and PO_4 reabsorption. Plasma t½ is 10 minutes, but its action lasts longer.

Preparation: Synthetic salmon calcitonin 100 IU/mL amp IM or SC (1/U = 4 µg)

Adverse effects: Nausea, flushing, tingling, bad taste.

Therapeutic uses of calcitonin

- Hypercalcemic states (hyperparathyroid, hypervitaminosis D): Osteolytic bony meta-stasis 4–8 IU/kg IM TBD to QDS × 2 days.
- Postmenopausal osteoporosis with vitamin D or as nasal spray (miacalcin). Nasal spray 2,200 IU/2 mL one spray in one nostril/day. Less effective than HRT and bisphosphonate.
- **Paget disease:** Bisphosphonate is the treat-ment of choice because calcitonin on prolong use produces resistance due to formation of antibodies.
- To diagnose medullary carcinoma of thyroid where there is high calcitonin.

Vitamin D

It is a group of sterols having common property to prevent rickets. Obtained from foods and produced in skin by ultraviolet rays. Vitamin D_2 and calcitriol are important physiologically. 25-OHD$_3$ is released from liver into blood and binds to vitamin D binding globulin which is

hydroxylated in kidney which is a rate limiting step, induced by Ca^{2+}/vit D deficiency, para-thormone, estrogen, prolactin while calcitrol inhibits it by feedback. It may be considered as hormone because:

- It is produced by specific organ skin.
- Transported in blood.
- Activated and acts on specific receptor and target tissues.
- Feedbackly inhibited by active level and Ca^{2+}.

Actions of Vitamin D

- Increases absorption of Ca^{2+} and PO_4 from intestine brought about by calcium-binding protein, calbindin. The calcitriol, like steroid hormone binds to cytoplasmic vitamin D receptor (VDR); translocate to the nucleus to increase the synthesis of specific mRNA to regulate the synthesis of specific protein. It may act quickly also which is not regulated by genes.
- Increases resorption of Ca^{2+} and PO_4 from bones, helps bone mineralization indirectly by maintaining normal plasma calcium and phosphate concentration helped by para-thormone. It is done by prompting the recruit-ment and differentiation of osteoclast precursor in bone remodeling units. Mature osteoclast lacks vitamin D receptor (VDR). It induces

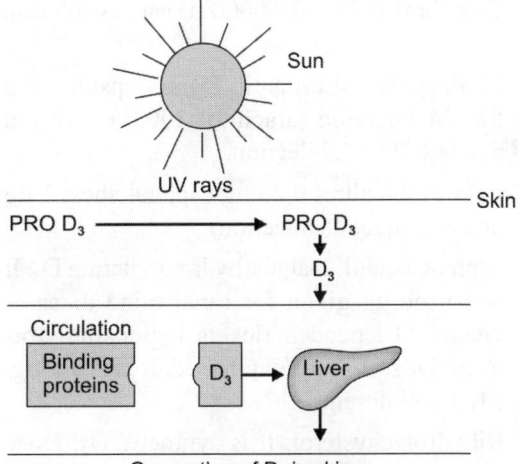

Fig. 83.1: Formation of vitamin D from UV rays of sun

RANKL in osteoblast which then activate osteoclast. The action of vitamin D is fascilitated by PTH.

- Enhances resorption of Ca and PO$_4$ from kidney.
- Acts on immunological cells and produces lymphokine, which helps in differentiation of epidermal cells, certain malignant cells and neuronal and skeletal muscle functions.

Deficiency in vitamin D produces rickets in child and osteomalacia in adult though osteoid is normal.

Hypervitaminosis of vitamin D produces elevated plasma calcium and its deposition in ectopic sites, weakness, vomiting, polyuria, nephrocalcinosis, growth retardation and hypertension.

Treatment of hypervitaminosis D

- Stop vitamin
- Low calcium diet
- Corticosteroid
- Plenty of fluids

Pharmacokinetics: Orally absorbed (D$_3$ form) bound to globulin stored in adipose tissue, hydroxylated in liver to active and inactive metabolites.

Preparations of vitamin D

- Calciferol as 25000–50000 IU cap; as solution in oil.
- Cholecalciferol (vitamin D$_3$ as capsules and for IM injection (arachitol 300,000 IU and 600,000 IU/mL injection.
- Calcitriol (caltrol 0.25 µg cap; calcibest 1 µg in 1 mL aqueous injection).
- Alpha-calcidol: 1-alpha-hydroxyvitamin D$_3$, It is a prodrug given for renal bone disease, vitamin D dependent rickets, hypoparathyroidism. Dose 1–2 µg/day for adult and 0.5 µg/day for children.
- Dihydrotachysterol. It is synthetic D$_2$. Dose 0.25–0.5 mg/day used for renal bone disease and hypoparathyroid condition.

Therapeutic uses of vitamin D

- Prophylaxis of vitamin D deficiency.
- Rickets:
  a. Vitamin D resistant ricket: PO$_4$ or calcitriol or α-calcidol is used.
  b. Vitamin D dependent ricket: Calcitriol or α-calcidol is used.
  c. Renal ricket: Calcitriol or α-calcidol or dihydrotachysterol is used.
- Senile osteoporosis
- Postmenopausal osteoporosis
- Hypoparathyroidism
- Fanconi syndrome. It can raise phosphate level.
- For skin cancer and immunological used systemetically
- Topically in psoriasis. Calcipotriol available as daivonex 0.005% oint. This is a nonhypercalcemic analogue of vitamin D.
- Doxercalciferol and paricalcitol are analogs of calcitrol used to treat secondary hyperpara thyroidism in chronic renal discuss.

Interactions of vitamin D: Phenytoin and phenobarbitone reduce responsiveness of target tissues to calcitriol. Liquid paraffin and cholestyramine reduce its absorption.

Some other hormones influencing calcium hemostasis:

- Glucocorticoids producing osteoporosis.
- Estrogen prevents osteoporosis.
- Androgen decreases Ca^{2+} excretion.

Other agents influencing calcium hemostasis:

- **Selective estrogen receptor modulators (SERMs): Raloxifene** used for postmenopausal osteoporosis.
- **Calcium-sensing receptors (CaSRs)**, higher calcium level blcoks PTH by sensing CaSR. *Cinacalcet* is approved for treatment of secondary hyperparathyroidism in chronic renal failure.
- **Stromtium ranelate** blocks osteoclast differentiation and promotes its apoptosis to prevent bone resorption and is used for osteoporosis.

- **Savelamer hydrochloride** is a phosphate binding gel used to treat hyperphosphatemia along with calcium.

- **Thiazide diuretic** reduces calcium excretion.

- **Fluoride:** It is incorporated in bone to produce fluorapatite making the bone denser earlier, but on prolong use it decreases its mechanical strength.

- **Denosumab:** This monoclonal antibody inhibits osteoclast differentiation and its function and promotes its apoptosis used for postmenopausal osteoporosis.

Fibroblast Growth Factor 23 (FGF-23): It is 251-amino acid with single chain protein. It inhibits $1, 25\text{-}(OH)_2D_3$ production and phosphate resorption *via* sodium phosphate cotransporters in kidney NaPi-2a and NaPi-2c causing hypophosphatemia and low circulating $1, 25\text{-}(OH)_2D_3$. It inhibits synthesis and decreases calcium and PO_4 absorption by intestine and PO_4 excretion by kidney.

In brief PTH raises Ca^{2+} and reduces PO_4^{2-}. Vitamin D raises Ca^{2+} and PO_4^{2-}. FGF-23 decreases serum PO_4^{2-}. Calcium is the principal regulator of PTH secretion.

84

Bisphosphonates (BPNs)

Bisphosphonates are pyrophosphate analogues where carbon atom replaces oxygen of POP skeleton structure of pyrophosphate, and they inhibit bone resorption. Following bisphosphonates are available, grouped into generation according to their chronology and potency.

1st generation
- Etidronate, Tiludronate (not marketed in India)

2nd generation
- Pamidronate
- Alendronate
- Ibandronate (not marketed in India)

3rd generation
- Risedronate
- Zoledronate

Used for
- Osteoporosis
- Paget's disease
- Hypercalcemia of malignancy
- Osteolytic bone metastasis

INDIVIDUAL BISPHOSPHONATES

Etidronate (Dronate OS 200 mg tab or 300 mg/inj. Dose 5–7.5 mg/kg/day). Used for Paget's disease. May cause osteomalacia. May be given IV or orally.

Pamidronate (Aredia 15, 30; 60 mg inj). Given IV over 2–4 hours weekly. Used for Paget's disease, hypercalcemia of malignancy. Thrombophlebitis, bone pain, fever, leukopenia, flu-like reaction due to cytokine release may occur.

Alendronate (osteophos 5, 10, 35, 70 mg tab): Orally active, prevents osteoporosis, given in empty stomach with a glass of water. Patient should not lie down or take food for ½ hour to prevent its contact with esophagus to prevent esophagitis. Its absorption is interfered by Ca, Fe, antacid, mineral water, tea or coffee, fruit juices. Headache, flatulence, retrosternal pain, bodyache and fall in serum calcium may occur.

Risedronate (risofo 35 mg tab): 3rd generation potent BPN used for osteoporosis and Paget's disease used weekly.

Zoledronate (zobone 4 mg/vial): Highly potent 3rd generation BPN, used for hypercalcemia, Paget's disease, for bone metastasis. 4 mg diluted in 100 mL of saline or glucose infused over 15 minutes, may be repeated after 7 days and then at 3–4 weeks.

Other Drugs Used for Hypercalcemia

- **Gallium nitrate:** Used for resistant hypercalcemia given by continuous infusion daily × 5 days. It is nephrotoxic so used as a reserve drug. It depresses ATP depressant proton pump of ruffled osteoclast.

- **Glucocorticoids** in high doses decrease calcium absorption and enhance its excretion.

- **Mithramycin (plicamycin):** This cytotoxic drug is used for non-responsive cases of hypercalcemia in Paget's disease.

- Saline diuresis with furosemide
- Bisphosphonate

- Calcitonin
- **Phosphate:** Used if other method fails. It fastest and surest. It may cause hypocalcemia, ectopic calcification, hypotension, renal failures. Available as oral and intravenous forms of Na or K salt.

Hyperphosphatemia: Occurs with renal failure, hypoparathyroidism (pseudo, idiopathic, surgical), vitamin D toxicity. For emergency treatment, dialysis is required for glucose and insulin infusion. Other methods for treatment:

- Dietary restriction
- Phosphate binding gel-like Savelamer
- Calcium supplementation

Hypophosphatemia: Occurs with hyperparathyroidism; vitamin D deficiency, Fanconi's syndrome, idiopathic hypercalciuria, overuse of phosphate binder and parenteral nutrition with inadequate phosphates.

Hypophosphatemia interferes with hemoglobin to tissue oxygen transfered by decreasing 2, 3-diphosphoglycerate and may cause rhabdomyolysis. It also decreases intracellular ATP.

Muscle weakness and osteomalacia may occur as long-term effects. Oral phosphate may be used to treat it.

85

Male Sex Hormones

Cushing established the role of pituitary in regulating the gonadal functions. Gonads produce steroidal hormones which have androgenic, estrogenic and progestational activities. The gametogenic function of testes is controlled by FSH of pituitary. Locally, high concentration of testosterone is required for production of sperms in seminiferous tubules. Sertoli cells of testes can also synthesize activin and inhibin. Activin stimulates FSH release. Inhibin in conjunction with testosterone and dihydrotestosterone inhibits FSH release.

ANDROGENS

Natural: Testosterone is responsible for secondary sex characters in castrated male. It was isolated, synthesized and its structure was established in 1935. Testes of adult male produce 3–12 mg of testosterone, converted to dihydrotestosterone, more active form by enzyme 5-alpha reductase. Total is 0.25–0.5 mg/day. Adrenal cortex produces weak androgens (dehydroepiandrosterone and androstenedione). Ovaries in female produce small quantities of testosterone. Other sources of testosterone are adrenals. Total is 0.25–0.5 mg/day in female. Cholesterol is precursor of all natural androgens.

Synthetic androgens

- Methyltestosterone
- Fluoxymesterone
- Resistant to first pass metabolism so orally active.
- Testosterone undecanoate

- Mesterolone. Testosterone and Mesterolone are also orally active.

Lipid-soluble esters of testosterone in oily vehicle, given by injection, absorbed slowly for prolonged action.

Regulation of secretions: Interstitial cells of Leydig, under influence of LH from anterior pituitary secretes testosterone. High concentration of testosterone inhibits LH secretion. Inhibin (a protein) produced by testes inhibits FSH may be acting as feedback mediator.

Testosterone level in human

- 0.3–1 µg/dL in male
- 20–60 ng/dL in female

Functions of Testosterone

1. **On sex organs and secondary sex characters:**
   - Growth of genitals (penis, scrotum, prostate, seminal vesicles)
   - Male pattern distribution of hairs like pubic, axillary, beard, moustache, chest hairs and body hairs.
   - Voice deepens, behavioral effects (physical vigour, aggressiveness, penile erection, *i.e.* all changes in puberty in male are due to androgens).

   Tests: Testosterone is required for normal spermatogenesis and maturation of spermatozoa.

2. **Skeleton and skeletal muscle:** Responsible for skeletal spurt (in length and thickness).

Large doses may cause fusion of epiphysis. Inhibits bone resorption and may be helpful in osteoporosis.

- Helps in muscle building
- Retention of nitrogen, minerals (Na, K, Ca, P, S)
- Body weight increases
- Appetite improves
- Stimulates erythropoiesis by stimulating erythropoietin secretion.

Mechanism of action: Testosterone reduced to dihydrotestosterone binds to cytoplasmic receptor combines with DNA; after such combination DNA transcription is enhanced leading to modification of protein synthesis. So testosterone may be considered as prohormone in circulation.

Pharmacokinetics: Testosterone is metabolized first passly in the liver, therefore, not effective orally. Methyltestosterone and fluoxymesterone are given orally. Bound to globulin, sex hormone binding globulin (SHBG) and albumin. Metabolized products are androsterone and etichol-anolone excreted through urine as conjugate with glucuronic acid and sulfate.

Preparation

Oral

- Testosterone undecanoate 40 mg (nuvir), 1–3 caps daily for osteoporosis or male hypogonadism.
- Mesterolone 25 mg tab (provironum), 1–3 tabs daily in case of androgen deficiency.
- Fluoxymesterone 5 mg (ultandren), 25–50 daily.
- Methyltestosterone 25 mg OD. Sublingually.

Parenteral

- Testosterone free 25 mg IM in fortnight (aquaviron 25 mg/mL).
- Testosterone propionate 25–50 mg IM twice a week (testoviron).
- Testosterone phenyl propionate 50–100 mg IM in 1–2 weeks.

- Testosterone cypionate 50–100 mg in 1–2 weeks.
- Testosterone enanthate 200 mg IM in 2–4 weeks.

Transdermal androgen: Dihydrotestosterone 25 mg/gm gel (Andractim). 100 gm tube applied over non-scrotal skin once daily in hypogonadism and impotence. It bypasses hepatic first pass metabolism and produces uniform round the clock blood level.

Therapeutic Uses of Testosterone

Replacement therapy

- Hypogonadism
- Male climacteric

Pharmacological therapy

- Osteoporosis in elderly
- Carcinoma of breast in female
- Anabolic agent
- Impotency
- Refractory anemia
- Suppression of lactation
- Menopausal syndrome
- Hereditary angioneurotic edema

Testosterone is contraindicated in

- Carcinoma prostate
- Carcinoma of male breast
- Liver and kidney diseases
- Pregnancy should be used with caution
- In CCF
- Migraine
- Epilepsy

Adverse Effects of Testosterone

Male: Sustained errection, may be painful, subsides spontaneously, oligospermia, precocious puberty, early closure of epiphysis.

Female: Virilization, menstrual irregularities and voice changes.

Male and female both: Acne, edema, cholestatic jaundice, hepatic carcinoma, gynecomastia.

86

Anabolic Steroids

Though testosterone has potent anabolic effects, it is not used as anabolic steroid because of its equally effective androgenic effects. Anabolic steroids have less virilizing properties.

Pharmacological Effects of Anabolic Steroids

- Euphoria
- Anabolic effects—retention of N, P, H_2O, K, and Na
- Anticatabolic effects—decreases N excretion in urine, used in uremic condition.
- Stimulation of erythropoiesis
- Stimulation of fibrinolysis
- Bone: Normalizes calcium level and helps in bone synthesis.
- Excitation of endogenous insulin secretion
- Fluid and electrolyte disturbances: Retention of Na and water may lead to edema.
- Virilization associated with androgenicity.
- Progestational effect: May produce break through bleeding.
- Anterior pituitary inhibition: Prolonged and continued use may result in inhibition of GH LH, FSH and ACTH.

Therapeutic Uses of Anabolic Steroids

- Promotion of anabolism
- Uremia
- Osteoporosis
- Anemia (hypoplastic or renal failure, leukemia, lymphoma)
- Recurrent metastatic cancer of breast
- Endometriosis

- Lactation suppression
- Aging of man
- Antithrombotic: Orabolin has been used with phenformin like hypoglycemic agents with encouraging results in prevention of thrombotic episodes in diabetes.
- Accelerating growth in children
- Chronic pancreatic insufficiency
- Diseases of muscle's insufficiency
  (a) Progressive muscular, dystrophy with glucocorticoids
  (b) Polio
- **Miscellaneous:** Chronic degenerative heart disease, diabetes retinopathy, hyperthyroidism (restores nitrogen balance without changing BMR). Certain inborn errors of metabolism (*viz.* De-Toni, Fanconi syndrome decrease in cystinuria with variable results). One should weigh the therapeutic benefit versus risk.

Adverse Effects of Anabolic Steroids

A. Non-hormonal
- Cholestatic jaundice
- Hepatocellular adenocarcinoma
- Local intolerance
  (a) Anorexia
  (b) Nausea
  (c) Diarrhea
- Leukemia, oral preparation may accelerate leukemic process
- Drug interactions commonly encountered with oral anabolic steroids and warfarin.

- Urinary retention in male (use short acting anabolics)
- Premature fusion of epiphysis.

B. Hormonal

- Virilization
- Female used in first trimester may cause virilization of female fetus.
- Precocious sex development
- Continued use may arrest spermatogenesis
- Fluid retention
- Interferes in diagnostic test of thyroid, hematocrit and plasma cholesterol concentration.

Mechanism of Action of Anabolic Steroids

Action on androgen-sensitive target cells: Combines with cytoplasmic receptor and reaches the nucleus, where it activates RNA polymerase and helps synthesis of new protein.

Action on androgen-insensitive target cells: Such as skeletal muscle lacks androgen receptor. It competes for cytosolic receptors for glucocorticoids.

For practitioner where not to use anabolic agents

- For period more than 4 weeks, LFT should be done regularly as 2–4 weeks.
- Routine use as tonic.
- Premature infants specially female.
- Fracture in young patient.
- Athletes (it is a doping agent)
- Young female with menstrual irregularities.
- Decompensated heart failure
- Hepatocellular damage
- Cancer prostate
- Pregnancy
- Estrogen-dependent breast cancer.

Preparation and doses

- Methandiendone 2–5 mg OD or BD oral, children 0.04 mg/kg/day (Anabolex 2–5 mg tab, 2 mg/mL drops and 25 mg/mL inj)
- Nandrolone phenyl propionate (durabolin 10, 25 mg/mL inj) 10–50 mg/IM weekly.
- Nandrolone decanoate (decadurabolin 25, 50, 100 mg/mL inj, 25–100 mg IM every three weeks)
- Oxymetholone (adroyd 5 mg tab) 5–10 mg children 0.1 mg/kg OD
- Ethylestrenol (orabolin 2 mg tab) 2–4 mg, 2 mg/mL drops in children 0.06 mg/kg
- Oxandrolone 5–10 mg (anavar)
- Stanozolol 2–6 mg; (stroamba; emstro) 2 mg tabs
- Norethandrolone (nilevar) 10–30 mg daily.

> Combination drugs with anabolic steroid is banned in India.

Some drugs used by sports person (Doping agent):

- **Anabolic steroids**: Discussed with the appropriate chapter. Detected in urine but erythropoietin is difficult to detect because of shorter t/2.

- **Erythropoietin**

- **Human growth hormone:** Increases body mass but decreases fat and hastens healing of tissue injury. Blood testing distinguises from exogenous variety.

- **Insulin with glucose,** as from exogenous variety.

- **Salbutamol** as bronchodilator to increase oxygen uptake.

- **Propranolol** by shooters, gymnastics to reduce tremor.

- **Ephidrine, Amphetamine, Cocaine:** Increase muscle strength use by swimmers, sprint eventers as doping agent.

- **Thiazide and Frusamide:** To reduce body weight before weighing.

- **Codeine morphine:** Masks injury pain.

- **Other prohibited** drugs for athletes are **methylphenidate, Nikethamide Amiphenazole, Fenfluramine.**

87

Impeded Androgens

Superactive GnRH agonists are most potent inhibitors of gonadal function. They inhibit LH and FSH release and loss of androgen secretion. Some testosterone and progesterone derivatives act as a partial agonist and antagonist to androgen receptors. Ketoconazole in high doses inhibit testosterone production. Cimetidine and spironolactone have weak anti-androgenic action. Progesterone is a weak androgen receptor blocker.

Danazol (danazol 50, 100, 200 mg caps): Dose 200–800 mg/day—orally active ethisterone derivative with:
- Weak androgenic
- Progestational
- Mild anabolic activity.

Suppresses secretion of gonadotropin from pituitary and gonadal functions directly and indirectly by inhibiting steroidogenic enzymes. Its t½ 12–18 hours.

Therapeutic uses of danazol

- Endometriosis
- Menorrhagia
- Fibrocytic breast disease
- Hereditary angioneurotic edema
- Gynecomastia
- Infertility: It is given for 3 months and then withdrawn, increases fertility in women.
- Precocious puberty in boys.

Adverse effects: Hirsutism, acne, voice changes. weight gain, loss of libido, hot flushes, muscle cramps, night sweat, GI side effects. Complete amenorrhea, if large doses given for long time.

Cyproterone acetate (Androcur 50 mg; dose 50–100 mg/day): Chemically related to progesterone. Posessses mild progestational activity which inhibits LH release and augments its antiandrogenicity. It competes with dihydrotestosterone for androgen receptor to inhibit its binding. Larger doses suppress gonadotropin release, spermatogenesis. May produce gynecomastia.

Clinically trialed for

- Precocious puberty in boys
- Inappropriate sexual behavior in man
- Hirsutism in women male type boldness
- Acne (boys and girls)
- Carcinoma of prostate

Flutamide (Prostamid 250 mg, 1 tab TDS): Antiandrogenic, its active metabolite 2-hydroxy-flutamide competitively blocks androgen action on accessory sex organ and pituitary. Plasma testosterone level increases and partially overcome the direct antiandrogenic action.

Used for palliative treatment in prostate carcinoma.

It is also used with GnRH agonist after castration and for suppressing LH and testosterone.

Tried for female hirsutism with OCP.

Bicalutamide (Biprosta 50 mg OD): Long acting potent congener of flutamide. It is less hepatotoxic than flutamide, used once daily for metastatic prostate carcinoma.

ADR: Flash, chill, edema, loose stool, raised hepatic transaminase (stop the drug, if it is doubled the normal).

Finasteride (Fincar 5 mg OD): Competitively inhibits 5α-reductase type 2 isoenzyme responsible for conversion of testosterone to more active dihydrotestosterone particularly predominating in male urogenital tract. Used to treat benign prostate hypertrophy to relief obstructive features. Orally active, metabolized in liver, excreted in urine and feces. Skin rash, swelling of lips, libido may decrease, impotence and volume of ejaculate may decrease. It is also used for male type baldness, acne, prostate cancer.

Dutasteride (Duprost 0.5 mg OD): This congener drug of finasteride inhibits type I and type II 5α-reductases and reduces dihydrotestosterone level. Long acting, metabolized by CYP3A4. Used for prostate cancer and baldness.

Drugs for Erectile Dysfunction (ED)

Sexual arousal increases blood flow to penis, relaxes cavernous sinusoids to fill it up with blood to make the penis errect, rigid and elongated. Nitric oxide from parasympathetic, non-adrenergic, non-cholinergic nerves; and vascular endothelium is the transmitter involved in the relaxation of smooth muscles of corpus cavarnosum. ACh and PG are also involved. Amongst the different mechanical/prosthetic or drug therapies the later is more commonly used. The different drugs are:

- Androgens
- Phosphodiesterase-5 inhibitors like sildenafil tadalafil and verdenafil
- Papeverine/phantolanine induced penile erection (PIPE therapy)
- Prostaglandin E.

Androgens: In androgen deficiency, parenteral testosterone or transdermal testosterone therapy may improve libido to improve ED.

Phosphodiesterase-5 inhibitors (PDE-5 inhibitors): Inhibition of PDE-5 inhibitor leads to accumulation of cGMP and potentiation of NO action. NO causes smooth muscle relaxation by generating intracellularly dephosphorylation of myosin light chain kinase (MLCK) so that myosin fails to interact with actin.

Sildenafil (penegra 25, 50 and 100 mg tabs): Inhibits PDE-5 to enhance NO action on corpus cavernosum to increase penile tumescence during sexual activity. Dose 50 mg OD 1 hour before intercourse. Effective even in diabetic neuropathy, but ineffective for ED due to nerve or cord defect. It lowers pulmonary artery pressure, also used for pulmonary hypertension to improve arterial oxygenation. **ADR:** Headache, nasal congestion, dizziness, BP may fall, flushing, impairment of color vision (blue green discriminations) due to iso-PDE-6 inhibition in retina, non-arteritic ischemic optic neuropathy (NAION), potentiation of vasodilatation of nitrates, BP fall and MI precipitation (contraindicated for CAD patients).

In patient of leukemia or sickle cell anemia or myeloma, it should be used with caution. CYP3A4 inhibitors like erythromycin and ketoconazole may potentiate its action.

Tadalafil (Megalis 10, 20 mg tabs): Long acting, potent faster, t½ 18 hours, congener of sildenafil. Visual disturbance is less. Should not be used with nitrates.

Vardenafil (Dose 10–20 mg): Congener of sildenafil, weak inhibitor of PDE-6, but may produce photosensitivity. Prolongs QT interval.

Papaverine/phentolamine penile errection therapy (PIPE therapy): Used only if PDE-5 inhibitors or PGE (alprostadil) are ineffective. Dose of papaverine 3–20 mg with or without phentolamine 0.5 mg injected into corpus cavernosum.

Prostaglandin E1: Alprostadil PGE is directly injected in corpus cavernosum by fine needle or in urethra as small pallets, produces penile erection for 1–2 hours. Penile fibrosis and priapism are lesser than PIPE therapy. Used where PDE-5 inhibitors fail.

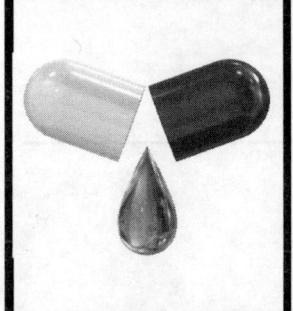
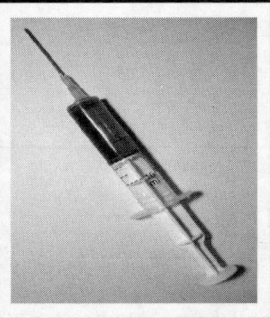
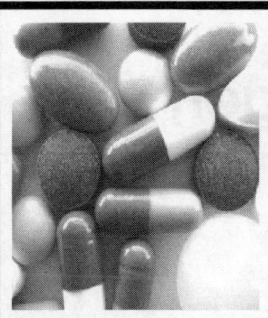
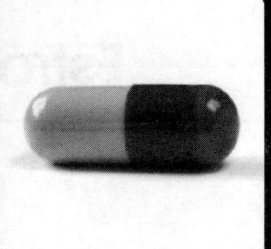

SECTION 12

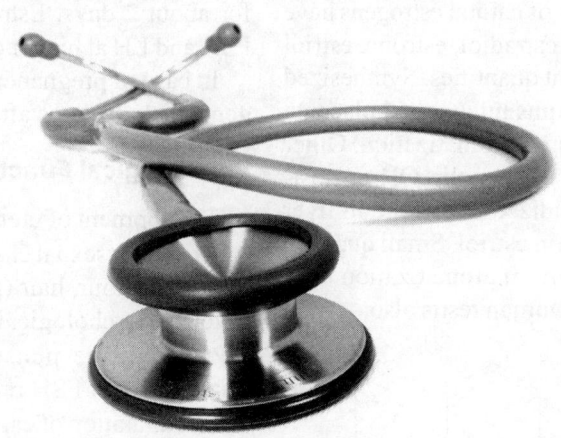

FEMALE HORMONES AND DRUGS OF PREGNANCY AND LACTATION

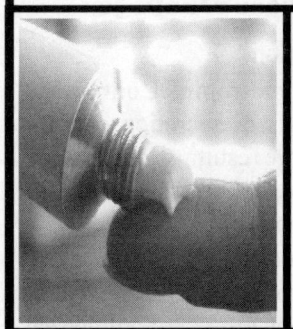
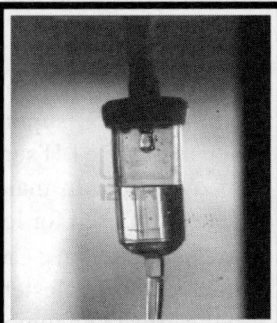
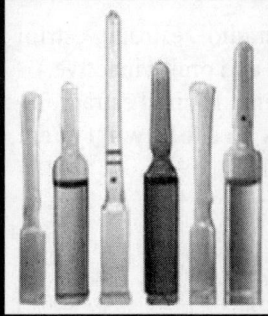
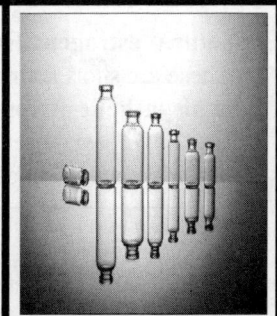

88

Estrogen

It is a naturally occurring female sex hormone. In the normal non-pregnant females, estrogens are secreted in major quantities by the ovaries, and only minute quantity by adrenal cortex. In pregnancy, it is produced by placenta.

Three different types of natural estrogens have been isolated of which estradiol, estrone, estriol are present in significant quantities. Synthesized in graafian follicle, corpus luteum and placenta from cholesterol by ring A aromatization. Other distinguishing feature is phenolic OH at position 3. Estradiol is oxidized to estrone in liver and hydroxylated to form estriol. Small quantity of estradiol is derived from aromatization of A of testosterone ring in human testis also.

Estrone

Classification of Estrogens

- **Natural estrogen:** Estradiol, estrone, estriol (These are short acting and orally inactive.)
- **Semisynthetic estrogens:** Ethinyl estradiol
- **Synthetic estrogens are of two types:** Steroidal, non-steroidal

Steroidal	Non-steroidal
• Mestranol	• Stilbesterol (Orally used)
• Tibolone	• Hexestrol ⎤
• Ethinylestradiol	⎟ (Used topically)
	• Dienestrol ⎦

Regulation of estrogen secretion: Its secretion varies in menstruating women which starts in graafian follicle under the influence of FSH. It rises modestly in preovulatory FSH surge. After ovulation corpus luteum continues to secrete it for about 2 days. Estrogen feedbackly inhibits FSH and LH at higher concentration in pituitary.

In case of pregnancy, placenta secretes estrogen which declines after delivery.

Physiological Functions of Estrogen

- Development of uterus, fallopian tube, vagina
- Secondary sexual characters of female: Breast, body contour, hair (pubic and axillary), skin, voice, psychological and emotional get up.
- Proliferative phase of endometrium and inhibition of FSH release.
- Vasodilatation of capillaries and endometrium
- Fusion of epiphysis and metaphysis (both osteoblast and osteoclast cells have estrogen receptors.)
- Na and water retention and keeping cholesterol low than that of males.

Pharmacological Actions of Estrogen

- For normal menstruation
- Suppression of gonadotropin: Continuous administration suppresses secretion of FSH and mid-cycle LH surge resulting in inhibition of ovulation. In male, suppresses spermatogenesis, if used for long time.
- Metabolic actions: Causes Na and water retention, lowers cholesterol level, have weak anabolic effect and inhibits growth of epiphyseal cartilage.

- Carcinogenicity: It is potentially carcinogenic.
- Antiandrogenic: Useful in prostate cancer.

Pharmacokinetics: Absorbed orally and transdermally. Natural estrogens are inactive orally because of their metabolism in liver. Natural estrogens are protein-bound (globulin and albumin). Estradiol esters are injected IM, absorbed slowly and produce prolong action. It is converted to estrone in liver. All conjugate with glucuronic acid and sulfate and excreted in bile, and urine. Enterohepatic circulation occurs.

Ethinylestradiol and stilbesterol are more active, metabolized slowly, orally active.

MECHANISM OF ACTION OF ESTROGEN

Estrogen receptor (ER) for the hormone has been detected in estrogen responsive tissues (female reproductive organ, breast, pituitary, hypothalamus). Estrogen first bound with high affinity to a cytoplasmic receptors in target cells. The ER like other steriod receptor: Agonist binds to ligand binding domain causing receptor dimerization and interacts with "estrogen response element (ERE)". Gene coactivation of target gene transcription is promoted by protein. Co-repressor protein inhibits gene transcription.

Estrogen receptors (ER) are of two types ERα and ERβ. Most tissues contain two subtypes. ERα predominates in uterus, vagina, breast, hypothalamus and blood vessels. ERβ predominates in prostate of male and in ovary of female. Estradiol binds to ERα and ERβ both. ERα and ERβ interact differently with coactivator or corepressor. These effects of estrogen can be blocked by inhibitors of RNA synthesis (dactinomycin) or protein synthesis (cyclohexamide).

Therapeutic Uses of Estrogen

1. Oral contraceptive
2. Menopausal syndrome

The common symptoms of menopausal symptoms
- **Osteoporosis:** Conjugated enquine estrogen or transdermal estrogen patched in cyclic manner. Alternatively raloxifene
- Vasomotor symptoms

- Cardiovascular symptoms with altered lipid profile
- Urogenital atrophy
- Insomnia, fatigue, etc.

Tibolone is a good alternative to hormone replacement therapy.

3. Hormone replacement therapy (HRT)
4. Senile or atropic vaginitis
5. Kraurosis vulvae
6. Delayed puberty in girls (Turner's syndrome, hypopituitarism)
7. Dysmenorrhea cyclic estrogen therapy is given. PG inhibitors are firstline drugs.
8. Dysfunctional uterine bleeding. It has adjuvant value protection in important.
9. Failure of ovarian development
10. Acne: Because it suppresses ovarian androgen production.
11. Hirsutism
12. Prevention of heart attack
13. Osteoporosis
14. Suppression of lactation
15. Prostate cancer. It has palliative role in metastatic Ca breast.
16. Atropic rhinitis and atropic skeletal changes.

Preparation and Dosage of Estrogen

- Estradiol benzoate (ovocyclin P 5 mg inj; progynon depot 10 mg/mL), dose 2.5–10 mg IM.
- Conjugated estrogen (premarin 0.625 mg, 1.25 mg tab). Dose 0.625–1.25 mg orally daily.
- Ethinylestradiol (Iynoral 0.01–0.05 mg tab) 0.02–0.2 mg/day used for menopausal syndrome.
- Mestranol (ovulen 0.1 mg tab + ethynodiol diacetate 1 mg) 0.1–0.2 mg/day. It is converted to ethinylestradiol in body.
- Estriol succinate (evalon 1–2 mg tab, 1 mg/gm cream) 4–8 mg to start with then 1–2 mg/day for menopause. Cream is applied for atropic vaginitis.
- Polyestradiol phosphate (estradurin 40 and 80 mg inj) 160 mg IM per month for cancer of prostate.
- Diethylstilbesterol (stilbesterol 1.5 mg tab,

5 mg/mL inj.) 0.5–5 mg/day oral or IM.

- Fosfestrol tetrasodium (Honvan 120 mg tab 60 mg/mL in 5 mL ampoule). Dose 600–1200 mg slowly IV for 5 days then 120–240 mg/day orally.
- Dienestrol (dienestrol 0.01% vaginal cream).
- Transdermal estradiol patches 25, 50 and 100 µg/24 hours are also available (Estraderm MX)
- Recently combined estradiol 50 µg + norethisterone acetate 0.25 mg patch estragest TTS is also available in some countries.
- Estradiol gel 3 mg/5 mg in 80 gm tube to apply over arms in HRT.

Adverse Effects of Estrogen

- Suppression of libido, gynecomastia in male
- Growth suppression
- Increases chances of vaginal and cervical cancers and endometrial carcinoma, breast cancer, benign hepatoma.
- Gallstones may occur, migraine and endometritis may aggravate.

Nausea, vomiting, diarrhea may occur with oral preparation which can be avoided by starting with low doses.

Tibolone (Livial 2.5 mg tab; 1 tab daily): Recently introduced, possesses estrogenic and progestational and weak androgenic activities (dose 2.5 mg daily). No endometrial stimulation occurs and extra progestin are required. Urogenital atrophy, psychological symptom, osteoporosis are improved in menopausal symptoms. CVS risks are less like other HRT. Weight gain, hirsutism, vaginal spotting may be noted. It should not be used in undiagnosed cancers of breast and uterus and thromboembolic patient, epilepsy, migraine, liver disease patients.

89

Antiestrogens

Theoretically—androgens, certain estrogens in low doses, progesterone. Non-steroidal compounds, clomiphene citrate and tamoxifen bind to intracellular estrogen receptor and produce antagonistic, partial agonistic and agonistic actions depending upon species and target organs.

a. **Clomiphene citrate (Fertomid; clomid 25, 50 mg tab):** Stimulates gonadotropin release from pituitary by blocking estrogen's feedback inhibitions. It is orally absorbed, deposited in adipose tissues, metabolized and excreted with bile.

Adverse effects: Multiple pregnancy, gastric upset, visual disturbances multiple cyst of ovaries.

Therapeutic uses of clomiphene citrate
- Infertility
- Oligospermia
- To aid *in vitro* fertilization

Fulvestrant: Selective estrogen receptor downregulator (SERD) or pure estrogen antagonist used for metastatic ER positive breast cancer in postmenopausal women who has stopped responding to tamoxifen. It is given IM monthly. It is slowly absorbed.

b. **Tamoxifen citrate (10 mg tab; 10–20 mg OD or BD):** It is selective estrogen receptor modulator (SERM) and partial agonist, orally effective, less toxic amongst other anticancer drugs used for breast cancer and male infertility. Hot flushes, vomiting, menstrual irregularity, dermatitis, anorexia, leukopenia, depression are frequent side effects.

Toremifene: This new congener is similar to tomoxifen in all respects. Doloxifen is structurally related to it.

Cyclofenil (ondomid 100 mg tab): Given 500–800 mg/day for 5–10 days cyclically to induce ovulation. It does not exert peripheral anti-estrogen effects like clomiphene.

Raloxifene (Bonmax 60 mg tab; dose 60 mg OD): It is selective estrogen receptor modulator (SERM). Estrogen partial agonist in bone and CVS but antagonist in breast and endometrium. Used to treat osteoporosis of bone with Ca^{2+} and vitamin D. It has high affinity for ERα and β with distinct DNA target "raloxifene response element (RRE)". It reduces LDL, but no response on HDL and TG. It reduces chance of breast cancer. It does not stimulate endometrial proliferation. No effect on vasomotor symptoms or menopausal symptoms. Orally absorbed, but low bioavailability due to first pass effect of glucuronidation.

ADR: Hot flush, leg cramps, vaginal bleeding, deep vein thrombosis can occur.

Ormeloxifene (Sevista 60 mg): SERM acting as estrogen antagonist, suppresses endometrial proliferation *via* ER. Used for DUB. Nausea, headache, weight gain, rise in BP, prolong menstrual cycle may occur as ADR. Dose 120 mg biweekly × 2–3 months.

Aromatase inhibitors (AIs): The A ring of testosterone is aromatized to produce estrogen. Aminoglutethmide is a first generation AI. The newers like letrozole, anastrozole, exemestane are other aromatase inhibitors.

Letrozole (Letoval 2.5 mg tab; dose 2.5 mg BD): Nonsteroidal compound, orally active, 100% bioavailable. Used for ER (+ve) early breast cancer and advanced breast cancer.

ADR: Nausea, diarrhea, dyspepsia, hot flush; joint pain, bone loss and thinning of hair can occur. Lipid profile not changed.

Anastrozole (altraz 1 mg tab; dose 1 mg OD): Reversible; nonsteroid AI; potent; single daily dose used for ER +ve breast cancer. Tomoxifen resistant cases may respond to it.

ADR: Hot flush, vaginal dryness and bleeding, nausea, diarrhea, arthralgia, thinning of hair and osteoporosis may occur.

Newer SERM is Bazedoxifene.

Exemestane: Steroidal and irreversible type I AI. It has weak androgen activities. Used for early breast cancer. Used orally. ADR are like other AI.

Other aromatase inhibitors are fadrozole and vorarole which are orally active triozole (nonsteroidal).

90

Progesterone

First isolated by Corner and Allen (1930) from corpus luteum. The distinguishing feature of progesterone is that it is 21 carbon containing steroid with ketone group at 3 position.

Physiological Function of Progesterone

- **Uterus:** It promotes uterus into secretory changes in the endometrium. Cytoplasm and stromal cells increase. Lipid and glycogen deposits also increase, thickness of endometrium doubles, blood supply increases proportionately required for food to implanted ovum (uterine milk).
- **Fallopian tube and vagina** undergo secretory changes to provide nutrition of fertilized ovum. It produces change in vaginal secretion and epithelium.
- **Breast:** Promotes alveolar cell proliferation, alveoli to enlarge and secretory in nature. Milk is only secreted after the prepared breast further stimulated by prolactin from anterior pituitary. It causes breast to swell up which is partly due to increased fluid and partly due to subcutaneous fat itself.

- **Fluid and electrolyte balance**—Na and H_2O are retained like aldosterone, but potency is less.
- **Raises midcycle basal** body temperature.
- It is a weak inhibitor of Gn secretion and decreases the frequency of LH pulse by hypothalamic pulse generator, but increases amount of LH secreted per pulse.

Classification of progestins: It may be classified by many ways, but simplest are:
- Pure progestin: Progesterone, dehydroprogesterone, esters of 17-α-hydroxyprogesterone, chlormadinone, megestrol.
- True progestin with possible androgenic effects: Medroxyprogesterone, norgestrel.
- Progestins with androgenic effect—norethisterone
- Progestins with estrogenic effect—norethynodrel.
- With uncertain status—ethynodiol diacetate. Newer compounds like desogestrel, norgestimate, gestodene.
- Spironolactone analogue—drospirenone.

Pharmacological Actions of Progesterone

Prepares uterus for nidation and maintenance of pregnancy by decreasing uterine motility and preventing immunorejection of fetus.
- **Uterus:** Produces secretory changes in estrogen primed uterus. Lack of progesterone support produces menstruation, whereas continued action brings decidual change and decrease sensitivity to oxytocin.

- **Cervix:** Cervical secretion becomes viscid, scanty and hostile to sperm penetration.
- **Vagina:** Viginal mucosa becomes cornified, infiltrated with leukocyte.
- **Breast:** Acting with estrogen, it prepares breast for lactation, prolactin is released when these hormones are withdrawal after delivery from pituitary to start milk secretion.
- **CNS:** High progesterone during pregnancy has sedative action. Body temperature: Resets thermostat center to raise body temperature at 0.5 °C higher.
- **Respiration:** Stimulated by progestin during pregnancy.
- **Metabolism:** Impairs glucose tolerance, lowers HDL, levels Na and water retention.
- **Pituitary:** Inhibits gonadotropin release; prevents ovulations.

Mechanisms of Action of Progesterone

Acts on progesterone receptor (PR) present in female genital tract, breast, CNS, pituitary. Binds to specific receptor in target cells. Progesterone on binding to PR undergoes dimerization and attaches to progesterone response element (PRE) of target genes which regulates the target genes through coactivator. Antiprogestin also binds to receptor PR, but produces opposite effects produced by interacting with corepressor. PR existing in two isoforms, short PR-A and longer PR-B having different activities, but agonist and antagonist for them are same. Estrogen increases progesterone receptor density, but progesterone represses estrogen receptor.

Pharmacokinetics: Not effective orally because of high first pass metabolism in liver. Given by injections in oily solution. Rapidly inactivated in liver, major product is pregnanediol, conjugates within glucuronide and sulfate, excreted with urine. Synthetic progesterones are metabolized slowly and orally active.

Preparation and Doses of Progesterone

- Progesterone (proluton 50 mg/mL) 10–100 mg IM OD.

- Hydroxyprogesterone caproate (maintane 250 mg IM, proluton depot 125–500 mg IM in 2–14 days gap)
- Medroxyprogesterone acetate (farlutal 5 mg, Provera 10 mg tab, depot provera 150 mg/mL inj) 5–10 mg and 50–150 mg/IM in 1–3 months interval.
- Dihydroprogesterone (duphaston 5 mg tab) 5–10 mg BD orally.
- Norethindrone (primolut N 5 mg tab) 5–10 mg OD or BD orally.
- Ethinylestrenol (orgametril 5 mg tab) 5–10 mg OD orally.
- Allylestrenol (gestanin, maintane 5 mg) 10–40 mg OD orally.
- Levonorgestrel (duoluton L)
- Ethynodiol diacetate 1 mg + mestranol 0.1 mg (Ovulen), 1 tab OD 1–21 days of cycle.
- Desogestrel 150 µg + ethinylestrenol 30 µg (Novelon) tab for 21 days cycle.

Therapeutic Uses of Progesterone

- Contraceptives
- Hormone replacement therapy
- Dysfunctional uterine bleeding
- Premenstruation tension
- Endometriosis
- Endometrial carcinoma
- Suppression of postpartum lactation
- Threatened and habitual abortion
- Dysmenorrhea
- Amenorrhea
- To postpone menstruation
- Medroxyprogesterone used to treat precocious puberty.

Adverse effects of progesterone therapy

Rise of temperature, breast engorgement, edema, headache, esophageal reflux, acne, mood swings, promotes atherogenesis, glucose intolerance, masculinization of fetus and congenital anomalies, if used in pregnancy (used for pregnancy diagnosis is contraindicated).

Antiprogestin

Mifepristone: Chemically 19-norsteroid. Having antiprogestational and antiglucocorticoid, antiandrogenic, partial agonist for both A and B forms of progesterone receptor (PR). In absence of progesterone, it exerts progesterone activity.

Action in follicular phase: Attenuates mid-cylce Gn surge of pituitary resulting follicular development and delay and failure of ovulation.

Action in luteal phase: Prevents secretory changes brought about by progesterone and late stages block progesterone support to endometrium; sensitizes myometrium to PG.

Therapeutic Uses of Mifepristone

- Termination of pregnancy. Orally active, metabolised in liver by $CYP3A_4$ and excreted with bile [Mifegest 200 mg tab) T-pill is Mifepristone 200 mg (3 tabs) +Misoprostol 200 µg 2 tab for MTP up to 49 days. 3 tab ofT-pill on day one and then 2 tabs on alternate day.
- Contragestational
- Induction of labor
- Inoperable Cushing's syndrome
- Other uses under evaluation are endometriosis, fibroid, breast cancer, meningioma.

- Postcoital contraceptives: Mifepristone 600 mg given within 72 hours.

The recently developed antiprogestins are onapristone and gestinone. Onapristone is a pure antagonist and gestinone is more effective in endometriosis.

Selective progesterone receptor modulator (SPRM): Its agonist activity is more where coactivator predominates and antagonist activity is more where corepressor activity predominates some drugs of this group are *ulipristal acetate, anoprishil* (procellex). Proellex is undergoing trial leiomyoma, endometriosis. Asoprisnil for uterine fibroid and ulipristal for emergency contraception.

Principles of hormone therapy

Hormones are used for the purpose of:
- Substitution
- Inhibition of function: Estrogen, androgen and progesterone inhibit anterior pituitary.
- Cortisone therapy inhibits ACTH of anterior pituitary.
- Stimulation of function: Gonadotropin stimulates ovarian functions, *etc.*

Hormonal Contraceptives

Population burst is one of the major problems of the world, particularly for the developing countries.

Oral contraceptive is safe, effective and reversible and one of the most extensively studied medications ever used by human being for delaying pregnancy.

Hormonal contraceptive currently in use/or under study may be classified as follows:

a. Oral pills

- Combined pill
- Progesterone only pills (mini-pills)
- Postcoital pill (emergency)
- Once a month long acting pill
- Male pills.

b. Depot slow release formulation

- Injections
- Subcutaneous implants
- Vaginal rings

   i. Combined pills: Contain estrogen and a progestin. The second generation OCP contains less amount of estrogen and progesterone with sound efficacy with less complication and side effects. The 3rd generation pill contains desogestrel. Estrogen is either ethinylestradiol or mestranol, 30 µg of ethinylestradiol is threshold. Progesterone used is generally, 19-nortestosterone 400 µg or levonorgestrel 60 µg, or desogestrel 60 µg, norgestimate 200 µg or gestodene 40 µg. One tablet taken from 5th day of cycle for 20–22 days. Calendar packs are available.

   ii. Sequential pills: 1–15 days estrogen then progesterone is added.

   iii. Phased regimen: Estrogen dose kept constant and dose of progesterone is increased gradually in second and third phases recommended for women over 35 years where risk factors are higher.

   iv. Progesterone-only pills: Low dose progesterone taken daily without gap to eliminate long-term complications of estrogen. Efficiency is lower (96–98%) as compared to combined pill.

   v. Postcoital pills: Levonorgestrel 0.5 mg + Ethinylestradiol 0.1 mg taken within 72 hours of unprotected intercourse may be repeated after 12 hours (Yuzpe method). Levonorgestrel 0.75 mg twice alone may serve the purpose. Mifepristone 600 mg an antiprogestin taken within 72 hours used in China. Used for rape patient, condom rupture.

   vi. Once a month (long acting): Long acting oral pill quinestrol estrogen with short progesterone is given, but results are disappointing.

Mechanism of Action of OCP

- Inhibits ovulation through suppression of FSH and LH.
- Hampering implantation through alteration in uterine secretion and endometrial thinning.

- Thickening cervical mucosa which interferes sperm transport.
- Postcoital pill dislodge the just implanted blastocyst or hamper fertilization.

OCP theoretically is 99% effective, but actually 97% effective. Factors which have impact on actual effectivity of OCP.

- Method failure
- Service provider
- Vomiting and diarrhea
- Client factor
- Drug interaction
- Expired pills.

Failure rate declines as duration of use and age of user increases.

Centchroman (Saheli: Centron 30 mg tab): Nonsteroidal estrogen antagonist developed by CDRI probably inhibits implantation. Failure rate 1–3%. Endocrine function does not alter. Dose 30 mg biweekly for 3 months then once a week so long pregnancy is not required. If pregnancy occurs with centchroman it should be terminated.

Adverse Effects of OCP

a. *Less serious side effects:* Nausea, vomiting

b. *Serious side effects*

- **Cardiovascular:** BP rise; myocardial infarction, cerebral and venous thrombosis (particularly in smokers).
- **Increased risk of cervical cancer** (risk increases with the duration of use of OCP).
- **Metabolic:** Decreases HDL, impaired glucose tolerance and decreased clotting factors, chloasma.
- **Liver:** Hepatocellular adenoma and gallbladder disease, cholestatic jaundice.
- Adversely affect constituents of breast milk and premature lactation suppression.
- **Subsequent fertilities:** Slight delay in conception (prolong use more than 5–10 years affects subsequent fertility). Ectopic pregnancies are common with progesterone pills, the birth defects are not substantiated.

Breast tenderness, weight gain, headache and migraine, breakthrough or spotting in early cycles, pruritis valvae, mood swings, abdominal distension, chloasma, carbohydrate intolerance.

Contraindications of OCP

a. **Absolute:** Cancer of breast and genitalis, history of liver disease and thromboembolism, cardiac disease, hyperlipidemia, undiagnosed uterine bleeding, porphyria, impending surgery, malignancy.

b. **Relative contraindications:** Special problems requiring medical surveillance—age over 40, smokers, hypertension, kidney disease, epilepsy, migraine, diabetes mellitus, gallbladder disease, nursing mother in first 6 months, history of infrequent bleeding, amenorrhea, varicose vein.

Depot formulations

A. Injectable contraceptives are of two types

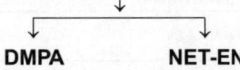

DMPA   NET-EN

- **Depot medroxyprogesterone acetate (DMPA):** 150 mg IM every 3 months protects for 3 months. Some countries does not allow DMPA because of effects on subsequent pregnancies.
- **Nor-ethisterone enanthate (NET-EN):** 200 mg IM every 60 days. Failure rate slightly higher than DMPA.
- **Long acting progestin + long acting estrogen:** Given once in a month with combination of medroxyprogesterone acetate and estradiol cypionate allowing reasonable menstrual bleeding. Long acting estrogen is more hazardous.

  Administration: The initial injections should be given during first 5 days of the cycle to rule out pregnancy in gluteus maximus. The site should not be massaged.

B. • **Subdermal implants:** Norplant-6 silastic (silicone rubber capsules) containing 36 mg each of levonorgestrel, more recent devices comprise fabrication of levonorgestrel into 2 small rods.

- **Norplants:** These are inserted beneath the skin of the forearm provide contraception for 5 years or which reverse after withdrawal of the implants. Requirement of surgical procedure and irregular menstrual bleeding are the main disadvantages.

C. Vaginal ring: Vaginal ring containing levonorgestrel has been found to be effective. Absorbed hormones through vaginal mucosa bypass digestive system and liver, so less doses are required. Ring kept in vagina for three cycles and removed in the fourth.

Etonogestrel + Ethinylestradiol (Nuva ring) contains estrogen and progestogen and protects pregnency for month. It is non-biodegradable, flexible and colorless. It does not protect HIV or STD.

Table 92.1: Some female oral contraceptives preparation available in market

Trade name	Contains
Combined pills	
Mala N	Norethisterone acetate 1 mg + ethinyl-estradiol 0.03 µg
Mala D	Norgestrel 0.30 mg + ethinylestradiol 30 µg
Orgalutin	Lynesternol 2.5 mg + ethinylestradiol 50 µg
Ovral G	Norgestrel 0.5 mg + ethinylestradiol 50 µg
Ovral	Levonorgestrel 0.25 mg + ethinyl-estradiol 50 µg
Ovral L	Levonorgestrel 0.15 mg + ethinyl-estradiol 30 µg
Novelon	Desogestrel 0.15 mg + Ethinylestra-diol 30 µg
Phased pills	
Triquilar	Levonorgestrel 50–75–125 mg + ethinylestradiol 30–40–30 µg (6 + 5 + 10 tabs)
Mini pills	
Micronor	Norethindrone 0.35 mg
Ovrette	Norgestrel 75 µg

Advantages and Disadvantages of OCP

Advantages

- Highly effective, if taken correctly.
- Safe for most women
- Reversible
- Independent of coitus
- Significant non-contraceptive benefit (protects ovarian and endometric cancer and PID)
- Reduce risk of functional ovarian cyst, fibroadenoma and ectopic pregnancy.

Disadvantages

- Require regular and dependable supply
- Client motivation
- No protection for STD and HIV
- Not appropriate for lactating mother
- Expensive
- Minor side effects in first 3 months. Amenorrhea, nausea, breast tenderness, headache, weight gain, depression may occur.

Different Male Pill Approaches Are

- Prevent spermatogenesis
- Interferes with sperm storage and maturation
- Prevent sperm transport
- Alter constituents of seminal fluds.
- Cytotoxic drug: Nitrofurans; indoles, cadmium suppress spermatogenesis.
- Estrogen and progesterone by inhibiting Gn release (may cause feminizations).
- Androgen: Will decrease Gn, but not reliable.
- Superactive GnRH inhibits Gn release, but also suppresses testosterone release.

Gossypol: Obtained from cotton seed oil, non-steroidal, orally effective male contraceptive, suppresses spermatogenesis and motility. Fertilization restores after several months of discontinuation. Dose 20 mg/day × 3 months followed by 40–60 mg/weekly.

Edema, diarrhea, breathlessness, neuritis, muscular weakness due to K loss may occur.

93

Drugs in Lactating Mother

Administration of drugs to lactating mother may have ill-effects on suckling infant or may affect the lactation, depending upon entry of drug in milk in pharmacologically significant amounts.

There are various ways to minimize the effect of medication in lactating mother:

- Prescribe safer alternatives
- Avoid breastfeeding at times of peak medication level in the blood, *i.e.* complete breastfeeding and take the medicine.
- Temporarily withheld drug, if it is contraindicated then express out of milk to maintain production in the mother.
- **Breastfeeding contraindicated for:** Gold salts, anticancer and radioactive substances (stop breastfeeding temporarily)
- **Monitor baby for possible adverse drug effects**
- Psychiatric drugs and anticonvulsants.

- **Alternatives should be used, if possible:** Metronidazole, quinolone, antibiotics, tetracycline, chloramphenicol.
- **Monitor baby for jaundice:** Dapsone, sulfonamide, cotrimoxazole fansider.
- **Drugs which may affect milk production:** Thiazides, ergometrine, estrogen and estrogen containing contraceptives.
- **Monitor baby for these drugs** are most commonly used drugs like analgesic, antipyretic, otherwise safe. Paracetamol, aspirin, morphine, pethidine, cough and cold remedies, antibiotics (ampicillin, cloxacillin and penicillin) antileprotic, antitubercular, erythromycin, antimalarial (except mefloquine), antihelminth, antifungal, bronchodilator (salbutamol), corticosteroid, antihistaminics, antacids, antidiabetics, antihypertensives, digoxin, nutrition, supplement of iodine, iron, vitamins.

94

Drugs Acting on Uterus and Oxytocin

The myometrium of uterus supplied by sympathetic and parasympathetic divisions of automatic nervous system and the drug affecting them can affect motility of the uterus. The most important group of drugs affecting endometrium are estrogen and progesterone.

UTERINE STIMULANTS

The drugs which increase the uterine motility also called *oxytocics, ecbolics, abortifacients.*

It can be classified as follows:

Oxytocics (All ergots are not oxytocics)

a. Ergot alkaloids
  - Amino acid alkaloids (ergotamine, ergosine)
  - Dihydrogenated amino acid alkaloid (dihydroergotamine, hydergine)
  - Amine alkaloid (ergometrine)
b. Posterior pituitary hormone
  - Oxytocin
c. Prostaglandins
  - PGE$_2$
  - PGF$_2\alpha$
  - 15-methyl-1-PGF$_2\alpha$
  - Misoprostol
d. Miscellaneous
  - Ethacridine
  - Quinine
  - Spartine sulfate
  - Hypertonic saline.

ERGOT ALKALOIDS

Ergot or *Claviceps purpura* is a fungus grown in rye or other grains, consumption of which may cause dry gangrene, stillbirth or abortion (saint Anthony's fire). It is a storehouse of pharmacological constituents like histamine, tyramine, acetylcholine, steroids, quarternary ammonium bases and acids.

Levorotatory alkaloids are pharmacologically active.

Pharmacological Actions of Ergot

- **Uterus:** All ergots stimulate uterus and response depends upon uterine maturity and stages of gestation. The amine alkaloid (ergotamine) is devoid of significant adrenergic blocking, vasoconstrictor, and emetic activity. Orally active. They increase tone of cervix in contrast to oxytocin which decreases it.

- **Vascular action:** Adrenergic blocking (except in amine alkaloids), peripheral vasoconstrictor

- **GI tract:** Ergotamines increase peristalsis and potentiate the action of neostigmine.

- **Miscellaneous:** Amine and amino acid ergot are 5HT antagonists. Methysergide is an ergometrine derivative, used clinically as 5HT antagonist.

Amino acid alkaloids, dehydrogenated derivative alkaloids are erratically absorbed from GI tract. Amine alkaloids are orally absorbed and their uterine stimulate effect starts 10–15 minutes of oral; 3–5 minutes of SC and 1–2 minutes of IV administration.

Probably they are metabolized in liver and degradation product excreted through kidney.

Adverse reactions: Ergometrine and methyl ergometrine are less toxic than ergotamine and hardly produces any complication.

Nausea, vomiting, rise in BP, milk secretion decrease. It should be used with caution in vascular disease, hypertension, toxemia, liver and kidney diseases. Contraindicated in pregnancy before 3rd stage of labor.

Treatments of Toxicities of Ergots

- Withdrawal of ergotamine
- Antiemetics
- Vasodilators like tolazoline and Na- nitroprusside
- Anticoagulants like heparin.

Therapeutic Uses of Ergot

- Postpartum hemorrhage
- After cesarean section or instrumental delivery to prevent uterine atony
- Uterine involution (ergometrine is used)
- Migraine (ergotamine is used)
- Hypertension (dihydrogenated derivatives are used)
- Bromergocryptine (2-bromo-α-ergocryptine), a semisynthetic ergot alkaloid has dopaminergic agonist, inhibits lactation. Oral dose 2.5 mg 2–3 times daily, uses are discussed earlier.

Preparation: Ergometrine 0.5 mg tab; 0.5 mg/mL methylergometrine (methregine, metharone) 0.125 mg tab, 0.2 mg/mL inj.

Oxytocin: Oxytocin is an octapeptide hormone of posterior pituitary secreted along with ADH. Both are synthesized in supraoptic, paraventricular nucleus of hypothalamus and transported to posterior pituitary through nerve ending for storage. Oxytocin is released on stimuli such as coitus, parturition, suckling.

Carbetocin: It is a long acting oxytocin analogue used after cesarean section or after PPH.

Physiological Roles of Oxytocin

Labor: It is released during labor to play a facilitatory role. PG and PAF are complementary to it in labor. Oxytocin acts on G-protein coupled oxytocin receptor which causes depolarization of muscles fiber due to influx of Ca^{2+} ions. IP_3 also mediates rise of intracellular calcium. The receptor for oxytocin increases in later part of pregnancy. Distinct types of oxytocin receptors present in myometrium and endometrium. Progesterone decreases its sensitivity.

Milk let down reflex: Myoepithelial cells are sensitive to oxytocin in milk let down process.

Neurotransmission: It appears in functioning as a peptide neurotransmitter in hypothalamus and brain stem.

Pharmacological Actions of Oxytocin

Uterus: It increases frequency and force of contraction, basal tone which increases with higher doses. Estrogen sensitizes uterus to oxytocin and progesterone decreases it. The fundus and body are contracted, but lower segment relaxes.

Breast: Oxytocin contracts myoepithelial cells to contract and helps in milk let down process.

CVS: Higher doses cause vasodilatation and brief fall in BP, tachycardia, flushing. These effects are blocked by vasopressin. It constricts umbilical vessels.

Kidney: Urine output decreases because of constriction of renal cortical vessels in presence of estrogens.

Pharmacokinetics: Has to be given IM or IV or by intranasal spray. Orally not absorbed because it is a peptide. It is degraded in liver. Pregnant uterus and placenta elaborate aminopeptidase called oxytokinase to inactivate it.

Adverse Reactions of Oxytocin

- Water intoxication
- Maternal and fetal soft tissue injury, rupture uterus. Fetal asphyxia due to violent uterine contraction. Pituitary shock is due to vasopressin by the use of posterior pituitary extract, not due to oxytocin.

1 IU of oxytocin = 2 μg of pure hormone (oxytocin, syntocinon 2 IU/2 mL or 5 IU/mL inj.)

Uses of Oxytocin

Available as oxytocin 2 IU/2 mL and 5 IU/mL. 1 IU = 2 μg of pure hormone used IV or IM because it is peptide ineffective orally.

- Induction of labor: 5 IU diluted in 5% dextrose or saline (10 milli IU/mL) infusion at slow rate, increased gradually to induce labor in post-maturity, toxemia, placental insufficiency, diabetic mother, erythroblastosis. Before infusion note that presentation is correct, no placenta previa, no fetal distress or cepha-lopelvic disproportion.
- Uterine inertia
- Postpartum hemorrhage (ergometrine preferred), if hypertensive or ergometrine is contraindicated.
- Abortion
- For breast engorgement intranasal spray is given.
- Oxytocin challenge test to determine utero-placental insufficiency where infusion of oxytocin markedly increase fetal heart rate.

Desamino oxytocin used as buccal formulation (Buctocin 50 IU tab) used for induction of labor, 50 IU tab every ½ hour max up to 10 tabs; uterine inertia 25 IU tab every ½ hour; breast engorgement 1 tab before breastfeeding; uterine involution 25–50 IU 5 times for 7 days.

PROSTAGLANDINS

They stimulate uterine contraction at any stage of pregnancy. PGF2α, E1 and E2 are used.

Nausea, vomiting, diarrhea, vasodilatation, headache, fever may occur.

Uses of Prostaglandins as Ecbolics

- Induction of labor
- Therapeutic abortion

Ethacrydine (vecredil; emcreidil): 50 mg/ 50 mL used by extra-amniotic infusion for medical termination of pregnancy (3–20 weeks of pregnancy).

Quinine: Not used therapeutically as ecbolics.

Spartein sulfate: Alkaloid obtained from flowering broom, apart from antiarrhythmic activity, has oxytocic property. Administered IM 100–600 mg. Inactivated quickly. Uterine contraction does not stimulate oxytocins. Fetal injury, cervical laceration can occur.

Hypertonic saline: Intra-amniotic adminis-tration of 100–250 mL of 20% hypertonic saline is introduced after withdrawing equal amount of amniotic fluid through transabdominal approach. Induces labor in 24–36 hours. Used for MTP in 13–20 weeks of pregnancy.

Hypertonic (40%) urea aminofusion used for MTP. Should not be used in kidney disease patient.

95

Uterine Relaxants

Drugs decreasing uterine motility are called tocolytics used for delaying labor, threatened abortion or dysmenorrhea.

Drugs are

- **Adrenergic agonist** (Ritodrine, yutopar, ritodine 10 mg/mL amp or 10 mg tab). Started with 50 mg/min IV, increases gradually till uterine contraction ceases or maternal HR increases to 120/min. Delivery can be postponed by it in 70% of cases by week. Hypotension, anxiety, restlessness, headache, neonatal hyperglycemia, pulmonary edema, hypokalemia may occur. Salbutamol, and terbutaline fenoterol, orciprenaline may be used as tocolytics. Isoxsuprine used orally or IM to prevent or stop threatend abortion.
- **Prostaglandin synthesis inhibitors:** Aspirin, indomethacin, *etc.,* but may lead to intrauterine closure of ductus arteriosus and oligohydramnios.
- **Magnesium sulfate:** Given IV to control convulsion and hypertension in eclampsia 2–4 gm over 10–20 minutes followed by 1–2 gm/hour, reduces uterine contraction, but may produce muscular paralysis, cardiac arrhythmia, CNS and respiratory depression of mother and neonate.
- **Calcium channel blocker:** Nifedipine relaxes uterus and postpones labor. Tachycardia and hypotension may occur. Reduces placental perfusion to cause fetal hypoxia.
- **Progesterone:** Decreases sensitivity of uterus to oxytocin, used for habitual abortion.
- **Ethyl alcohol:** 10% of alcohol 0.8 gm/kg/hour IV delays labor. CNS depression and fetal hypoxia may occur.
- **Miscellaneous:** Nitrates, diazoxides, anticholinergics, general anesthetics, phenothiazine, *etc*. are used to reduce uterine contraction. Halothane used as general anesthetic which relaxes uterus also used for external and internal versions. Oxytocin receptor antagonist, **atosiban** peptide analogue has been found to reduce uterine contraction.

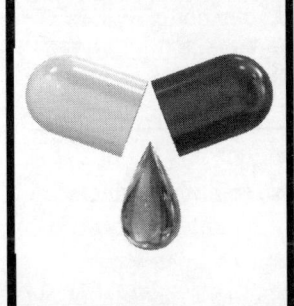
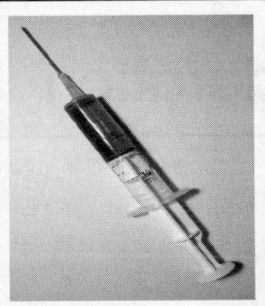
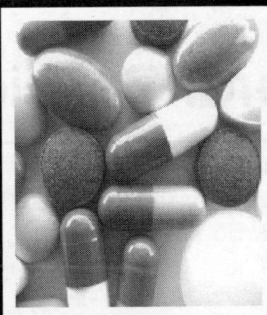
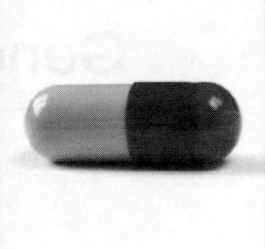

SECTION 13

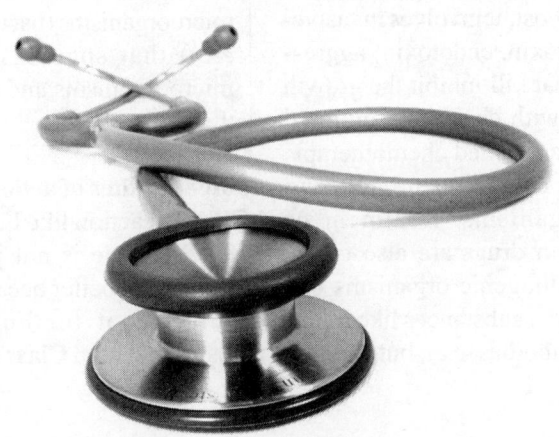

ANTIMICROBIALS
AND CHEMOTHERAPY

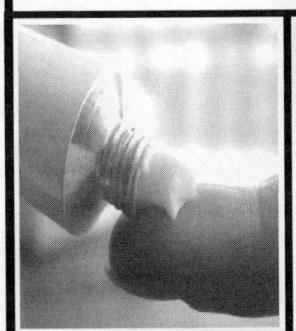
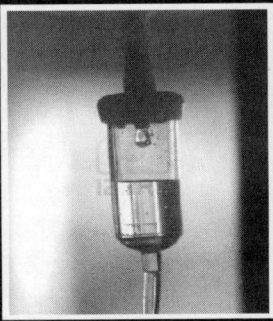
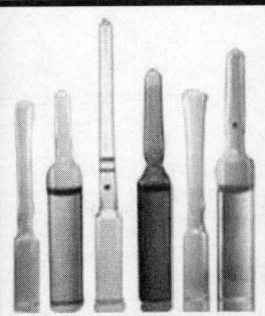
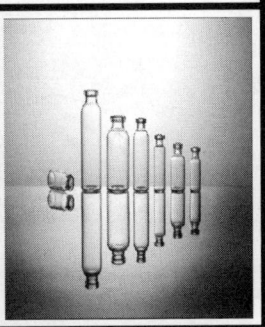

96

General Consideration

The history of antibiosis, *i.e.* substances obtained from one living organism can kill another in very low concentration is as old as microbiology. Microbes are greatest threat to mankind, because of their virulence [is the capacity of pathogenic bacteria to damage the host, it involves invasiveness and toxicity (exotoxin, endotoxin) aggressiveness]. The drugs that kill/inhibit the growth of infecting organism with or without minimal effect on the recipient are called chemotherapy. Because of similarity of malignant cells and pathogenic microorganisms, treatment of neoplastic diseases with drugs are also called chemotherapy. The pathogenic organisms can also produce other natural substances like H_2O_2, lactic acid, ethanol, antibodies, *etc.*, but they are

required in higher concentration and are not designated as antibiotics.

> By definition, antibiotics are chemical substances produced by various species of microorganisms (bacteria, fungi, actinomyces, *etc.*) that suppress the growth of other microorganisms and may eventually destroy them.

Potential sites of action of antibacterial drugs: **Class I** reaction like Emden-Meyerhof pathway of TCA cycle is not promising site. **Class II** reaction are better because some are specific for bacteria not for human calls, *viz.* folate biosynthesis and **Class III** reaction which is good

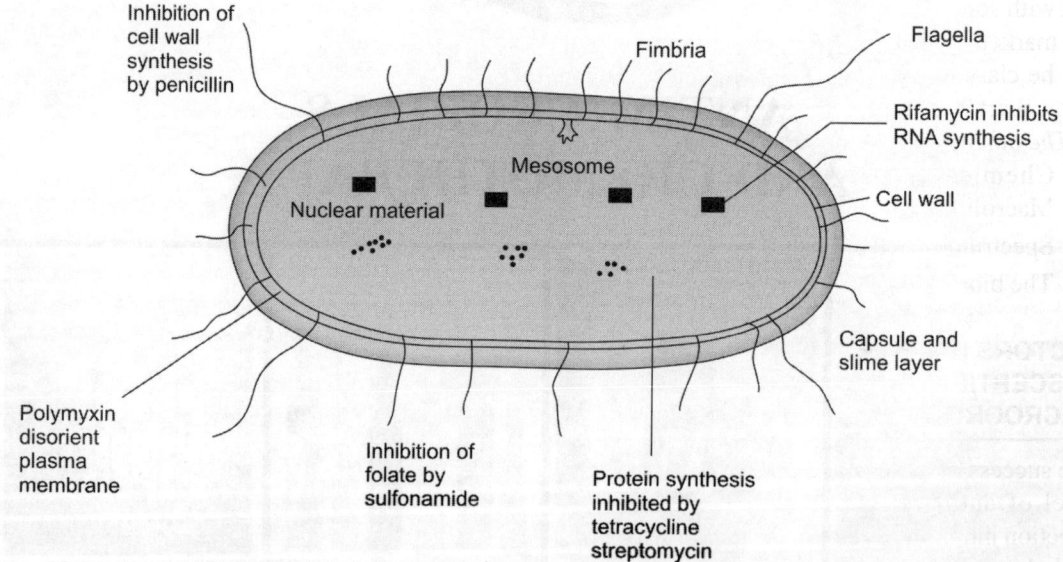

Fig. 96.1: Structure of a bacteria and site of action of different antimicrobials

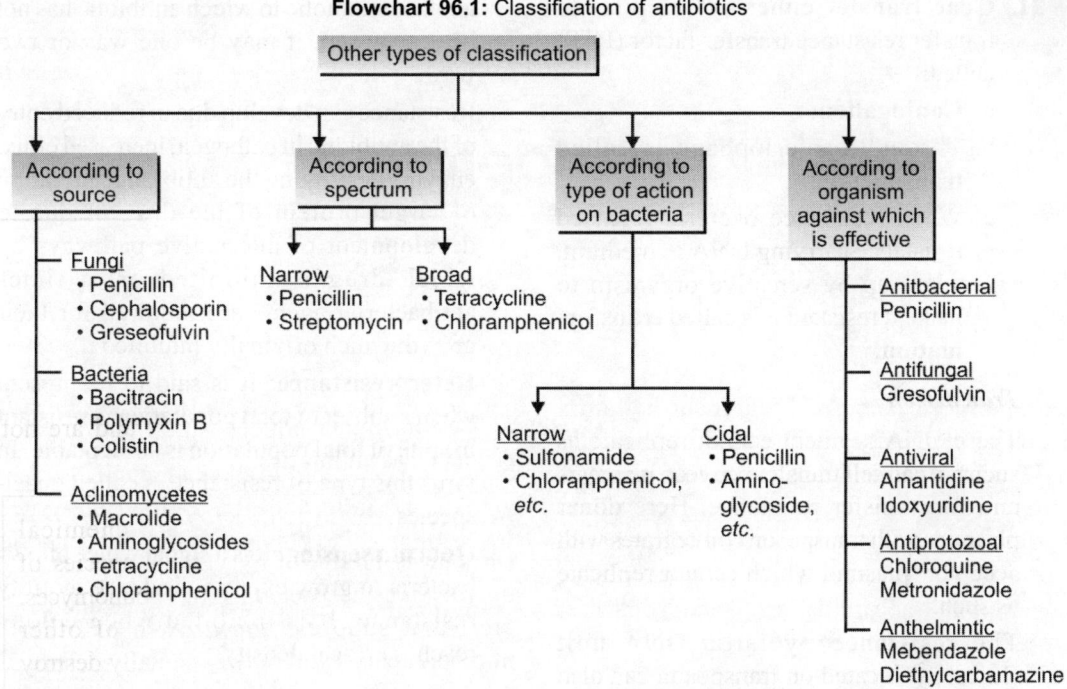

Flowchart 96.1: Classification of antibiotics

Other types of classification

According to source
- Fungi
  - Penicillin
  - Cephalosporin
  - Greseofulvin
- Bacteria
  - Bacitracin
  - Polymyxin B
  - Colistin
- Aclinomycetes
  - Macrolide
  - Aminoglycosides
  - Tetracycline
  - Chloramphenicol

According to spectrum
- Narrow
  - Penicillin
  - Streptomycin
- Broad
  - Tetracycline
  - Chloramphenicol

According to type of action on bacteria
- Narrow
  - Sulfonamide
  - Chloramphenicol, etc.
- Cidal
  - Penicillin
  - Amino-glycoside, etc.

According to organism against which is effective
- Anitbacterial Penicillin
- Antifungal Gresofulvin
- Antiviral Amantidine Idoxyuridine
- Antiprotozoal Chloroquine Metronidazole
- Anthelmintic Mebendazole Diethylcarbamazine

target *viz* synthesis of peptidoglycan by bacteria not by eukaryotes.

Antibiotics are the greatest contribution to the medical therapeutics, and about 30% of all hospitalized patients receive one or more course of antibiotics and unfortunately they are the common abused drugs. There are about 100 antibiotics or chemotherapeutics at the market and with some 100 are in pipeline to come up in the market. For the sake of convenience, they can be classified in one of the following ways (Flowchart 96.1).

The other way of classification are:

i. Chemical structure, *viz*. Betalactam, Macrolide, *etc.*

ii. Spectrum of activity .

iii. The biochemical pathway it interfere.

FACTORS DETERMINING SUSCEPTIBILITY AND RESISTANCE OF MACROORGANISMS TO ANTIMICROBIALS

The success of antibiotic therapy depends upon level of antibacterial activity at the site of infection inhibiting bacteria in a manner that tips the balance in favor of host.

1. **Acquired resistance**: The spectrum of antibiotic activity gradually decreases or lost because of ingenious alterations that allow them to survive in presence of antibiotics is called **resistance**. Some organisms are always resistant to a particular antibiotics, *viz.* penicillin never effective against gram-negative organism called **natural resistance**. Acquired resistance is a clinical problem when antibiotics are no more effective in an organism in which it was effective before, is called **acquired resistance** which may develop quickly or gradually, gonococci develop resistance to sulfonamide quickly and penicillin gradually.

Resistance develops due to

I. **Mutation:** Sudden change in gene either by single step or multiple steps by insertion, deletion or substitution of one or more nucleotides within the genome which may persist or be corrected by organism. One example of rifampicin resistant M tuberculosis when rifampicin is used as single antituberculous drug.

II. Gene transfer either by sex pilus to transfer resistance transfer factor (RTF) called:

  a. **Conjugation**

  b. Through bacteriophage is called **transduction**.

  c. When resistance bacteria released resistance carrying DNA in medium, taken up by sensitive organism to make it resistant it is called **transformation**.

Transposon

These DNA segment cannot replicate as such but can self transfer between plasmids and can transfer resistance. Here donar plasmids with transposon cointegrates with acceptor plasmid which cannot replicate as such.

The resistance by large DNA unit (Integron) located on transposon can also occur. Transposon can only transfer resistance genes only in present of integron as integron lacks transporter genes.

Resistant organism can be

- **Drug tolerant:** When affinity for target microorganisms start liberating enzymes to destroy the antibiotics, *viz.* gonorrhea by β-lactamase or efflux of the drug is increased.

- Permeability of drug into bacteria is lost. Through specific channel called 'porins'.

Five major systems of efflux pumps which are relevant to antimicrobials.

  i. **MATE:** Multidrug and Toxic compound extruder.

  ii. **MFS:** Major facilitator super family transporters.

  iii. **SMR:** Small multidrug resistance system.

  iv. **RND:** Resistance nodulation division exporters.

  v. **ABC:** ATP binding cassette transporters.

Cross-resistance is a condition when resistance to one antibiotic confers resistance to another antibiotic to which antibiotic has not been exposed, it may be one way or two ways.

Resistance can develop due to reduced entry of the antibiotic in pathogen, increased efflux, enzyme destroying the antibiotic, alteration of target protein of the drug or due to development of alternative pathways by which drug is inhibited or at times antibacterial agents are required for their growth which originally inhibited it.

Heteroresistance: It is said to be present when a subset of total population is resistant in spite of total population is susceptable. In virus this type of resistance is called quasi-species.

Quorum sensing: It is a signal which allows bacteria to grow express virulence motility resistance. It is inhibited when colony reaches critical density.

Antibiotics resistance can be prevented by

• Discriminate use of antibiotics with adequate antibiotics for right period.
• Preference should be made for rapid acting, selective narrow spectrum antibiotics.
• Notorious to produce antibiotic resistance producing organism should be treated with multiple drugs.

2. **Superinfection:** Normal flora contributing host defence by elaborating bacteriocin may be lost by the use of antibiotics, producing new infection. More common with broad-spectrum antibiotics and indiscriminate use of antibiotics for trivial, self-limiting or untreatable (viral) infections or unnecessary prolonging antibiotic therapy. Super-infections are common in:

- Simultaneous corticosteroid therapy
- AIDS
- Agranulocytosis
- Diabetes and DLE
- Leukemia and other malignant conditions.

3. **Nutritional deficiency:** Antibiotics may alter the intestinal flora which produces

vitamin B complex and vitamin K causing their deficiency. Neomycin may cause steatorrhea.

4. **Pharmacokinetic factors:** Success of antibiotic therapy depends upon minimal toxicity to the host which depends upon several pharmacokinetic factors.

The location of infection to a large extent may dictate the choice of drugs and routes of administration; *viz.* Levofloxacin is better penetrated in urine than respiratory and skin so most effective in UTI.

- **Minimal inhibitory concentration (MIC):** Lowest concentrations of antibiotic that prevent visible growth at 18–24 hours of incubation is called MIC.
- **Minimal bactericidal concentration (MBC):** Lowest concentration that results in 99.9% decline in bacterial numbers or that sterilizes the medium is known as minimal bactericidal concentration (MBC).

    The minimal drug concentration achieved at infected site should be equal to MIC for the infecting organism. Some advice 4–8 times of this concentration.

- **Access of antibiotics** increases in some pathological conditions and may favor antibiotic therapy, *e.g.* in meningitis, permeability of drug through blood-brain barrier to CNS for penicillin increases.

Antibiotic penetrating infection site is proportional to free drug concentration of extracellular fluid. The protein-bound drugs do not penetrate to the same extent. There are controversies whether antibacterial activity at the site of infection by constant level is superior to that of peak concentration followed by subinhibitory activity by pulse therapy.

5. **Routes of administration:** Oral route is preferred except for unconscious patient or antibiotics not effective orally (streptomycin).

6. **Host factors:** At times prime determinants of antibiotic therapy along with dose are route of administration, risk and nature of untoward effects and therapeutic effectiveness.

7. **Age:** Certain antibiotics should be avoided in childhood, *viz.* chloramphenicol (may produce gray baby syndrome); tetracycline may accumulate in bones and teeth of growing children.

8. **In disease states of liver (organ for metabolism) and kidney (organ of excretion),** caution for dose adjustment or its use should be avoided which involves these two organs for their metabolism or excretion.

9. **Local factors:** Pus, which contains PABA decreases efficiency of sulfonamide. Penicillin, tetracycline, cephalosporin, *etc.* bind to hematoma and they foster growth of bacteria, therefore, decrease their efficiency. Local penetrating barrier, as in prostate, hampers access of antibiotics.

10. **Pregnancy:** Intelligentsia should be applied in selection of antibiotics in pregnancy. Penicillin and cephalosporin are safe. Rest all have risk to the fetus or mother.

11. **Genetic factors:** Nitrofurantoin, sulfonamide produce hemolysis in glucose $6PO_4$-deficient patient.

12. **Organism-related factors:** Clinical diagnosis and bacteriological effect direct the choice of antibiotics. Bacteriocidal, less toxic, less expensive antibiotics are preferred.

Combination of antibioitic therapy

Purposes

- To achieve synergism
- To reduce adverse effects
- To prevent resistance
- To broaden spectrum
- To reduce cost of therapy
- For reducing chances of superinfection
- In mixed bacterial infection.

Generally, the bacteriocidal drugs are effective in multiplying bacteria, a bacteriostatic drug may reduce its efficiency. It is postulated, if a bacteriostatic drug is added to the bacteriocidal drug, two things may occur.

Flowchart 96.2

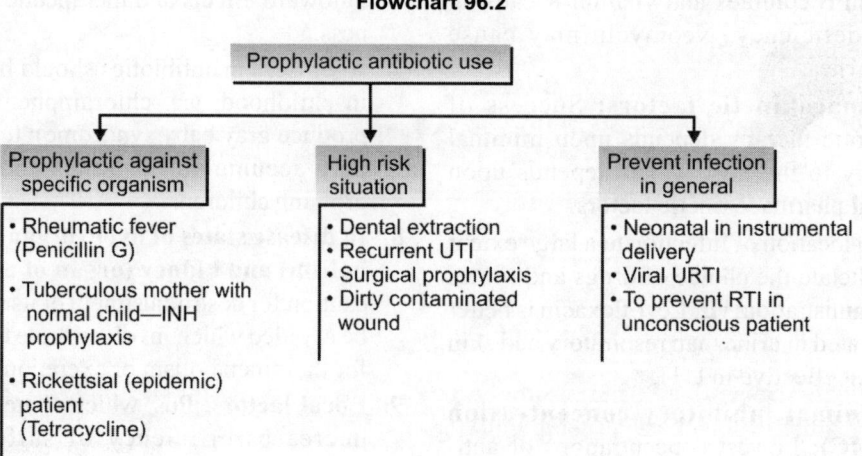

- If organisms are highly sensitive to bactericidal drugs, antagonism may occur.
- If the organism is relatively resistant to bacteriocidal drug, additional action may occur.

Combination of two bacteriocidal drugs among themselves produces synergism. However, clinical data regarding combination of antibiotics are limited. **Synergism:** The concentrations are less than 25% of MIC of each drug acting alone to produce inhibitions shown by concave curve.

$$FIC = \frac{MIC \text{ of } A \text{ with } B}{MIC \text{ of } A \text{ alone}} + \frac{MIC \text{ of } B \text{ with } A}{MIC \text{ of } B \text{ alone}}$$

or vice versa

FIC = Fractional inhibiting concentration

Table 96.1: Antibiotics inhibiting bacterial protein synthesis by acting on 30s and 50s ribosomal subunits

30s subunits	50s subunits
Aminoglycoside	Chloramphenicol
Tetracycline	Erythromycin
Spectinomycin	Macrolide
	Spiramycin
	Pristinamycin
	Fusidic acid
	Virginiamycin
	Clindamycin

Addition: Half of the concentration required to produce inhibition shown by straight line.

Antagonism: More than half of each drug is required to produce inhibition shown by convex curve (Fig. 96.2).

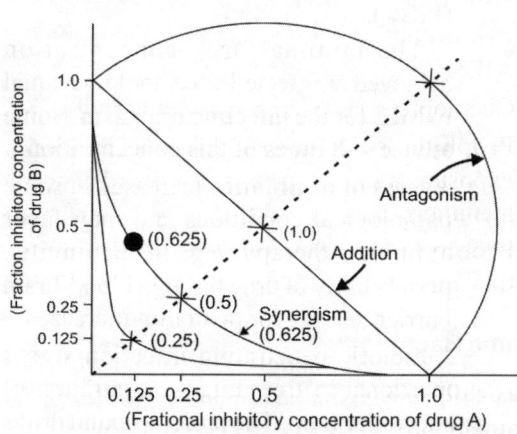

Fig. 96.2

Risk of antibiotic combination

- Increased risk of superinfection
- Emergence to resistance to multiple drugs
- Increased risk for toxicity
- Sense of false security may lead to incomplete and inadequate therapy.
- Increases cost of therapy.

Antibiotic Prophylaxis

Though the prophylactic use of antimicrobial may produce resistance or superinfection it is given in the following situations (Flowchart 96.2).

Failure of chemotherapeutics: Failure of chemotherapeutic may occur in the following conditions:

• Treatment began late with improperly selected antimicrobial, through improper route, in wrong dose for wrong duration.

• Poor host defence or infection is behind the barrier.

• Trying to treat untreatable (viral, malignant or collagen) fever with antimicrobial.

• Altered organism may produce relapse

• Drain abscess otherwise there will be failure of antimicrobial therapy.

• **Prophylactic therapy** of antibiotic therapy can also groups an follows:

• **Prophylactic** in immune compromised or AIDS.

• Chemoprophylaxis in surgical procedure.

• Prophylaxis in healthy person, *i.e.* post exposure, *viz.* rifampicin in meningococcal meningitis contacted people.

• Prophylaxis in mother to child from transmission of HIV.

Some Bacteriostatic and Bactericidal Drugs

Basically bacteriostatic drugs: Sulfonamide, Trimethoprum, Sulfones, Tetracyclines, Chloramphenicol, Linocomycin, Clindamycin.

Some basically bactericidal drugs: Cotrimoxazole, Penicillin, Cephalosporin, Streptomycin, Bacitracin, Vancomycin.

Concentration dependent effect: INH, Erythromycin, Novabiocin.

Principles of antibiotic dosing: Folloiwng four characteristics influence the antibiotic dosing: (i) Minimum inhibitory concentration (MIC), the definition of which given earlier, (ii) concentration dependent killing effect (CDKE). Some antibiotics are more effective in higher concentration (CDKE), (iii) Time dependent killing effect (TDKE) in some antibiotics are more effective if given for a longer period and (iv) post-antibiotic effect (PAE) which is suppression of bacterial growth after brief period of antibiotic exposure.

The different groups are:

Group I : Agents showing CDKE and prolonged PAE are given at higher dose with wider dose intervals, *viz.* gentamicin.

Group II : Time dependent killing effect with shorter PAE—they require frequent dosing, *viz.* penicillin.

Group III : Showing time dependent killing effect with prolong PAE—here the killing effectiveness is not compromised, if concentration falls below MIC as because they have longer PAE, *viz.* longer acting macrolides like clarithromycin or azithromycin.

97

Sulfonamides

Sulfonamides were first antibacterial agents effective against pyogenic infection. Domagk first cured his daughter with prontosil suffering streptococcal septicemia. All sulfonamides may be considered to be the derivatives of sulfanilamide, para-amino benzene sulfonamide $-SO_2-NH_2$ group. Chemically, antibacterial activity depends on:

$$NH_2 - \bigcirc - SO_2 - NH_2$$

- Potentially free para-amino group
- Direct link of the sulfur atom of the sulfonamide group with benzene ring.

The individual member differs in the nature of N-substitution which governs solubility, potency and pharmacokinetic properties.

Sulfonamides are effective against variety of gram-positives and gram-negatives. Chlamydia infections like *Strepto, Staphylo, Gono, Pneumo, H. ducreyi, Vibrio, E. coli, P. pestis, Shigella, Donavania, Nocardia, Actinomyces, Toxoplasma, Chlamydia, Trachoma, Psitacosis.*

Mechanism of action: It competetively inhibits bacterial folate synthetase, being the structural analogue of PABA, with pteridine residue to form dihydropteroic acid which conjugates to glutamic acid to produce dihydrofolic acid. It may get incorporated to form an altered folate, which is metabolically injurious. Bacteria as well as sexual forms of malaria cannot use preformed folic acid. Tetrahydrofolic acid is essential for bacterial

Flowchart 97.1

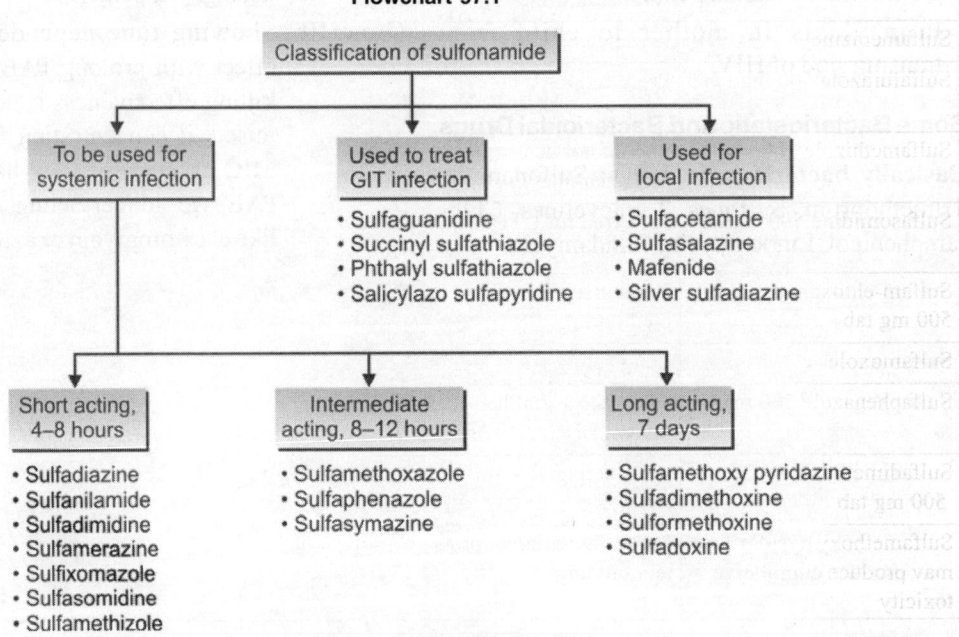

growth and one carbon transfer in nucleic acid synthesis.

Resistance: Occurs due to mutations, producing increased PABA, decreased affinity for sulfonamide to folate synthetase or follow alternate path for folate metabolism.

Pharmacokinetics: Sulfonamides intended for systemic use are rapidly absorbed from GI tract. Absorption from abraded skin, respiratory tract or vagina is variable. They are protein-bound which determines its period of activity. Free sulfonamides attain same concentration in all tissues including CSF and placenta. They are acetylated by non-microsomal enzymes in liver (some are slow and some are fast acetylators according to pharmacogenetic). It is excreted in urine. Acidic urine produces crystalluria, so urine has to be alkalized to avoid its deposition.

Adverse effects of sulfonamide: Nausea, vomiting, epigastric pain, crystalluria, hyper-sensitivity (arthritis, serum sickness, polyarthritis nodosa) photosensitization, Stevens-Johnson syndrome. Exfoliative dermatitis, hepatitis, hemolysis in glucose $6PO_4$-deficient patient, neutropenia, blood dyscrasia, kernicterus in premature babies.

Therapeutic uses of sulfonamides: UTI, streptopharyngitis, trachoma, lymphogranuloma venerium, malaria (combined with pyrimethamine), toxoplasmosis, nocardiosis, burns (topical silver sulfadiazine), bacillary dysentery.

Therapeutic utility of sulfonamide is determined by

• Absorption from GIT.
• Degree of protein binding
• Rate of renal excretion
• Host resistance, presence of pus
• Type of pathogenic organism
• Toxic potential and cost of therepy.

Table 97.1: Some commonly used sulfonamides

Name	Properties	Adult dose	Children dose
Sulfadiazine	50% protein-bound, CSF penetration good	2–3 gm/day then 1 gm 6 hourly	150 mg/kg/day in 4–6 devided doses
Sulfadimidine	Acetyl derivative, soluble in urine	2–3 gm/day then 1 gm 6 hourly	–
Sulfamerazine	Less potent	–	–
Sulfafurazole 500 mg tab	Preferred for UTI	Start with 3 gm/day then 1.5 gm 6 hourly	60 mg/kg then 30 mg/kg 6 hourly
Sulfamethizole 100 mg tab	Should not be used with methenamine	0.1–0.2 gm 4–6 hourly	30–40 mg/kg/day in 4 divided doses
Sulfasomidine 500 mg tab	Preferred for UTI	Initially 3 gm then 1.5 6 hourly	1 gm then 0.25 gm 6 hourly above 10 years
Sulfam-ehtoxazole 500 mg tab	Combined with tri-methoprim	1–2 gm BD	–
Sulfamoxole	Long acting	0.5–1 gm BD	–
Sulfaphenazole 500 mg tab	Start with 1 gm then 0.5 gm BD	65 mg/kg then 30 mg BD	
Sulfadimethoxine 500 mg tab	Long acting, 0.5 gm/day	1 gm/day then 15 mg/kg	30 mg/kg
Sulfamethoxy pyridazine may produce cumulative toxicity	Long acting due to protein binding	1 gm OD then 0.5 gm OD	30 mg/kg followed by 15 mg/kg

Contd...

Table 97.1: Some commonly used sulfonamides (*Contd...*)

Name	Properties	Adult dose	Children dose
Sulformethoxine bound	Highly protein-bound	2 gm/week	–
Sulfaguanidine 500 mg	Not absorbed from GIT. Used for intestinal infection	3 gm/6 hourly	150 mg/kg in 24 hours
Succinyl-sulfathizole 500 mg tab	May impair vit. K synthesis. Do not absorbed from GIT.	10–20 gm/day	250 mg/kg/day
Phthalyl sulfathizole	Do not absorbed from GIT	5–10 gm/daily every 24 hours	50–100 mg/kg
Sulfasalazine	Used for ulcerative colitis	0.5–1 gm 6 hourly	–
Sulfacetamide 30% eye-drop or 6% eye oint	Used as 10%; 20%	–	–
Mafenide eye, nose, throat infections	Used topically in cellulose and 10% cream	It has 2.5% carbonic anhydrase inhibition properties	–
Silver sulfadiazine	1% cream in burn patient	–	–

Table 97.2: Injectable preparation of sulfonamide

Sulfadiazine Na	250 mg/mL	Dose (100 mg/kg IV)
Sulfadimidine	1 gm/3 mL (IM or IV)	2 gm/day
Sulfafurazole diolamine	400 mg/mL (IV or SC)	Dose same as oral

Cotrimoxazole
(Septran, Bactrim, Supristol)

Fixed dose combination of sulfamethoxazole and trimethoprim in the ratio of 5 : 1 is called **cotrimoxazole**, causes sequential block of folate metabolism. MIC of each component may be reduced by 3–6 times, additional organisms covered by combinations are *Salmonella, Serratia, Klebsiella, Enterobacter; Yersinia enterocolitica, Pneumocystis jiroveci, entero-pathogenic E. coli. H. infiuenzae, Gonococci and Meningococci, Staph, Strepto, Shigella.* Resistance occurs through mutation or plasmid-mediated DHFase. Combinations are less likely to produce resistance.

Mechanisms of action of cotrimoxazole

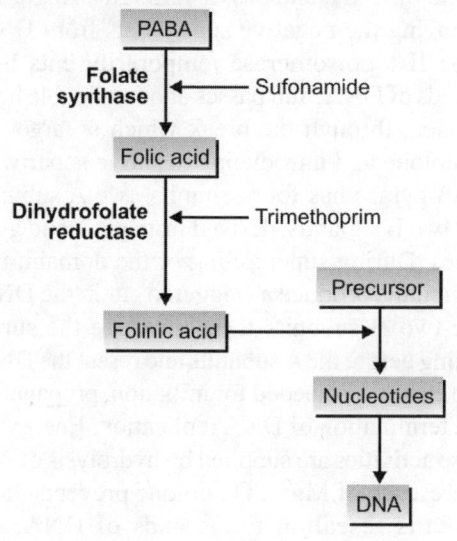

Cotrimazine (trimethoprim + sulfadiazine) (triglobe, ultrox): Mechanism and spectrum similar to cotrimoxazole.

Adverse effects: Nausea, vomiting, stomatitis, headache, rashes, folate deficiency, bone marrow, depression, thrombocytopenia, if given with diuretics.

Trimethoprim (tuliprim 100 and 200 mg tab): Used for UTI and prostatitis (because concen-trated in prostate). Some claims it is equally effective as combinations. Dose 100–200 mg BD.

Drug interactions of sulfonamide: Being protein-bound drug, it displaces other protein-bound drugs like phenytoin, warfarin, tolbuta-mide to increase their toxicities.

Pyrimethamine with sulfonamide combi-nation: Used for leishmaniasis; toxoplasmosis and for malaria. Dose interval should increase from 12 to 24 hours, if creatinine clearance is less than 30 mL/min and it should not be used, if less than 15 mL/min.

Therapeutic uses of cotrimoxazole: UTI; RTI; typhoid; bacterial diarrhea and dysentery; *Pneumocystis jiroveci;* chancroid. **Iclaprim** is a trimethoprim analogue given IV. It is better tolerated to trimethoprim and equally effective.

Fluoroquinolones

The second half of 20th century saw truly remarkable advances in antibacterial therapy, but unfortunately bacteria began to fight back in developing resistance towards antibacterial agents particularly by gram-negative bacteria and *Staphylococci*. Development of the entirely synthetic fluoroquinolone agents are active against many of these resistant organisms showing advancement towards fighting infection and they penetrate well into tissues and cells.

The first member, nalidixic acid discovered during the synthesis of chloroquine in 1962 by Hescher *et al.*

Fluoroquinolones: The first generation fluoroquinolone was introduced with one fluoro substitution in quinolone derivatives. Now a series of fluoroquinolones are in the market. These are bactericidal antimicrobial agents.

The quinolones are now classified on the basis of generation: The *1st generation* quinolones include nalidixic acid and cinoxacin are effective in gram-negative, but not to pseudomonas patients. *2nd generation* quinolones are Norfloxacin, Lomefloxacin, Enoxacin, Ofloxacin, Ciprofloxacin. Their spectrums include gram-negative including pseudomonas, some gram-positives like *Staph aureus*; *Strepto, Pneumoniae*. *3rd generation* quinolones are Levofloxacin, Sparfloxacin, Gatifloxacin, Moxifloxacin. Its spectrum is like second generation plus expanded gram-positive coverage and penicillin resistant *S. pueumoniae*. *4th generation* quinolones are Pazufloxacin, Grepafloxacin, Sitafloxacin, Clinafloxacin, Trovafloxacin. Their spectrums are like third generation plus anaerobic coverage.

MODE OF ACTION OF QUINOLONES

Quinolones selectively inhibit bacterial DNA synthesis by acting on the enzyme DNA gyrase. The enzyme is one of a group of topoisomerases which insert negative supercoils into DNA (*i.e.* against the normal direction of the DNA helix). The bacterial chromosomes comprise a molecule of DNA 1300 mm in length compressed in a cell of 1×2 mm in size. DNA strand intertwined 400,000 times have to be interwind during replication. Topoisomerase alters the linking number without changing the DNA molecule itself. All living cells contain two types of topoisomerase. Type I topoisomerase breaks one strand of DNA, and passes through a single gap removing the negative supertwists from DNA. Type II topoisomerase temporarily cuts both strands of DNA, and passes another double helix segment through the break which is target for quinolone and introducing negative supertwist. DNA gyrase has four subunits, two A subunits and two B subunits, derived from gyrA and gyrB genes. During supercoiling of the domain, two A subunits produce a staggered cut in the DNA. The two B subunits then introduce the supercoiling before the A subunits and reseal the DNA. The enzyme is needed for initiation, propagation and termination of DNA replication. Energy for these activities are supplied by hydrolysis of ATP in presence of Mg^{2+}. Quinolone prevents the A subunits resealing the strands of DNA, the compaction is reversed and the incorporation of precursors is stopped. The cells form filaments and the exposed breaks in the DNA promote the activity of exonucleases leading to cell death.

Quinolones bind more strongly to denatured and negatively supertwist DNA than to normal double strand DNA.

Resistance to quinolones: Not related to plasmids, drug inactivation or target modification due to chromosomal mutation or due to alteration of the quantity of type of porins in the outer membrane of gram-negative bacteria or due to reflux pump. Mutation in gyrA produces resistance to all quinolones. The resistance may occur unrelated to quinolones such as chloromycitin, tetracycline or β-lactam.

Nalidaxic acid (Gramoneg 0.5 mg tab, 0.3 gm/5 mL syr). Effective against gram-negative bacteria *E. coli, Proteus, Klebsiella, Shigella, Pseudomonas, Enterobacter.* Orally absorbed, plasma protein-bound, metabolized in liver, excreted in urine so effective for UTI.

Adverse effects: Rare GI upset, rashes, neurological toxicities (like headache, drowsiness, vertigo, seizure in children, parkinsonism), leukopenia, biliary stasis, hemolysis in G-6PD deficient patient, phototoxicity may occur. Used for UTI in sensitive patient. Nitrofuration antagonizes it. Also used for *Proteius, E. coli. Shigella, Salmonella* producing diarrhea. It is contraindicated in infants. Dose 0.5–1 gm TDS.

Norfloxacin: Used for urinary and genital tract infection and bacterial diarrhea. Single 800 mg dose recommended to cure gonorrhea. Not used for respiratory and other systemic gram-positive infection.

Ciprofloxacin: Second generation fluoroquinolones effective against *E. coli, Klebsiella, Salmonella, Shigella, Proteus, Neisseria gonorrhoeae* and *meningitides, Haemophilus (influenzae, ducreyi), Campylobacter; Yersinia, Vibrio* moderately sensitive to *Pseudomonas aeroginosa, Staph. aureus, Staph. epidermidis, Legionella, Listeria, Mycobacterium tuberculosis.*

Orally absorbed, food interferes with absorption. High tissue permeability in lung, sputum, bone, prostate, muscle. Urinary and biliary concentrations are higher than plasma.

Adverse effects: Nausea, vomiting, bad taste, dizziness, headache, anxiety, insomnia, confusion, tremor, seizure, rash, pruritis, photosensitivity, urticaria, tendonitis, cartilage damage. Withdrawal required in less than 1.5% of patient.

Drug interaction: Antacids, iron and sucralfate reduce its absorptions. NSAID increases chances for seizures. Inhibits metabolism of theophylline, caffeine, warfarin by increasing their plasma level.

Therapeutic uses: UTI, STD (gonorrhea, chancroid), *Shigella, Salmonella, Campylobacter jejuni* induced gastroenteritis, typhoid, gynecological soft tissue infection, osteomyelitis by susceptible bacteria, respiratory tract infection by *Mycoplasma, Leginonella, H. influenzae,* some *Streptococcal, Pneumococal* infection besides gram-negative organisms, tuberculosis, gram-negative septicemia, meningitis. Topically used to treat gram-negative organism producing conjunctivitis, prophylactically for infection in neutropenic and susceptible patients.

Pefloxacin (PELOX 400 mg tab, 400 mg/5 mL to be diluted in 100–250 mL glucose): More lipid-soluble, completely absorbed orally, passage to CNS is better, so preferred for meningitis. It is metabolized partly to norfloxacin. Spectrum of activity is like norfloxacin.

Ofloxacin (Tarivid 100–200 mg/tab or 200 mg/100 mL IV infusion): More potent than ciprofloxacin for gram-positive organism. Used to treat *Chlamydia, Mycoplasma, M. tuberculosis, M. leprae.* Less interfering with theophylline, used for chronic bronchitis, respiratory and ENT infections.

Lomefloxacin (Lomef 400): Longer acting, single day therapy, less interaction with theophylline spectrum similar to ciprofloxacin.

Sparfloxacin (Acespar; Sparquin 200 mg tab): Active against *Strep. pneumoniae, Staph, Enterococcus, anerobes, mycobacteria,* therefore, used for pneumonia, chronic bronchitis, sinusitis, ENT infection. No interaction with warfarin and theophylline. Phototoxicity and QT prolongation may occur. Single day therapy. Withdrawn from market.

Levofloxacin (Levoday 500 mg tab or 500 mg/ 100 mL): Single day therapy and levoisomer ofloxacin. Orally absorbed. Interaction with theophylline, zidovudine is less. Used for pneumonia, chronic bronchitis, sinusitis, pyelonephritis, skin and soft tissue infections. It is a levoisomer of ofloxacin.

Gatifloxacin (Gatiflox 200, 400 mg tabs): Orally absorbed, can be given without regard to food, 20% protein-bound. Unlike to alter pharmacokinetics of drugs like midazolam, cyclosporine, warfarin, theophylline, excreted unchanged in kidney. It may produce hyperglycemia in diabetic or hypoglycemia in patient receiving antidiabetic.

Its concentration increases when used within probenecid. Antacids reduce absorption.

QTc prolongation may occur, so should not be used with class Ia, III antiarrhythmics. It is withdrawn from market in the USA in 2006.

Therapeutic uses: Chronic bronchitis, due to *Strepto, Pneumoniae, Haemophilus influenzae, Moraxella catarrhalis, Staph. aureus, Mycoplasma, Legionella,* Community-acquired pneumonia, acute sinusitis, complicated and uncomplicated UTI by *E. coli, Klebsiella, Proteus,* pyelonephritis, uretheral and cervical gonorrhea, uncomplicated rectal infection in female.

Contraindicated in pediatrics, pregnant, lactating mother. Symptomatic hyper- or hypoglycemia may occur with patient receiving concurrent hypoglycemics.

Moxifloxacin (Moxif 400 mg tab, 400 mg/250 mL IV 0.5% eyedrops): 3rd generation fluoroquinolone. Less interaction with theophylline, superior to levofloxacin, gatifloxacin. Used for skin infection, chronic bronchitis, sinusitis, community-acquired pneumonia. It is not a good drug for UTI. Dose 400 mg OD × 5 days. Seizure or QTc prolongation may occur.

Fluoroquinolone may damage growing cartilage causing arthropathy (may be reversible) so not recommended below 18 years except in few cases for treatment of pseudomonal infection in cystic fibrosis. In adults, it causes tendonitis even its rupture.

Advantages of newer quinolones

- Greater clinical efficacy
- Greater safety less toxic
- Less tendency to develop resistance
- Better patient compliance
- Better oral absorption and tissue distribution
- Longer t½
- Better entry in phagocytic cells
- Excellent urinary concentration on oral administration.

Newer Quinolones

A. **Balofloxacin (Baloflox 100 mg tab):** Relatively effective against *Staph, Strepto, E. coli, Citrobacter, Kliebsiella pneumoniae, Enterobacter, Proteus, Morganella morganii, Bacteroides fragllis* used for uncomplicated UTI. Dose 100 mg BD.

   ADR: Hypersensitivity, seizure, tendonitis, QTc extension. Not recommended for pediatric, pregnancy and lactation.

B. **Trovafloxacin:** 50% is conjugated in the liver and 43% excreted in feces used for LRTI; skin and soft tissue infections, prostatitis, sinusitis, community-acquired pneumonia PID; intra-abdoiminal infection, hospital-acquired pneumonia (use is reserved for lifethreatening infection)

   ADR: Dizziness, hepatotoxicity. It is available as oral tablet and as prodrug alatrofloxacin as an intravenous formulation, dose 100–200 mg/day orally.

INDICATIONS OF QUINOLONES

1. **UTI:** Nalidixic acid, Norfloxacin, Ciprofloxacin, Levofloxacin, Ofloxacin, Gatifloxacin.

2. **Lower RTI:** Lomefloxacin, Ofloxacin, Ciprofloxacin, Trovafloxacin.

3. **Skin infection:** Ofloxacin, Ciprofloxacin, Levofloxacin, Trovafloxacin.

4. **Gonococcal urethral:** Norfloxacin, Gatifloxacin, Ciprofloxacin, Ofloxacin, Trovafloxacin.

5. **Urethral clamydial infection**: Ofloxacin; Trovafloxacin

6. **Bone and joint infections:** Ciprofloxacin by gram-negative.

7. **Diarrhea infection:** Ciprofloxacin

8. **Typhoid:** Ciprofloxacin

9. **Prostatitis:** Norfloxacin, Ofloxacin, Trovafloxacin

10. **Sinusitis:** Ciprofloxacin, Levofloxacin, Gatifloxacin. Trovafloxacin.

11. **Bronchitis acute:** Levofloxacin, Gatifloxacin, Sparfloxacin, Moxifloxacin, Trevafloxacin

12. **PID:** Trovafloxacin

13. **Nosocomial pneumonia:** Trovafloxacin.

NB: After post-marketing surveillance following quinolones are withdrawn from the US market.

- Levofloxacin and sparfloxacin for phototoxicity and QTc prolongation
- Gatifloxacin for hypoglycemia
- Temafloxacin for immune hemolytic anemia.
- Trovafloxacin for hepatotoxicity
- Grepafloxacin for cardiotoxicity
- Clinafloxacin for phototoxicity
- Most quinolones are cleared by kidney and their dose should be adjusted. Moxifloxacin and pefloxacin are metabolized by liver and none of them are removed by dialysis (hemo- or peritoneal).

Nitrofurans

Dodd and Stillman first found antibacterial activity of nitrofuran. Bacteriostatic, effective against *Staph, Strepto, E. coli, Salmonella, Shigella.* Probably inhibits anaerobic steps of pyruvate metabolism of susceptible bacteria. They are bacteriostatic, but may be bactericidal in higher doses. It undergoes enzymatic reduction producing reactive intermediate which damages DNA.

Pharmacokinetics: Nitrofurantoin is orally absorbed, metabolized in liver, excreted in urine. Resistance develops slowly. Probenacid inhibits its tubular secretion and interferes with its action.

Adverse effects: Nausea, vomiting, skin rash, anemia in G-6PD patient, antabuse reaction, polyneuritis, pulmonary interstitial fibrosis, deafness, tinnitus, increased sensitivity to MAO-I to exogenous catecholamine.

Preparations

- **Nitrofurantoin (furadantin):** Used as urinary antiseptic 50 mg TDS. May be given for 1 year.
- **Furazolidine (furoxone):** Used for vaginal and GIT infections (bacillary dysentery, giardiasis, trichomonal vaginitis) 100 mg QDS × 5–7 days.
- **Nifuroxime:** Used locally for vaginal fungal infection *(Candida albicans).*
- **Nitrofurazone (Furacin):** 2% solution used for skin infection and for trypanosomiasis 500 mg TDS × 7–10 days. Systemic allergic reaction may occur with topical therapy. Generally used over burn and skin grafting dressing.

Penicillins and β-Lactam Antibiotics

In 1928 at St. Marys Hospital, London, Fleming noticed culture of *Staphylococci* when became contaminated with mould and the filtered broth of mould had lethal effect on gram-positive organism. It was named as penicillin by Fleming because mould produced the lethal effect on *Staphylococcus* growth belonging to genus *Penicillium*. Florey of Oxford University, revived interest on Fleming observation. Chain *et al.* isolated crude sample of penicillin from *Penicillium notatum*. When Fleming was first presenting his paper hardly 10 persons were there and most of them were sleeping.

Later it was found *P. chrysogenum* as richer source of penicillin. In penicillin, a thiazolidine and β-lactam ring fused together to produce penicillin nucleus (Fig. 101.1) (6-aminopenicillinic acid, 6APA). When penicillin is added to a growing sensitive culture bacteria swells up and brusts. Penicillin interferes with cell wall synthesis by inhibiting peptide cross-linkage (*i.e.* transpeptidation reaction) in the final stage of cell wall synthesis (Fig. 101.2). The rigid cell wall of bacteria covers cytoplasmic membrane

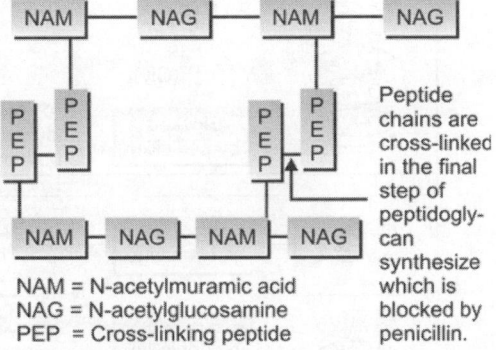

NAM = N-acetylmuramic acid
NAG = N-acetylglucosamine
PEP = Cross-linking peptide

Peptide chains are cross-linked in the final step of peptidoglycan synthesize which is blocked by penicillin.

Fig. 101.2: Bacterial cell wall and site of action of penicillin

of bacteria maintains shape and prevents its lysis in high osmotic pressure.

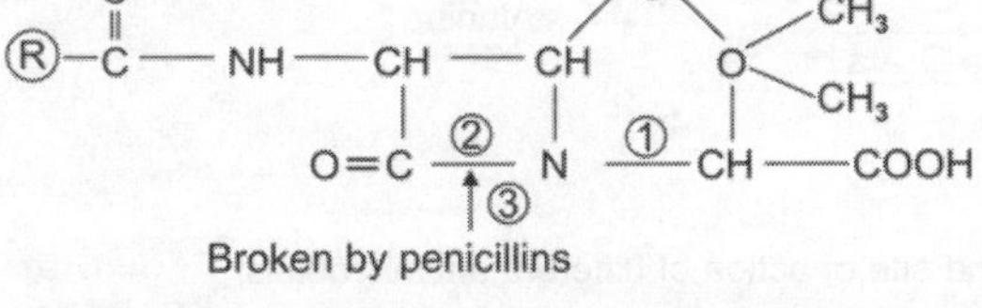

Some bacteria produce degradative enzyme autolysin which remodels bacterial cell wall. In presence of penicillin and the action of autolysin proceeds in absence of cell wall synthesis, *i.e.* it destructs existing cell wall by autolysin. Penicillin and cephalosporins kill the bacteria when they are actively growing.

Gram-positive bacteria have more peptide cross-linkage than gram-negative, so penicillin is more active on them. It is bactericidal. Blood, pus or tissue fluids do not interfere with its antibacterial action.

Structure of Penicillin (Fig. 101.1)

1. Thiazolidine
2. β-lactam
3. Bond is broken by Penicillinase

The nature of R group which determines the drugs stability to enzymatic or acidic hydrolysis

Broken by penicillins

① Thiazolidine; ② β-lactam and ③ Bond is broken by Penicillinase. The nature of R group which determines the drugs stability to enzymatic or acidic hydrolysis and may alter its antibacterial spectrum.

Fig. 101.1: Structure of penicillin

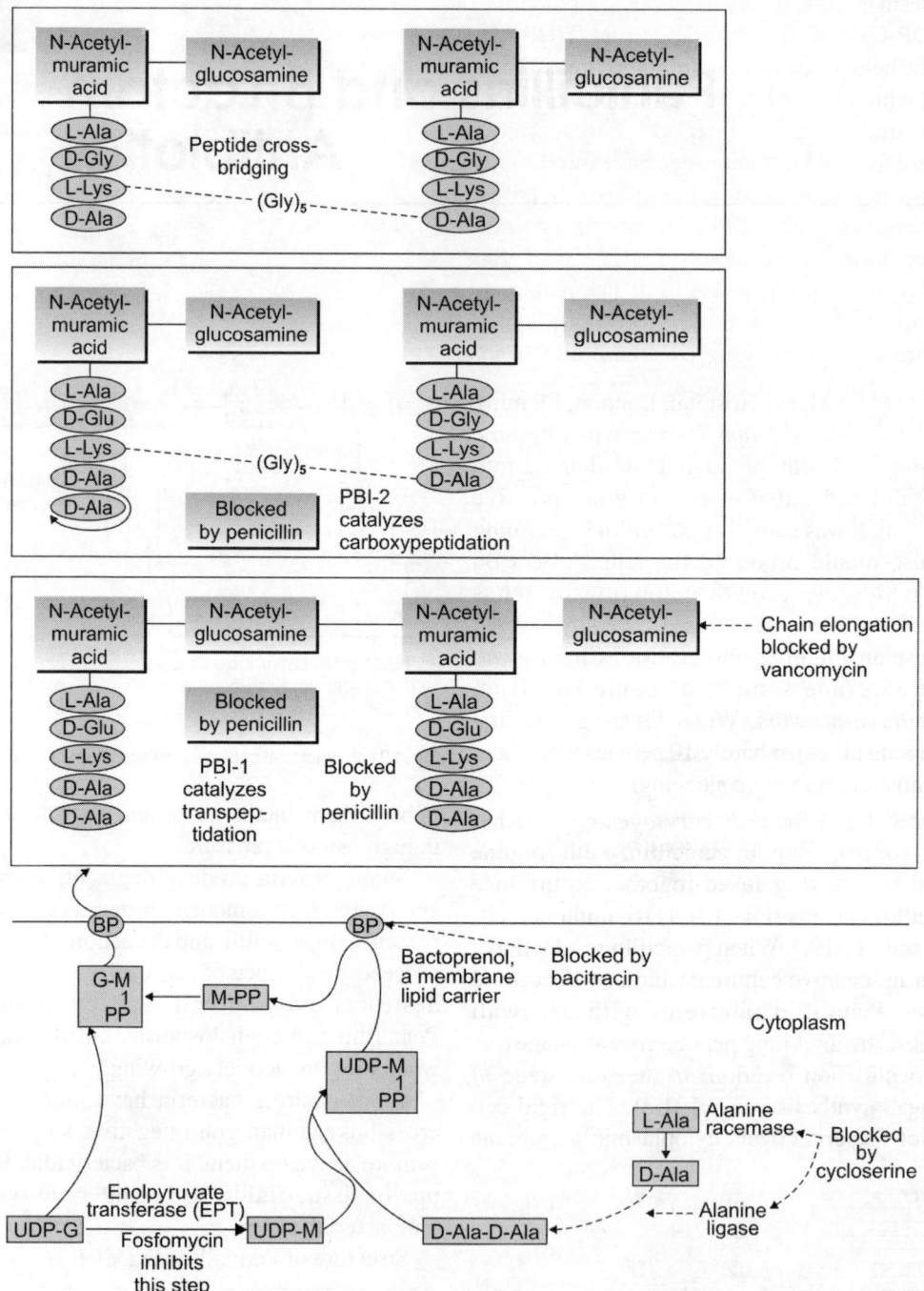

Fig. 101.3: Synthesis of bacterial cell wall and site of action of different antimicrobials

and may alter its antibacterial spectrum. Penicillin interferes with cell wall synthesis by inhibiting peptide cross linkage *i.e.* transpeptidation reaction.

Bacterial cell wall synthesis: Bacterial cell wall is a peptodoglycan consisting of N-acetyl-muramic acid and N-acetylglucosamine, and pentapeptide. Synthesis of cell wall starts at cytoplasm by conversion of N-acetylglucosamine G (UDP-G) to N-acetylmuramic acid (UDP-M) with the help of enzyme enolpyruvate transferase (EPT) which is blocked by fosfomycin. UDP-M then acquires the pentapeptide. Pentapeptide units are formed by alanine racemase and alanine ligase which is blocked by cycloserine. UDP is then removed from UDP-M, a membrane lipid carrier called bactoprenol (BP) and N-acetylglucosamine is added to it. The resulting molecule is now transported through plasma membrane with the help of membrane lipid carrier, bactoprenol. Bacitracin causes dephosphorylation of bactoprenol. Peptido-glycan chain elongates with the help of enzyme, transglycosylase. Cross-linking which provides strength to peptidoglycan chain is provided by the enzyme transpeptidase. Transglycolase is blocked by vancomycin. (Fig. 101.3)

Mechanism of action of penicillin: Bacteria utilize supportive structure round the cell to withstand osmotic changes which is high outside and low inside osmotic pressure. Bacterial thick cell wall confers their stability and rigidity which are composed of peptidoglycan, *i.e.* two parallel glycan (polysaccharide) chains crossed linked by peptide chains. Polysaccharide chains are alternate units of amino sugars N-acetylmuramic acid and N-acetylglucosamine-pentapeptide chains are cross-linked from one acetylmuramic acid to other by pentoglycine. Cross-linking provides strengthening and the process is called transpeptidation catalyzed by penicillin-binding protein (PBP).

Penicillin inhibits transpeptidation and forms imperfect cell wall which cannot withstand osmotic changes so the bacteria swells up and brust to die.

There are three types of penicillin-binding proteins, PBP-1 cleaves the terminal D-alanine to produce imperfect cell wall, PBP-2 is carboxy-peptidase which hyrolyzes D-alanine on adjacent pentapeptide and when it is inhibited and produces spherical bacterial cell and PBP-3 is endopeptidase and splits cross-linking in bacterial septum. Its inhibition produces filamentous formation of bacteria and bacteria cannot seperate. Gram-positive bacteria's cell wall consists of thick peptidoglycan layer and it is accessible to β-lactam, so β-lactam antibiotics are more effective in gram-positive bacteria.

In gram-negative bacteria there is cytoplasmic membrane and outer membrane of lipopolysac-charide with narrow porin channels. Porin channels act as a barrier to β-lactam antibiotic so they are resistant to it. β-lactam Ampicillin and Amoxycillin can penetrate porin channel of gram-negative bacteria to reach pepti-doglycan layer and is effective on them. (Figs 101.4A and B).

β-lactam weakens the bacterial cell wall and facilitates penetration of aminoglycosides into bacteria so they together act synergistically.

Therefore, it may be concluded that the cell wall synthesis of bacteria is targeted by anti-bacterial agents in the follwing steps, if their mechanism of action targets cell wall synthesis.

• β-lactam targets transpeptidase.

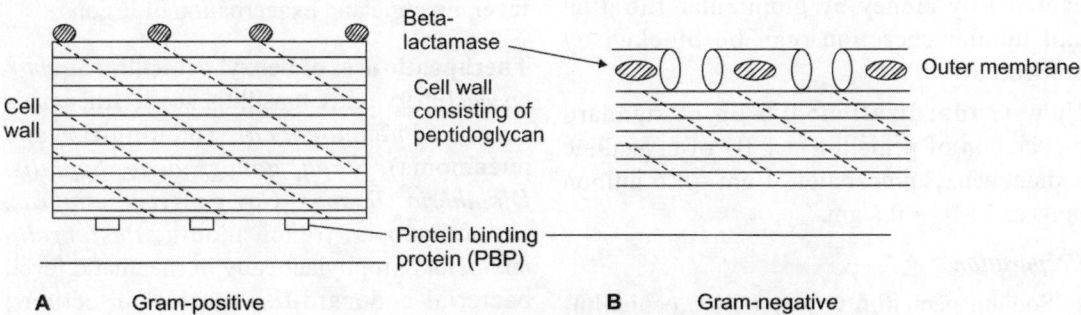

Figs 101.4A and B: Cytoplasmic membrane

- Vancomycin targets transglycolase.
- Cycloserine targets alanine racemase and alanine ligase.
- Bacitracin targets dephosphorylation of bactoprenol.
- Fosfomycin targets enolpyruvate tranferase.

Benzyl penicillin (penicillin G): Effective against gram-positive and gram-negative cocci and some gram-positive bacillus. Group D streptococci are not sensitive, *Gonococci, Diphtheria, Clostridium welchi* are moderately sensitive. *Treponema pallidum* is highly sensitive, but *Leptospira* responds moderatively.

Bacterial resistance: Acquired resistance occurs due to production of penicillinase which breaks β-lactam ring. Penicillinase is produced by *Staph, Gonococci, B. subtilis, H. influenzae, E. coli, Staphylococci.* Penicillinase is acquired by plasmid and propagated by selection through conjugation or transduction. The other mechanisms of resistant to penicillin are modification of target PBP. Less penetration of drug to PBP as in gram-negative organism and efflux pump. Efflux pump consists of cytoplasmic and periplasmic proteins.

In gram-negative bacteria, there are porins. Permeability of β-lactam antibiotics through these porins differs (*viz.* Ampicillin crosses it). Alteration to porin channels makes bacteria resistant to it.

Pharmacokinetics of benzyl penicillin: Benzyl penicillin is destroyed by gastric acid. Absorption from IM site is good, distributed extracellularly, CSF and serous sac penetration is poor, but in inflammation increases. Protein-bound, rapidly excreted by kidney by glomerular filtration and tubular secretion (can be blocked by probenecid).

Unit standardization: 0.6 µg of standard preparation of penicillin = 1 IU of crystalline sodium benzyl preparation. 1 gm = 1.6 million units or 1 MU = 0.6 gm.

Preparation

1. Sodium penicillin G (crystalline penicillin) [Crystapen 0.2–0.5 MU, dose 0.5–5 MU IM

or IV 6–12 hourly] (to be dissolved in distilled water)
2. Potassium penicillin 2–8 lac unit QID before food. (Pentid)
3. Repository penicillin G: Insoluble salts, given deep IM not IV.

- Procaine penicillin G, 0.5–1 MU IM given 12–24 hourly.
- Fortified procaine penicillin G (Crys4) contains 3 lac U procaine penicillin + 1 lac U sodium penicillin.
- Benezathine penicillin (penidure LA, longacillin 0.6, 1.2, 2.4 MU dry powder in vial) 0.6–2.4 MU every 2–4 weeks used for prophylactic purposes.

Adverse effects of benzyl penicillin: Non-toxic, may be used up to 100 MU without toxicity. Adverse effects observed are local irritation, nausea, vomiting, injection thrombophlebitis, toxicity may be manifested as confusion, twitching, coma, arachnoiditis and spinal cord degenerative changes when given intrathecally.

Hypersensitivity, rash, urticaria, fever, wheeze angioedema, serum sickness, anaphylaxis (course is unpredictable), procaine itself is allergic so its incidence is high with procaine penicillin, scratch test should be done before hand, but it can itself produce anaphylaxis.

Superinfection rare because it is a narrow spectrum.

Jarisch-Herxheimer reaction: Particularly in secondary syphillis due to sudden release of spirochetal lytic product manifested as shivering, fever, myalgia and exacerbation of lesions.

Therapeutic uses of benzyl penicillin: *Streptococcal* (pharyngitis, tonsillitis, scarlet, rheumatic fever). *Pneumococcal* (meningitis and pneumonia), *Staph, gonorrhoeae, Syphilis, Diphtheria, Tetanus, Gas gangrene, Anthrax,* actinomycosis, trench mouth, *Pasteurella multocida,* prophylactically in rheumatic fever, bacterial endocarditis, surgical infections, agranulocytosis patient with aminoglycosides.

SEMISYNTHETIC PENICILLIN

Produced to overcome the following drawbacks of benzyl penicillin. The major drawbacks of benzyl penicillin are:

- Inactivation by gastric HCl
- Short duration of action and poor penetration into CSF
- Mainly active against gram-positive organism.
- Possibility of anaphylaxis
- Development of resistant staphylococci.

a. Acid resistant

- Potassium phenoxymethyl penicillin (Kaypen 125–250 mg tab, 125 mg/5 mL dry syr) given 6 hourly, orally active (250 mg = 4 lac U).
- Potassium phenoxyethyl penicillin (Phenethicillin)
- Propicillin (brocillin, ultrapen). More plasma protein-bound.

b. Penicillinase-resistant penicillin

- **Methicillin (Staphcillin):** Penicillinase-resistant, not acid-resistant, hence given IM or IV. In case of methicillin resistance, linezolid (a oxazolidinone) is a drug of choice, but vancomycin or ciprofloxacin can also be used. Hematuria, albuminuria, reversible interstitial nephritis may occur. 1–2 gm dissolved in 50 mL of normal saline for IV or 1–2 gm IM 2–6 hourly.
- **Cloxacillin (Klox 0.25; 0.5 gm and 125 mg/3 mL dry syr):** Penicillinase- and acid-resistant. Incompletely absored from GIT, 90% protein- bound and excreted through kidney. **Oxacillin, flucloxacillin** not marketed in India. All these are isoxazolyl penicillin *Dicloxacillin* which is a derivative of cloxacillin gives better blood level on oral routes, now it is available in Indian market.
- **Nafcillin (Unigen):** Penicillinase-resistant, but partial acid-resistant, therefore, oral absorption unreliable. Indicated for servere *Staphylococcus* infection by parenteral route. May produce hepatitis and neutropenia. It is highly protein-bound. Dose oral like

cloxacillin, parenteral 0.5–1 gm, 4–6 hourly and 25 mg/kg for children BD.

Effective Against Gram-positive and Gram-negative Organisms (Extended spectrum)

I. Aminopenicillin

- **Ampicillin (Roscillin 250 and 500 mg caps; 125–250 mg/5 mL dyr syr; 100 mg/mL paed drops; 250 mg, 500 mg, 1 gm vial):** Effective against organisms sensitive to penicillin G, *H. influenzae, E. coli, Proteus, Salmonella, Shigella, Strep. viridans, Enterococci, Pneumococci, Gonococci, Meningococci.*

  Orally absorbed, excreted in bile and kidney. Dose 0.5–2 gm oral/IM/IV used for UTI, RTI, meningitis, gonorrhea, typhoid, bacillar dysentery, cholecystitis, endocarditis, septicemia.

  Adverse effects are diarrhea, rash specially in AIDs or leukemia, Ebstein virus infection.

  Probenecid retards its excretion, contraceptive failure with OCP because of its deconjugation and enterohepatic circulation of OCP.

- **Talampicillin:** Carboxylic esters of ampicillin, rapidly absorbed from GIT hydrolized by tissue esterases in intestinal wall to release ampicillin into circulation. Dose 250–500 mg TDS or QDS. Other prodrugs of ampicillin are **Pivampicillin, Hetacillin**.

- **Bacampicillin (Penglobe 200–400 mg tab):** This ester of ampicillin completely absorbed from GIT. Diarrhea is less common. Dose 400–800 mg BD.

- **Amoxicillin:** Congener of ampicillin, but not prodrug of ampicillin, orally better absorbed, less chances of diarrhea, but less active against *Shigella* and *H. influenzae*. Preferred by physicians for typhoid, bronchitis, UTI, gonorrhea, bacterial endocarditis (Mox 125 mg/5 mL; 125–250, 500 mg cap, 500 mg/vial).

Note: Talampicillin, pivampicillin, hetacillin, becampicillin are prodrugs of ampicillin.

II. *Carboxy Penicillin*

- **Carbenicillin:** This penicillin congener effective against *Pesudomonas aeruginosa, Proteus.* Less active against *Salmonella, E. coli and Enterobacter.* Inactive orally, given IM 1–2 gm 4–6 hourly as sodium salt marketed as pyopen, carbelin 1–5 gm vial. Higher doses may cause Na overload leading to water retention, may be dangerous for CCF patient. It may interfere with platelet function. It is neither penicillinase nor acid-resistant. Superinfection with *Aerobactor aeruginosa* may occur. Used for UTI, burn or septicemia.

- **Carbenicillin indanyl and carbenicillin phenyl** are acid stable esters of carbenicillin hydrolyzed in body to active drugs. Orally active. Dose 0.5–1 gm 6 hourly for *Pseudomonas* or *Proteus.*

- **Ticarcillin:** More potent than carbenicillin used for *Pseudomonas.*

III. *Ureidopenicillin*

- **Mezlocillin:** Given parenterally to treat enteric bacilli.

- **Piperacillin (Piprapen 1–2 gm vial):** 8 times potent than carbenicillin for *Pseudomonas.* Dose 100–150 mg/kg/day in three divided doses.

- **Mecillinam (Amdinocillin):** Semisynthetic penicillin given parenterally for gram-negative *E. coli, Salmonella, Klebsiella, Enterobacter,* but not for *Pseudomonas.* Dose 500 mg 4–6 hourly.

IV. β-*lactamase Inhibitors*

β-lactamase opens up β-lactam ring to inactivate penicillin. They are effective against Ambler class of β-lactamases, *i.e.* plasmid encoded transposable element produced by *Staph, H. influenzae, N. gonorrhoea, Salmonella, Shigella, E. coli, K. pneumoniae.* Beta lactamases are classified on molecular basis (Amber classification) or on type of substrate (Bush classification. A, C, D of Amber classification requries serine and B contains Zinc.

Class A : Confers resistance to penicillin, 3rd generation cephalosporin.

Class B: It destroys all beta lactams except aztreonam.

Class C: Aztreonam and 2nd and 3rd generation cephalosporin are inactivated by it.

Class D: Cloxacillin degrading enzyme.

Class A and D can be inhibited by beta lactamase inhibitors.

Two inhibitors of this enzyme are:

i. Clavulanic acid and Tazobactam

ii. Sulbactum

They do not possess antibiotic effect *per se.*

- **Clavulanic acid:** Progressive, suicide (because it is inactivated after inhibiting the enzyme) inhibitor of b-lactamase. Orally absorbed. Distribution matches with amoxicillin, eliminated by glomerular filtration, hydrolyzed and decarboxylated before excretion. It establishes activity of amoxicillin against *H. influenzae, N. gonorrhoeae. E. coli, Proteus, Klebsiella, Shigella, Salmonella, B. fragilis* producing b-lactamase. Available as amoxicillin 500 mg + Clavulanic acid 125 mg or Amoxicillin 250 mg + Calvulanic acid 125 mg. Amoxicillin 125 mg + Clavulanic acid 32 mg/5 mL dry syr. Used 1–2 tabs TDS.

  Amoxicillin 1 gm + Clavulanic acid 200 mg injection vial, dose vial IM or IV; TD to QD.

  Adverse effects: Intolerance, *Candida* stomatitis, glossitis, vaginitis, hepatic damage. It is obtained from *Streptomyces clauvuligerus.*

- **Sulbactam:** Semisynthetic β-lactamase inhibitors, less potent than clavulanic acid. Orally inconsistently absorbed. Given parenterally, but its complex salt with ampicillin-sultamicillin tosylate is orally absorbed. Used for penicillinase producing gonorrhea (sulbactam *per se* inhibits gonorrhea), mixed aerobic and anaerobic infections.

  Pain at injection site, rash. Diarrhea, thrombophlebitis may occur.

Available as ampicillin 1 gm + sulbactam 0.5 gm 1 vial IM or IV, TD or QD.

- **Tazobactam:** Similar to sulbactam combined with piperacillin because its pharmacokinetics matches with it. 0.5 gm of tazobactam combined with 4 .gm of piperacillin injected IV over 30 minutes 8 hourly.

V. *Cycloserine*

Produced by *Streptomyces orchidaceus*. It is unstable in acidic pH. Since it is structurally similar to D-alanine it inhibits alanine racemase which converts D-alanine-D-alanine ligase and incorporation of D-alanine into peptidoglycan pentapeptide. It inhibits many gram-positive and gram-negative organisms, but reserved as 1st drug in firstline resistant anti-tubercular drug. It produces side effects of headache, tremor, psychosis, *i.e.* neuropsychiatric symptoms and seizure. For tuberculosis its dose of 0.5–1 gm/day in two or three divided doses. The CNS dose related toxicity is less, if dose is 0.75 gm/day.

102

Cephalosporins

Cephalosporin was first isolated from Sardinian sea coast by Brotzu from *Caphalosporium acremonium*. Cephalosporin C consists of side chain derived from D-α-aminoadipic acid condensed with a dihydrothiazine β-lactam ring sytem (7-aminocephalosporinic acid) Fig. 102.1. Modification at position 7 of β-lactam ring associated with alteration in antibacterial activity and substitution of postion 3 of dihydrothiazine associated with change of pharmacokinetic properties. Cephamycin have a methoxy group at position 7 of β-lactam ring of the 7-amino-cephalosporinic acid nucleus.

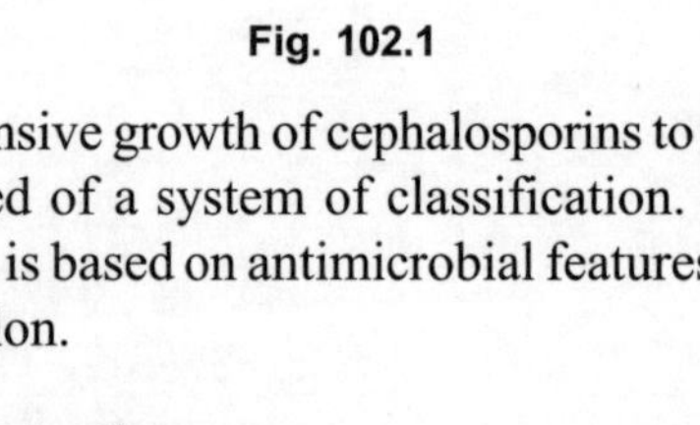

Fig. 102.1

Extensive growth of cephalosporins to memorize need of a system of classification. Classification is based on antimicrobial features called generation.

1st Generation

Good activity against gram-positive and moderate activity against gram-negative *(E. coli, Klebsiella pneumonia, Pr. mirabils)*.

Oral

• Cephalexin
• Cepharadine
• Cefadroxil

Cephalexin and cepharadine are given 250–500 mg QDS (15–30 mg/kg/day) and dose of cefadroxil for adult is 500 mg BD. Dose should be less in renal impaired patient since they are excreted via kidney by glomerular filtration and tubular secretion.

Parenteral

• Cephalothin   • Cefazolin
• Cephaloridine

The dose of cefazolin IV 500 mg–2 gm every 8 hours for adult. It can also be given IM. Dose adjustment required for renal impaired patient.

2nd Generation

More activity against gram-negative, but less than third generation.

Oral

• Cefaclor   • Cefuroxime axetil
• Cafprozil

Parenteral

• Cefoxitin   • Cefotetan
• Cefuroxime   • Loracaref
• Ceforanide   • Cefonicid

Should be given IV because IM route may be painful. Dosing depends upon agents because of their difference in t½ and protein binding.

3rd Generation

Activity against gram-positive organism is less

than 1st generation. Active against *Entero-bacteriacea* including penicillinase producing strains, also effective against *Pseudomonas aeruginosa*. Some of them are able to cross blood-brain barrier.

Oral

- Cefixime
- Cefdinir
- Cefpodoxime proxetil
- Ceftibuten
- Cefditoren pivoxil

Parenteral

- Cefotaxime
- Ceftriaxone
- Cefoperazone
- Ceftizoxime
- Ceftazidime

4th Generation

Antibacterial activity similar to 3rd generation, but highly resistant to β-lactamase. **Cefepime** and **cefpirome** both are used parenterally. All cephalosporins are bactericidal with mechanism of action like penicillin. Resistance occurs due to:

- Impermeability of antibiotics to bacteria
- Elaboration of β-lactamase (cephalosporinase by bacteria)
- Alterations of target proteins affinity to antibiotics.

Adverse effects: Well-tolerated, but more toxic than penicillin. Diarrhea, hypersensitivity (rash, anaphylaxis, angioedema, asthma, urticaria, cross-hypersensitivity with penicillin and other cephalosporin may occur, skin test unreliable), pain, thrombophlebitis at injections site, bleeding, nephrotoxicity, neutropenia, antabuse-like reaction with some cephalosporins.

Ceftobiprole is a 5th generation cephalosporin effective in MRSA and pseudomonas.

INDIVIDUAL DRUGS OF CEPHALOSPORINS

1st Generation

Oral

Cephalaxin (Sporidex 250, 500 cap; 125 mg/5 mL dry syr, 100 mg/mL drops): Dose 0.25–1 gm 6 hourly (25–100 mg/kg/day).

Cephradine (Ceftad): Orally and parenterally used and dose 0.25–1 gm 6–12 houry oral or IM or IV.

Cefadroxil (Cefadrox 250, 500, 125 mg/5 mL syr): Dose 0.5–1 gm BD. It has good tissue penetration.

Parenteral

Cephalothin: Given IV 1–2 gm 6 hourly partly metabolilzed, used for penicillinase producing *Staph* infection.

Cefazolin (Alcizon 0.25 gm, 0.5 gm; 1 gm/vial) given 8 hourly IM or IV.

Cephaloridine: Nephrotoxic so withdrawn from some countries.

2nd Generation

Oral

Cefaclor (Keftor 250 mg cap, 125 mg tab, 125 mg/5 mL syr): Orally active, more active than first generation compounds. More susceptible to β-lactamase hydrolysis.

Cefuroxime axetil (Ceftum 125, 250, 500 mg tab, 125 mg/5 mL syrp): Esters are orally effective and activity depends upon hydrolysis and release of cefuroxime.

Cefrozil and lorcarbef: Usual adult dose is 10–15 mg/kg/day in two to four divided doses. For children, dose is 10–40 mg/kg/day.

Parenteral

The IM route is painful so should be given IV. Dose interval depends upon individual agent; t½ and on protein binding.

Cefoxitin: 1–2 gm IM/IV every 6–8 hours in treatment of anaerobic and mixed obstetric, surgical infections, lung abscess. It is resistant to β-lactamases, produced by gram-negative bacteria. Cefoxitin 2 gm IM + Probenacid 1 gm oral is effective for penicillinase producing gonococcal urethritis.

3rd Generation

Oral

Cefixime (topeef 200, 400 mg tab): Active

against *Enterobacteriaceae, H. influenzae, Strep. pyogens, Strep. pneumoniae*. Dose 200–400 mg BD for respiratory, urinary and biliary infections.

Parenteral

Cefotaxime (0.25, 0.5, 0.1 gm/vial Omnatax): Potent action on aerobic gram-negative and gram-positive, dose 1–2 gm IM or IV 12 hourly 50–100 mg/kg/day for children. Deacetylated in body.

Ceftizoxime (cefizox 0.5–l gm/vial): Similar to cafotaxime, but not metabolized. Dose 0.5–l gm IM or IV 8–12 hourly.

Ceftriaxone (monocef 0.25 gm, 0.5 gm; 1 gm/vial): Dose 1–2 gm IV or IM/day. For meningitis 4 gm followed by 2 gm IV (children 75–100 mg/kg) and for typhoid 4 gm IV × 2 days followed by 2 gm/day till 2nd day after fever subsides. Used for meningitis, typhoid, UTI. Abdominal sepsis and septicemia, hypoprothrombinemia may occur. It is secreted in bile.

Ceftazidime (Fortum 0.25 and 0.5 1 gm/vial): 0.5–2 gm IM or IV 8 hourly for children, for typhoid 30 mg/kg/day). Active against *Pseudomonas*.

ADR: Neutropenia, thrombocytopenia, rise in blood urea, plasma transaminases may occur.

Cefoperazone (Magnamycin 1–2 gm IM or IV 12 hourly): Effective against *Pseudomonas, S. typhi, B. fragilis*. Used for urinary, biliary, respiratory, meningitis, skin and soft tissue infections and septicemia. It is secreted in bile.

ADR: Hypoprothrombinemia and antabuse-like reaction may occurs. Hypoprothrombinemia can be treated with vitamin K_1 10 mg twice weekly.

4th Generation

Cefepime: Resistant to β-lactamase, effective against *Pseudomonas aeruginosa* plus other bacteria of 3rd generation.

Cefpirome (Cefrom 1 gm, 1–2 gm IM or IV 12 hourly): Used for hospital-acquired infection and septicemia RTI. Zwitter ion in character, penetrates better through gram-negative bacterial porins.

5th Generation

Ceftobiprole is effective against MRSA and pseudomonas is called 5th generation cephalosporin.

The active metabolite of **cefteroline** a prodrug cefteroline fosamil is active against MRSA. Used for skin, soft tissue infection.

MONOBACTAM

Aztreonam (0.5–2 gm IM or IV 6–12 hourly): Active against gram-negative, enteric bacillus, *H. influenzae, Pseudomonas*. No cross sensitivity with other β-lactamase. Occasionally skin rash, rise in serum aminotransferase may occur. Here there is only one ring, so they are monobactam.

CARBAPENEMS

Imipenem: New broad-spectrum β-lactam antibiotic effective against gram-positive cocci, *Pseudomonas, Enterobacteriaceae, Listeria, Bact. fragilis, Cl. difficile*. Resistant to β-lactamase.

Rapidly hydrolyzed by dihydropeptidase I in brush border of renal tubular cells, which can be overcome by its combination with cilastatin (reversible inhibitors of dihydropeptidase I). Used for hospital-acquired infection, neutropenic patients and AIDS patients with infection.

Other *Carbapenems* are *Ertapenem, Doripenem* and *Meropenem.*

Dose: Imipenem 0.25–0.5 gm IV 6–8 hourly. Meropenem 1 gm 8 hourly IV and ertapenem 1 gm/day IM or IV.

They may produce nausea, vomiting, diarrhea, skin rash, seizure perticularly with imipenem. Patients allergic to penicillin may be allergic to carbapenem also.

Meropenem, doripenem and **ertapenem** are not metabolized by renal dihydropeptidase I and less prone to produce seizure.

Faropenem (Faronem 100, 200 mg tab): Orally active carbapenem effective against gram-positive, gram-negative anaerobes, *Staph. phenmoniae, H. influenza, Moraxella catarrhalis.*

ADR: Diarrhea, pain in abdomen, nausea and rash. Dose 200–300 mg oral TDS.

103

Aminoglycosides

Streptomycin, gentamicin, tobramycin, amikacin, neomycin, netilmicin, sisomicin, kanamycin, framycetin, paromomycin belong to amino-glycoside antibiotics.

Common properties of aminoglycosides

- Contain aminosugar in glycosidic linkage.
- Orally poorly absorbed and penetration in CSF is poor.
- Excreted by kidney on filtration.
- Bacteria develop resistance rapidly and exhibit cross-resistance.
- Their spectrum of toxicity is same, *viz.* oto- and nephrotoxic.
- Spectrum of activity same (mainly gram-negative bacilli).
- They act by interfering bacterial protein synthesis.
- All are produced from soil actinomycetes.

Mechanisms of Action of Aminoglycosides

Protein systhesis of bacteria is done by 70s ribosome which consists of two units 30s and 50s. The 50s has got acceptor site (A) and peptadyl site (P). Nascent peptide chain attaches to P site. tRNA with complementary base pairs transports next amino acid to the A site. A new peptide bond is formed with peptide chians and newly attahed amino acid by enzyme peptidyl transferase and nascent peptide chain shifts from P to A site. A side should be free for further elongation of peptide chian which is carried by translocation of peptide from A to P site and the steps go on repeating till it terminates.

All other drugs which inhibit protein synthesis are bacteriostatics except aminoglycosides and streptogramins. Aminoglycosides transport through cell wall and cytoplasmic membrane and binds to ribosome 30s, resulting in inhibition of protein synthesis. Cidal action of these drugs are based on secondary changes to the integrity of bacterial cell membrane which become perme-able to ions, amino acids and even protein leak out followed by bacterial death. Its cidal action is concentration dependent, *i.e.* using in higher concentration kills increase number and rapid killing and its activity persisting beyond its presence in body called postantibiotic effect.

Mechanisms of Resistance of Aminoglycosides

- Cell membrane bound inactivating enzyme which conjugates the antibiotic will phos-phorylate or acetylate or adenylate. The con-jugated antibiotics do not bind to ribosomes.
- Mutation decreases binding of aminoglyco-sides (particularly in *E. coli*).
- Aminoglycosides are less permeable through the pores of bacteria, *i.e.* decreased trans-porting mechanism.

Common Toxicities of Aminoglycosides

- **Ototoxicity:** Vestibular and cochlear divisions of VIII cranial nerve and hair cells undergo dose-dependent destruction. Deafness is permanent. Tinnitus disappears gradually. Vomiting, nystagmus, vertigo and ataxia occur due to vestibular damage. Concurrent diuretic therapy aggravates these toxicities.

Aminoglycosides accumulate in internal ear and ototoxicity occurs with persistently elevated plasma drug concentration. It is largely irreversible due to progressive destruction of vestibular or cochlear cells. Neomycin, kanamycin and gentamicin are more vestibulotoxic. The initial symptoms may be reversible with patient receiving either high or prolonged aminoglycosides, but those patients should be carefully monitored. Deafness may occur after the therapy is discontinued.

- **Nephrotoxicity:** 6–26% of patients receiving aminoglycosides develop mild renal impairment which is almost reversible. Manifest as loss of urinary concentration capacity, nitrogen retention, albuminuria casts, but these are reversible, if drug is withdrawn promptly. Prostaglandins may be responsible for nephrotoxicity.

  Other drugs like cisplatin, vancomycin, ACE-1, Amphotericin-B, cyclosporine, *etc.* and volume depletion and hypokalemia may aggravate aminoglycoside-induced nephrotoxicity. Neomycin, gentamicin, tobramycin are most nephrotoxic.

- **Neuromuscular blockade:** Reduces acetylcholine release from motor end plate and decreases sensitivity of motor end plate to it. Can be reversed by IV calcium. Neostigmine has unpredictable reversing action. In myasthenic patient or in neuromuscular blockade, it should be used with caution.

INDIVIDUAL DRUGS

Streptomycin: Obtained from *Streptomyces griseus,* oldest aminoglycosides effective against *H ducreyi, Brucella, Y. pestis, M. tuberculosis, Tularenesis, Nocardia;* moderately sensitive to *Staphylococcus, Streptococcus, D. pneumoniae, V. cholerae, Salmonella.*

It is effective in alkaline pH.

Streptomycin dependence: Certain mutants grown in presence of streptomycin cause misreading of the genetic code of the organisms become dependent on it, which is of clinical significance particularly in tuberculosis.

Resistance and cross-resistance: Subinhibitory concentration of streptomycin encourage resistance by several mechanisms explained earlier which is usually permanent. Cross-resistance with dihydrostreptomycin is also seen.

Pharmacokinetics: Not absorbed from GIT, highly ionized rapid absorption occurs from injection site of muscle and distributed extracellularly. Low concentration is achieved in synovial, pleural, CSF, aqueous humor. Not metabolized, excreted by glomerular filtration unchanged in urine.

Adverse effects

- **Local irritation:** Oral streptomycin may produce nausea and vomiting, sterile abscess at injection site.
- **Intolerance:** Skin rash, eosinophilia, lymphadenopathy, angioedema, anaphylactic shock, pericarditis, thrombocytopenic purpura, agranulocytois.
- **CNS:** Vestibulocochlear damage.
- **Skeletal muscle:** Curaromimetic like neuromuscular blockade.
- **Superinfection:** With *Staph. aureus* and *Candida,* endocarditis due to *Candida* may be fatal.
- **Nephrotoxicity**

Preparation: Streptomycin sulfate (Ambistryn-S 0.75 and 1 gm powder) for acute infection, 1 gm IM BD × 7 days; for tuberculosis 1 gm (above 50 years), 0.75 g IM OD or twice weekly × 30–60 days.

Uses: Tuberculosis, bacterial endocarditis, plague, tularemia. For UTI, peritonitis, septicemia, newer aminoglycosides are preferred.

Do not use in pregnancy, concurrent use with high ceiling diuretics, minocycline (ototoxicity); amphotericin B, vancomycin cephalothin, cyclosporine, cisplatin (nephrotoxicity) and with muscle relaxants.

Gentamicin

(Genticyn, garamycin 20, 60, 80 mg/vial, 0.3% eye- and eardrops, 0.1% skin cream). Obtained from *Micromonospora purpurae.* Effective against *Pseudomonas, Proteus, E. coli, Klebsiella, Enterobacter* and *Serratia*. Ineffective against *M. tuberculosis* and *Strep. pyogens*. Bactericidal resistance is slowly developed. Cross-resistance to kanamycin and neomycin occur. Dose 1–1.5 mg/kg IM or IV 8 hourly.

Adverse effects: Skin reaction, photosensitivity on topical application, oto- and nephrotoxicities.

Therapeutic uses: Cheapest aminoglycosides, locally used to treat burn with pseudomonas, bed sores, systematically used to treat susceptible bacteria in RTI, UTI, septicemia, meningitis, subacute bacterial endocarditis.

It is additive with ampicillin, tetracycline and chloramphenicol. With cephalosporin acute tubular necrosis may occur. Gentamicin polymethyl methacrylate (septopal) chain used for osteomyelitis. Here acrylic beads with 7.5 mg gentamicin threaded over surgical grade wire implanted in bone marrow for 10 days with good cure rates.

Tobramycin (Tobacin 20, 60, 80 in 2 mL inj; 0.3% eyedrops): Obtained from *Streptomyces tenebrarius*. Spectrum of activity is like gentamicin, but more active against *Ps. aeruginosa*. Toxicities are like gentamicin. Administered IM 1–5 mg/kg/day in 3–4 divided doses.

Amikacin (Amicin 100, 250, 500 mg/2 mL injection): Semisynthetic, specially active against gentamicin resistant *Ps. aeruginosa, Klebsiella, E. coli, Proteus*. Reserved for hospital-acquired gram-negative infection. Effective for tuberculosis. Dose 15 mg/kg/day in 1–3 doses, for UTI 7.5 mg/kg/day. It is resistant to bacterial aminoglycosidase inactivating enzyme. Hearing loss common.

Sisomicin (Sisocin 50 mg and 10 mg/mL): Obtained from *Micromonospora inyoensis*. More potent on *Pseudomonas* and gram-negative bacilli, β-hemolytic *Streptococci* used with penicillin for bacterial endocarditis.

Verdamycin (Under evaluation)

Kanamycin (Kancin): Used for fulminating UTI with septicemia by *E. coli, Proteus, P. aeruginosa, Klebsiella*. Dose 0.5 gm IM BD to TDS. Its use has declined because of its limited spectrum of activity.

Netilmicin (Netromycin 10, 25, 50, 100 mg/ mL): Semisynthetic derivative of sisomicin, more active against *Klebsiella, Enterobacter, Staphylococci*. Useful for critically ill patient, dose 4–6 mg/kg/day in 1–3 divided doses. It is relatively resistant to aminoglycoside inactivating enzyme.

Neomycin: Source is *Streptomyces fradiae*. Highly oto- and nephrotoxics so not used systematically. Dose 0.25–1 gm QID oral and 0.3–0.5% topical.

Topically used for infected wound, ulcer, burn, external ear infection, conjunctivitis, ophthalmia neonatorum. Orally for preoperative bowel preparation, hepatic coma, oral neomycin has damaging effect on intestinal villi. Potentiate warfarin by decreasing vitamin K production by colonic bacteria, superinfection with *Candida* may occur.

Paromomycin (Humatin): Obtained from *Streptomyces rimosus*. Spectrum of activity as like neomycin. Also effective for *E. histolytica*. Oral therapy may produce headache, emesis, diarrhea, skin rashes, superinfection with *Candida*.

Dose 4 gm followed by 2 gm in 2 divided doses. Also used for bacillary dysentery, preoperative bowel preparation, hepatic coma.

Framycetin (Soframycin 1% cream, 0.5% eyedrop): Obtained from *Streptomyces lavendulae*. Toxic for systemic use. Used topically on skins, eyes.

Spectinomycin: It is an aminocychitol antibiotic, structurally related to aminoglycosides used solely for drug-resistant gonorrhea or patient allergic to penicillin. It is given IM 40 mg/kg up to 2 gm. Pain, fever, nausea, anemia, nephrotoxicity may occur.

104

Macrolide Antibiotics

Macrolide antibiotics contain a large macrocylic lactone ring usually with 14–16 atoms to which deoxy sugars are attached in its chemical structure. Erythromycin, oleandomycin, triacetyloleandomycin, spiramycin, roxithrormycin, clarithromycin, azithromycin belong to these groups.

Erythromycin: Isolated from fermentation of fungus, *Streptomyces erythreus.* Here sugars are desosamine and cladinose. Stable in 4 °C, but looses activity at 20 °C and acid pH. It may be bacteriostatic or cidal depending upon concentration. Sensitive bacteria accumulates erythromycin intracellularly by active transport. Acts on 50s ribosomal subunits and inhibits bacterial protein synthesis by inhibiting translocation of peptide chain from A stie to P site. Acts on mostly gram-positive and few gram-negative. Effective against *Staphylococcus, Streptococcus, Pneumococci, Neisseria;* some strains of *H. influenzae, Rickettisias, Listeria, Treponema, Campylobacter, Legionella, Branhamella catarrhalis, Gardnerella vaginalis, H. ducreyi, B. pertussis, Chlamydia trichomatis, Corny, diphtheriae, Helicobacter.*

Resistance occurs because of some mechanisms in bacterial cells impermeable to it. Like:
• Active efflux
• Production of esterases hydrolyzing it and alteration to ribosomal binding for plasmid encoded methylase enzyme and change in 50s ribosomal mutation. Cross-resistance with other macrolide and chloramphenicol has been observed.

Adverse effects: Epigastric pain, increases gastric contraction by stimulating motilin receptors, rare hypersensitivity, hepatitis, raises plasma level of theophylline, carbamazepine, valproate, warfarin, cisapride, terfenadine.

Pharmacokinetics: It is given in enteric coated tablet to protect it from gastric acid, food delays its absorption, distributed in bodies (including serous membrane, placenta, prostate) protein bound, metabolized in liver and excreted in bile.

Therapeutic uses: Streptococcal pharyngitis, tonsillitis, RTI caused by *Pneumococci, H. influenzae,* prophylactic for rheumatic fever, bacterial endocarditis, diphtheria, tetanus, syphilis, pneumonia by mycoplasma, legionnaire pneumonia, whooping cough, campylobacter enteritis, chancroid, *chlamydia trachomatis.*

Preparation: Erythromycin base (erysafe 125, 250, 500 mg), erythromycin stearate (erythrocin 100, 250, 500, 100 mg/5 mL), erythromycin estolate (Athrocin 250, 500, 125 mg/5 mL or 250 mg/5 mL dry syr), erythromycin ethyl succinate (erynate 100 mg/5 mL dry syr), erythromycin ointment (gery ointment), erythromycin ethylsuccinate, glycoheptonate for IM use, lactobionate for IV parenteral use in treating pneumonia by *Legionella* sp.

Oleandomycin and triacetyloleandomycin: Oleandomycin obtained from *Streptomyces antibioticus.* Triacetyloleandomycin is semisynthetic, but less potent and not commonly used.

Spiramycin (Rovamycin): Macrolide antibiotic obtained from *Streptomyces ambofaciens.* Spectrum similar to erythromycin, but weaker in action. Available as 1.5 MU and 3 MU tabs.

Dose 6 MU/day. Used for *Toxoplasma gondii* infection. GI irritation, nausea, diarrhea, rash may occur.

Roxithromycin (Rockcin 150, 300 mg, roxibid 150 mg; 50 mg): Semisynthetic, long acting, stable macrolide, more potent for *Branh. catarrhalis, Gard. vaginalis, Legionella*. Well-absorbed orally, less prone to produce drug interaction with terfenadine and cisapride. Used for respiratory, ENT, genital tract, soft tissue infections.

Clarithromycin (Claribid 250 and 500 mg tabs): Macrolide antibiotic with spectrum like that of erythromycin plus *Mycobacterium avium* complex. More active against *Moroaxella, Legionella, Helicobacter pylori, Mycoplasma pneumoniae*. Orally absorbed, but food delays absorption, first pass metabolism makes 50% available, excreted through kidney.

Indicated for RTI, sinusitis, otitis media, AIDS patient with *Mycobacterium avium* complex (MAC), *H. pylori* infection.

Gastric tolerance better, pseudomembranous enterocolitis may occur.

Azithromycin (Azithral 250 mg cap and 250 mg/5 mL dry syr): More active against *H. influenzae, Mycoplasma, Chlamydia, Legionella, Moraxella, Campylobacter, H. pylori, N gonorrhoeae, Mycobact. avium complex*. It is 15 atoms lactone macrolide derived from erythromycin by adding a methylated nitrogen to lactone ring.

Orally absorbed, acid stable, high concentration in macrophages, fibroblast. Used for pharyngitis, tonsillitis, sinusitis, otitis media, bronchitis, skin infection, chlamydial, pulmonary and genital infections, gonorrhea, AIDS with MAC infection, *H. pylori,* typhoid, toxoplasmosis, in malaria its activity being tried.

KETOLIDES

These are semisynthetic macrolides where a 3-keto group is substituted for neutral sugar 1-cladinose of erythromycin. Telithromycin is approved for clinical use. Oral bioavailability and intercellular penetration is good. Metabolized in liver and excreted by kidney. Daily dose is 800 mg for RTI including community-acquired pneumonia, bronchitis, sinusitis, pharyngitis. May prolong QT interval because it inhibits CYP34. Liver failure has been reported.

Streptogramin: Quinupristin–Dalfopristin (synercid) are the combination of streptogramin B and A in the ratio of 30 : 70. It is bactericidal except for *Enterococcus faecium* which kills slowly. They are approved for treatment of infection by *Staphylococcus* or by vancomycin resistant strain of *E. fascium*. Dose 7.5 mg/kg 8–12 hourly, requires its adjustment for renal failure or patient on dialysis. Drug interactions with warfarin, cisapride, terfenadine diazepam occur, because it inhibits CYP3A4. It is effective against MRSA and some VRSAs; vancomycin resistant enterococci.

OXAZOLIDINONES

Synthetic antibiotic, **Linezolid** is an oxazolidinone, active against *Staph, Streptococcus, Enterococcus, Corynebacteria, Listeria, M. tuberculosis*. It acts by 23s and 50s ribosomal subunits to inhibit protein synthesis. It is used in MRSA and VRSA *Staph. aureus*.

Thrombocytopenia may occur. Orally effective. Dose 600 mg BD orally or IV indicated for community-acquired pneumonia, complicated skin infection, vancomycin-resistant *E. faecium,* nosocomial pneumonia. Trade name lizolid 600 mg tab; linox 600 mg tab, 200 mg/100 mL IV.

Tedizolid phosphate is prodrug of **tedizolid** is next generation of oxazolidinone is effective against gram positive bacteria, MRSA used for skin, soft tissue infection.

105

Tetracycline

Tetracyclines are naphthacene derivatives made up by fusion of four partially unsaturated cyclohexane rings. Chlortetracycline is obtained from *Streptomyces aureofaciens*. They are bacteriostatic, inhibit protein synthesis by binding 30s ribosomes in susceptible organism in which it enters by energy-dependent active transport and in gram-negative bacteria it enters through porin channel. The lipid-soluble tetracycline may enter by passive diffusion.

Bacterial protein synthesis and site of action of some antibiotics: The 70s ribosomal mRNA is shown with its 50s and 30s subunits (step I), charged tRNA binds to acceptor site on 70s ribosome. The peptidyl tRNA at donor site (P) with amino acid binds the growing amino acid called transpeptidation (step 2). The uncharged tRNA is released at donor site (step 3). New amino acid with its tRNA shifts to the peptidyl site called translocation. Fig. 105.1

- Aminoglycoside binding with 30s and 50s subunits freezes initiation polysome formation.
- Tetracycline (T) binding 30s ribosome interferes with aminocyl tRNA attachment to acceptor site (A), *i.e.* it blocks step 1.
- Chloramphenicol (Ch) binds to 50s subunits and blocks transfer of amino acid from donor site (P), *i.e.* it blocks step 2.
- Macrolides (M) binds to 50s ribosome and hinders translocation of elongated peptide chain, so peptide synthesis is prematurely terminated.

The carrier involved in active transfer of tetracycline is absent in host cells. They chelate cations of calcium and magnesium, important for integrity of enzyme system. Tetracyclines are sensitive to all gram-positive and gram-negative cocci, *viz. Pneumococci, Gonococci, Clostridium, H. influenzae, H. pertusis, H. ducreyi, Brucella, K. pneumoniae, V. cholerae, Donovania granulomatis;* moderately sensitive *to E. coli, Aerobactor, Salmonella, Shigella, B. anthracis, P. tularensis, P. pestis, Fusibacterium, Listeria monocytogenes, Borrelia recurrentis, Mycoplasma pneumoniae, Leptospira ictohemorrhagica, T. pallidum.* It inhibits *Entamoeba histolytica* and *plasmodium* in high concentraction. Resistance to tetracycline occurs due to:
- Decreased concentrating power within the bacterial cell.
- Synthesis of protection protein which protects binding to ribosomes. Cross-resistance occurs between different tetracyclines and partial cross-resistance with chloramphenicol.
- Enzymatic inactivation.

Pharmacokinetics: Orally absorbed and taken ½ hour before meal. Tetracyclines are also available as IM. Ointments, creams are also available, but they produce sensitization.

Adverse effects of tetracyclines: Epigastric pain, nausea, vomiting, esophageal ulceration, thrombophlebitis when used IV, liver damage, kidney damage, phototoxicity, staining of teeth and depress bone growth, antianabolic effect. Increased intracranial pressure. Vestibular toxicity with minocycline, hypersensitivity (skin rash, urticaria, glossitis, pruritus ani and valve, exfoliative dermatitis), superinfection. Demeclocycline antagonizes action of ADH. It should

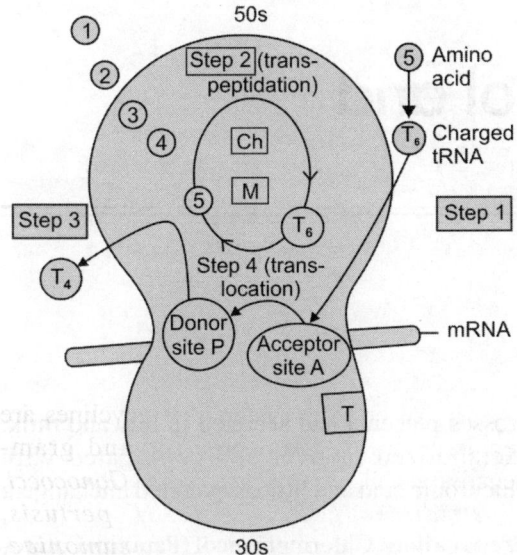

Ch = Chloramphenicol ⎫ Blocks step 2, i.e.
M = Macrolide   ⎬ transpeptidation
T = Tetracycline blocks step 1 and blocks incoming of charged tRNA

Fig. 105.1: Site of action of some antibiotic inhibiting protein synthesis

never be used in pregnancy, lactation and in children. Avoid with diuretics, kidney and liver damages. Use before expiry date, do not give it intrathecally. Do not mix penicillin and injectable tetracycline.

Therapeutic uses of tetracycline

- Rickettsial infections, drug used is tetracycline, 2–3 gm 1st day then 1–2 gm till recovery.
- Granuloma inguinale, drug used is tetracycline, 2 gm daily × 14 days.
- Primary atypical pneumonia
- Cholera
- Chlamydia infection
- Bacillary infections. Tetracycline 0.5 gm QDS × 2 weeks.
- Venereal deseases
- UTI
- Plague, tetracycline 4–6 gm daily orally for 1st 48 hours.
- Acne vulgaris ⎫
- Anthrax   ⎬ Penicillin is a preferred drug.
- Actinomycosis ⎪
- Yaws ⎭

- Relapsing fever
- Leptospirosis
- Amoebic dysentery and *Balantidium coli* dysentery
- Diagnosis for neoplastic cells of sputum. Gastric lavage in which they are accumulated and exhibit brilliant yellow-gold fluorescence to ultraviolet light.
- Demeclocycline is used for inappropriate secretion of ADH.
- Minocycline is used prophylactically in meningococcal meningitis epidemics. Rifampicin is a preferred drug.
- *H. pylori* infection of peptic ulcer
- Brucellosis
- Malaria

Different preparations of tetracycline

- Chlortetracyclilne (aureomycin 250, 500 mg caps; 3% skin oint; 1% eyedrop).
- Oxytetracyline (terramycin 250, 500 mg caps, 50 mg/mL 10 mL vial, 3% skin oint, 1% eye- or eardrop).
- Tetracycline (Idilin 250, 500 mg cap. 100 and 250, 500 mg vial for IV use, 3% skin oint, 1% eye- or eardrop and ointment).
- Dimethyl chlortetracycline (Demeclocycline, Ledermycin 150, 300 mg caps).
- Doxycycline (Tetradox 100 mg cap)
- Minocycline (cyanomycin 50, 100 mg caps)
- Rolitetracycline (Roverin 250–500 mg BD) used IV and IM
- Methacycline (rondomycin)
- **Lymecycline:** 150 mg of Lymecycline is equivalent to 250 mg of tetracycline made soluble by combining it with lysine.
- **Tigecycline:** Broad-spectrum; glycylcycline, Spectrum: Coagulase negative *Staph,* methicilline-resistant *Staph. aureus,* gram-positive rods, *Enterobactericeae, Rickettsia, Chlamydia, Legionella, Mycobacteria.* Dose 100 mg IV loading then 50 mg every 12 hours used for intra-abdominal and skin infections. Not effective in UTI as its concentration in urine is low.

Chloramphenicol and Thiamphenicol

Originally obtained from *Streptomyces venezuelae,* now prepared synthetically. Thiamphenicol is one of the derivatives of chloramphenicol which was used therapeutically, but was very toxic so withdrawn. It attaches itself to 50s ribosome and inhibits bacterial protein synthesis. It inhibits peptidyl transferase which results in inhibition of peptide bond formation and transfer of peptide chain from P to A site (Fig. 106.1). At higher doses mammalian mitochondrial protein synthesis particularly in bone marrow is inhibited. It is bacteriostatic. Active against gram-positive, gram-negative, *Rickettsiae, Chlamydia, Mycoplasma*. More active against *Salmonella, H. infiuenzae, B. pertusis, Klebsiella, Bact. fragilis*.

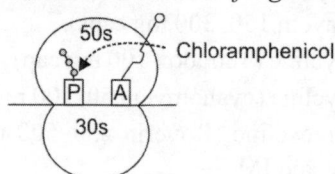

Fig. 106.1

Resistance develops through transfer of R factors which prevent to bind it with ribosomes and inactivates chloramphenicol. Partial cross-resistance with erythromycin, clindamycin, tetracycline has been noted.

Pharmacokinetics: Orally absorbed, plasma protein-bound, penetrates BBB, serous cavities, crosses placenta and secreted in bile and milk. Metabolized in liver and conjugated with glucuronic acid and little is excreted unchanged.

Preparation: Chlormphenicol (Paraxin, Enteromycetin 250–500 mg cap, 125 mg/4 mL oral syr, 0.5% eyedrop, 5% eardrop, 1% applicaps). Dose 250–500 mg 6 hourly; 25–50 mg/kg/day,

Chloramphenicol sodium succinate used parenterally.

Adverse effects: Rash, fever, glossitis, hypersensitivity (bone marrow depression, nausea, vomiting), superinfection, Gray baby syndrome—when given in high doses in children blocks electron transport in liver, myocardium and skeletal muscle leading to cardiovascular collapse.

Therapeutic uses: Enteric fever, *H. influenzae* meningitis, intraocular infection, secondline drug for brucellosis, cholera, rickettsia, chlamydia, whooping cough, *Meningococcal, Pneumococcal, Shigella*, dysentery, UTI. Topically used for conjunctivitis and ear infections.

It should be used with caution. Chloramphenicol inhibits metabolism of tolbutamide, warfarin, cyclophosphamide. Phenytoin, rifampicin, phenobarbitone induce chloramphenicol's metabolism.

Other Antibiotics

Lincomycin and clindamycin: Lincomycin is produced by growth of *Streptomyces lincolnensis*. Clindamycin is 7-chloro-7-deoxy-lincomycin derivative. It binds to 50s ribosomal subunits and inhibits amino acids synthesis of bacteria. It inhibits most gram-positive cocci, *C. diphtheriae, Nocardia. Actinomyces. Toxoplasma, Bact. fragilis* and ineffective against gram-negative.

Lincomycin is partially absorbed from gut, food interferes with absorption, penetrates serous sacs, skeletal and soft tissues, crosses placenta, but not blood-brain barrier.

Rash, urticaria, abdominal pain, impaired liver function, pseudomembranous enterocolitis due to *Clostridium difficile* superinfection. Lincomycin is available as 500 mg cap; 600 mg/2 mL inj. Dose 500 mg TDS or 600 mg IM or IU.

Clindamycin is essentially absorbed from gut but side effects are similar. Dose - 300 mg/2 ml/ lincomycin (lynx 500 mg cap; 125 mg/5 ml syr 300 mg/1 and 2 ml amp). Clindamycin is available as dalcap 150–300 mg caps. QID or 200–600 IV 8 hourly.

Vancomycin (Vancocin CP 150 mg tab and 500 mg/vial): Glycopeptide antibiotic, mol. wt. 1500. It targets transglycosylase enzyme of bacterial cell wall synthesis. Vancomycin resistance occurs due to modification of D-alanine-D-alanine binding site of peptidoglycan replaced by D-lactate. Effective against *Strep. viridans, Enterococcus, C. difficile.* Inhibits cell wall synthesis. Not absorbed orally. After IV administration widely distributed in serous sacs,

inflamed meninges. Excreted by glomerular filtration, so dose reduction required in kidney diseases. Not removed by hemodialysis. Given orally for pseudomembranous colitis and IV for methicillin-resistant *S. aureus,* dialysis patient, sepsis or endocarditis. Penicillin-resistant *Pneumococcal* infection and diphtheroids. While given by infusion it can cause "red man" or "red neck" syndrome due to flushing, caused by histamine release, which can be largely prevented by increasing dose interval and infusion time.

Teicoplanin (Targocid 200 mg/vial): Glycopeptide antibiotic can be given IV or IM once daily because of long t½, mechanism and is like vancomycin. Dose 400 mg 1st day then 200 mg daily.

Dalbavancin: It is semisynthetic lipoglycopeptide derivative of teicoplanin, but with improved action against gram-positive methicillin-resistant and vancomycin intermediate *S. aureus.* It how long t½ co-11 days so used weekly by IV route.

Telavancin: It is also semisynthetic lipoglycopeptide derivative of vancomycin. It apart from inhibiting cell wall synthesis also targets bacterial cell membrane causing disruption of membrane potential and increasing membrane permeability. It is approved for skin, soft tissue and hospital acquired pneumonia.

Daptomycin: Cyclic lipopeptide, fermentation product of *Streptomyces roeseosporus.* It appears to bind to cell membrane *via* calcium-dependent insertion in its lipid tail and depolarize it to efflux potassium and causes its death. Dose 4–6 mg/kg for skin infection and bacterial endocarditis. It causes myopathy so CPK should be monitored. Should not be used for pneumonia as it is antagonized by surfactant. In renal failure dose of interval should be increased.

Fosfomycin: It inhibits early stages of bacterial cell wall synthesis, *i.e.* targeting enol pyruvate transferase. Effective against gram-positive and gram-negative. Both oral and parenteral preparations are available. May be combined with aminoglycosides, β-lactam or fluroquinolones. Safe in pregnancy. Used for lower UTI. Dose single, 3 gm orally or parenterally.

Viomycin and capreomycin: Produced by *Strep guiseus var purpureus* and *Strep. carpreolus* respectively, are polypeptide antibiotics. Act against protein synthesis of mycobacteria, as tuberculostatic. Kidney damage and deafness may occur. Administered by IM route, because of poor oral absorption.

Virginiamycin or staphylomycin: Obtained from *St. virginiae,* active against gram-positive and some gram-negatives (gonorrhea). Orally absorbed, excreted through kidney, probably inhibits 50s ribosomal induced protein synthesis.

Spectinomycin: Obtained from *Strep. spectabilis.* Active against some gram-positives *(Staph)* and gram-negatives *Brucella, Klebsiella, Proteus, Pseudomonas* and *Niesseria.* Acts on 30s ribosome to inhibit protein synthesis. Side effects are urticaria, fever, CNS symptoms. Specially indicated for penicillinase producing gonococcal infection allergic to penicillin in pregnancy when fluoroquinolones are contraindicated. It is used as 1 gm IM as single dose.

Fusidic Acid (Fucidin leo 2% unit and cream): Steroidal antibiotic, active against penicillinase producing gram-positive bacteria. Topically used.

Bacitracin (Nebasulf 250 U/gm powder): Polypeptide antibiotic obtained from certain strains of bacteria, *Bacillus subtilis* and *Bacillus licheniformis.* Active against gram-positive *Staphylococci;* hemolytic and nonhemolytic *Strepto, Clostridium, Corynebacterium, Treponema* and gram-negative *Neisseria.* It inhibits cell wall synthesis. Nephrotoxic, polyuria, albuminuria, anorexia, nausea, pain at injection site may occur. Parenterally rarely used under strict supervision because of toxicity. Externally used on skin, nose, eye in susceptible organism.

Ristocetin: Produced by *Actinomycetes and Nocardia luridie* used for severe *Staphylococcus* infection not responding to other antibiotics, but rarely used because of its adverse effects of hypersensitivity, blood dyscrasia, diarrhea, thrombophlebitis. Mechanism of action is like vancomycin.

Polymyxin B and Colistin: Obtained from *Bacillus polymyxa* and *B. colistinus* respectively. Effective against gram-negative except *Proteus, Sarrtia, Neisseria.* Colistin is more effective on *Pseudomonas, Salmonella* and *Shigella* are more bactericidal, act as detergent, leading to leaking out of amino acids from bacterial cells. Resistance develops quickly, topically applied. Adverse reactions are rare. Rash, nausea, vomiting may occur with oral preparation. Colistin sulfate 25–100 mg TDS (Walamycin 125 mg/ 5 mL dry syr).

Used topically to treat burns, otitis externa. conjunctivitis, corneal ulcer caused by gram-negative organism. Orally colistin (Walamycin 25,000 IU/5 mL dry powder) is used in infants to treat diarrhea. Polymyxin is also used intrathecally.

Tyrothricin: Obtained from *Bacillus bravis* is a mixture of gramicidin and tyrocidin. Active against gram-positive and few gram-negative bacteria. Acts on cell membrane and uncouples oxidative phosphorylation. Toxic for systemic use and orally not absorbed. Topically used, (tyrodem 0.5 mg/gm skin cream; prothricin 0.2 mg/mL solution).

Novobiocin: Obtained from *Streptomyces niveus.* Highly toxic, not used routinely.

Bacteriostatic drug. Fever, dermatitis, hemolytic anemia, leukopenia, bone marrow depression, kernicterus in infants, superinfection with fungus and yeast may occur. Used for *Staphylococcus* infection resistant to other antibiotics.

Dose: 0.5–1 gm 8–12 hourly; children 30 mg/kg/day.

Mupirocin (T-Bact 2% w/w oint): Obtained from *Pseudomonas fluorescens,* inhibits bacterial protein synthesis. Effective against *Staphylococcus* MRSA and many other gram-negative organisms like *Clostridium, Haemophillia, Proteius, Klebsiella.* Should not be applied on face, eye and nose. Itching, sensitization may occur. Topically used.

Urinary Tract Infection (UTI)

DRUGS EFFECTIVE IN UTI

Urinary tract infection (UTI) is a common disorder in all ages and sexes. Majority of the UTI are due to gram-negative bacilli *E. coli;* other offending organisms are *Proteus, Klebsiella, Pseudomonas, Enterococci, Streptococcus* and *Staphylococcus.* Normal urinary tract except distal urethra is sterile. Commonly, UTI is diagnosed by culture and sensitivity with colony count. Colony count about 10^5/mL is significant bacteriuria and below that is insignificant bacteriuria. Following drugs are usually used for UTI.

- Sulfonamide*
- Cotrimoxazole*
- Nitrofurantoin*

- **Methenamine mandelate (Mandelamine):** Rapidly absorbed from GIT and excreted in urine at low pH of 5. Methenamine liberates formaldehyde which is bactericidal to gram-negative pathogens and *C. albicans.* $N_4(CH_2)_6 + 6H_2O + 4H^{(+)} \rightarrow 4NH_4 + 6HCHO.$ Acidic urine is must for its action, maintained by

Table 108.1: Favourable urinary pH for antibacterial action in UTI

pH does not effect	Alkaline pH	Acidic pH
Chloramphenicol	Sulfonamide	Nitrofurantoin
Ampicillin	Cotrimoxazole	Methenamine
Colistin	Aminoglycosides	Methicillin
Amoxycillin	Fluoroquinolone	Cloxacillin

administering organic acid or ascorbic acid. It should not be used with sulfamethazole with which it produces insoluble precipitates. Fluid restriction ensures adequate concentration in urine 0.5 to 1 gm tab TDS dose. Other drugs effective for UTI are:

- ◆ Fluoroquinolone*(Norfloxacin, ciprofloxacin)
- ◆ Ampicillin*
- ◆ Cloxacillin*
- ◆ Piperacillin/carbenicillin*
- ◆ Cephalosporin/gentamicin*
- ◆ Chloramphenicol*
- ◆ Tetracyclines*
- ◆ Methicillin*
- ◆ Cephalothin*

Some newer quinolones and newer drugs are also used.

Prophylactic Antibacterial Therapy for UTI

- Following instrumentation of urinary tract
- Indwelling catheter in bladder
- Uncorrectable congenital anomalies of urinary tract
- Asymptomatic bacteriuria: Sulfonamides, ampicillin, nitrofurantoin are used for the purposes.

Phenazopyridine (Pyridium 200 mg; 1 tab TDS): It has no antibacterial property, gives symptomatic relief to burning pain, dysuria, urgency by acting as urinary analgesic. Nausea, epigastric pain may occur.

---

*Discussed in detail in individual chapter.

Treatment of Sexually Transmitted Diseases

The WHO reports 250 million new cases of sexually transmitted diseases (STD) each year of which 1 million are HIV/STD categorized by symptomatology.

Genital ulcer

- Syphilis
- Chancroid
- Herpes
- Human papilloma
- Lymphogranuloma venereum (LGV)
- Granuloma inguinale

Vaginal discharge

- Gonorrhea
- Chlamydia
- Candidiasis*
- Trichomoniasis*
- Bacterial vaginosis*

Other STD infections are HIV, hepatitis B, scabies, lice.

Urethral discharge

- Gonorrhea
- Chlamydia

Lower abdominal pain

- Pelvic inflammatory diseases

TREATMENT

Syphilis

Benzathine penicillin

2.4 MU IM 1–3 weekly or procaine penicillin G 1.2 MU IM × 10 days

Alternatively

Doxycycline 100 mg BD × 15 days
or ceftriaxone 1 gm IM × 7 days
or erythromycin 500 mg QID × 15 days

Table 109.1: Safe and unsafe sexual activities		
Safe	Probably safe	Unsafe
• Touching, hugging, massage • Masturbation alone or with partner • Rubbing bodies together • Talking about sex • Kissing or licking the body (no oral contact with genitals or open sores)	• Vaginal intercourse with condom • Oral intercourse with a condom • Anal intercourse with condom • French kissing	• Vaginal intercourse without condom • Oral and anal intercourse without condom • Sharing objects inserted into vagina or anus • Any activity allows blood to blood contact.

---

*Not always STD.

Gonorrhea

Amoxycillin	3 gm
or ampicillin	3.5 gm + 1 gm probenecid
Penicillinase	Ceftriaxone 250 mg IM or
producing	Cefuroxime 250 mg IM

Alternatively

Cefixime 400 mg once orally
Doxycycline 100 mg BD × 7 days
Erythromycin 500 mg oral or
Norfloxacin 800 mg oral
Pefloxacin 400 mg or ofloxacin orally 200 mg

Chancroid (*H. ducreyt*)

Cotrimoxazole 960 mg BD × 7 days
or Erythromycin 500 mg QDS × 7 days

Alternatively

Tetracycline 500 mg QDS × 7 days
or ciprofloxacin 500 mg BD × 3 days
or ceftriaxone 250 mg IM.

Chlamydia Trachomatis

Tetracycline 500 mg QDS × 7 days
or Doxycycline 100 mg BD × 7 days

Alternatively

Sulfamethoxazole 1 gm BD × 7 days
or erythromycin 500 mg QDS × 7 days

Granuloma Inguinale

Doxycycline 100 mg BD × 3 days
Tetracycline 500 mg QDS × 10 days

Alternatively

Co-trimoxazole 960 mg BD × 14 days
or erythromycin 500 mg QDS × 21 days

Trichomoniasis

Metronidazole 400 mg TDS × 7 days
or Tinidazole 600 mg × 7 days (treat both partner)

Alternatively

Cotrimazole 100 mg intravaginal every night × 2 weeks

Herpes

Acyclovir 5% ointment 6 times × 10 days
Acyclovir 200 mg 5 times × 10 days orally for late cases.

110

Chemotherapy of Tuberculosis

Tuberculosis is an infectious disease producing chronic granulomatous lesion produced by several species of mycobacteria collectively termed as Tubercle bacilli. It is a disease which indicates social welfare barometer. It has been described as king of disease in Vedas as mentioned by Charaka and Sushruta. Robert Koch discovered the bacilli in 1882.

Principles of treatment of tuberculosis
- Rest
- Nutrition
- Chemotherapy
- Adequate prolonged follow-up gives 100% cure rate.

Aims of treatment of tuberculosis
- To cure patient with least interference with their activities.
- To prevent death in seriously ill-patient.
- To prevent complication and extensive damage.
- To prevent relapse.
- To prevent development of resistance.
- To prevent family and the community from infection.

Resistant to Antitubercular Drug

Primary resistance: Right from beginning of therapy.

Secondary resistance: During therapy due to:
- Incorrect treatment
- Two drugs are given, but patient is resistant to one of them.
- Patient failing to take drug regularly.

Resistant to antituberculosis drug occurs due to:
- **Bad doctor**—not giving adequate doses.
- **Bad patient**—not accepting right advice.
- **Bad luck**—resistance to drug right from beginning.

Microbiologically and clinically confirmed TB patient are also classified according to: (i) anatomical site viz. (a) Pulmonary and extrapulmonary. Miliary TB is pulmonary (ii), based on history (a) New cases (b) previously treated recurrent TB treatment failure cases, treatment with loss of follow up transfered in patients, (iii) based on drug resistance as mono resistance (MR); (b) poly drug resistance (PDR) (c) Multi drug resistance (MDR) and (d) Rifampicin resistance (RR) (e) Extended drug resistance (XDR) resistance to fluoroquonolone and injectable anti TB drug second line (Kanamycin, capreomycin, amikacin, etc).

Tuberculosis is difficult to treat because
- Caseation necrosis keeps tuberculosis remain dormant.
- Caseation blocks the blood vessels supplying necrotic area making penetration of antitubercular drug difficult.
- Organism develop resistance quickly.
- Tubercle bacilli remain viable inside macrophages where most of antitubercular drugs could not penetrate.

A big list of drugs effective against tuberculosis is discovered in last 60 years. They are categorized into two groups (Table 110.1):

Table 110.1: List of antitubercular drugs

1st line drugs	2nd line drugs	Newer drugs
Isoniazid (H) (1952)	Thiacetazone (Tzn)	Ciprofloxacin
Rifampicin (R) (1962)	Para-aminosalicylic acid (PAS)	Ofloxacin
Pyrazinamide (Z)	Ethionamide (Etm)	Sparfloxacin
Ethambutol (E) (1962)	Morphazinamide	Clarithromycin
Streptomycin (S) (1947)	Cycloserine (Cys)	Azithromycin
	Kanamycin (Kmc)	Rifabutin
	Amikacin (Am)	Rifapentine
	Capreomycin (Cpr)	Linezolid
	Clofazinamide	Bedaquiline clofazomine, co-amoxyclav

Isoniazid (H): Excellent tuberculocidal drug, if there is no rsistance or patient can tolerate it. Most probably effects are on nucleic acid and glycolysis, and affects membrane lipids and inhibits synthesis of mycolic acid unique to mycobacterial cell wall.

INH is a prodrug activated by KatG, the mycobacterial catalase peroxidase. Overexpression of INH A produces low level INH resistance and cross-resistance to ethionamide. KatG mutant expresses INH resistant, but not always cross-resistant to ethionamide.

At least two active drugs should be prescribed to treat active tuberculosis to avoid resistance development.

Combined with other antitubercular drug. Prevents resistance to other drug and cross-resistance.

INH is orally absorbed and enters all body tissues, *viz.* placenta, meninges. Metabolized by acetylation in liver (some are fast acetylators and some are slow). Dose 300 mg/day or 5 mg /kg/day.

ADR: Hepatitis, peripheral neuropathy, optic neuritis, convulsions, difficulty in micturition, tremor, hyperreflexia, pellagra, hemolytic reaction in glucose-6PO_4-deficient patient, granulocytosis, arthralgia, SLE. Pyridoxine should be given simultaneously to prevent neuropathy. ADR common with slow acetylators.

Drug interactions of INH

• Antacids prevent its absorption

• Phenytoin, carbamazepine, diazepam, warfarin level increase because their metabolisms are inhibited.

• PAS inhibits INH metabolism and increases t½.

Rifampicin (R) (R-cin 150, 300, 450, 600 mg caps or mg/mL): Semisynthetic derivative of rifamycin B, obtained from *Streptomyces mediterranei* effective against gram-positive, gram-negative and tuberculocidal to all subpopulation of Tubercle bacill. Other derivatives are refabutin and rifapentine. Inhibits DNA dependent RNA polymerase, stopping expression of bacterial gene. Its resistance to tuberculosis is low and cross-resistance does not occur. Dose below 50 kg body wt. is 450 mg, above 50 kg is 600 mg or 10 mg/kg daily for intermittent therapy (600–900 mg biweekly). It is bactericidal. Given in empty stomach.

Orally absorbed and penetrates placenta, caseous masses, meninges. Eliminated through feces, so can be used safely in renal dysfunction.

ADR: Nausea, vomiting, red man syndrome, jaundice, hepatitis, osteomalacia, pseudomembranous colitis, pseudoadrenal crisis, flu-like syndrome, thrombocytopenia, hemolytic anemia, renal failure, light chain proteinuria, eosinophilia.

It is an liver enzyme inducer, therefore, doses of oral contraceptive pills, digoxin, oral hypoglycemics, anticoagulants, dapsone, cyclosporine, ketoconazole, phenobarbitone should be adjusted.

Other uses of rifampicin

- Leprosy (fastest acting drug)
- Prophylaxis of meningococcal and *H. influenzae* meningitis, and carrier state
- Methillin-resistant *Staph, Diphtheroids, Legionella* infections
- In brucellosis with doxycycline
- To enhance effect of amphotericin B in fungal infection.

Pyrazinamide (Z) (pyzina 05, 75, 1 gm or 0.3 gm kid tab or 250 mg/5 mL): Chemically related to thiosemicarbazones and nicotinamide. Effective in acidic medium and intracellular bacilli. Developed parallel to INH in 1952 with sterilizing effect on *T. bacilli* of human. Effect in first two months, when inflammatory changes are present against intracellular bacteria. Resistance develops quickly, absorbed orally, CSF concentration is equal to plasma.

Dose below 50 kg body wt. 1.5 gm/day; above 50 kg bdoy wt. 2 gm/day or 35 mg/kg/day or 50 mg/kg triweekly.

ADR: Hepatotoxicity, arthralgia (increases absorption of urates), anorexia, sideroblastic anemia, porphyria, photosensitivity.

Ethambutol(E) (mycobutol 0.2, 0.4, 0.6, 1 gm tabs): Dextroisomer of butanol, bacteriostatic but susceptible to many atypical mycobacteria and fast multiplying bacteria. Mechanism not known, may be interfering of mycolic acid incorporation in cell wall and inhibits RNA synthesis. Orally absorbed, widely distributed, CSF penetration 20%, RBC acts as depot for it, excreted with urine. Dose 15–25 mg/kg/day.

ADR: Retrobulbar neuritis, arthralgia, peripheral neuropathy, paresthesia of limbs, anaphylactic shock, nausea, vomiting, anorexia, confusion, headache, allergic reaction.

Streptomycin (S): Antibiotics obtained from *Streptomycin greseus.* Dihydrostreptomycin is more stable, but more ototoxic. Effective against *M. tuberculosis, Shigella, E. coli, Proteus, Pseudomonas, H. influenzae, H. ducreyi, P. pestis, Brucella, Actinobacillus, Listeria, Nocardia,* moderately sensitvie to *Staph.* and *Strepto. pyogenes and faecalis, D.pneumoniae, Vibro cholera.* It is bactericidal.

It enters bacteria through porin channels, carrier mediated linked to electron transport chain which is favored by alkaline pH. Inside the cell, they bind to 30s ribosomes (other aminoglycosides bind to 50s ribosomal subunit) and freeze protein synthesis. The cidal effect of streptomycin is concentration-dependent. Develops resistance quickly.

It has to be given IM and CSF penetration is poor. Dose 0.75–1 gm/day.

ADR: Hypersensitivity, ototoxicity, renal damage, neuromuscular blockage, rarely hemolytic anemia, thrombocytopenia. It is a cause of concern for TB and HIV programs in view of risk of transmission by HIV contaminated needle.

Thiacetazone (Tzn) (50, 150 mg tab): Thiosemicarbazone derivative, first ATD drug tested. Bacteriostatic, low efficacy, highly toxic drug, orally active. Excreted unchanged with urine.

ADR: Cutaneous reactions, Stevens-Johnson syndrome, vertigo, agranulocytosis, thrombocytopenia, cerebral edema. Do not give in liver disease or renal failure patient. Dose 150 mg/day or 4 mg/kg/day.

Para-amino salicylic acid (PAS): Chemically sulfonamide derivative. Bacteriostatic, mechanism is similar to sulfonamide, PAS and PABA may be having receptor in Tubercle bacilli making it effective for tuberculosis, but not for other sulfonamide derivatives. Resistance develops slowly. Orally absorbed, distributed widely except CSF and acetylated which may competes with INH. Absorption of rifampicin is interfered. Dose 10–12 gm in 2 divided doses.

ADR: GI upsets, malabsorption syndrome with folic acid deficiency, megaloblastic anemia, acute renal failure, goiter, diffuse pulmonary opacities with eosinophilia may occur.

Ethionamide (ETm) (Ethinex 125 and 250 mg tabs): Tuberculostatic drug, effective against both typical and atypical bacilli, quickly develops resistance, believed to inhibit protein synthesis in cell. Orally absorbed and cross-resistance to thiacetazone may occur, distributed throughout body, completely metabolized.

ADR: Anorexia, metallic taste, psychotic disturbances, hypoglycemia, menstrual disturbances, gynecomastia, impotence, peripheral neuropathy. Dose 0.5–0.75 gm/day or 10–15 mg/kg/day,

Cycloserine (Cys): Obtained from *S. orchidaceus,* tuberculostatic and inhibits cell wall synthesis. Useful to treat gram-positive organism. Orally absorbed, diffuses all over including CSF, metabolized in liver and excreted with urine. Dose 250 mg BD.

ADR: Dizziness, slurred speech, convulsion. headache, tremor, insomnia, *i.e.* neurosymptoms preventable with pyridoxine. It should be avoided in epilepsy, anxiety state or alcoholism. Safety profile in pregnancy not known.

Capreomycin (Cm): Used for those not responding to classical ATD or atypical tuberculosis. Dose 1 gm/day. Oto- and nephrotoxicities, decreases K, Ca, Mg level of blood.

Viomycin: Weak antitubercular drug rarely used.

Kanamycin and amicacin: Reserve for rare cases not responding to usual therapy and for atypical mycobacteria. Highly toxic not combined with streptomycin or between them.

Quinolones (ciprofloxacin, ofloxacin, sparfloxacin): Sparfloxacin is eight times more potent than ciprofloxacin, penetrate cells and kill mycobacteria, lodged in macrophages. They are better tolerated and active against *M. avium* complex, so their use is increasing in multidrug-resistant tuberculosis.

Macrolides (roxithromycin, azithromycin, clarithromycin): They are good accompanying drug in multidrug-resistant tuberculosis.

Rifabutin: More effective than rifampicin for MAC and its t½ is also more (45 hours) than rifampicin (4 hours). Less enzyme inducing and its metabolism is inhibited by clarithromycin and fluconazole.

Rifapentine: This is an analog of rifampicin, so cross-resistant possible, inhibits bacterial polymerase. Dose 600 mg or 10 mg/kg weekly. It should not be used in HIV patient because it produces rifampicin-resistant organism. It is more lipophilic and longer acting.

Linezolid: This oxazolidinone derivative is used in the dose of 600 mg daily for adult as 2nd and 3rd line drugs to treat tuberculosis. Long-term use may depress bone marrow or may cause peripheral or optic neuropathy.

Indications of corticosteroids in tuberculosis
- Allergic reaction to drugs.
- Pleural, peritoneal, pericardial effusions
- To reduce fibrosis of eye, larynx, ureter
- Tuberculous meningitis
- Tuberculous Addison's disease

Short-term therapy (Long-term, 12–18 months treatment is replaced by: 2 RHSZ + 4 HR or 2 RHZE + 2 HR).

Short-term therapy advantagses
- Rapid bacteriological conversion
- Low failure rate
- Reduce frequency of drug resistance
- Improved patient compliance.

Home treatment is best but isolation of patient is required for:
- Teacher and other in contact with children.

Table 110.2: Clinical types of TB bacteria and their sensitivity to different ADTs			
Rapidly growing	*Slow growing*	*Spurter grow in*	*Dormant*
With high bacillary load susceptible to H > R, E and S	Intracellular, grows at low pH. Susceptible to Z less than H; R; E	Low oxygen, low pH, caseous meterial sensitive to R and insensitive to S	Inactive to ATD drug
There is continuous shifting of bacilli between these subpopulation			

Table 110.3: Indicates the treatment regimen, type of patients and regimen prescribed

Treatment group	Type of patient	Regimen* Intensive phase (IP)	Regimen* Continuation phase (CP)
New	Sputum smear-positive Sputum smear-negative Extrapulmonary Others	$2H_3R_3Z_3E_3$	$4H_3R_3$
Previously treated	Smear-positive relapse Smear-positive failure Smear-positive treatment after default Others	$2H_3R_3Z_3E_3S_3/1H_3R_3Z_3E_3$	$5H_3R_3H_3$

*Regimen for New cases treatment consists of total 78 doses and for previously treated cases consists of 102 doses.

Regimen for	IP Blisters	IP Doses	Extended IP blister and doses	CP Blisters	CP Doses
New cases (Cat-I)	24	24	12	18	54
Previously treated cases (Cat-II)	36	36	12	22	66

- Getting immunosuppressive till sputum turns negative.
- Only resistant tuberculosis.
- Home treatment is best.

Hospitalization required in

- Massive hemoptysis
- Massive effusion
- Pneumothorax
- No one to look after in home.

Biology of tuberculosis infection

Depending on environmental condition they

Table 110.4: Categorization of tuberculous patients

Category-I	Category-II	Category-III	Category-IV
New smear (+) PTD failure	Smear-positive PTD with failure relapse	Smear-negative remaining	Chronic cases positive after full treatment
New smear (−) with patient parenchymal involvement	Interrupted treatment or failure	Parenchymal involvement ion	
TB, meningitis, peritonitis, pericarditis, etc.			

Table 110.5: Treatment according to category

	Category-I	Category-II	Category-III	Category-IV
Initial phase	2 (HRZE) (S)	2 HRZE (S) + 1 HRZE	2 (HRE)	Therapy depends upon drug used in earlier regimen and associated conditions of AIDS/diabetes/leukemia, etc.
Continuation	4 HR	5 (HRE)	4 HR	
Total duration	6 months	8 months	6 months	

multiply in aerobic conditions can be categorized into following groups (Table 110.2): Category 1 (New cases), Category 2 (Previously treated patient)

Tuberculosis in pregnant woman: 2 months HRZ + 4 months H + R treatment. Should not be delayed or withheld for pregnancy; breastfeeding should be continued. Infant should be protected with BCG and isoniazid.

Drug reaction: In case of hepatitis, rifampicin is withdrawn, streptomycin and ethambutol is started. Fluoroquinolone may be added.

HIV and tuberculosis: Are deadly duo, because it can make latent risk factors overt and the adverse effects of ATD are more in HIV patient. The regimens are same. For *Mycobacterium avium* complex (MAC), clarithromycin or azithromycin + ethambutol may be used. Ciprofloxacin/clofazamine/rifabutin/ethionamide/cycloserine may be added.

HIV patients require life long prophylaxis with rifabutin.

Drugs for Atypical Mycobacteria

M.kanasii susceptible to rifampicin and ethambutol.

M. avium complex: Azithromycin 500 mg or clarithromycin 500 BD + ethambutol 15–25 mg/kg/day or ciprofloxacin 750 mg BD or rifambutin 300 mg OD.

New drug **Bedaquiline fumarate** is approved for Multidrug resistant tuberculosis (MDR-TB) in adults aged above 18 years but may be considered in children, HIV infected, pregnant woman, extapulmonary TB if effective treatment cannot be provided. It specifically targets mycobacterial ATP synthetase.

Nausea, vomiting, anorexia, dizziness arthralgia, myalgia, headache raised serum transaminases, rash may occur.

It is given after meal.Patient should abstain from alcohol and hapatotoxic drug. Another new

drug **Delamanid** is uses for multi drug resistant tuberculosis. It inhibits mycolic acids synthesis.

A Drug sensitive regimen:

i. **New Tb cases intensive phase** (IP) INH; Rifampicin pyrazinamide, Ethambutol. In continuation phase pyrazinamide in stopped.

ii. **For previously treated cases,** Streptomycin, INH; Pyraznamide Rifampicin, Ethambutol in intensive phase of 12 weeks. Streptomyncin is stopped after 8 weeks; rest drug for four weeks. In continuation phase pyrazinamide in stopped and rest of the drug continues for 20 weeks as daily doses. The continuation phase may be extended by 12-24 weeks in TB of CNS, bones, dessiminated TB.

MDR/RR TB Cases

6–9 months of intensive phase with Kanamycin, levofloxacin, ethambutol, pyrazinamide, ethionamide and cycloserine. Continuation phase for 18 months with levofloxacin. ethambutol, ethionamide, cycloserine. Appropriate modification done in presence of additional resistance.

XDR TB treated with capreomycin injection, moxifloxacin linezolid, PAS, clofazimine, high dose INH and Co-amoxyclav the intensive phase is 6–12 months. The continuation phase is 18 months when injectables are stopped.

Physician should consult the latest guidelines for tuberculosis treatment always.

Extensively drug-resistant (XDR) TB

Patient of TB who are resistant to at least four cidal drugs with or without any number of other drugs are called extensively drug resistant (XDR) TB. They are virtually untreatable with high mortality, particularly if with HIV patient.

111

Chemotherapy of Leprosy

Causative organism of leprosy is *Mycobacterium leprae* discovered by Hansen in 1873, is obstinate disease, has prolong treatment. It is difficult to transmit leprosy in animals though recently it has been cultivated successfully in foot pad of mice and successfully transmitted to some species of armadillo, providing model for human leprosy.

DISEASE OF LEPROSY

Types

Clinically

- Tuberculoid
- Borderline tuberculoid
- Borderline lepromatous
- Borderline
- Lepromatous

According to bacterial load

- Multibacillary leprosy (MBL)
- Paucibacillary leprosy (PBL)

Classification of Antileprotic Drugs

- **Sulfones:** Dapsones (DDS), 4, 4-diacetyl-diamino-diphenylsulfones, diaminodiphenylthiourea (thiambutosone).
- **Phenazine derivatives:** Clofazamine.
- **Antitubercular drugs:** Rifampicin, ethionamide.
- **Other antibiotics:** Ofloxacin, moxifloxacin minocycline, clarithromycin.
- **Mercaptan compounds:** Diethyl dithiolisophthalate (ditophal).
- **Chaulmoogra and hydnocarpus oil.**

Sulfones: Diamino-diphenylsulfones are oldest, cheapest, chemically related to sulfonamide.

They inhibit PABA incorporated into folic acid (specific for *M. leprae*).

Orally absorbed, well-distributed, 70% plasma protein-bound, concentrated specially in lepromatous skin, muscle, liver and kidney. Acetylated and conjugated with glucuronide and sulfate, excreted in urine. It is cumulative in nature. Resistance may develop (either primary or secondary) like tuberculosis, (dapsone, novaphone 25, 50, 100 mg. There is color coding for tablet strength).

Repository sulfones (4, 4-diacetyldiamino-diphenylsulfones, DADDS) given IM (225 mg) gives effective blood level of DDS for 70–80 days.

Other sulfone derivatives like glucosulfone sodium (promin), sulfoxone sodium (diasone), thiazole sulfones (promizole), promacetin are also used. But offer no advantage. Adverse reactions to sulfones are anorexia, nausea, vomiting, dermatitis, skin sensitization, hepatitis, exfoliative dermatitis, blood dyscrasia, goiter, methemoglobinemia, hematuria, hemolysis in glucose-6PO$_4$-deficient patient.

Diaminodisphenylthiourea: (Thiambutosine) as thiosemicarbazide derivative usually given orally, may be by injection (oral 0.5 gm daily) IM [20% suspension in arachis oil 1 mL (200 mg of drug) weekly]. Rapidly develops resistance, useful for those patients who are not able to tolerate dapsone. Adverse reactions are anorexia, nausea, vomiting, dermatitis, anemia, blood dyscrasia.

Clofazamine (Hansepran 50, 100 mg cap): Phenazine dye, retained in tissues of RE system, leprostatic and weak anti-inflammatory and 2nd line drug in sulfone-resistant leprosy.

Apart from skin discoloration, conjunctival pigmentation, itching, nausea, loose stool, abdominal pain, anorexia, weight loss can occur.

Rifampicin: Leprocidal, rapidly makes leprosy patient non-contagious, resistant develops. Antileprotic dose is relatively nontoxic. Included in multidrug therapy, rifampicin congener rifabutin is also leprocidal, but not superior to it.

Ethionamide: Antitubercular drug has anti-leprotic activity used as alternative to clofaza-mine.

Fluoroquinolones: Ofloxacin, moxifloxacin pefloxacin, sparfloxacin have antileprotic activity. Ofloxacin includes in MDT has better clinical and biological response. Dose 400 mg/day.

Minocycline (100 mg/day): Bactericidal, lipophilic, active against *M. leprae.*

Clarithromycin: Macrolide antibiotic has lepro-cidal; 500 mg/day kills 99% bacteria in 8 weeks.

Chaulmoogra and hydnocarpus oil: Obtained from seeds of trees of genus *Hydnocarus* used in India, Burma, Thailand, Malaya. Chemically, both oils are indentical, unsaturated fatty acids chaulmoogric acid and hydrocarpic acid, used as or by local intradermal injection.They are not recommended now.

MULTIDRUG THERAPY (MDT) IN LEPROSY

Advantages

- Effective in dapsone resistance
- Prevents dapsone resistance
- Quick relief and makes patient non-contagiousness and short duration of action
- Efficacy, safety and acceptability excellent, lepra reaction less
- Resistance to rifampicin develops less

MDT regimens for leprosy patient

Children should get proportionate less dose.

Multibacillary leprosy

Dapsone 100 mg/day (self)

Rifampicin 600 mg/month (supervised)
Clofazamine 300 mg/months (supervised), 50 mg daily for 1 years.

Paucibacillary leprosy

Dapsone 100 mg/day (self)
Rifampicin 600 mg/month (supervised) for 6 months.

Lepra reaction: Usually occurs at initiation of therapies like Jarish Herxheimar (Arthus) type of reaction, due to liberation of antigens from killed bacteria, may be mild or severe like **erythema nodosum leprosum** (generally with lepromatous leprosy), develops 4–6 weeks of dapsone therapy called sulfone syndrome, chara-cterized by fever, malaise, lymph node enlarge-ment, with crops of bright, erythematous nodules and red patches with existing lesion becomes worse.

Treatment: Discontinue treatment of dapsone temporarily and start after 2 weeks. Clofazamine 200 mg daily.

Analgesic, antipyretic, antibiotics, chloro-quine, corticosteroid and thalidomide in rare cases.

Reversal reaction: Occurs with tuberculoid leprosy, is delayed type of hypersensitivity reac-tion. It is treated with clofazamine and cortico-steroid. Manifests with cutaneous ulceration, nerve involvement with pain and tenderness.

Some Alternative Regimens

They are used in case of rifampicin resistance or when standard multidrug therapy is unadvisable.

- Clofazamine 50 mg + ofloxacin 400 mg/ minocycline 100 mg × 6 months.
- Clofazamine 50 mg + minocycline 100 mg + clarithromycin 500 mg × 6 months.
  followed by clofazamine 50 mg + ofloxacin 400 mg daily × 18 months.
- Clarithromycin 500 mg + minocycline 100 mg + sparfloxacin 200 mg + rifampicin 600 mg for 3 months.
- ROM regimen: **R**ifampicin 600 mg + **O**flox-acin 400 mg + **M**inocycline 100 mg, single dose for solitary lesion of paucibacillary lesion. Once a month for 3–6 months for PBL and 12–24 months for BML.

112

Antimalarial Drugs

Malarial parasites are globally present, but in tropical zones it is endemic. It is caused by *Plasmodium vivax, Plasmodium falciparum, Plasmodium malariae, Plasmodium ovale,* pass their life cycle asexually in man (intermediate) and sexually in anopheline female mosquitoes (definitive) host.

Man is the natural reservoir of malarial parasite infected by sporozoites, injected by mosquito bite through proboscis along with anticoagulant in saliva, has to enter liver cell, because sporozoites survive in blood for one hour only. In the liver cells it multiples (pre-erythrocytic stage) to produce thousands of uninucleated merozoites, which are liberated. Some of the merozoites recycle the process of development (para-erythrocytic or exoerythrocytic phase) (this para-erythrocytic phase is absent in *P. falciparum*). However, recrudescencer (*i.e.* persistence of blood infection) occurs with *P. falciparum* without relapse. The merozoites released, enter RBC. *P. falciparum* causes RBC to agglutinate causing capillary obstruction specially in brain and kidney.

Some merozoites undergo sexual differentiation to become haploid female gametocyte (macrogametocyte) and male gametocyte (microgametocyte) sucked by mosquitoes. Male gametocyte divided thrice to produce eight microgametes. A single microgamete fused with female macrogamete to produce zygote. Motile zygote (ookinete) penetrates in stomach, rests outside in spherical shape called oocyst. In oocyst multiple fission (sporogony) occurs to produce sporozoites. Oocyst brusts into body cavity and moves forward towards salivary gland, and thus cycle is completed (Fig. 112.1).

CLASSIFICATION OF ANTIMALARIAL DRUGS

Various stages of life cycle of malaria susceptable to different group of drugs and can be classified accordingly.

Clinical Classification

- **True casual prophylactic:** Destroying sporozoites, no drug available.
- **Casual prophylactic:** Prevents maturation in hepatocytes, primaquine, pyrimethamine, proguanil, tetracycline.
- **Suppressives:** Inhibit erythrocytic schizogony; mepacrine, proguanil, pyrimethamine. Tissue phase of *P. vivax* may cause relapse because they do not affect *P. vivax* tissue phase. Suppressive can cure *P. falciparum* because it does not have erythrocytic phase.
- **Clinical cure:** Malarial episodes can be terminated by erythrocytic, schizonticide halofantrine, lumefentrine, atovaquone, artemisinin (all these are fast acting), proguanil, pyrimethamine, sulfonamide, tetracycline (all these are slow acting).
- **Radical cure:** Eradication of both erythrocytic and para-erythrocytic schizogony. For *P. vivax* of primaquine. Suppressives are radical cure agent for *P. flaciparum.*
- **Gametocidal drugs:** Mostly act against gametocytes of *P. vivax.* Proguanil and

427

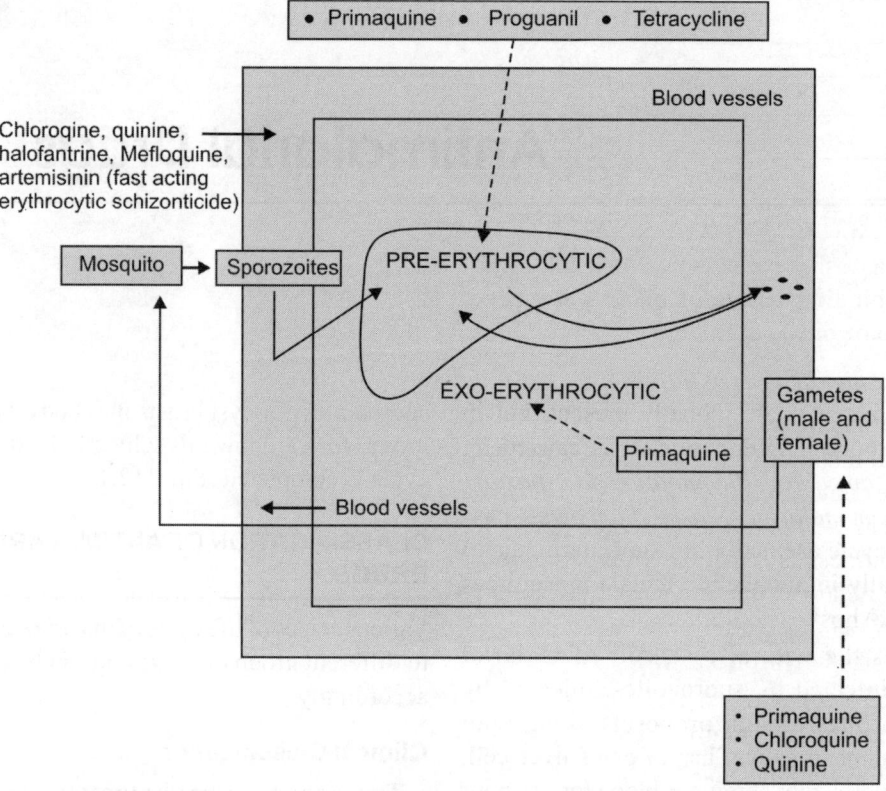

Fig. 112.1: Target of different antimalarial drugs in different stages of life cycle

pyrimethamine prevent development of gametocytes in mosquitoes.

Chemical Classification

- **Cinchona alkaloids:** Quinine, quinidine.
- **4-aminoquinolines:** Chloroquine, amodiaquine, piperaquine,
- **8-aminoquinolines:** Primaquine, pentaquine, pamaquine, bulaquine, tafenoquine
- **Quinoline:** Mefloquine
- **Acridine:** Mepacrine (atabrine, quinacrine)
- **Biguanides:** Proguanil, chlorproguanil
- **Diaminopyrimidine:** Pyrimethamine, trimethoprim
- **Sulfonamide and sulfone:** Sulfadoxine, sulfamethopyrazine, dapsone.
- **Tetracycline:** Tetracycline, doxycycline.
- **Amino alcohol:** Halofantrine, lumefantrine
- **Sesquiterpene lactone:** Artesunate, artemether, arteether

- **Mannich base:** Pyronaridine
- **Naphthaquinone:** Atovaquone.

QUININE

Quinine is an alkaloid obtained from bark of cinchona tree. Active against chloroquine-resistant malaria, erythrocytic schizonticidal against all species of malaria. It binds to DNA and inhibits synthesis of plasmodial nucleic acid, since it is sequestered by erythrocyte it is possible that it inhibits heme polymerase. It has no effect on pre-erythrocytic state.

Other actions of quinine: General protoplasmic poison, local anesthetic, local irritation, increases gastric secretion, analgesic, antipyretic, effects in vision and hearing. IV quinine falls BP, decreases excitability of heart and motor end plates.

Cinchonism is featured by: Ringing of ears, nausea, vomiting, tinnitus, vertigo, blurred vision,

Table 112.1: Oral dose for *Plasmodium vivax* of chloroquine				
Dose	Oral dose for Plasmodium vivax of chloroquine			
	1st day	*6 hours after*	*2nd day*	*3rd day*
Adult	600 mg	300 mg	300 mg	300 mg
Child	10 mg/kg	5 mg/kg	5 mg/kg	5 mg/kg
IM dose of base: 10 mg/kg or 2.5 mg/kg/6 hourly				

amblyopia, rash, respiratory failure, fall of BP. Hemoglobinuria feature of black water fever appears to be due to quinine.

Some therapeutic uses of quinine

• Resistant falciparum malaria.
• Cerebral malaria: 10 mg/kg quinine dihydrochloride diluted in 200–500 mg of 5% dextrose infused in 2–3 hours, repeat every 8 hourly till consciousness is regained. When consciousness is regained quinine sulfate 10 mg/kg/8 hourly × 7 days (orally).
• Diagnosis of myasthenia gravis
• Myotonia congenita
• Nocturnal muscle cramp
• Spremicidal vaginal cream
• As sclerosing agent injected with urethane causes thrombosis and fibrosis of varicose vein.
• Babesiosis: Quinine is used in combination of clindamycin.

AMINOQUINOLINES

During World War II many members are synthesized by Russia, German and French; but chloroquine, amodiaquine and hydroxychloroquine are most effective.

Chloroquine: Erythrocytic schizonticide against all species. It stacked base pairs of DNA by interclating with purine base (adenine and guanine). It produces toxic heme in RBC which damages plasmodial membrane. Chloroquine response is due to ability of parasite to accumulate chloroquine. Verapamil has been shown to restore chloroquine sensitivity in chloroquine resistance cases. Oral dose of chloroquine vide in Table 112.1.

IV dose of base (constant slow infusion) 10 mg/kg—1st 8 hours followed by 15 mg/kg/8

hours × 3 doses, *i.e.* total 25 mg/kg in 72 hours or 5 mg/kg/6 hours × 5 doses, *i.e.* total 25 mg/kg in 30 hours diluted in 5% dextrose slowly.

Chloroquine is orally absorbed, plasma protein-bound, has affinity for melanin, concentrated in liver, spleen, kidney, lungs, skin, erythrocyte, retina. Chloroquine-resistant with *P. falciparum* is quite common and its resistant to *P. vivax* is also coming up. It is due to slow accumulation of chloroquine in parasite. Verapamil may restore concentrating ability and sensitivity of chloroquine. *P. falciparum* mdr1 gene appears to play role in chloroquine resistance which is responsible for chloroquine transporter glycoprotein in *P. falciparum*.

Adverse reactions: Nausea, vomiting, epigastric pain, vision disturbances, parenteral use may cause cardiac depression, arrhythmia, lenticular opacity, retinopathy, graying of hair, attacks of porphyria, psoriasis, myopathy, photoallergy. It is safe in pregnancy without teratogenic and abortifacient effects.

Uses of Chloroquine

• Malaria (clinical cure + suppressive prophylaxis)
• Extraintestinal amoebiasis
• Rheumatoid arthritis
• DLE
• Lepra reaction
• Photogenic reaction
• Infectious mononucleosis.

Hydroxychloroquine: Similar in action, but less toxic to chloroquine.

Amodiaquine (Camoquin 250 mg): 25–35 mg/kg over 3 days. Suppressive to attack of malaria. GI disturbance, headache, photosensitivity or agranulocytosis may occur. It is also available as 150 mg base/5 mL susp. The WHO suggests amodiaquine + artesunate for *P. falciparum,* and amodiaquine + sulfadoxine pyrimethamine, if artemisinin is not available.

Piperaquine: Developed in China, bisquinolone congener of chloroquine, long acting, high efficacy, erythrocytic schizonticide, more active against chloroquine resistant *P. falciparum.* It is combined with dihydroartemisinin in 8:1 ratio.

- Pyronaridine is structurally related to amodiaquine used for *P. vivax* and *P. falciparum.*

8-AMINOQUINOLINES

Primaquine (PMQ-INGA or malirid 7.5; 15 mg tab): Effective against erythrocytic schizonticidal of *P. vivax* and pre-erythrocytic and sexual form of *P. vivax* and *P. falciparum.* Along with 4-aminoquinoline, it can produce radical cure. It has no effect on schizonts of *P. falciparum.* They exert antimalarial activity by binding plasmodial DNA, mitochondria of plasmodium swells and vacuolated.

Orally absorbed, concentrated in liver, lung. Oxidized in liver and excreted in urine.

Epigastric distress, abdominal cramps (take after food or antacid), anemia, methemoglobinemia, cyanosis, leukopenia, intravascular hemolysis with glucose-6-phosphate dehydrogenase deficiency due to oxidant property of primaquine. Used for relapsing malaria, dose 15 mg/day × 14 days (adult) and 0.25 mg/kg/day or 0.75 mg/week (children) for 2½ months with 300 mg of chloroquine weekly. Other 8-aminoquinolines are pentaquine, pamaquine used mainly in Russia.

Primaquine and clindamycin combinations are used for pneumocystis.

Bulaquine: Developed in India; primaquine congener, partly metabolized to primaquine, better tolerated by G-6-PD deficient individuals. Dose 25 mg/day for 5 days starting on 2nd day of chloroquine treatment. Used for antirelapse of *P. vivax.*

- Tafenaquine is new long acting primaquine-like drug.

QUINOLINE METHANOL

Mefloquine (meflotas 250 tab): Erythrocytic schizonticidal, rapid acting, single dose of 15 mg/kg, max 1 gm. Orally absorption is good, plasma protein-bound, concentrated in liver, lungs and intestine.

ADR: Nausea, vomiting, bradycardia, neuropsychiatric reactions. Safe in pregnancy except in 1st trimester. May produce QTc prolongation or cardiac arrest, if used with halofantrine or quinine.

- Used for multidrug-resistant malaria.
- Travelers as prophylactic visiting endemic zone of multidrug-resistant malaria.

ACRIDINE DERIVATIVE

Mepacrine (Chlorguanidine in the USA) [Maladin 100 mg tab]: Schizonticidal against *P. vivax,* and it prevents development of gametes encysted in the gut wall of mosquitoes. It inhibits dihydrofolate reductase thereby blocking thymidine and purine syntheses of plasmodia. Resistance develops quickly. Adequately and slowly absorbed, partly metabolized and excreted in urine. Used for prophylaxis. Dose 600 mg/week. Other uses are taeniasis, giardia, *Trichomonas vaginalis,* DLE, cutaneous leishmaniasis. Rarely used.

BIGUANIDES

Chlorproguanil: Causal prophylactic. Dose 20 mg weekly. Cross-resistance with proguanil may occur.

Cycloguanil: Given as suspension in oil (5 mg/kg IM). Protects from *P. vivax* and *P. falciparum* for 3 months.

Proguanil (Laveran 100 mg tab): Slow acting schizonticidal and causal prophylactic.

DIAMINOPYRIMIDINE

Pyramethamine (Daraprim, 25 mg tab): Effective schizonticidal against *P. vivax* and pre-erythrocytic *P. falciparum.* Inhibits dihydrofolate reductase of plasmodium. Also effective against

Toxoplasma gondii and *Pneumocystosis* in higher doses. Absorbed from GIT, concentrated in liver, lung, spleen, kidney. Relatively safe, may produce rash, nausea, vomiting. Cross-resistance may occur with proguanil. Used as prophylactic 25 mg weekly. It is used in combination with sulfones or sulfonamides for treatment of *P. falciparum*. It is also used for polycythemia vera.

Trimethoprim: Basically antibacterial, has antimalarial action.

SULFONAMIDE AND SULFONES

They possess inhibitory influence on erythrocytic phase specially of *P. falciparum*. Some popular combination of India are sulfadoxine 500 mg + pyrimethamine 25 mg (malaprime); sulfamethopyrazine 500 mg + pyrimethamine 25 mg (Metakelfin). The prophylactic use of these combinations is no longer recommended.

TETRACYCLINES AND OTHER ANTIBIOTICS

Tetracycline and doxycycline are weak erythrocytic schizonticidal. Never used alone to treat malaria. Inhibit pre-erythrocytic stage of *P. falciparum*. Clindamycin, azithromycin have also antibacterial activity so do some fluoroquinolones. Other antibiotics which are effective in malaria are Clindamycin, azithromycin, fluoroquinolones. Most of them are slow acting erythrocytic schizonticidal.

Artemisinin Derivatives

Used in China as traditional medicine (quinghaosu) of plant *Artemisia annua,* effective against *P. falciparum* where all drugs are resistant, now it is used world-wide.

Artemisinin derivatives are chemically sesquiterpene lactone endoperoxides, potent schizonticidal. Artemisinin is poorly soluble in water and has several derivatives, but artemether soluble in oil. Arteether and artesunate are marketed in India. Artesunate and artemether are prodrugs.

The mechanism of action of artemisinin is not exactly known, most likely the endoperoxide bridge in its molecule interacts with heme in the parasite and the iron-mediated cleavage of the bridge releases free radicals which bind membrane proteins causing lipid peroxidation as a damaging and inhibiting protein synthesis of ER, causing malarial parasites lysis.

α/β arteether (E-mal 150 mg/2 mL) is developed in India, used 1M for three days in complicated and cerebral malaria.

Artemisinin-based Combination Therapy (ACT)

Advantages

- Good tolerance
- Rapid parasitological cure
- Low rate of resistance development

Table 112.2

	Adult		Pediatric	
Artemether (Rezart M) 80 mg/amp IM	1.6 mg/kg, 1st day BD	1.6 mg/kg/day once 2–5 days	1.6 mg/kg BD (day 1)	1.6 mg/kg/day once
40 mg cap oral	1.6 mg/kg BD	1.6 mg/kg/day once	1.6 mg/kg BD	1.6 mg/kg once 5 mg/day, 2–5 days
Arteether (Rezart E) 150 mg/amp IM	150 mg	150 mg/day, 2–3 days	3 mg/kg	3 mg/kg/day, 2–3 days
Artesunate (Rezart S) 60 mg/vial IV or IM	2–2.4 mg/kg followed by 1–1.2 mg/kg after 12 hours	1–1.2 mg/kg/day, 2–5 days	2–2.4 mg/kg followed by 1–1.2 mg/kg after 12 hours	1–1.2 mg/kg/day, 2–5 days
Tab 60 mg oral	4 mg/kg	2 mg/kg/day	4 mg/kg	2 mg/kg/day

Table 112.3: Treatment of malaria

Uncomplicated	Complicated P. falciparum
P. vivax: Chloroquine + primaquine	Artesunate or
If chloroform-resistant:	Artemether or
Quinine + doxycycline + primaquine *P. falciparum* or quinine + primaquine	Arteether or
or sulfadoxine + pyrimethamine + primaquine	Quinine dihydrochloride
Chloroquine-resistant *P. falciparum:*	
Artesunate + sulfadoxine + pyrimethamine or quinine + doxycycline	

Some ACT combinations

- Artesunate + sulfadoxine + pyramethamine
- Artesunate + mefloquine
- Artemether + lumefantrine
- Dihydroartemisinin + piperaquine
- Artesunate + amodiaquine
- Artisunate + pyronaridine
- Artesunate + chlorproguanil + dapsone
- Arterolane + piperaquine

Arterolane is a trioxolane congener of artemisinin synthetically prepared.

Mechanism of action not known.

Adverse effects: Nausea, vomiting, itching, bleeding, ST changes, QT prolongation, leukopenia have been reported, which are reversible on withdrawal of drugs. With terfenadine, tricyclic antidepressant, antiarrhythmic, increases the risk of cardiac conduction defect, when used simultaneously. Use should be restricted for severe acute attacks of malaria *(P. falciparum)* resistant to multidrug and cerebral malaria.

AMINO ALCOHOL

Halofantrine is blood schizonticidal: Comparable to mefloquinine, cross-resistant develops with it. Available as 250 mg tab. Dose 2 tabs on 8 hours interval for *P. falciparum* and *P. vivax;* resistant to chloroquine, sulfapyrimethamine. Its oral absorption is erratic. Abdominal pain, diarrhea, rash, rise of serum transaminases, QT prolongation may produce arrhythmia.

Lumefantrine: A fixed dose combination of lumefantrine with artemether marked as coartem is recommended for *P. falciparum* in African countries.

NAPHTHYRIDINE

Pyronaridine: Mannich base, erythrocytic schizonticidal. Mechanism of action is like chloroquine. Used as fixed doses combination with artesunate 3:1 for multidrug resistance *P. falciparum* and *P. vivax.*

ADR: Abdominal pain, vomiting, headache, dizziness, palpitation, ECG changes (transient may occur).

NAPHTHAQUINONE

Atovaquone: Synthetic naphthaquinone derivatives is erythrocytic schizonticidal for *P. falciparum.* Also used for *Pneumocystis jeroveci; Toxoplasma gondii.* It interferes mitochondrial ATP production of plasmodium.

Clindamycin: This antibiotic has got erythrocytic schizonticidal property, use with quinine.

Doxycycline among tetracycline used with quinine antibiotics are slow acting erythrocytic schizonticidal.

Guidelines to Treat Malaria in the USA

- Chloroquine for non-falciparum or non-chloroquine-resistant *P. falciparum* patient.
- Quinine for *P. falciparum* cases. Other drugs are melfloquine; halofantrine and artemisinin derivatives.

Antiamoebic and Some Antiprotozoal Drugs

Amoebiasis is caused by *Entamoeba histolytica,* and is distributed world-wide.

Clinical Classification of Antiamoebic Therapy

Clinical classification (Fig. 113.1)

- **Used in intestinal amoebiasis:** Emetine bismuth iodide, halogenated oxyquinolines, pentavalent organic arsenicals. Antibiotic, diloxinide furonate, chlorphenoxamide, kurchi.

- **Used for intestinal and extraintestinal amoebiasis:** Emetine, dehydroemetine, metronidazole, phanquone.

- **Used for extraintestinal amoebiasis:** Chloroquine.

Emetine Group

Alkaloid obtained from root plant of *Caphalis ipecacuanha,* targets trophozoites which show degeneration of nucleus, arrest of division and subsequently phagocytosis. It also arrests translocation of tRNA. Though absorbed orally, given by deep IM because of irritant nature. Concentrated in liver, excreted through kidney.

Local pain, stiffness, abscess may occur. Oral administration may produce vomiting, diarrhea, headache. The CVS side effects are tachycardia, precordial pain, myocarditis, invert T wave, QT and PR prolongations, ST and QRS changes. Patient should get bed rest to avoid it. May produce neuritis, should be avoided in heart patient, renal damage and pregnant woman. Dose

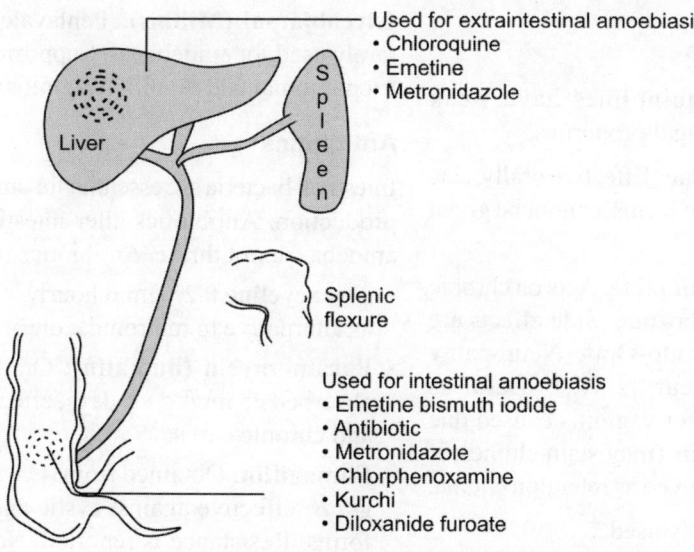

Used for extraintestinal amoebiasis
- Chloroquine
- Emetine
- Metronidazole

Spleen

Liver

Splenic flexure

Used for intestinal amoebiasis
- Emetine bismuth iodide
- Antibiotic
- Metronidazole
- Chlorphenoxamine
- Kurchi
- Diloxanide furoate

Fig. 113.1: Site of action of different antiamoebic drugs

Table 113.1: Classification of chemically antiamoebic drugs

Emetine group	Quinoline derivative	Organic arsenicals	Antibiotics	Miscellaneous
Emetine	Diiodohydroxy-quin	Carbarsone	Tetracycline	Diloxanide furoate
Dihydroemetime	Amodiaquine	Glycobiarsol	Parmomycin	Chlorphenoxamine
Emetine bismuth iodide	Chiniofon sodium		Fumagillin	Niridazole
				Metronidazole
	Broxyquinoline			Ornidazole
	Chlorohydroxy-quinoline			Tinidazole
	Chloroquine			Phanquone
				Kurchi
				Bialamicol
				Secnidazole
				Ornidazole

30–60 mg daily. It is also used for *Paragonimus westermoni* (lung fluke) and Fasciola hepatica.

Dihydroemetine: Semisynthetic, less toxic, dose 1 mg/kg IM for 6–10 days. Useful for giardiasis, cutaneous leishmaniasis. Dihydroemetine resinate is slow release preparation for oral use 50 mg daily × 10 days.

Emetine bismuth iodide (60 mg), NF: Orally effective, mild astringent effect due to bismuth, may produce iodism, other toxicities are like emetine. Dose 60–200 mg after evening meal × 12 days.

Quinoline Derivatives

All halogenated oxyquinolines have weak antibacterial and antifungal properties.

Diiodohydroxy quinoline: Effective orally, acts on cystic and trophozoite forms, cannot be given by retention enema.

Iodo-chlorohydroxy quinoline: Acts on chronic cyst carrier and on trophozoite. Side effects are myelitis, Sub-acute **M**yalo-**O**ptic **N**europathy (SMON), peripheral neuritis. Also useful as antifungal cream (3%) for vaginitis caused due to *Trichomonas vaginalis* (may stain clothes, if used topically). Can be given as retention enema.

Chinifon sodium: Rarely used.

Broxyquinoline (Intestopan): No special advantage over hydroxyquinoline.

Chlorhydroxyquinoline (Halquinal): 0.25–0.5 gm QDS similar to other quinoline derivative.

Chloroquine: Orally well-absorbed, selectively concentrated in liver so effective for hepatic amoebiasis, but not for intestinal amoebiasis. Other uses are discussed earlier with antimalarial drugs.

Organic Arsenicals (Rarely used)

Carbarsone: Effective against trophozoite and cystic form. Inhibits sulfhydryl enzyme of parasite. Dose 250 mg BD × 10 days. Also useful for vaginitis caused due to *Trichomonas vaginalis*.

Glycobiarsol (Milibis): Pentavalent arsenical rarely used for amoebiasis. Suppository used for trichomonial and monilial vaginitis.

Antibiotics

Intestinal bacteria are essential for amoebic lesion production. Antibiotics alter intestinal flora so amoeba cannot thrive. Antibiotics used are:

- **Tetracycline** 0.25 gm 6 hourly × 15–20 days as alternative to metronidazole.
- **Paramomycin (humatin):** Orally not well-absorbed 25 mg/kg × 5 days, effective in acute and chronic cases.
- **Fumagillin:** Obtained from *Aspergillus fumigatus,* effective against cystic and vegetative forms. Resistance is reported. Not useful for extraintestinal amoebiasis. It is a cyclic polyene macrolide antibiotic.

Adverse effects: Desquamation of skin, headache, vertigo, muscular pain, granulocytopenia.

Diloxanide furoate (Furamide 500 mg TDS × 10 days): Useful in cyst passers, not useful in extraintestinal amoebiasis, relatively safe, flatulence, skin reaction may occur.

Nitazoxanide: Prodrug, congener of niclosamide. Used for *E. histolytica; T. vaginalis, Cryptosporidium, H. pylori, Ascaris, H. nana.* Dose 500 mg BD × 3 days and for children 7.5 mg/kg BD.

Chlorphenoxamine (mebinol): 500 mg TDS × 8 days. Limited value in intestinal amoebiasis. Eradicate cysts.

Niridazole (ambilhar): Antischistosomial, used in amoebiasis (intestinal and hepatic). Adverse effects include GI disturbances, insomnia, headache, epistaxis, epilepsy, ECG changes like emetine, hemolysis in glucose-6PO_4-deficient patient, also useful in guinea worm infestation. Also possesses immunosuppressive action.

Phanquone (Entobex): 150 to 300 mg in divided doses × 5 to 10 days. Orally absorbed, used for intestinal and extraintestinal amoebiasis, alternative to emetine has antibacterial properties. Dizziness, GI disturbances, dark-yellow urine may occur.

Bialamicol: Has been tested for its antiamoebic properties.

Kurchi: Alkaloids of bark of *Holarrhena antidysentrica* 1% w/v, causes mild toxicity of nausea and vomiting, has mild antiamoebic effect in intestinal amoebiasis.

Metronidazole (Flagyl and Metrogyl): Useful in all forms of amoebiasis, retatively safe.

Mechanism of Action: Selective toxicity to anaerobic microaerophilic microorganism for anoxic or hypoxic to cells. Nitro group as electron acceptor for flavoproteins of mammalian cells and ferrodoxin in bacteria. Nitroreductase catalyses reaction of flavin radical with nitro compound in later case, reduction is catalyzed by iron-sulfur complex. Sources for electron reduction is endogenous NADPH or sulfide.

Chemically reactive reduced form of the drug produces biochemical lesion and death of cells. Earlier it was established to inhibit DNA synthesis in *T. vaginalis, Cl. bifermentans.*

Adverse effects: Anorexia, metallic taste, abdominal cramps, headache, glossitis, dry mouth, dizzines, neutropenia, rash, seizure, neuropathy.

Antabuse-like reaction with alcohol decrease renal clearance of lithium.

Used for: Amoebiasis, giardiasis, trichomonas vaginitis, anaerobic infection, ulcerative gingivitis, pseudomembranous enterocolitis, trench mouth, helicobactor gastritis and acid peptic disease, guinea worm infestation. Dose 400 mg TDS × 7 to 10 days.

Tinidazole: Congener of metronidazole, used for trichomoniasis, giardiasis, prophylactic in anaerobic infection in colorectal surgery, *H. pylori* gastritis. Differs from metronidazole in following ways. More efficacious, slowly metabolized, better tolerated.

Secnidazole (secnil): Congener of metronidazole, orally active, single dose therapy. Dose 2 gm, single dose or 30 mg/kg.

Ornidazole (dazolic): Spectrum of activity similar to metronidazole.

Satranidazole (satrogyl): Nitroimidazole derivative better tolerated, no antabuse reaction, does not produce carcinogen. It is also devoid of metalic taste and neurological adverse effects.

Balantidial Dysentery

Balantidium coli is a largest protozoa infests human from pig or domestic animals. Treatment—oxytetracycline or diiodohydroxyquinoline.

Pneumocystis carinii

Pear-shaped protozoa, usually closed in mucus cyst, transmitted by droplets, produces pneumonitis in immunocompromised host. Treatment is difficult. Some success with pentamidine isoethionate or with pyrimethamine plus sulfadiazine.

Drugs used for Giardiasis

- Metronidazole/tinidazole/secnidazole
- Mepacrine 100 mg TDS × 5 days
- Quiniodoclor 250 mg TDS × 7 days
- Furazolidone (Furoxone) 100 mg TDS × 7 days also effective in *Salmonella, Shigella, Trichomonas*. **ADR:** Nausea, headache, dizziness may occur, turns urine orange.
- Nitazoxanide: This prodrug inhibits pyruvate-ferredoxin oxyreductase (PFOR) enzyme. Used for giardiasis, *E. histolytica, C. carvum*. Dose 500 mg BD and for children 7.5 mg/kg BD × 3 days.

Drugs for Trichomoniasis

Trichomonas vaginalis is a flagellate protozoan producing vulvovaginitis.

Drugs used are

Oral route

- Metronidazole 400 mg TDS × 7 days
- Tinidazole 600 mg OD × 7 days

- Nimorazole 2 gm single dose (flosogyn)

Vaginal route

- Diiodohydroxyquin (floraquin 100 mg) 200 mg intravaginally at HS × 1–2 weeks
- Quiniodochlor (gynosan 200 mg). Intravaginal at HS. 1–3 weeks.
- Natamycin (25 mg). Intravaginal × 10 days
- Povidone iodine (betadine vaginal 400 mg). Intravaginal at HS × 2 weeks.
- Furazolidine, sodium lauryl sulfate, triclobisonium, dioctyl sodium sulfo succinate.

Drug of choice for some other protozoal infections

- *Balantidium coli*—Tetracycline
- Cryptosporidium—Paramomycin
- Chagas disease—Nifurtimox
- Cyclospora—Cotrimoxazole
- *T. gondii* during pregnancy—Spiramycin
- *T. gondii*—Pyrimethamine + Clindamycin
- African trypanosomiasis—Suramin (early cases); Melarsoprol in late CNS cases

114

Antileishmanial Drugs

Leishmania donovani is a causative parasite of visceral leishmaniasis or kala-azar, was discovered by Leishman from London, and Donovan from Chennai, endemic in many places in India, China, Africa and South America. Morphologically the parasite exists in two forms,

- Amastigote or leishmanial form persents in man
- Promastigote or leptomonal form occurs in sand fly or artificial culture.

Characterized by fever (may be double rise), splenomegaly, may be hepatomegaly, lymphadenopathy (in African and Chinese forms), malaise, apathy, good appetite, epistaxis. Dermal lesions—warty eruption, dry, rough and pigmented.

Drugs Used to Treat Leishmaniasis

a. Pentavalent antimonials
- Urea stibamine
- Sodium stibogluconate
- Ethyl stibamine

b. Diamidine derivative
- Dihydroxystilbamidine isethionate
- Pentamidine isethionate

c. Miscellaneous
- Amphotericin
- Allopurinol
- Paromomycin
- Ketoconazole
- Miltefosine

a. Pentavalent antimonial compounds are drugs of choice in kala-azar, possibly they are reduced to trivalent antimony compounds in body. Trivalent antimonials are no longer used.

- **Urea stibamine:** Produced by interaction of stibanic acid with urea contains 38 to 42% antimony, undergoes chemical changes when exposed to air. Dose 50–200 mg IV on alternate days for 4 weeks. Usually given with sodium stibogluconate in resistant case. Prepared in India.

- **Sodium antimony gluconate (abanate):** Contains 30–34% antimony. 2 gm of the drug contains 600 mg of antimony in 6 mL, given IV or IM after skin testing then 15 mL daily or alternate days with a break of 10 days after 5th or 6th injection till 120 mL is reached. Liposome incorporated preparations for IV use are available.

- **Ethyl stibamine:** Contains 40–44% antimony, less toxic, 5–25% freshly prepared given IV or IM on alternate days. 100 mg 1st dose then 200 mg then 300 mg till 3–4 gm for curation and relapse cases. It is a complex mixture of para-aminobenzene stibonic acid, para-acetyl-aminophenylstibonic acid, antimonic acid, diethyl amine.

Adverse reactions: Metallic taste, nausea, vomiting, giddiness, delirium, muscular pain, fall of temperature, hematuria, blood dyscrasia, anaphylactic shock.

b. Diamidine derivatives: Reserved for resistant cases of antimonial chemotherapy, more toxic. Also used to treat *T. gambiense* and Rhodesian trypanosomiasis.

- **Dihydroxystilbamidine isethionate:** 250 mg daily IV × 10 days, pause for 2 weeks, total 7.5 gm in 4–5 weeks.
- **Pentamidine isethionate (Iomidine):** Supplied by Govt agencies only. Effective against *L. donovani, Trypanosomes, Pneumocystis jiroveci,* interacts with DNA and inhibits topoisomerase II or interferes with aerobic glycolysis. Dose 4 mg/kg deep IM or IV slowly over 1 hour on alternate days for 5–15 weeks, till it becomes leishmanial negative in splenic aspirates in 2 weeks apart. Antihistaminics should be given beforehand to check headache, fever, rigor. Other adverse effects are hypotension, circulatory collapse, urticaria, angioedema may also occur.

c. **Miscellaneous**
- **Amphotericin B:** Antifungal antibiotic useful for mucocutaneous leishmaniasis in the dose of 0.5 mg, increase by 0.5 mg/kg by slow IV on alternate days and total 15–20 mg/kg is given.
- **Ketoconazole:** Antifungal shown in limited clinical trials in the dose of 600 mg/day × 4 weeks gives encouraging results in dermal leishmaniasis.
- **Allopurinol:** Xanthine oxidase inhibitor incorporated with RNA of leishmania, interferes protein synthesis and competes with ATP has been trialed for kala-azar in India and Africa, 4–12 mg/kg TDS × 3 to 4 weeks.

- **Nifurtimox:** Dose 8–10 mg/kg/day orally in 3–4 divided doses used to treat Chagas' disease.
- **Nitromidazole:** Benzidazole derivative. Effective in Chagas' disease.
- **Miltefosine:** An alkylphosphocholine analog, in the dose of 2.5 mg/kg orally × 28 days for visceral leishmaniasis.
- **Suramin:** Sulfated naphthylamine used in East African trypanosomiasis.
- **Melarsoprol:** Arsenical compound used for advanced CNS trypanosomiasis in East Africa.
- **Paramomycin:** Used for visceral leishmaniasis orally.
- **Eflornithine:** New drug registered for African trypanosomiasis. It is ornithine decarboxylase inhibitor.

The other drugs which are approved for Kala-azar are fluconazole, metronidazole; for cutaneous leishmaniasis, sitamaquine is used orally for visceral leishmaniasis.

Drugs Used for Dermal Leishmaniasis

- **Sodium stibogluconate:** 2 ml infiltered around sore.
- **Mepacrine:** 100 mg dissolved in 2 mL is infiltered around sore. They are painful and takes time to heal.
- **Paramomycin oint:** To apply locally. Multiple and severe lesions should be treated by systemic drugs. Antibiotic required for secondary infections.

115

Chemotherapy of Infestations by Multicellular Organisms

The main multicellular parasites of human being are either worms of the group helminth, nema-thelminth or platyhelminth. Worm infestations are one of the major global public health problems particularly in tropical countries as illustrated by Stoll in 1947.

An anthelminthic which kills the worm is called vermicide and which expels the worm is called vermifuge.

Commonest parasites observed in India are roundworms, hookworms, threadworms, tape-worms, guinea worms, filarial worms, *etc.*

Criteria of an ideal anthelminthic

- Should have broad-spectrum of action
- High percentage of cure with a single dose
- Should not be absorbed
- Should be cheap and palatable
- No toxic effects
- Should not require purgatives.

Drugs for Tapeworms

- Mepacrine
- Camoquine
- Paramomycin
- Male fern
- Chloroquine
- Niclosamide
- Dichlorophen

Mepacrine: Useful for *T. saginata, T. solium, H. nana, D. latum.* is vermifuge. Nausea, vomi-ting can be tackled by antiemetic. Patient given bland low residue diet for 3–4 days. 1 gm mepa-crine is given in 3 divided doses which may be followed by saline purgative, frequent sips of water is given for passage of drug into jejunum. Stools are examined for scolex. It may be given by duodenal tube. May be repeated after 1–2 weeks.

Chloroquine: 2 gm given in empty stomach followed by saline purgative, is effective for fish tapeworm. Comoquin 0.6–0.8 gm is also effective.

Niclosamide: Vermicidal for *T. saginata, T. solium, H. nana.* Patient kept on low residue

Table 115.1: Helminth			
Platyhelminth		*Nemathelminth*	
Cestodes	*Trematodes*	*Intestinal*	*Somatic*
Taenia saginata	*Schistomes haematobium*	*Ascaris lumpbricoidis*	*Wuchereria brancrofti*
Taenia solium	*Schistomes mansoni*	*Ancylostoma duodenale*	*Oncheocerca volvulus*
Diphyllobotrium latum	*Schistomes japonicum*	*Necator amerecanes*	*Loa loa*
Echinococcus granulosus	*Fasciola hepatica*	*Enterobius vermicularis*	*Dracunculus medinensis*
Hymenolepsis nana	*Fasciolopos buski*	*Trichuris trichura*	
Paragonimus westermani	*Strongyloides stercoralis*		
Clonorchis sinensis	*Trichinella spiratis*		

diet 1 gm of drug is chewed and repeated after 1 hour followed by saline purge. *H. nana* requires prolong therapy.

Paramomycin: 1 gm 4 hourly × 4 doses effective against *T. saginata, T solium, D. latum, H. nana.*

Dichlorophen: Used as veterinary medicine, also given to humans, 6 gm for adults, 2–4 gm for children for two successive days. After purge may be given. Effective for *T. solium* and *T. saginata.* Nausea, vomiting, diarrhea, urticaria, jaundice may occur.

Male fern: Oldest remedy for taeniasis and not used because of its toxicity.

Drugs for Roundworms

• Piperazine	• Pyrantel pamoate
• Tetramisole	• Bephenium hydroxy-naphthoate
• Thiabendazole	
• Mebendazole	• Albendazole
• Diethyl carbama-zine	• Santonin
	• Dithiazanine

Piperazine: Causes flaccid paralysis of the worms which are expelled by peristaltic movements. A considerable portion of the drug is absorbed. Nausea, vomiting, diarrhea, vertigo, muscular incoordination, ataxia (worm wobble), paresthesia, blurring of vision, convulsion may occur but effect disappears rapidly. Adult dose for ascariasis of piperazine is 4 gm.

Pyrantel pamoate (Nemocid 250 mg tab or 50 mg/mL): Effective against *E. vermicularis,* roundworm, ancylostoma. Causes activation of nicotinic receptors, resulting in persistent depolarization producing spastic paralysis. Piperazine antagonizes its action. Only 10–15% absorbed. Anorexia, vomiting, diarrhea, abdominal pain, headache, drowsiness, rash, SGPT may be raised. No purging or other preparation required (dose 10–15 mg/kg max 1 gm).

Tetramisole (decaris)/Levamisole (50–100 mg tab): Effective in the doses of 2.5–5 mg/kg tab for ascariasis. No purgative required, non-competitively blocks acetylcholine response of ascaris. Partly absorbed, nausea, vomiting,

abdominal pain, diarrhea, giddiness, drowsiness may occur. Levamisole restores depressed T cell function, so used for rheumatoid arthritis and in adjunct in malignancies.

Bephenium hydroxynaphthoate (Alcopar): Effective against roundworm, hookworm moderately effective against *Trichostrongylus orientalis,* produces contracture of parasite muscles, which are expelled by peristaltic movements. Should be given with sugar in children because of its bitter taste. Nausea, vomiting, diarrhea may occur. May be given to pregnant woman. Adult dose 5 gm in empty stomach; no purgation required.

Thiabendazole (mintezol): It is a benzimidozol derivative, effective against roundworm, threadworm, strongyloides, trichinosis, dracontiases. Interferes with metabolic pathway of helminths. Partly absorbed and metabolized in liver and excreted via kidneys. Anorexia, nausea, vomiting, epigastric distress, dizziness, fever may occur. Dose 25 mg/kg twice daily for 3 days.

Mebendazole (mebex): Orally effective, not much absorbed, broad-spectrum antihelminth (ascariasis, enterobiasis, trichuriasis, hookworm, strongyloides), slow acting. Dose 100 mg BD × 3 days. Probably blocks glucose uptake in the parasite and depletes glycogen of parasites. Hatching of the parasite egg and larva is also inhibited.

Albendazole (*zental, alminth* 400 mg tab 200 mg/5 mL): Broad-spectrum anthelmintic, single oral dose. Moderately absorbed from GIT, first pass metabolism. Produces albendazole sulfoxide which is active and enters brain. No preparation, fasting or post-drug purging required. Prolong use in case of cysticercosis and hydatid. Produces headache, fever, alopecia, jaundice.

Diethylcarbamazine (discussed with filariasis)

Santonin and dithiazanine iodide no longer used for availability of better drugs.

Drugs for Hookworm

• Tetachloroethylene	• Mebendazole
• Bephenium	• Pyrantel
• Bitoscanate.	

Tetrachloroethylene (tetracap): Effective against *N.americanus*. Probably produces reversible paralysis of it, purgation required for expulsion. Orally less absorbed, irritancy may produce nausea, vomiting, fat enhances its systemic absorption. For ancylostomiasis 1 mL of the drug is given as gelatin capsules. Patient should be advised to take high carbohydrate and protein and low fat diet, alcohol and other food should be avoided and patient should remain in bed. May be repeated after 10 days. Rarely used now.

Bitoscanate (joint): Equally effective for *A. duodenale* and *N. americanus*, 200 mg in two divided doses and 100 mg in second day is the dose for adult. Dizziness, nausea, vomiting may occur.

Drugs for Threadworm

• Viprynium	• Piperazine
• Tetracycline	• Gentian violet
• Mebendazole	• Pyrantal

Viprynium: Cyanine dye, effective against *E. vermicularis,* strongyloidosis. Probably inhibits cellular oxidation within worms. Orally administered dose is 7.5 mg/kg to be repeated every 2–3 weeks. Nausea, vomiting, photosensitization may occur.

Piperazine: Discussed earlier.

Oxytetracycline: 1–2 gm daily × 10 to 15 days, cures oxyuriasis and rarely used because of cost and side effects.

Gentian violet: 60 mg daily × 16 days cures, oxyuriasis.

Drugs for Schistosomiasis

• Lucanthone	• Hycanthone
• Trivalent antimony compounds	• Amphotalide
	• Niridazole
• Metrifonate	• Dichlorovos.

Lucanthone (miracil-D): Effective against *S. mansoni, S. hematobium,* interferes with their egg productions. Orally absorbed, metabolized in liver and excreted in urine. Nausea, vomiting,

anorexia, dark-skin people tolerate it better. 1 gm thrice daily for 3 days to be repeated after 1 month.

Hycanthone: Metabolite of lucanthone, less toxic, 4 mg/kg × 4 days orally or as sulfamate or methanesulfonate IM 2–3 mg/kg. Loss of body weight, jaundice may occur.

Trivalent Antimony Compounds

• **Antimony dimercaprosuccinate:** Dose 30–50 mg/kg in 5 divided doses, IM. Injection at biweekly interval for *S. haematobium*.

• **Antimony sodium tartrate 2% solution:** 30 mg daily IV, effective against all varieties of schistosomes. Also used for leishmaniasis and lymphogranuloma inguinale.

Amphotalide: 400 mg/kg orally in divided doses for 5–15 days effective in *S. haematobium*.

Niridazole (ambilhar): 25 mg/kg orally × 7 days. Effective for amoebiasis, *S. japonicum, S. mansoni* and guinea worm.

Metrifonate: Organophosphorus, orally effective in the dose 5–7.5 mg/kg × 10 days in morning followed by 12 hours fast. Effective for trichuriasis, hookworm, roundworm, S. *haematobium. Transienty* lowers plasmacholinesterase.

Drugs for Guinea Worm

• Niridazole 25 mg/kg/daily
• Metronidazole or
• Thiobendazole 100 mg/kg for 1 day

Drugs for Filariasis

Diethylcarbamazine (Hetrazan): Orally absorbed, metabolized in the body and excreted in urine. Anorexia, nausea, vomiting, headache, drowsiness, allergy may occur. Used for filariasis, tropical eosinophilia, onchocerciasis, larva migrans, *Loa loa.*

Ivermectin: Semisynthetic derivative obtained from *Streptomyces avermitilis,* now marketed in India, drug of choice for *O. volus, W. bancrofii, B. malayi, Ascaris, Enterobius, Trichuris* and visceral larva migrans. Orally also effective for scabies and pediculosis.

Praziquantel (Cysticide 500 mg tab): Rapidly taken up by susceptible worms (schistosomes, trematodes, castodes) causing leakage of intracellular calcium from membrane, causing contracture and paralysis. Orally absorbed, high first pass metabolism, limits bioavailability. Nausea, abdominal pain, headache, dizziness, sedation, itching, urticaric, rash may occur. Used for tapeworm, *T. saginata. T. solium, H. nana, D. latum, Neurocysticercosis,* schistosomes, *Fasciola hepatica.*

Doxycycline: It has significant microfilaricidal effect.

MISCELLANEOUS

Bithionol: Used to treat fascioliasis (sheep liver fluke) and pulmonary parigonimiasis. Dose 30–50 mg/kg in two or three divided doses

orally after meals on every alternate days for 10–15 doses.

ADR: Diarrhea, abdominal cramps, anorexia, vomiting, dizziness, headache, skin rash.

Doxycycline: It has got action against filaria; onchocerciasis.

Oxamniquine: Alternative to praziquantel to treat *S. monsoni.*

Anthelmintic classified according to mechanism of action:

- Causing spastic paralysis through NN receptor: Levamisole; Pyrantel pamoate
- Causing Flaccid paralysis: Piperazine, Ivermetin.
- Polymerization of β-tubulin: Mebendazole, Albendazole, Thiobendazole.
- Uncoupling oxidative phosphorylation: Niclosamide, Bithional.
- Causing influx of calcium: Praziquantel.

116

Chemotherapy of Neoplastic Diseases

Disease cancer is characterized by shift of control of cell survival, proliferation and differentiation. A small subpopulation of cells may be called tumor. Stem cells undergo repeated proliferation and colonize in other organs or sites called metastasis.

Basic character of cancer cells

- Excessive cell growth
- Undifferentiated cells
- Invasiveness
- Ability to metastatize
- Acquired heredity
- All cancer cell progenies retain cancerous properties.
- Shift of metabolism for increased cancerous cell building with increased carbohydrate catabolism for energy.

Causes of cancer: Sex, age, race, genetic predisposition, exposed to environmental carcinogens (radiation, tobacco, smoking, azo dyes, aflatoxin, asbestos, benzene, radon) and viruses are responsible for its genesis.

Effects of cancer

- Local pressure effect
- Destructive effects
- Generalized deleterious effects

Specificity of chemotherapy: Generally non-specific. In choriocarcinoma, Burkit's lymphoma, Wilms' tumor, Hodgkin's disease, testicular tumor, it is specific.

Causes of non-specificity of cancer chemotherapy

- Target cell similar to host cell (*cystic fibrosis* bacteria *vs* host cells)

- No different biochemical pathways between normal and cancer cells (exception aspergine).
- No different structural characteristics
- No differential host defence mechanism, hence chemotherapy depends only on rapidly proliferating cells.

Effects of cancer chemotherapy is governed by following factors:

- Post-treatment survival is inversely proportional to tumor cell burden.
- **Log kill hypothesis**, *e.g.* drug A which kills 90% of cells in one cycle of treatment will leave 10% of viable cells, *i.e.* 10^9 cells are reduced to $10^8 = 1$ log kill. Though 90% kill will reduce tumor size, but for a cure 10^9... $10^8 10^2$ ... 9 cycles of treatment are required.

To show observable effect in one treatment cycle, drug should have at least 2 log kill potency.

Solid tumor does not follow this and their growth fraction decrease exponentially with time. Maximum growth fraction when tumor is 37% of its maximum size and the model is called Gompertzian model.

- Differential log kill—normal cells should not be effected then only 9 cycles of treatment will be tolerated by the body.
- Regrowth of survival cells in intermittent cycle period, survived cells keep on growing so more than nine cycles of treatment will be required.
- We should have drugs which acting on both resting and proliferating phases (Fig. 116.1).

Cytotoxic drugs: These act on cycling proliferating cells.

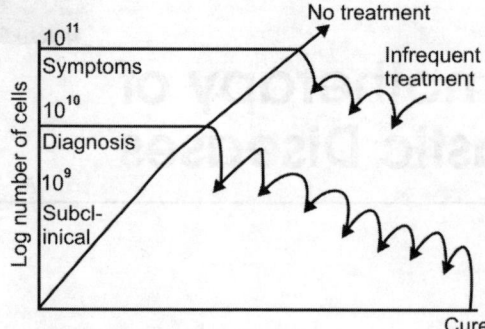

Fig. 116.1: Log kill hypothesis of anticancer drugs

CCNS (cell cycle non-specific) drugs

- Nitrogen mustard, cyclophosphamide
- Chlorambucil
- Carmustine
- Dacarbazine, 5FU, L-asparaginase
- Cisplatin, procarbazine
- Actinomycin D

CCS (cell cycle specific) drugs. Act on specific phase of a cell cycle.

- G1 = Vinblastine
- S = Mtx, cytarabin, 6TG, doxorubicin, 6MP Pemetrexed, Hydroxyurea, mitomycin C, doxorubicin,
- Daunorubicin, Antimetabolite
- G2 = Daunorubicin, bleomycin, etopoxide, Topotecan
- M = Vincristine, vinblastine, paclitaxel, Docetaxel, Ixabepilone, Estramustine (Fig. 116.2).

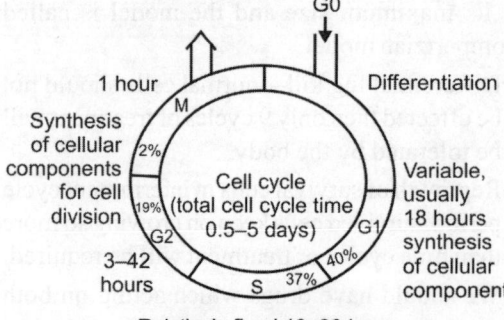

Fig. 116.2: Cell cycle

To Achieve Highly Effective Chemotherapy

Should have several log kill potencies, killing those cells which are both proliferating and resting, which is possible by multipronged attack by combining drugs having different mechanisms of action and acting on different sites of cell growth cycle. (Fig. 116.1)

GENERAL EFFECTS OF ANTICANCER DRUGS

Inhibit rapidly multiplying tissues

A. Malignant tissues
- Regression

B. Normal tissues

Bone marrow
- Agranulocytosis
- Anemia
- Lymphocytopenia

GI tract
- Denudation
- Hemorrhage

Gonads
- Oligospermia
- Inhibition of ovulation

Miscellaneous
- Alopecia

Embryo
- Teratogenic
- Abortion

C. Immunosuppression
- More infection
- Used in autoimmune disorder
- Inhibits transplant rejection

D. Miscellaneous
- Carcinogenesis
- Mutation
- Some other effects
- Nausea, vomiting (most drugs)

CNS depression
- Procarbazine
- L-asparaginase
- Hexamethyl melanamine
- Neuropathies

CNS stimulation
- Vincristine

Myopathies
- Vincristine
- Vinblastine

Hepatitis
- BCNU
- Mithramycin
- L-asparaginase

Renal toxicity
- Cisplatin

Cardiotoxicity
- Daunorubicin
- Daunomycin

Pulmonary fibrosis
- Bleomycin

Pancreatitis
- L-asparaginase

Fluid retention
- Steroids, masculization and feminization

Ototoxicity
- Cisplatin

Hyperuricemia
- Secondary to massive cell destruction

CLASSIFICATION OF ANTICANCER DRUGS

- A. Cytotoxic drugs
- B. Altering hormonal milieu
- C. Miscellaneous group

A. Cytotoxic drugs
  I. Alkylating agents
   a. Nitrogen mustard
   - Mechloroethamine
   - Cyclophosphamide
   - Ifosfamide
   - Chlorambucil
   - Melphalan
   b. Ethyleneamines
   - Thio-TEPA
   - Hexamethylmelamine (Altretamine)
   c. Alkyl sulfonate
   - Busulfan

d. Nitrosoureas
- Cramustine
- Lomustine
- Semustine

e. Triazines
- Dacarbazine
- Procarbazine
- Temozolamide
- Bendamustine

(*These are non-classical alkylating agents*)

II. Antimetabolites
  a. Folate antagonists
  - Methotrexate
  - Pemetrexed
  - Pralatrexed
  b. Purine antagonists
  - 6-mercaptopurine
  - 6-thioguanine
  - Azathioprine
  - Fludarabine
  - Cladribine
  c. Pyrimidine antagonists
  - Cytarabine
  - 5-fluorouracil
  - Capecitabine
  - Gemcitabine

III. Natural products
  a. Vinca alkaloids
  - Vincristine
  - Vinblastine
  - Vinorelbine
  b. Taxanes
  - Paclitaxel
  - Cabazitaxel
  - Docetaxel
  c. Camptothecins
  - Topotecan
  - Irinotecan
  d. Epipodophyllotoxins
  - Etoposide
  - Teniposide
  e. Antibiotics
  - Actinomycin D
  - Bleomycin

- Doxorubicin
- Mitoxantrone
- Mithramycin
- Dactinomycin
- Epirubicin
- Idarubicin
- Daunorubicin

(*These are anthracyclines*)

f. **Enzymes**
- L-asparaginase

B. **Altering hormonal milieu**

I. **Hormones**

a. **Corticosteroids**
- Glucocorticoids
- Prednisolone

b. **Estrogens**
- Diethylstilbesterol
- Ethinylestradiol

c. **Antiestrogens**
- Tamoxifen
- Doloxifen
- Toremifen
- Fulvestrant

d. **Androgens**
- Testosterone
- Fluoxymesterone

e. **Progesterones**
- Medroxyprogesterone
- Hydroxyprogesterone

f. **Antiandrogens**
- Flutamide
- Bicalutamide
- Nilutamide

g. **Gonadotropin-releasing hormone analogues**
- Leuprolide
- Gosereline
- Nafarelin
- Busurelin
- Histerelin

h. **Aromatase inhibitors**
- Aminoglutethimide
- Anastrozole
- Formestane
- Letrozole

- Exemestane
- Vorozole
- Cetrozole

i. **GnRH antagonists**
- Cetrolix
- Ganirelix
- Abarelix

j. **Adrenal cortex suppressant**
- Mitotane

C. **Miscellaneous**

1. **Hydroxyurea**
2. **Procarbazine**
3. **Platinum compounds**
   - Cisplatin
   - Carboplatin
   - Oxaliplatin
4. **Growth factor receptor inhibitors**
   - Cetuximab-Pazopanib
   - Gefitimib
   - Erlotinib
   - Bevacizumab
   - Panitumumab
   - Sorafenib
   - Sunitinib
5. **Asparaginase**
6. **Retinoic acid derivative tretinoin**
7. **Arsenic trioxide**
8. **Adenosine deaminase inhibitor**
   - Pentostalin
9. **Monoclonal antibodies**
   - Rituximab
   - Trastuzumab
10. **Biological response modifiers**
    - Recombinant 1L-2 (aldesleukin)
    - GMM-CSF (Sargramostim)
    - G-CSF (Filgrastim)
11. **Tyrosine kinase inhibitors**
    - Geftinib
    - Erlotinib
    - Imatinib
    - Dasatinib
    - Nilotinib, Bosutinib etc

Combined Therapy

Each drug should have unique mechanism:

1. Sequential or two consecutive blocks

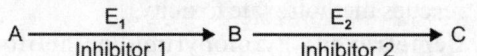

$$A \xrightarrow[\text{Inhibitor 1}]{E_1} B \xrightarrow[\text{Inhibitor 2}]{E_2} C$$

Azathioprine + 6MP → inhibition of purine synthesis

2. Concurrent block

Two parallel path block

6-thioguanidine + cytarabin

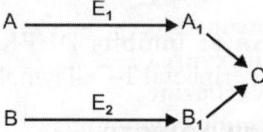

(Purine synthesis) + pyrimidine synthesis blocker = Nucleic acid synthesis block.

3. Complementary block: Two different paths are blocked.

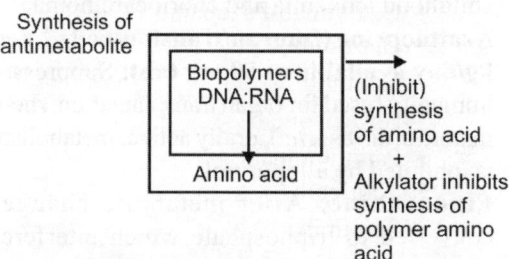

Principles of combined blocks

- Each drug should have a clinically desirable effect.
- Any drug having 25–30% of response considered as potential candidate for combined treatment.
- Each drug should be administered in a dose schedule comparable to that utilized as a single agent.
- Each drug should be given as intermittent treatment at regular intervals to maximize antitumor effect and minimize immunosuppressive effect.

Resistance to antimalignancy agents

Sometimes responses of chemotherapy are below the expected levels. It may be primary resistance, *i.e.* resistance since first exposure or acquired resistance in drug-sensitive tumors. The mechanism of resistance identified as follows:

a. Insufficient uptake by the neoplastic cells methotrexate

b. Insufficient activation of the drug 6MP, 6FU

c. Increased activation, *viz.* cytosine arabinoside

d. Increased utilization of an alternative biochemical pathway.

Antimetabolite

e. Rapid repair of drug-induced lesion—alkylating agents

f. Decreased requirement for a specific metabolic product.

L-asparaginase resistance is due to

g. Genomic instability

h. MDRI gene for cell surface glycoprotein responsible for drug efflux.

- **Individual drugs of alkylating agents:** Alkylating agents have radiominatic actions, resulting in cross-linking/abnormal basepairing/scission of DNA. They produce highly reactive carbonium ion intermediates which transfer alkyl groups to cellular macromolecules forming covalent bonds especially at position 7 of guanine residues in DNA. These are cell cycle non-specific.

- **Mechlorethamine (Mustine):** First nitrogen mustard, highly reactive, should be given IV 0.1 mg/kg/IV × 4 days, available as 10 mg dry powder/vial.

- **Cyclophosphamide (ENDOXAN):** Transformed into active metabolites. Chloramphenicol retards its metabolism. It is immunosuppressant. Alopecia and cystitis are common. 2–3 mg/kg/day orally or 10–15 mg/kg IV or IM every 7–10 days.

- **Ifosfamide (Haloxan):** 1 gm vial useful in bronchogenic, breast, testicular, bladder, head and neck carcinoma, lymphoma, osteogenic sarcoma. Hemorrhagic cystitis is bothersome and can be prevented by mesna which binds vesicotoxic metabolites.

- **Chlorambucil (Leukeran 2 and 5 mg tab):** Drug for CLL, Hodgkin's disease. It has immunosuppressant property, dose 0.1–0.2 mg/kg daily for 3–6 weeks and then 2 mg daily for maintenance.

- **Melphalan (Alkeran):** Used in multiple myeloma, causes bone marrow depression. Dose

6 mg/day for 2–3 weeks. Available as 2, 5 mg tabs or 50 mg/vial.

- **Thiotepa:** Seldom used because of toxicity. Dose 0.3–0.4 mg/kg IV.
- **Busulfan (Myleran 2 mg tab):** Dose 2–6 mg/day used for CML; pulmonary fibrosis is a common side effect.
- **Nitrosurea:** Lipid-soluble so crosses blood brain-barrier, used for meningeal leukemia and brain tumors.
  - ◆ Carmustine (BCNU) 50–200 mg/sq. m BSA IV over one hour.
  - ◆ Lomustine (CCNU) 100–130 mg/sq. m BSA orally. Repeat after 6 weeks
  - ◆ Methyl (CCNU) 100–200 mg/sq. m BSA orally.

TRIAZINES

These are non-classical alkylating agents.

- **Procarbazine:** Used in combination therapy of Hodgkin's and non-Hodgkin's lymphoma and brain tumor. Its carcinogenic potential is high.
- **Bendamustine** used for Hodgkin's and non-Hodgkin's lymphoma, multiple myeloma, breast cancer.
- **Dacarbazine:** Inhibits RNA and protein synthesis used in malignant melanoma and for Hodgkin's disease. Dose 3.5 mg/kg/day IV for 10 days to be repeated after 4 weeks.
- **Antimetabolite:** Analogues of normal components of DNA or coenzymes for nucleic acid synthesis, competes for normal substrate or involved in dysfunctional macromolecules.

Folic acid antagonists

- **Methotrexate (Neotrexate 2.5 mg tab; 50 mg/2 mL inj.):** Inhibits DHFRase, so inhibits conversion of DHFA to THFA, essential coenzyme for one carbon transfer reaction in purine synthesis. It is cell cycle specific (S phase). Orally absorbed, 50% plasma protein-bound. Toxicities of methotrexate can be overcome by folinic acid and thymidine. Used for choriocarcinoma and remission of leukemia; 15–30 mg/day for 5 days. Other uses are rheumatoid arthritis, psoriasis, immunosuppressants, folinic acid rescues methotrexate toxicity.
- **Pemetrexed:** Pyrolopyrimidine antifolate analog acts on S phase of cell cycle, targets dihydrofolate reuctase (DHFR) involved in purine synthesis. It may be combined with cisplatin for treating mesothelioma and single in non-small cell lung cancer. Causes myelo-suppression, skin rash, mucositis, diarrhea, fatigue.
- **Pralatrexate:** Inhibits DHFR. Used for refractory peripheral T-Cell lymphoma.

PURINE ANTAGONISTS

- **Mercaptopurine and thioguanine:** Inhibit conversion of inosine monophosphate to adenine and guanine nucleotides used for childhood leukemia and choriocarcinoma.
- **Azathioprine (Imuran/transimune 1–2 mg/kg/day available as 50 mg tab):** Suppresses immunity (used for organ transplantation, rheumatoid arthritis, *etc.*), orally active, metabolism is inhibited by allopurinol.
- **Fludarabine:** After metabolic changes converted to triphosphate which interferes DNA synthesis and repaired by inhibiting DNA polymerases a and b. It also induces apoptosis. Used for CLL and low grade non-Hodgkin's lymphoma. It is given parenterally. Since it is an immunosuppressor so leads to opportunistic infection of fungi, herpes, *Pneumocystis jiroveci.* Dose 25 mg/m^2/day × 5 days slowly IV every 4 weeks.
- **Cladribine:** Inhibits DNA synthesis and repairs like fludarabine. Used for hairy cell leukemia, CLL, low grade non-Hodgkin's lymphoma. It is given by infusion continuosly for seven days. Dose 0.09 mg/kg/day × 7 days IV with saline.

PYRIMIDINE ANTAGONISTS

- **5-fluorouracil** converted in body 5-fluoro-2'-deoxyuridine-5'-monophosphate, which inhibits thymidylate synthase and blocks conversion of deoxyuridilic acid and deoxythymidylic acid. Used for breast, colon, bladder, liver tumors. Topical application for basal cell carcinoma 250 mg caps or 250 mg/5 mL or 1% topical application. 1 gm orally in alternate days × 6 doses, then 1 gm weekly.

- **Cytarabine:** Triphosphate of cytarabine is an inhibitor of DNA polymerase and blocks formation of cytidylic acid, it impairs DNA repair (cell cycle specific of phase S), used for remission of leukemia in children and Hodgkin's disease (100 mg/5 mL), dose 1.5–3 mg/kg IV. Main toxicities are GI bleeding and bone marrow depression.

- **Capecitabine:** Used for metastatic breast cancer either alone or with taxane and also used for colorectal cancer. It produces diarrhea, hand-foot syndrome, mucositis, nausea, vomiting, myelosuppression. Dose 1250 mg/m^2 BD orally × 14 days.

- **Gemcitabine:** Used for pancreatic cancer, non-small cell lung cancer, non-Hodgkin's lymphoma, bladder cancer. Myelosuppression as neutropenia is the main toxicity. Dose 1000 mg/m^2 IV weekly for 7 weeks.

- **Ftorafur (Furator 200 mg cap):** Used orally 0.8–1.2 gm/day, 5FU congener, used for breast and gastrointestinal cancers.

CAMPTOTHECINS

These natural products are obtained from *Camptotheca acuminata*. It inhibits topoisomerase I enzyme responsible for cutting and religating DNA strands.

- **Topotecan** is used for ovarian cancer and small cell lung cancer.

- **Irinotecan** is a prodrug, used for metastatic colorectal cancer. Topotecan is excreted by kidney whereas irinotecan is excreted by bile and feces. It causes diarrhea and myelosuppression. Early diarrhea is treated by atropine occurring within 24 hours, but late diarrhea after 2–10 days may cause electrolytic imbalance and dehydration. Dose of topotecan 1.5 mg/m^2 IV × 5 days and irinotecan 125 mg/m^2 IV weekly.

VINCA ALKALOIDS

These are alkaloids obtained from periwinkle plant *Vinca rosea*.

These are mitotic inhibitors bind to microtubular protein and disrupt mitotic spindle, cell cycle specific for M phase.

- **Vincristine (Oncovin):** Used for leukemia, Hodgkin's disease, Wilms' tumor, lymphosarcoma, Ewing's sarcoma, lung carcinoma, 1 mg vial inj. Dose 1.5 mg/m^2 IV weekly.

- **Vinorelbine:** Semisynthetic vinca alkaloid, used for non-small cell lung cancer and breast cancer. It inhibits mitosis in M phase by inhibiting tublin polymerization. Dose 20 mg/m^2 IV weekly.

- **Vinblastine:** Used for Hodgkin's disease, testicular carcinoma. Bone marrow depression is common. Dose 0.1–0.15 mg/kg IV weekly × 3 doses (10 mg/vial).

EPIPODOPHYLLOTOXINS

- **Etoposide (Peltasol; lastet):** Semisynthetic derivative from plant glycosides. It arrests G$_2$ phase, breaks DNA by inhibiting DNA topoisomerse II. Used in testicular tumor, Hodgkin's and other lymphoma, bladder cancer, lung cancer (100 mg/5 mL vial). Dose 50–100 mg/m^2 IV or oral × 5 days.

  Other epipodophyllotoxins is a teniposide which is semisynthetic.

- **Taxanes and related drug:** Paclitaxel is an alkaloid of *Taxus brevifolia* and yew used for solid tumors like ovarian, non-small-cell breast and small-cell lung, prostate, esophagus, bladder, esophagus, kaposi sarcoma. It is mitotic spindle poison. Albumin-bound paclitaxel formulation is Abraxane. Docetaxel is semisynthetic taxane and ixabepilone though not taxane inhibits microtubule and used for breast cancer.

ANTIBIOTICS

Generally, they intercalate DNA and interfere their template function.

- **Actinomycin D:** Used for Wilms' tumor, rhabdomyosarcoma, choriocarcinoma. Dose-15 µg/kg/IV daily for 5 days.

- **Daunorubicin:** Effective in leukemia and solid tumors. It is **cardiotoxic** (arrhythmia, hypotension, ECG changes) cardiomyopathies. Dose, daunorubicin 30–50 mg/m^2 IV daily × 3 days is repeated weekly.

- **Doxorubicin:** 60 mg/m^2 IV every 3 weeks 10 mg/mL vial. It is cardiotoxic.

- **Idarubicin:** Semisynthetic anthracycline glycoside analog of daunorubicin is approved to treat AML in combination with cytarabine for induction therapy. Dose 12 mg/m^2 IV × 3 days.

- **Epirubicin:** Analog of doxorubicin used for node positive breast cancer and gastric cancer.

- **Mitoxantrone (Oncotron 20 mg/10 mL):** Dose 12 mg/m^2 single IV used in leukemia; Non- Hodgkin's lymphoma. It is an analogue of doxorubicin with lower cardiotoxicity because it does not produce quinone type free radical.

- **Dactinomycin:** Anticancer antibiotic obtained from *Streptomyces* organism, binds to double stranded DNA through intercalation and inhibits all forms of DNA-dependent RNA synthesis. Used for pediatric tumor, *viz.* Wilms' tumor, Ewing's sarcoma; rhabdomyosarcoma and gestational trophoblastic disease. Dose 0.04 mg/kg IV × 3 days.

- **Bleomycin (Bleocin):** Chelates of copper or iron, produces superoxide and intercalates DNA, leading to chain scission and inhibits repair. Effective in testicular tumor, squamous cell carcinoma of skin genitourinary, esophageal cancer, Hodgkin's lymphoma. Important toxicities are mucocutaneous toxicity, pulmonary fibrosis. Dose 30 mg biweekly IV, total 300–400 mg.

- **Mitomycin C:** Used only in resistant cases of stomach, cervix, colon, rectum and bladder cancers, because of its toxicity. Acts on G$_1$ and M phases. It is obtained from *Streptomyces caespitosus*. Dose 10 mg/m^2 IV every 6 weeks.

- **Mithramycin (Plicarnycin):** Used in embryonal testicular, disseminated cancers, acts by intercalating DNA. Highly toxic dose 25 µg/kg slowly IV daily or alternate days, 8–10 doses.

MISCELLANEOUS

- **Hydroxy urea (Hydrea 500 mg caps):** Blocks conversion of ribonucleotide to deoxyribonucleotide, inhibiting enzyme ribonucleoside diphosphate reductase. Used for CML and polycythemia vera. Dose 20–30 mg/daily.

- **Procarbazine:** After metabolic activation it depolymerizes DNA, leading to chromosomal damage, weak MAO inhibitor, used for brain tumors, Hodgkin's and non-Hodgkin's lymphoma (MOPP regimen), Oat cell carcinoma of lung. 1–2 mg/kg/day for maintenance.

- **Dacarbazine:** Synthetic agent, acts like alkylating agent following activation by liver enzymes. Diazomethane generates methyl carbonium which appears to cytotoxic. Used for melanoma, soft tissue sarcoma and Hodgkin's disease. Myelosuppression, nausea, vomiting are important side effects. Dose 3.5 mg/kg/day IV for 10 days.

Bendamustine

Cross-links with DNA leading to inhibition of DNA synthesis induces mitotic catastrophe used for chronic lymphocytic leukemia.

- **Altretamine:** Biotransfered in liver by demethylation to pentamethylmelamine and tetramethylmelamine. It is given orally. It may produce neurotoxicity, nausea, vomiting and myelosuppression. Used for ovarian cancer. Dose 10 mg/kg/day × 3 weeks.

Enzymes

- **L-asparaginase (Leunase):** Obtained from *E. coli,* degrades L-asparagine to L-aspartic acid depriving leukemic cells of an essential metabolite. Used in childhood acute leukemia, it is short lasting. Dose 50–200 KU/kg/IV daily for 2–4 weeks 10,000 KU per vial.

Platinum Compounds

- **Cisplatin (aquaplat 10 mg/10 mL):** Cis-isomer of platinum complex, hydrolyzed intracellularly to produce reactive moiety, cross-linking DNA. Also reacts with SH groups in proteins, radiomimetic properties. Hydration, reduces nephrotoxicity, 50–100 mg/m^2

every 3–4 weeks slowly IV used for testicular and ovarian cancer emesis, kidney damage. Shock may occur.

- **Carboplatin (oncocarbin):** 2nd generation platinum with less oto-, nephro- and neuro-toxicities, used in squamous cell carcinoma, seminoma, small-cell lung cancers.
- **Oxaliplatin:** This is a third generation platinum analog used for metastatic colorectal cancer along with 5-fluorouracil and leucovorin. It produces neurotoxicity either dose dependent or worsened by cold. Dose 85 mg/m^2 every two weeks.
- **Aromatase inhibitors:** Aminoglutathimide used for metastatic breast cancer. Anastrozole, letrozole and exemestane all are used to treat breast cancer. All drugs of this group inhibit corticosteroid synthesis in first step involving cholesterol to pregnenolone.

HORMONES

- **Glucocorticoids:** Used in lymphoma and leukemia.
- **Estrogen:** In carcinoma prostate, life is prolonged, used in carcinoma of male breast, relapse occurs. Fosfesterol (Honvan 120 mg tab, 300 mg/5 mL inj) is phosphate derivative of stilbesterol used for calcium prostate, 600–1200 mg IV then 120–240 mg as maintenance.
- **Estrogen and androgen inhibitors (tomoxifen):** It is an estrogen antagonist, used in breast cacinoma in older patient when surgery and other chemotherapy not possible in woman.
- **Flutamide and bicalutamide:** They bind to androgen receptor to inhibit its effect. Used in prostate cancer.
- **Androgen:** Used in premenopausal breast cacinoma in woman.
- **Progesterone:** Gives temporary remission in recurrent (after surgery and chemotherapy) advanced metastatic endometrial carcinoma and metastatic hormone-dependent and breast cancer.
- **Miscellaneous anticancer drugs:** Imatinib, dasatinib and nilotinib are approved to treat CMI.

Growth factor receptor inhibitors, panitumumab and cetuximab: They are chimeric monoclonal antibodies act against epidermal growth factor receptors, used for metastatic colorectal cancer.

- **Bevacizumab:** This recombinant monoclonal antibody acts against vascular endothelial growth factor, used for metastatic colorectal cancer. **ADR:** Hypertension, TIA, CAD, delayed wound healing, GI perforation, proteinuria.
1. **Sorafenib:** Approved for advanced renal cell cancer and hepatocellular cancer.
2. **Sunitinib:** Approved for advanced renal cell cancer and gastrointestinal stromal tumor.
3. **Gefitinib and erlotinib:** Inhibit tyrosine kinase associated with epidermal growth factor receptor, used for non-small-cell lung cancer.
- **Retinoic acid derivatives (tretinoin):** Cause remission of acute promyelocytic leukemia.

   ADR: Vitamin A toxicity, retinoic acid syndrome with fever, leukocytosis, dyspnea, pleural and pericardial effusion, raised cholesterol, dizziness, anxiety, depression, diarrhea, abdominal pain, teratogenicity.
- **Arsenic trioxide:** Given IV to treat acute promyelocytic leukemia.

   ADR: Fatigue, QT prolongation, arrhythmia, fever dyspnea, skin rash, fluid retention and weight gain.

Amelioration of Toxicities of Anticancer Drugs

- Folinic acid rescues normal cells from methotrexate.
- Systemic mesna and irritating bladder with acetylcystine reduces cystitis of cyclophosphamide and ifosphamide.
- 5HT3 antagonist: Ondansetron, granisetron and palonosetron decrease vomiting.
- Lithium carbonate stimulates bone marrow with myelosuppressive drugs.
- Allopurinol and alkalization prevent gout formation.

- Rasburicase also prevents hyperuricemia from tumorlysis.
- Aprepitant, an antagonist to NK-1 used to reduce cisplastin-induced delayed vomiting.
- Pilocarine reduces xerostomia.
- Palifermin is a keratinocyte growth factor to prevent mucositis.
- Pamidronate and zolendronate to treat hypercalcemia of malignancy.
- Platelet or granulocyte transfusion to prevent bleeding or infection.
- Biological response modifiers like GM-CSF/G-CSF hastens recovery from drug-induced bone marrow depression or bone marrow transplantation to rescue myelosuppressant therapy.
- Erythropoietin and darbopoietin to treat anemia.
- Dexrazoxane: Iron chelator prevents cardiotoxicity of anthracyclinc antibiotics.
- Oprelvekin: IL-11 for thrombocytopenia.

Strategy for Developing Drug Regimen for Specific Tumors

Following knowledge is important for choosing drug for tumors.

Knowledge of specific tumors

- Is the growth fraction high?
- Whether most of the cells in G0 phase?
- Are the majority of tumors composed of hypoxic stem cells?
- Whether they are under hormonal control?
- Knowledge of receptor expression of tumor cells, *viz.* for breast cancer expression of estrogen or progesterone receptor or overexpression of HER-Z receptor.

Knowledge of specific drugs

- Whether the tumor cells sensitive to the drug intended to use?
- Drug is cell cycle specific or not?
- Whether the durg is activated in normal tissue or activated in tumor cell itself?

DRUGS USED FOR DIFFERENT CANCER CONDITIONS

- **Childhood leukemia:** Methotrexate, 6-mercaptopurine, cyclophosphamide, vincristine, daunorabicin, asperginase, corticosteroid.
- **Adult acute myeloid leukemia (AML):** Cytorabine + Anthracycline
- **Chronic myeloid leukemia (CML):** Imatinib.
- **Chronic lymphocytic leukemia (CLL):** Chlorambucil and cyclophosphamide with prednisone or Cyclophosphamide + Vincristine + Prednisone, Bendamustine newest alkylating is approved for its treatments.
- **Hodgkin's lymphoma:** Mechlorethamine, Vincristine, Procarbazine, Predinisome (MOPP) or Doxorubicin, Bleomycin, vinblastine and Dacarbazine (ABVD).
- **Non-Hodgkin's lymphoma:** Cyclophosphamide + Hydroxydaunorubicin + Oncovin (Vincristine) + Prednisone (CHOP)
- **Multiple myeloma:** Melphalan + Prednisone or Lenalidomide + Dexamethasome or proteosome inhibitor Bortezomib + Prednisone Melphalan, Thalidomide for refractory or relapse cases.
- **Breast cancer:** Cyclophosphamide + Methotraxate + Fluorouracil (stages I and II).

  Stages III and IV: Anastrozole and Letrozole, Tamoxifen and exemestane as second-line treatment.
- **Malignant Melanoma:** Metastatic are treated with dacarbazine, temozolomide, cisplatin, Ipilimumab.
- **Prostrate Cancer:** Leuprolide, Goserelin (LHRH agonist). Flutamide, Bicalutamide, Nilutamide (Antiandrogen); Abiraterone (Steroid synthesis inhibitor).
- **Brain Cancer:** Carmustine or lomustine; Temozolomide (Alkylating agent). Bivacizumab for glioblastoma multiforme.

117

Antifungal Drugs

Fungi are known to cause human diseases earlier than bacteria. Its incidence has increased dramatically nowadays. It may even cause death in HIV; immunocompromised cancer therapy patient or organ transplant patient. It may be classified as those used **topically** and those used for **systemic** infections.

Topically effective: Tolnaftate, undecylenic acid, benzoic acid, quiniodochlor, sodium thiosulfate, ciclopirox olamine, butenafine.

INDIVIDUAL ANTIFUNGAL DRUGS USED FOR SYSTEMIC INFECTIONS

1. **Amphotericin B:** Obtained from *Streptomyces nodosus*. Amphotericin A obtained from it is not used. Amphotericin B obtained from it is polyene macrolide. Effective against *Histoplasma capsulatum, Cryptococcus neoformans, Coccidioides immitis, Candida albicans, Blastomyces dermatitidis, Rhodotorula, Aspergillus*. The polyenes have high affinity for ergosterol of fungal cell membrane and insert into it in such a way that they produce a micropore and cell permeability is markedly increased. Bacteria are insensitive to polyenes because they do not have ergosterol in their membranes. It also enhances immunity to immunocompromised patient.

   Orally poorly absorbed, IV amphotericin is widely distributed, binds to sterols and lipoproteins. Metabolized in liver and excreted in urine and bile.

   Administered orally for intestinal candidiasis, topically for vaginitis, otomycosis.

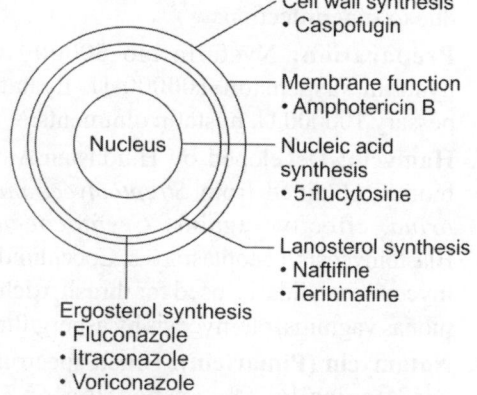

Fig. 117.1: Site of action of antifungal drugs

For systemic mycosis, it is given IV where dose is increased gradually. May be given intrathecal for fungal meningitis.

Liposomal amphotericin B: Here the drug is packaged into lipid delivery vehicles acting as its reservoir which has affinity for fungal ergosterol and this lipid vehicle serves as reservoir of amphotericin. By this drug delivery system larger doses can be given with less toxicity. Apart from this, some fungi contain lipase, which can liberate free amphotericin B at the site of infection.

Adverse effects: IV infusion may produce chills, fever, ache, pain, nausea, vomiting, thrombophlebitis which decreases gradually. Hydrocortisone may reduce infusion reaction.

Nephrotoxicity, reduced glomerular filtration rate (GFR), acidosis, anemia due to bone marrow depression. Intrathecal injection may produce headache, vomiting, nerve paralysis. Used as antifungal, leishmaniasis.

2. **Nystatin:** Obtained from S. *noursei.* It is polyene macrolide, effective against *Candida Histoplasma, Blastomycoses, Microsporum.* Depending upon concentration, it is fungistatic and fungicidal. It combines with cell membrane and interferes with respiration and glucose utilization. Oral administration produces much toxicity, but with topical applications adverse effects are rare. It is used orally due to monilial diarrhea due to superinfection.

   Preparation: Nystatin tab 500000 U, nystatin suspension 100000 U, nystatin pessary 100000 U, nystatin ointments.

3. **Hamycin:** Developed by Hindustan Antibiotics, obtained from *Streptomyces pimprina,* effective against *Cryptococcus,* Blastomycosis, histoplasmosis, Coccidioidomycosis, candidasis, used for thrush, trichomonas vaginitis, otomycosis by aspergillius.

4. **Natamycin (Pimaricin):** Broad-spectrum, used topically. 5% suspension or 1% ointment in eye in *Fusarium solani* keratitis, monilial and trichomonas vaginitis can be treated by natamycin (Pimafusin vaginal 100 mg tablets).

   The 1, 2, 3, 4 antifungal drugs mentioned above are polyene antibiotics.

5. **Griseofulvin:** Antifungal antibiotics obtained from *Penicillium griseofulvum* effective against dermatophytes (epidermophyton, trichophyton, microsporium). Resistance occurs due to loss of concentrating ability. It is fungistatic, arrests mitotis of fungi and interferes with nucleic acid synthesis of finer particles.

   Absorbtion is enhanced by fat in the diet, deposited in keratin precursors, and has greater affinity for diseased skin. Finer particles are better absorbed. Chemically, it is heterocyclic benzfuran.

   Adverse effects: They are epigastric distress, nausea, vomiting, paresthesia, peripheral neuritis, vertigo, psychomotor incoordination, lethargy, transient leukopenia, proteinuria, gynecomastia, pigmentation of skin, decreases anticoagulant activity of warfarin, antabuse-like reaction. Dose 500 mg daily in 2–4 divided doses.

6. **Flucytosine (5FC):** Pyrimidine antimetabolite inactive as such, converted to 5-fluorouracil then to 5-fluorodeoxyuridylic acid, inhibitor of thymidylate synthesis component of DNA. Mammalian cells except marrow cells have low capacity to convert 5FC. It is narrow-spectrum fungistatic against *Cryptococcus neoformans, Torula, Chromoblastomyces, Candida, Aspergillus.* Bone marrow toxicities like anemia, leukopenia, thrombocytopenia, toxic enterocolitis are some adverse effects. Dose 100–150 mg/kg/day in 4 divided doses.

   Imidazole and triazoles: Mostly used for topical application, fluconazole and itraconazole are used for systemic mycosis. Broad-spectrum antifungal covering *Candida, Nocardia* and some gram-positive anerobic bacteria, *viz. Staph. aureus. Strep. faccalis, Bac. fragilis, Leishmania.* They inhibit cytochrome P450 enzyme, lanosterol 14-demethylase, impair ergosterol synthesis leading to membrane abnormalities. First azole introduced was ketoconazole.

   Dose of itraconazole is 100–400 mg/day. Oral and parenteral preparations are available. Its availability is decreased with rifampicin. Fluconazole is more water-soluble and its CSF penetration is good, voriconazole is a newer triazole. Dose 400 mg/day. May be given orally or IM. Posaconazole is a newest triazole with broadest action against candida and aspergillus.

7. **Econazole (Econazole 1% oint; 150 mg vaginal tab):** Highly effective for dermatophytosis, oral thrush and otomycosis.

8. **Miconazole (Daktarin 2% gel and powder):** It is azole derivative used topically. Effective for tinea, pitriasis, versicolor, otomycosis, cutaneous and valvovaginal candidiasis. Irritation may occur.

9. **Clotrimazole (Surfaz 1% lotion, cream, powder, 100 mg vaginal tab):** Effective for athlete foot, otomycosis, oral cutaneous and vaginal candidiasis, also effective against skin *Corynebacteria.* Local irritation may occur in some patients. Oral clotrimazole troches are available to treat oral thrush.

10. **Ketoconazole (Fungicide; nizral 200 mg tab; niral 2% oint; shampoo):** Orally effective, gastric acidity facilitates absorption, bound to albumin and RBC, metabolized in liver and excreted in urine and feces. Not effective for fungal meningitis. Loss of hair, decrease in libido, oligozoospermia, menstrual irregularities, elevation of serum tramsaminase may occur.

    Rifampicin, phenytoin induce its metabolism. Reduction of gastric hydrochloric acid by H_2 blocker, proton pump inhibitors reduce oral absorption. Raises blood level of warfarin, sulfonylurea by inhibiting their metabolisms. Arrhythmia with terfenadine, cisapride and astermazole may occur. It decreases androgen production from testes and displaces testosterone from protein binding site.

    Used for dermatophytosis, systemic mycosis, also used for kala-azar and dermal leishmaniasis. Ketoconazole topical or shampoo is used to treat seborrheic dermatitis and tinea versicolor. High dose is used in Cushing's syndrome. It should not be used in pregnancy and lactation.

    ADR: Rash elevated hepatic enzymes, visual distrubances. Effective against *Candida* and dimorphic fungi and aspergillosis.

11. **Fluconazole (Forcan 50, 100, 150, 200 mg caps 200 mg/100 mL IV infusion):** Orally absorbed, excreted in urine, used to treat cryptococcal meningitis, systemic and mucosal candidiasis, sporotrichosis, histoplasmosis, coccidioidal meningitis (Co-drug of choice is amphotericin), 0.3% eyedrop (syscan) for fungal keratitis. Nausea, vomiting, abdominal pain, rash, headache may occur. Interacts with oral contraceptive, terfendine. Interaction with theophylline has not been reported.

12. **Itraconazole (canditral, itaspor 100 mg cap):** Orally active, fungistatic, broader-spectrum than ketoconazole and fluconazole, effective against *Aspergillus, Mucor.* Protein-bound, penetration in CSF is poor, accumulates in vaginal mucosa, skin, nails. Metabolized in liver, excreted through feces. Absorption is hampered by H_2 blocker. Omeprazole, rifampicin, phenytoin induce metabolism. Arrhythmia may occur with terfenadine, cisapride; phenytoin, digoxin, sulfonylurea, cyclosporine level may increase with its concomittant use.

13. **Voriconazole:** This is a new triazole, dose 400 mg/day orally absorbed, metabolized in liver.

14. **Posaconazole** active against mucomycosis. Dose 800 mg/day in 2–3 divided doses, given with fatty meal. Used also for aspergillosis, fungal infection during chemotherapy.

15. **Terbinafine (It is synthetic allylamine Sabifen 250 mg tab; 1% cream):** Topically used and orally effective fungicidal. In therapeutic doses it is non-competitive inhibitor of squalene epoxidase, producing ergosterol in fungus. Protein-bound, concentrated in sebum, nail and stratum corneum, metabolized and excreted through urine and feces. GI upset, taste disturbances, liver dysfunction, hematological disorders may occur. Topical use may cause itching, erythema, dryness, irritation. Dose 250 mg OD used for tinea pedis, corporis, captis and pityriasis versicolor, onychomycosis. Niftifine is an another topical allylamine.

Echinocandins: Caspofungin, micafungin and anidulafungin belong to this group, chemically large cyclic peptide linked to long chain fatty acid. Dose of caspofungin 70 mg loading then 50 mg daily.

Micafungin 150 mg/day; anidulafungin 100 mg 1st day then 50 mg/day × 14 days. All echinocandins are given intravenously.

They inhibit fungal cell walls β (1–3) glucan causing its disruption and death.

Nikkomycin: It inhibits fungal cell wall chitin synthesis.

TOPICAL ANTIFUNGAL DRUGS

Tolnaftate (Tinadern 1% lotion): Used for tinea cruris, corporis. Less irritating.

Cyclopirox olamine (Laprox 1% cream): Used for tinea pedis and other dermatophytoses, vaginal candidiasis, nappy rash. Irritation may occur.

Undecylenic acid: Generally used with zinc salt for tinea pedis and other dermatophytoses, nappy rash. Irritation and sensitization may occur.

Benzoic acid: Fugistatic, used with salicylic acid (as keratolytic). Whitfield ointment.

Chlorphenesin: Antibacterial, antifungal, antitrichomonial; used for prophylactic and treatment of dermatophytoses as 0.5% ointment or dusting powder.

Quinidochlor: Dermoquinol 4–8% topically, it has antifungal, antibacterial properties, used for dermatophytoses, sycosis barbae, seborrheic dermatitis, infective eczema, pityriasis versicolor. Orally luminal amoebicide.

Dithranol: 0.1 to 1% ointment used for psoriasis, ringworm; chronic dermatoses, skin test should be done to rule out hypersensitivity.

Chrysarobin: Obtained from wood of Andira araroba used for ringworm.

Ichthammol: 10% used for dermatomycosis.

Selenium sulfide: Used for dandruff and tinea versicolor.

Sodium thiosulfate (Karpin lot): Fungistatic used for *Malassezia furfur* infection.

Trichomycin and candicidin: These polyene antibiotics are used topically to treat vaginitis due to *Trichomonas* and *Candida*.

Other topical antifungals are nystatin, clotrimazole, miconazole, topical shampoo of ketoconazole, terbinafine naftifine.

118

Antiviral Drugs

VIRAL CHEMOTHERAPY

Pasteur (1884) failed to demonstrate bacteria in infected material from rabid dog was tempted to believe it was caused by small organism. Iwansky confirmed this through different disease TMVs.

Luria (1967) has defined viruses as entities whose genome is an element of nucleic acid (DNA or RNA) reproduces inside the cells and uses their virion which contain their viral genome and transfer it to other cells. Two cardinal features of this definition:

- They possess genetic control of virus itself.
- They are intracellular obligatory parasites.

Viral chemotherapy is difficult as it interferes with host cells. Drugs could target at attachment of virus to cell surface, uncoating reverse transcription, virus assembly and maturation (Fig. 118.1).

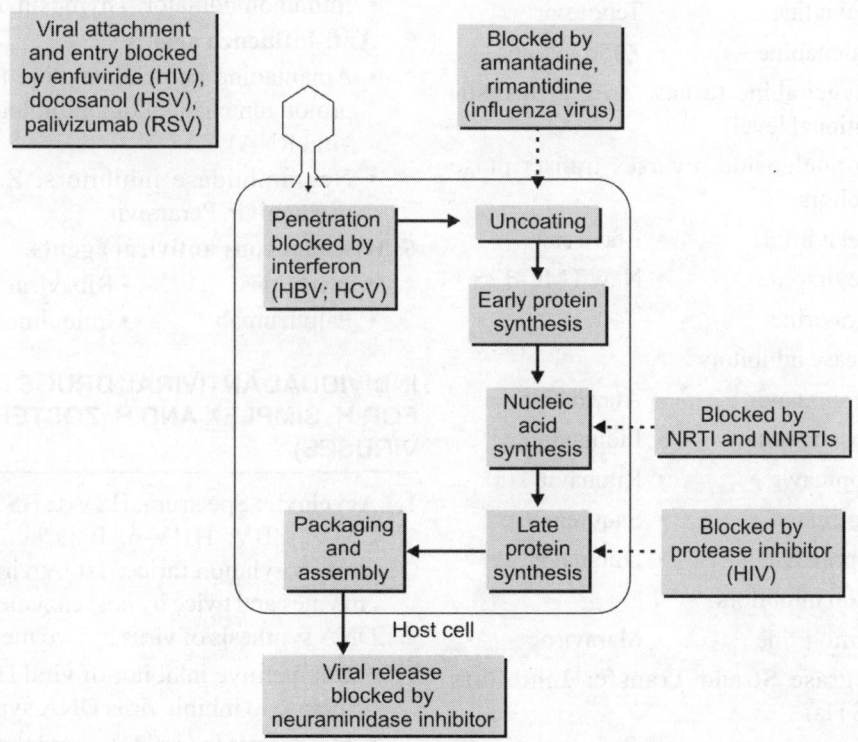

Fig. 118.1: Site of action of different antiviral drugs

ANTIVIRAL AGENTS

1. **Agents used for herpes simplex and herpes zoster viruses**
   - Acyclovir
   - Valacyclovir
   - Famciclovir
   - Penciclovir
   - Docosanol
   - Trifluridine
   - Valomaciclovir
   - 5-iododexyuridine and trifluorothymidine are used locally for Herpes keratitis as they are too toxic for systemic use.

2. **Agents used for cytomegalovirus**
   - Ganciclovir
   - Valganciclovir
   - Foscanet
   - Cidofovir
   - Maribavir at investingation level

3. **Antiretroviral agents**
   a. Nucleoside and nucleotide reverse transcriptase inhibtors
      - Abacavir
      - Didanosine
      - Emtricitabine
      - Lamivudine
      - Stavudine
      - Tenofovir
      - Zalcitabine
      - Zudovudine
      - Elvucitabine (a new drug at investigational level)
   b. Non-nucleoside reverses transcriptase inhibitors
      - Delavirdine
      - Efavirenz
      - Nevirapine
      - New TMC-125
      - Etravirine
   c. Protease inhibitors
      - Amprenavir
      - Atazanavir
      - Fosamprenavir
      - Indinavir
      - Lopinavir
      - Ritonavir
      - Nelfinavir
      - Saquinavir
      - Tipranavir
      - Duranavir
   d. Fusion inhibitors
      - Enfuvirtide
      - Maraviroc
   e. **In**tegrase **S**trand **T**ransfer **I**nhibitors (INSTIs)
      - Reltegravir
      - Elvitegravir
      - Dolutegravir

4. **Antihepatitis agents**

   Hepatitis B
   - Lamivudine
   - Adefovir
   - Entecavir
   - Interferon α and β
   - Tenofovir
   - Telbivudin
   - Drugs at investigational level: Emtricitabine, clevudine valtorlitabine pradefovir, Alamifovir, Thymosin α_1.

   Hepatitis C:
   - Sofosbuvir
   - Pegylated interferon alpha-2a
   - Ribavirin
   - Protease inhibitor: boceprevir, simeprevir, telapevir

   Inhibitors of HCV RNA polymerase:
   - Valopicitabine
   - Telaprevir (protease inhibitor)
   - Viramidine and merimepodib (amino phospholipid antibody)
   - Monoclonal antibodies against glycoprotein
   - Immunomodulator: Thymosin α_1

5. **Anti-influenza agents**
   - Amantadine and rimantadine (block M_2 proton ion channel to inhibit uncoating of viral RNA)
   - Neuraminidase inhibitors: Zanamivir; oseltamivir, Peramivir

6. **Miscellaneous antiviral agents**
   - Inerferons
   - Ribavirin
   - Palivizumab
   - Imiquimod

INDIVIDUAL ANTIVIRAL DRUGS (USED FOR H. SIMPLEX AND H. ZOSTER VIRUSES)

1. **Acyclovir:** Spectrum: HSV-1; HSV-2; VZV; CMV; EBV; HHV-6. It is activated by phosphorylation thrice. 1st by virus specifc enzymes and twice by host enzymes. Inhibits DNA synthesis of virus by two mechanisms.
   - Competitive inhibitor of viral DNA polymerase to inhibit virus DNA synthesis.
   - Incorporate in viral DNA and terminate the chain. Used topically; orally; IV (used for

HS encephalitis; neonatal HSV and for immunocompromise patient with VZV). Nausea, diarrhea, cystal nephropathy, tremor, seizure may occur.

2. **Valacyclovir:** L-valyl ester of acyclovir, converted to acyclovir, so serum level after oral dose is high. Confusion, headache, liver enzymes elevation, GI intolerance, thrombotic microangiopathy, hemolytic uremic syndrome may occur.

3. **Famciclovir:** A prodrug converted to penciclovir after oral administration used for HSV-1; HSV-2; VZV; EBV; HBV. Well-tolerated. Headache; diarrhea; nausea may occur.

4. **Penciclovir:** Metabolite of famciclovir used topically for herpes labialis.

5. **Docosanol:** This aliphatic alcohol prevents fusion of viral and plasma membrane. Used topically as 10% cream.

6. **Trifluridine:** This fluorinated pyrimidine inhibits viral DNA synthesis of HSV-1; HSV-2 and some adenoviruses. Used as 1% solution in treating keratoconjunctivitis; recurrent epithelial keratitis (used for cytomegalovirus).

7. **Valomaciclovir:** This drug inhibits DNA polymerase is under going clinical trial for zoster and EBV.

Used for Cytomegalovirus

1. **Ganciclovir:** It is phosphorylated for activation before inhibiting viral DNA polymerase (DNA elongation). Its activity includes CMV; HSV; VZV; Kaposis's sarcoma associated herpes virus (KSHV), human herpes virus 6. May be given orally, IV or as intraocular implant. Myelosuppression, nausea, rash, diarrhea, headaches, insomnia, neuropathy, confusion, seizure, hepatotoxicity, mitogenic, carcinogenic, embryotoxic. Dose 5 mg/kg/day.

2. **Valganciclovir:** Prodrug of ganciclovir. Mixture of two diastereomers used to treat CMV retinitis and in transplant patients to prevent CMV infection. Used orally. Dose 900 mg/BD and then 900 mg/day as maintenance.

3. **Foscarnet:** It inhibits DNA polymerase. RNA polymerase, HIV reverse transcriptase without requiring activation by phosphorylation. Used for HSV; VZV; CMV; EBV; HIV-1; HHV-6, KSHV. Renal impairment; hypo- or hypercalcemia; hypermagnesemia. Saline preloading prevents nephropathy; penile ulceration; nausea; vomiting; anemia; liver enzyme elevation. Headache, hallucination; seizure may occur. 60 mg/kg TDS for induction, then 90–120 mg/kg/day for maintenance.

4. **Cidofovir:** Spectrum CMV; HSV-1; HSV-2; VZV; EBV; HHV-6; KSHV; adenovirus; poxvirus; polyomavirus; papillomavirus.

   After phosphorylation, it inhibits DNA polymerase. Dose 5 mg/kg/week as induction and 5 mg/kg/14 days as maintenance. It causes dose-dependent nephrotoxicity (may be reduced by prehydration), neutropenia, GI intolerance, uveitis and acidosis.

5. **Maribavir:** It is benzimidezole riboside, on clinical investigational level for anti-CMV. It inhibits viral DNA assembly egress viral capsid from the infected cell's nucleus.

Targets of Various anti-HIV Drugs

The HIV virus enters the CD_4 cells. Viral GP_{41} fuses with CCR_5 or $CXCR_4$ receptor in human cells. The viral RNA is converted to DNA with the help of reverse transcriptase (RNA-dependent DNA polymerase). The viral DNA now integrates with human DNA with the help of enzyme integrase and form provirus. This proviral DNA can replicate and transcript to form RNA which forms protein *via* translation. Protein thus produced are inactive and activated by enzyme protease. The complete HIV virus, thus produced leaves CD_4 cells to infect other CD_4 cells.

Nucleoside and Nucleotide Reverse Transcriptase Inhibitors

• **Abacavir:** This is gnanosine analogue. Dose 300 mg BD. May produce hypersensitivity,

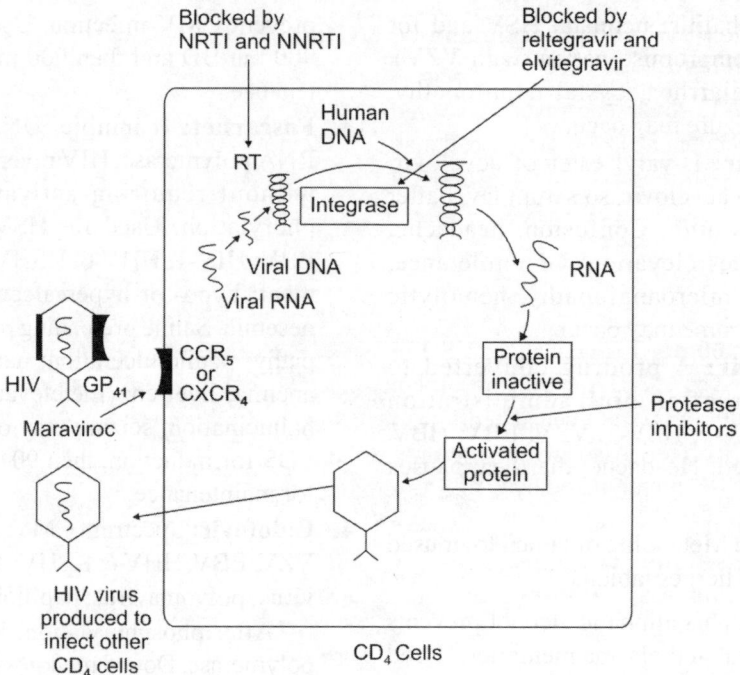

Fig. 118.2: Life cycle of HIV virus and site of action of different anti-HIV drugs

fever, malaise, nausea, diarrhea, dyspnea; pharyngitis, skin rash, pancreatitis, elevated serum aminotransferase; pancreatitis which disappeared on discontinuation. Resistance occurs due to mutation. Increases the risk of myocardial infarction.

- **Didanosine:** Synthetic analog of deoxyadenosine. Dose 250–400 mg daily as buffered powder solution or chewable tab or enteric coated as food decreases oral bioavailability. Resistance occurs due to mutation. It produces dose-dependent pancreatitis.

- **Emtricitabine:** Fluorinated analog of lamivudine. Dose 200 mg/day. Headache, diarrhea, nausea, asthenia, hyperpigmentation of palm and sole may occur. Lamivudine and emtricitabine are best tolerated NRTIs.

- **Lamivudine:** Cytosine analog. Dose 150 mg BD. Orally absorbed. Headache, insomnia, fatigue, GI discomfort may occur.

- **Stavudine:** Thymidine analog. Dose 30–40 BD. Neuropathy, pancreatitis, arthralgia, lactic acidosis, raised aminotransferase, hepatic steatotis may occur.

- **Tenofovir:** It is incorporated in DNA and competitively inhibits reverse transcriptase of HIV to cause chain termination. Tenofovir disopoxil fumarate is the prodrug. Its oral bioavailability increases after fatty meal. Dose 300 mg QDS. Dose adjustment required for renal insufficiency, nausea, diarrhea, headache, asthenia, acute renal failures, Fancony syndrome may occur as ADR. It is nucleotide RTI.

- **Zalcitabine:** High oral bioavailability, cytosine analog. Dose 0.75 mg TDS. Dose-dependent neuropathy. AUC of it increases with co-administration with cimetidine or probenecid.

- **Zidovudine:** Deoxythymidine analog, well-absorbed from gut and well-distributed. Dose 200 mg TDS. Adjust in renal insufficiencies. Myelosuppression, GI intolerance, headache, insomnia may occur.

All NRTIs are excreted *via* kidney. They may cause hepatomegaly, steatosis and lactic acidosis by inhibiting mitochondrial as DNA polymerase.

Non-nucleoside Reverse Transcriptase Inhibitors (NNRTIs)

It binds to HIV-1, reverse transcriptase and blocks RNA-dependent DNA polymerase. It may produce Stevens-Johnson syndrome and GI intolerance.

Individual NNRTIs

Drugs

- **Delavirdine (400 mg TDS):** Causes VSD in rats metabolized by CYP3A. Orally absorbed.
- **Efavirenz (600 mg OD):** Given at bedtime to minimize CNS effect. Also given in empty stomach. Long t½, metabolized by CYP3A to inactive hydroxylated form.

  ADR: Dizziness, insomnia, confusion, ammetic nightmare, nausea, vomiting, diarrhea, cystorrhagia, raised liver enzymes.
- **Nevirapine:** 90% absorbed orally, t½ 25–30 hours. Metabolized by CYP3A. Prevents transmission of HIV from mother to fetus. Rash, hepatotoxicity are important ADRs. Dose 200 mg/day single dose.
- **Etravirine:** Used in resistant cases of first generation NNRTI. Rash, nausea, diarrhea may occur. Triglyceride hepatic transaminase and glucose may rise.
- **Rilviprine:** Used with meal. Depression, headache, rise in trans-aminase may occur.

PROTEASE INHIBITORS

Protease inhibitors by preventing *Gag-Pol* gene products produce immature, non-infectious, viral particle.

Central obesity, breast enlargement, facial and peripheral wasting, causingoid appearance may occur.

- **Amprenavir (1400 mg BD):** Alcohol should be avoided, contraindicated to sulfa-sensitive patient.
- **Atazanavir (400 mg OD):** Orally absorbed. Inhibitors CYP3A4 and glucuronide enzyme.
- **Fosamprenavir:** Prodrug of amprenavir. Dose 1400 mg BD. Hydrolyzed by enzymes of intestinal epithelium.

- **Indinavir (800 mg TDS):** Given in empty stomach or with ritonavir. High CNS penetration. Nephrolithiasis, jaundice may occur.
- **Darunavir:** Coadministered with ritonavir. **ADR:** Dysdipidemia, increase in hepatic transaminase, rash, nausea, headache. Dose 600 mg BD with ritonavir 100 mg.
- **Lopinavir:** Taken with food. Nausea, vomiting, pain in abdomen may occur.
- **Ritonavir (400 mg BD + lopinavir 100 mg, licensed combination):** Ritovanir acts as pharmacokinetic enhancer of lopinavir by inhibting CYP3A, well-tolerated.
- **Nelfinavir (750 mg TDS or 1250 mg BD):** Higher absorption. Inhibitor of CYP3A. Diarrhea, flatulence may occur.
- **Saquiuavir (1000 mg soft gel capsules):** Nausea, diarrhea, dyspepsia may occur, soft gel capsules are better absorbed.
- **Tipranavir:** 500 mg cap BD with ritonavir 200 mg BD.

All protease inhibitors are metabolized in liver and can cause diabetes mellitus, hyperlipidemia, lypodystrophy, insulin resistance, rise in blood cholesterol. Atazanavir is devoid of these adverse effects.

ENTRY INHIBITORS

- **Enfuvirtide:** This syntheitc 36-amino acid peptide binds to GP_{41} subunits of viral envelop glycoprotein, producing conformational changes required for fusion of viral and host cell membrane. Given by SC route.
- **Maraviroc:** This is CCR5 coreceptor antagonist only effective in CCR5 tropic virus which predominates in early infection, given orally. Dose adjustment required, if given with delavirdine, ketoconazole or clarithromycin because it is a substrate for CYP3A4.
- **Raltegravir:** It is orally absorbed integrase inhibitor enzyme essential for viral replication of HIV-1 and HIV-2. New drug of this group is elvitegravir.
- **Dolutegravir:** Taken with or without food. Hypersensitivity, rash, aliver injury may occur.

Following antiretroviral may be recommended in pregnancy lamivudine, zidovudine, nevirapine, lopinavir, ritonavir, atazanavir.

- **Elvitegravir:** Used with cobicistat or ritonavir taken with food.

Following antiretroviral drugs may be recommended in pregnancy: lamivudine, zidovudine, nevirapine, lopinavir, ritonavir, atazanavir. Highly active antiretroviral therapy (HAART) is mentioned at last.

ANTIHEPATITIS AGENTS

For Hepatitis B

- **Lamivudine** 100 mg OD orally
- **Adefovir** 10 mg OD orally
- **Entecavir** 0.5 mg OD orally
- **Interferon alpha-2b** 5 million units OD IM or subcutaneously.
- **Telbivudine** 600 mg OD

Investigational level: Emtricitabine; Clevudine, Voltorcitabine, Pradefovir, Alamifovir.

Immunlogical modulator: Thymosin α_1.

For Hepatitis C

INF- used in multiple selerosis and INF - r for chronic granulomatous disease malignants melanoma.

- Pegylated interferon alpha-2a 180 mcg weekly SC with ribavirin.
- Pegylated interferon alpha-2b 1.5 mcg/kg weekly SC with ribavirin.
- Ribavirin 800–1200 mg OD orally.
- Paritaprevir
- Isatoribine
- Viramidine
- Monoclonal antibody against glycoprotein.

Investigational level

- **RNA polymerase inhibitor** of HCV, *viz.* valopicitabine, sifosbufir.
- **Protease inhibitor, *viz.* telaprevir**
- **Analogs of ribavirin**
- **Merimepodib**
- **Viramidine** (anti-aminophospholipid antibody)
- **Thymosin α_1** as immunomodulator.

ANTI-INFLUENZA AGENTS

Amantadine and its α-methyl derivative rimantidine block the M_2 proton ion channels of the virus particle and inhibit uncoating of viral RNA in host cell and prevent replication of virus. Effective in viral influenza only. Rimantidine causes less ADR due to dopaminergic neurotransmission than amantadine.

Amantadine is used in the dose of 100 mg BD. Used for prophylactic and treatment of influenza A and parkinsonism. Anorexia, nausea, insomnia may occur. It should not be used in CNS disease, epilepsy, gastric, wart and pregnancy.

Zanamivir and oseltamivir are neuroaminidase inhibitors, inhibit release of virus from infected host. Zanamivir is given by inhalation, but oseltamivir is given orally. It is a prodrug converted to active form by hepatic enzymes. Dose 75 mg BD × 5 days for treatment and 75 mg D for prevention. Zanamivir is anti-influenza A and B drugs, but oseltamivir is effective in swine and bird flu.

Newer drugs peramivir, laninamivir are neuraminidase inhibitor have action against influenza A and B virus.

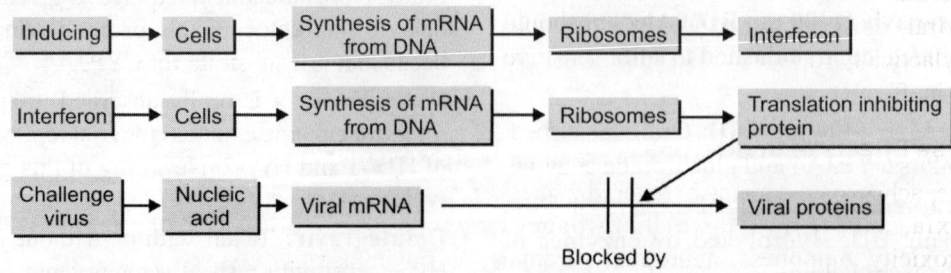

MISCELLANEOUS ANTIVIRAL AGENTS

Interferons (INF)

These are low molecular weight glycoprotein cytokines produced by vertebrate cells including sensitized lymphocytes. Both DNA and RNA viruses can produce to stimulate interferon, but differ in their inducing efficiency. Mol wt 30000 daltons, so readily released and diffused in extracellular space. They are three major classes of interferons α, β and γ. INF - α & β are acid stable whereas INF-γ is acid lable. INF α and β are more potent than INF- γ. INF α used for hairy cell leukemia, CML, malignant melanoma. Kaposis. Sarcoma, hepatititis B and C. Recombinant INF used clinically are non-glycosylated protein of MW 19500. INFα and β are produced by all cells in response to viral infection, cytokines (interleukin I; II; TNFα2). INFγ is produced by T lymphocyte and natural killer cells in resposne to antigenic stimuli mitogens and cytokines. INFα and β possess antiviral and antiproliferative actions. INFα possesses antiviral and immunoregulatory effects. INF inhibits most animal viruses, but DNA viruses are relatively insensitive. They have non-specific antiviral and complex effects on immunity and cell proliferation binds to specific cell surface receptors and affect viral replication at multiple steps, viz. penetration, synthesis of viral RNA and assembly of viruses.

It inhibits DNA and RNA viruses, but is host specific. Interferons α, β, γ are identified in human being and recently produced by recombinant DNA technology. Marketed in India as Reaferon powder.

Indicated for chronic hepatitis B and C, AIDS, hairy cell leukemia, *Condyloma acuminata* (papilloma virus), *H. simplex, H. zoster.* In rhinoviral, cold intranasal interferon is used prophylactically. It has to be given SC or IM. Orally ineffective.

Adverse Effects of Interferons

Fatigue, aches, pains, malaise, fever, dizziness, anorexia, visual and taste disturbances, neurotoxicity, numbness, neuropathy, tremor, convulsion, hypotension, transient arrhythmia, alopecia, liver dysfunctions, myelosuppression.

Nonviral Properties of Interferon

- Phagocytosis
- Antitumor activity of macrophages
- Production of lymphokines
- Cytotoxicity of cellular immunity
- Expression of cellular antigens

OTHER ANTIVIRAL AGENTS

Palivizumab: This human monoclonal antibody directed against epitope of A antigen site on the surface protein of RSV given to high-risk children (premature infants, congenital heart disease, *etc.*) reduces oxygen supplementation and recurrent hospitalization. URTI, fever, rhinitis, rash, diarrhea, vomiting, cough, otitis media, raised aminotransferase are potential adverse effects.

Imiquimod: This immune response modulator used for topical treatment of genital and perianal warts (*i.e.* human papilloma induced virus as 5% cream thrice weekly for 6–10 hours then it is washed off. Effective also for actinic keratosis and molluscum contagiosum. Adverse effects: Local pigmentary changes, fatigue and influenza like symptoms are systemic side effects.

Highly Active Anti-Retroviral Therapy (HAART) should be prescribed to all symptomtic patient or to asymptomtic patients where:

- CD_4 count is below 350 cells/mL.
- Viral load is more than 100,000/mL.
- With infectin of hepatitis B and C.
- Risk factors for non-AIDS related cancer.

Three anti-HIV drugs are prescribed. All regimens should have:

NRTI is back bone of HIV treatment used in pairs but didanosine and tenofovir is avoided for drug inter action.

- Lamivudine
- Two NRTIs + One NNRTI

The other NRTIs can be zidovudine or stavudine.

- One NNRTI can be chosen from nevirapine or efavirenz.
- Efavirenz is chosen in liver dysfunction patient, but not in pregnant lady.
- The three drugs should be from different groups: Some examples recommended by NACO.

     a. Lamivudine + Zidovudine + Nevirapine

     b. Lamivudine + Stavudine + Efavirenz

     c. Lamivudine + Tenofovir + Efavirenz

- Three NRTIs only for patient who are not able to tolerate efavirenz.

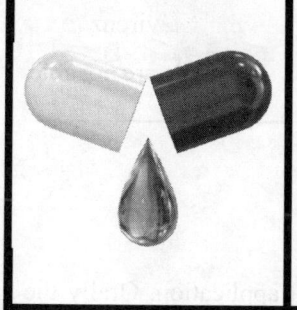
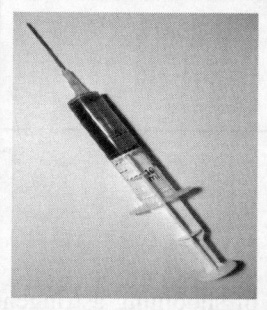
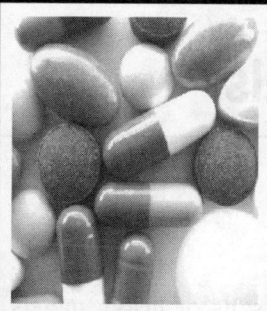
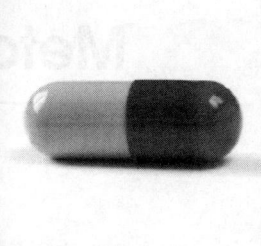

SECTION 14

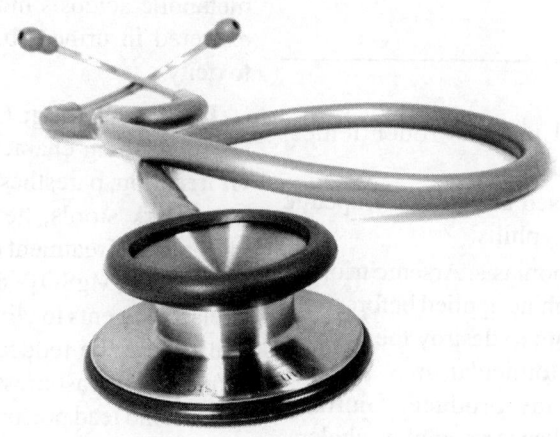

MISCELLANEOUS

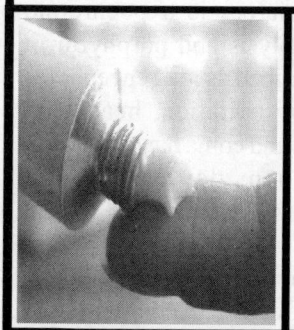
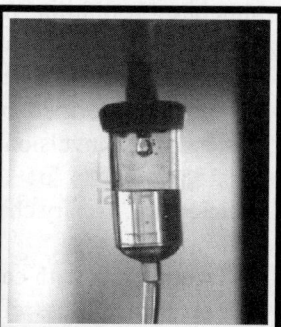
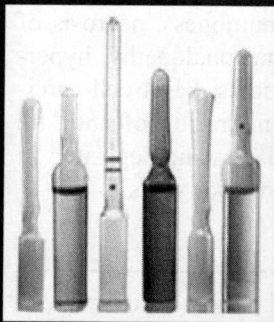
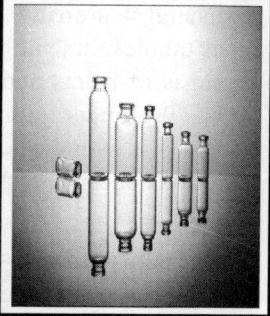

119

Metals

Organic and inorganic salts of heavy metals possess astringent, corrosive and caustic properties on local applications, protoplasmic poison, and lethal to gram-positive and gram-negative organisms called **oligodynamic action.** They are cumulative and potentially toxic.

ARSENIC (AS)

A Metaloid

- Inorganic arsenical used as rodenticides, herbicides, insecticides.
- Organic arsenic is used as chemotherapeutic in trypanosomiasis, syphilis.
- Amoebiasis, trichomoniasis. Arsenic trioxide with cocaine or morphine applied before to fill cavities of caries tooth to destroy the nerves.

Arsenic poisoning: Homicidal, may be accidental in children. May produce vomiting, diarrhea, circulatory collapse resembling cholera. Treatment aimed at correction of electrolyte imbalance, specific antidote (dimercaprol) and antibiotic. Chronic As poisoning causes loss of weight, anorexia, edema, hyperpigmentation of skins (eyelid, neck, nipple, axilla), dermatitis, hair loss, britle nail, jaundice, aplastic anemia, peripheral neuropathy, numbness, necrosis of renal tubules, arsenic encephalopathy, hyperkeratosis of palms and soles, basal cell carcinoma. Prolonged administration of antidote dimercaprol is indicated. Arsenic deposited in hairs and bones are retained for years.

LEAD

No therapeutic use, used only in industry. Lead subacetate is sometimes employed as constituent of shoothing astringent application. Orally the inorganic lead is absorbed, associated to RBC and deposited in the liver, kidney and subsequently deposited in bone in epiphysis.

High phosphate and vitamin D favor deposition, low PO_4, hypoparathyroidism, iodide and metabolic acidosis mobilize Pb from bone and excreted in urine. Pb in bone does not cause toxicity.

Lead poisoning: Generally, chronic. Acute lead poisoning characterized by metallic taste, GI irritation, paresthesia, muscle cramps, weakness, dark stools, hemolysis, anemia, hemoglobinuria. Treatment consists of gastric lavage. Purgatives ($MgSO_4$), calcium and PO_4 salts and chelating agents to eliminate it from circulation. Colitis may be reduced by antispasmodics, IV infusion and vasopressor to manage shock.

Chronic lead poisoning is due to sucking lead paints and toys, petroleum and printing industries. Symptomized by anorexia, constipations, abdominal pain and colics, lead line in gingivial margins, lead palsy due to degenerative change in motor neurons and impairment of high energy phosphate metabolism of affected muscle, punctate basophilia, microcytic hypochromic anemia, jaundice, hemolysis and porphyrin in urine, CNS effects described as lead encephalopathy characterized by irritation, headache, restlessness, convulsion and coma have mortality of 25% and ½ of them develop mental deficiencies, urinary changes are cast and protein in urine.

Treatment is with calcium disodium edetate. Dimercaprol is less effective. Antispasmodic, convulsion is treated by paraldehyde or diazepam. Intracranial tension treated by mannitol or by lumbar puncture.

ANTIMONY

Used as antimony potassium tartrate as emeties or IV of mycosis fungoides, filariasis, schistosomiasis, protozoal diseases. Toxicities are treated by dimercaprol, but its efficacy against inorganic antimony compound is doubtful.

Bismuth (Compounds used are carcanet subsalicylate, subnitrate, subgallate)

Bismuth subgallate is used to control fecal odour in patient of iliostomy. Bismuth is used for antidiarrheal, amoebiasis, peptic ulcer, lichen planus, local scleroderma, SLE, piles, condylomata acuminata. Intoxication rare, may lead to fever, urticaria, stomatitis, nephritis which can be treated with dimercaprol.

MERCURY

Salts are used as preservatives, antiseptics, spermicides and diuretics. Acute Hg poisoning is characterized by GI disturbances, electrolyte imbalance, arrhythmias. Treated by raw egg, and by medicated charcoal. Dimercaprol is effective antidote along with supportive treatment for shock. Chronic mercury poisoning is manifested with tremor, headache, stomatitis, colitis, electrolyte imbalance, treated symptomatically and with dimercaprol. Pink disease is systemic absorption of local mercury, present with swelling, erythema responds to acetyl penicillamine.

SILVER

Used as antiseptic. Applications may lead to argyria a bluish-black discoloration of skin disappears slowly.

CADMIUM

Used in manufacturing processses. Poisoning leads to GI irritation, shock. Inhalation of fumes cause cough, sore throat, vertigo, dyspnea, cyanosis, yellow pigmentation of teeth, emphysema. Calcium gluconate IV is treatment. 1% suspension of cadmium is used for seborrheic dermatitis. Do not give dimercaprol or EDTA as they may further damage kidney.

THALLIUM

Used for depilation, highly neurotoxic after systemic absorption. Treated with dimercaprol and dithiocarb.

120

Chelating Agents

Chelating agents form ring structures within their molecules and hold the metal like a crab's claw, generally used for heavy metal poisoning. The compounds produced with molecules are stable, non-toxic and easily excreted. Heavy metals exert toxic effect by combining with and inactivating the functional groups of the enzymes. Chelating agents compete with the heavy metals with varying affinity for different metals. They should have higher affinity for toxic metals than for Ca^{2+} and their distribution should correspond to the metal to be chelated.

Useful drugs for chelating agents

1. Dimercaprol or British anti-Lewisite (BAL)
2. Dimercaptosuccinic acid (succimer)
3. Disodium edetate
4. Calcium disodium edetate
5. Calcium disodium DTPA
6. Penicillamine
7. Trientine
8. Desferrioxamine
9. Deferiprone
10. Desferasirox
11. Prussian blue

British developed dimercaprol as antidote to arsenical poison in warfare against possible use of poisonous gas Lewisite. It is used by Soviet

Union, as aqueous solution for the same purpose. (BAL inj. 100 mg/2 mL in arachis oil): Two SH groups of dimercaprol bind to AS, Hg, Au, Bi, Ni, Sb and Cu. Dose 5 mg/kg stat followed by 2–3 mg/kg every 4–8 hours × 2 days. It protects the sulfhydryl containing enzymes. Urine should be made alkaline. It is used as adjuvant to calcium disodium edetate in lead poisoning and Cu poisoning in Wilson's disease. It is contraindicated to Fe and Cd poisoning because complex formed is toxic.

Adverse effects: BP may rise, tachycardia, sweating, tingling and burning, cramps, headache. In Wilson's disease dose is 300 mg IM × 10 days in every second month.

Succimer dimercaptosuccinic acid: Orally effective, less toxic with similar action used for As, Hg and Pb poisoning. May produce loose motion, vomiting, anorexia.

Disodium edetate: Given slow IV 50 mg/kg in 2–4 hours (to prevent tetany) in hypercalcemia but rarely because better drug (bisphosphanates) are available.

Calcium disodium edetate: Removes Pb, Zn, Cd, Mn, Cu and some radioactive elements. It is not absorbed orally, should be given parenterally, does not cross blood-brain barrier. Used for Pb poisoning, may be used for Fe, Zn, Cu and Mn radioactive metals, but not for Hg, because it is not accessible to Hg bound constituents in body. Renal tubular necrosis, fever, chill, bodyache, anaphylactoid reaction may occur (manifest as fall in BP and congestions in eyes and nose).

H H H
H—C—C—C—H + NaOAs=O→NaOAs
SH SH OH Sodium arsinate

S—CH₂
S—CH
HO—CH₂
Cyclic thioarsinate

Calcium disodium DTPA: Used to treat radioactive metals like uranium not responding to calcium disodium edetate.

D-penicillamine (Artamin 150; 250 mg cap): Selectively chelates Cu, Hg, Pb and Zn. l-isomer causes optic neuritis. Absorbed orally, slowly metabolized in body and excreted in feces and urine. Patient intolerant to penicillamine is given trientine captured agent. 2 gm for adult or 1.5 gm for children in 2–4 divided doses.

Penicillamine is used for
- Wilson's disease
- Cu and Hg poisoning
- Pb poisoning with $CaNa_2$ EDTA
- Cystinuria and cystine stone
- Scleroderma
- Rheumatoid arthritis.

Cutaneous reactions, itching, fever, long-term use may produce dermatological, hematological, collagen tissue renal toxicities.

Deferoxamine (Desferol 0.5 gm/vial): 1 gm. Chelates 85 mg of elemental iron. It removes loosely bound iron, and iron of hemosiderin and ferritin, but not iron of Hb. Used for iron poisoning, transfusion siderosis in thalassemia. Adverse reactions are histamine release (BP may fall, itching, urticaria), dysuria. It is isolated from *Streptomyces pilosus.*

Deferiprone (Kelfer 250, 500 mg cap; dose 50–100 mg/kg in 2–4 divided doses): Orally active, iron chelator, cheap and less adverse effects. Anorexia, vomiting, altered taste, joint pain, neutropenia, agranulocytosis may occur.

Deferasirox: Has high affinity for iron and low for Zn and Cu. Orally active used for iron overload due to transfusion, thalassemia, myelodysplastic syndrome.

Prussian blue: Used for radioactive cesium (Cs^{137}) and thalium toxicity. Used orally and diminishes gastrointestinal absorptions of those cations and hasten their elimination with feces.

Dithiocarb: Useful for nickel carbonyl, Wilson's disease and in thalium poisoning. IV 200 mg followed by oral dose of 2 gm daily × 7 days.

121

Vitamins and Antioxidants

(Vitamins K, B$_{12}$ and folic acid are dealt with hemopoietic system)

Vitamins are nonenergy producing, mostly exogenous, organic compounds required in small quantities for various metabolic functions of the body. They form important enzyme system catalyzing reactions for fat, carbohydrate and protein metabolism. Balanced diet does not require supplements, but deficiency may occur due to:

- Poor intake (poors not eating balanced diet)
- Inadequate absorption (diarrhea, obstructive jaundice, *etc.*)
- Interference with utilization (by drugs)
- In increased demands (pregnancy, lactations *etc.*)

Vitamins are overprescribed and overused with the myth they energize the body. They are classified into:

Fat-soluble vitamins: A, D, E and K. Cumulative, liable to cause toxicity.

Water-soluble vitamins (B complex and C): Excess is exerted, so less chance of toxicity.

FAT-SOLUBLE VITAMINS

Vitamin A (Retinol A1; Dihydroretinol A2): β-carotene is inactive *per se,* splits to produce 2 molecules of retinol. Retinyl palmitate hydrolyzed in the intestine, absorbed by carrier transport with the help of bile, circulates with chylomicron and stored in the liver. In biliary obstruction, its absorption is reduced.

Retinal obtained from oxidation of retinol is a component of *rhodopsin* (light-sensitive pigments) synthesized by rods during dark adoptation. Rhodopsin is bleached in dimlight to generate nerve impulse through G-protein called transductin. Retinal released is reutilized. Iodopsin produced in cone, responsible for bright light and color vision and dark adoptation. Vitamin A maintains intergrity of skin, promotes mucus secretion, prevents keratinization, retards malignant growth of skin and protects against infection.

Vitamin A deficiency is quite common. Manifested as in eye like xerosis, Bitot's spot, keratomalacia, nightblindness and in skin like phrynoderma, hyperkeratinization, atrophy of sweat glands (in others), respiratory tract infection, diarrhea, urinary stone formation, sterility, growth retardation. Daily requirement 5000 IU in adult and 3000 IU in children below 3 years.

Therapeutic uses: In infancy, pregnancy, lactation, steatorrhea, vitamin A deficiency, skin disease, acne, psoriasis, ithyosis, prevention of cancer. Transretinoic acid (tretinoin) used topically as comedolytic. It is also used to treat skin striae of Cushing's syndrome and acanthosis.

Regular use of liquid paraffin inteferes with its absorption.

Vitamin E promotes storage and utilization. Vitamin A toxicity is produced by intake of 100000 IU/day for a month producing nausea, vomiting, itching, erythema, exfoliative dermatitis, hair loss, bone and joint pain. Treatment is to stop vitamin A intake and supportive measure, and vitamin E.

Cellular retinoic acid binding protein (CRABP) is present in skin not in retina so it is not effective in visual cycle.

Preparation: Vitamin A tablet NF = 50000 IU, 1 tab OD or BD (Aquasol).

Vitamin A injection NF 100000 IU/mL, 1 mL weekly or biweekly.

Retinoic acid (Vitamin A acid): It has vitamin A activity on epthelial cells, but inactive on eye and reproductive organs. Transretinoic acid (tretinoin) is applied locally and 13-*cis*-retinoic acid (isotretinoin) is given orally for acne.

Retinoid receptors: Retinol and retinoic acid act through nuclear retinoid receptors like steroid receptor. Their activation results in modulation of protein synthesis in epithelial, gonadal and fibroblasts. Retinoid receptors till now identified are of two distinct families, *viz*. retinoic acid receptors (RARs) and retinoid X receptors (RXR) which have different affinities for different retinoids.

Vitamin E: Tocopherol, d-isomer more potent, prolong deprivation produces sterility in rats and abortion in female. May produce megaloblastic anemia, resistant to B_{12} and folic acid.

It is absorbed from intestine, circulates with β-lipoprotein, acts as antioxidant, protecting unsaturated lipids in cell membrane.

Therapeutic uses of vitamin E (mostly empirically)

- Glucose-6PO_4 deficiency increases survival time of RBC.
- Acanthicytosis
- Vitamin A toxicity
- Intermittent claudication
- Retrolental fibroplasia due to high concentration of oxygen
- Nocturnal muscle cramp
- Fibrocystic breast disease
- Sterility
- Toxemia of pregnancy
- IHD
- Cancer prevention
- Postherpetic neuralgia
- Scleroderma, degenerative lesions in skeletal muscle (depressed tendon reflex, position and vibration sense. Vitamin E acts as an anti-oxidant).

Large doses of vitamin E for long period rarely produce significant toxicity, but impairs wound healing, creatinuria, loose motion, pain in abdomen, lethargy can occur. It may interfere iron therapy.

WATER-SOLUBLE VITAMINS

B Complex

Thiamine (B_1) (Aneurine, B_1): Present in outer mesocarp layers of cereals, pulses, nuts, green vegetables, yeast, egg. Absorbed actively and in large dose by passive diffusion. Daily requirement 1–2 mg/day. Acts as a coenzyme (thiamine pyrophosphate) in carbohydrate metabolism. Hexose monophosphate shunts, decarboxylation of ketoacids, have some role in neuromuscular transmission. Pyrithiamine and oxythiamine and tea also contain thiamine antagonists. Deficiency manifests as dry beriberi with neurological symptoms and wet beriberi with cardiovascular symptoms.

Therapeutic uses

- Prophylactically (2–10 mg) in pregnancy, chronic diarrhea on parenteral alimentation
- Beriberi
- Chronic alcoholics
- Neuro- and cardiovascular disorders
- Hyperemesis gravidarium
- Obstinate constipation
- Parenteral administration may produce anaphylaxis otherwise it is non-toxic.

Riboflavin (B_2)

(Riboflavin tablet 2 mg, 1 to 2 tabs)

Riboflavin IP 10 mg/mL, daily requirement 1.5 to 3 mg FAD; FMN are coenzymes for oxidation–reduction reaction of carbohydrate and amino acid. Deficiency produces angular stomatitis, sore and raw tongue, lips, throat, ulcer mouth, dry skin, loss of hair, anemia. Natural sources are kidney, liver, meat, eggs, milk, yeast, green vegetables.

It is absorbed by intestine and phosphorylated.

Niacin (B₃)

Initially called pellagra preventing factor (PPF). Sources are cereals, pulses, liver, milk, egg, potato, vegetables, also synthesized from tryptophan. Daily requirement 15–20 mg. Maize eaters suffer pellagra because it contains B_3 antagonist. Readily absorbed from intestine and converted to NAD and NADP responsible in oxidation–reduction reactions, acting as hydrogen acceptor in electron transport chain in tissue respiration, glycolysis, fat synthesis. Nicotinic acid is vasodilator, deficiency produces pellagra (dermatitis, dementia, diarrhea).

Therapeutic uses: Pellagra, Hartnup's disease, carcinoid tumors, nicotinic acid in peripheral vascular disease and hyperlipoproteinemia.

Pyridoxine (B₆)

Pyridoxine, pyridoxal and pyridoxamine are natural pyridines obtained from yeast, cereals, legumes, milk, meat. All forms are absorbed from intestine, oxidized in body, little is stored and excreted as pyridoxic acid. Acts as coenzyme (pyridoxal phosphate) for amino acid decarboxylase and transaminase. Produces biological amines (catecholamine 5HT; GABA). Deficiency is generally associated with other vitamin B deficiency. Symptoms are seborrheic dermatitis, glossitis, growth retardation, convulsion, neuritis, anemia. INH therapy, oral pills, hydrallazine, cycloserine, penicillamine therapy intefere with pyridoxine utilization. 4-deoxypyridoxin is B_6 antagonist reduces efficacy of levodopa as antiparkinsonian drug.

Therapeutic uses: INH, cycloserine, hydrallazine, OCP, anemia (defective heme synthesis), convulsion in children and homocystinuria.

Pantothenic Acids

Converted into coenzyme A to produce physiological role in carbohydrate, fat steroid and porphyrin metabolism. Obtained from yeast, wheat, peanuts, cereals, livers. Normally, deficiency state not known. Absorbed from intestine. Used for streptomycin ototoxicity, postoperative paralytic ileus, rheumatoid arthritis, graying of hair. Dexpanthenol employed topically over burn wounds.

Biotin

Acts as coenzyme; normally deficiency states not encountered except by taking avidin present in raw egg. Deficiency produces seborrheic dermatitis, glossitis, muscular pain.

Ascorbic Acid (Vitamin C)

Sources are citrous fruits, tomato, green chillies, guava, human milk, cabbage, vegetable, amla. Absorbed from GIT, distributed extra- and intracellularly. It plays an important role in oxidative and other metabolic reactions, hydroxylation of proline and lysine residues of protocollagen, essential for formation of collagen helix, hydroxylation of carnitine, conversion of folic to folinic acid, biosynthesis of adrenal steroids, catecholamine, oxytocin, cyclic nucleotides and prostaglandin. Deficiency produces scurvy.

Therapeutic uses: Scurvy, postoperative patient to hasten healing, anemia, common cold, acid, urine and dental infections.

Folic acid and B₁₂ have been discussed with hematology.

Multivitamin combinations: Selective deficiency of a single vitamin is rare hence multivitamins are used prophylactically and indiscriminately to keep up the energy and strength and act as placebo are wasteful and harmful and costlier too which are washed with urine in drain.

The ICMR and WHO recommendations of various vitamins for adults.

Vitamin	ICMR	WHO
Thiamine	1.2–2.0 mg	1–1.5 mg
Riboflavin	1.3–2.2 mg	1.3–2.1 mg
Pyridoxine	–	1.5–2 mg
Niacin	16–32 mg	–
Vitamin B₁₂	1 µg	2 µg
Folate	100 mg	200 mg
Vitamin C	50 mg	30 mg
Vitamin A	750 µg	750 µg
Vitamin D	5 µg	2.5 µg

ANTIOXIDANTS

Oxidation is the removal of electrons; and is always coupled with reduction. Many oxidation occurs without molecular oxygen. Molecular oxygen has little capacity to oxidize other chemicals so it is first converted to active form called reactive species of oxygen, *i.e.* an oxidant. The free radicals are also produced during metabolism during process of phagocytosis and also from environmental pollutions, radiation, cigarette smoking and alcohol intake.

Free radical donates its unpaired electron to stabilizes itself. It is normally removed by antioxidant defense mechanism by several enzymes and non-enzymetics when it is given away body are in oxidation stress. A free radical has one or more unpaired electrons so has a tendency to acquire electrons from other substances. The reactive oxygen can damage most cell structure (*viz.* membrane lipid, protein, enzymes, nucleic acid) and the body has small mop-up mechanism to protect this damage.

Free radicals are involved in generation of cancer, diabetes, cardiovascular and neurological diseases. Consumption of cereals, pulses, fruits, vegetables are good source of antioxidants. Coenzyme Q10 (Ubiquinone) is fat-soluble antioxidant available as dietary supplements.

Some reactive oxygen species

O_2	Singlet oxygen
$O^{\bullet}$	Superoxide radical
$OH^{\bullet}$	Hydroxyl free radical
$RO^{\bullet}$	Alkoxyl free radical
$ROO^{\bullet}$	Peroxyl free radical
H_2O_2	Hydrogen peroxide
$LOOH$	Lipid peroxide

Oxidants produced in the body by

- Cyclooxygenation
- Lipoxygenation
- Lipid peroxidation
- Reperfusion of ischemic areas
- Neutrophils by microbes
- Xenobiotics in their metabolisms
- UV and ionization radiation

Free radicals in diseases

Free radicals involved in multiorgan diseases like rheumatoid arthritis, autoimmune diseases, alcohol toxicity carcinogenesis.

CNS	:	Parkinsonism, Alzheimer's diseases
CVS	:	Atherosclerosis and myocardial infarction.
Endocrine	:	Diabetes mellitus
GIT	:	Cirrhosis, pancreatitis
Eye	:	Cataract, retinopathy

Coenzyme Q10: This fat-soluble antioxidant sold as dietary supplement. Body also synthesize it. Its concentration declines with age. It generates ATP. Dose 100 mg/day. It is reported to benefit parkinsonism, CCF. Vomiting may occur and its use needs substantiation.

Pharmacological, *i.e.* exogenous auto-oxidants

Allopurinol xanthine oxidase inhibitor is an anti-gout and has antioxidant property to inhibit the process of superoxidation.

Selegline possesses free radical scavenging action.

Trace elements: Vitamin E, antioxidant properties are enhanced by selenium, zinc, copper and manganese which help in generating catalase, superoxide dismutase, glutathione peroxidase.

Some substances protecting body against oxidants

a. **Enzymes:** Catalases, superoxide dismutases, glutathione peroxydases.

b. **Antioxidants:** Coriander, clove, cardamom, vitamins A; C; E, selenium, flavonoids, fruits, amla, tea, garlic, carotinoids, melatonin, adenosine lactoferrin, nicotinamide, spirulina.

Agents augmenting endogenous antioxidants

N-acetylcysteine, ebselen, deferoxamine cerulo-plasmin.

Enzymes in Therapy

Enzymes are the biological catalysts which are protein in nature, to be given parenterally.

The enzymes may be simple protein or a complex enzyme with non-protein part called prosthetic group, here protein part of enzymes is called *apoenzyme* and prosthetic group is called *coenzyme*. The two portions collectively called *holoenzyme*.

Characteristics of enzymes

- They are proteins and follow the physical and chemical reactions of it.
- Water-soluble, but heat labile.
- Precipitated by protein precipitants like amonium sulfate or trichloroacetic acid.
- Contains 16% of nitrogen by weights.
- It ends with suffix of "ase" to the substrate, but earlier they are whimsically named like trypsin, chymotrypsin, *etc.*

May evoke allergic reactions. Pancreatin, diastase, pepsin and papain are used for certain gastrointestinal disturbances. (Fibrinolysin, thromboplastin, urokinase, streptokinase are used for thrombolytic therapy, asperginase as anti-cancer drug dealt in respective chapters).

Hyaluronidase (hyalase; roudase): Increases tissue permeability, administered subcutaneously, used to promote absorption of fluid and drugs, fluid in traumatic or postoperative edema or along with anesthetics. Contraindication in malignancy and should not be given around infection. May produce allergy.

Trypsin: Obtained from ox pancreas, active at pH 5–8, hydrolyzes natural proteins including respiratory mucin. Should be used with caution in renal and hepatic insufficiencies. 3–5 mg of enzyme/mL applied on small area every 15–30 minutes for wet dressing in every 3 hours, small gelatin capsules inserted in fistula, aerosol to liquefy excess bronchial secretion. Should not be given IV.

Chymotrypsin: Obtained from bovine pancreas, may be used as adjuvant to conventional treatment of traumatically induced inflammation either applied locally or given orally (usefulness doubtful). Tablets contain 50000 units of enzymes.

Alpha-chymotrypsin: Used to dissolve suspensary ligament of lens during cataract operation, called zonulolysis 0.2–0.5 mL, prepared freshly in 1 : 5000 solution. May produce transient glaucoma, wound disruption, retinal damage and loss of vision, if penetrates it.

Serratiopeptidase: It is a proteolytic enzyme, given orally, claimed to digest necrotic tissue, coagulated blood, promoted with NSAID group of drugs, the claiming is inadequately substantiated.

Collagenase: Obtained from *Cl. histolyticum* acts on denatured collagen, used for debridement of dermal ulcer or burns as local ointments.

Deoxyribonuclease: Recombinant human deoxyribonuclease is tried to reduce viscosity of sputum in cystic fibrosis given by inhalation as DNA released from neutrophils and fibrils produces viscous sputum in cystic fibrosis.

L-asparaginase: It is given parenterally. Used as antineoplastic drug (dealt with there).

Drugs Acting on Skin and Mucous Membrane

Skin is one of the major interfaces between body and environment, covers an area of 1.6–1.85 m² to a depth of 3–5 mm comprising 10% of body weight, equipped to deal with microbiological, chemical and physical assault. Important organ for sensory inputs and temperature regulation, consisting of two main layers, epidermis (with appendages, nails, hair, glands) and dermis.

Skin is unique for pharmacology because here target organ for diagnosis and treatment is directly accessible. It prevents absorption and loss of water and electrolytes. Drug molecule can penetrate skin by: (a) Intact stratum corneum, (b) sweat glands and (c) sebaceous follicles. Topical drugs with low molecular mass, easy water- and oil-soluble drugs and high partition coefficient mass easily penetrate skin. Water-soluble ions and polar molecules do not penetrate stratum corneum.

Drugs in the skin may be metabolized by CYPs, epoxide hydrolase and different transferases present in the viable epidermis.

Factors modifying drug absorption through skin

i. Altered barrier function in diseases, *viz.* psoriasis. Absorption of topical steroid may suppress hypothalamus, pituitary, adrenal axis.

ii. Hydration: Increases drug absorption (*viz.* occlusion with impermeable films, lipophillic occlusive vehicles like ointment, soaking skin before occlusion, *etc.*)

iii. Age: In children topical dose results greater systemic absorption.

iv. Intralesional drug used for inflammatory lesions, warts, keloids and neoplasm.

v. Frequency of applications: Stratum corneum acts as resorvoir.

Drugs acting on skin act primarily by virtue of their physical, chemical or mechanical actions.

Demulcents

Demulcents are high molecular weight substances applied as thick colloidal or viscous solution in water on denuded or inflamed skin produce foam with water, reduce surface tensions. Some demulcents are:

- **Gum acacia and gum:** Tragacanth used as emulsifying agent for oils and in lozenges.
- **Glycyrrhiza:** Obtained from liquorice root, used as lozenges, used to sooth throat and also to treat peptic ulcer.
- **Methyl cellulose:** Used as bulk purgative, nasal drops and contact lens solution. (Codilose 5% drops in 10 mL bottles).
- **Propylene glycol:** Used as cosmetics and dressing for ichthyosis.
- **Glycerine (50%):** Applied on dry skin, orally 50–75% or IV as 10% to reduce intraocular or intracranial tension.

Emollients

Applied on oily substances to restore elasticity in cracked dry skin like vegetable oils, petroleum products, *etc.*

Astringents

Precipitate protein without penetrating cells to decrease exudation from surface.

Drugs are

- **Tannic acid and tannins:** Used for bleeding gums (glycerine + tannic acid), bleeding piles (tannic acid suppository) and in alkaloidal poisoning.
- **Ethanol:** Used to treat bedsores and as aftershave. Methanol is also a good astringent.
- **Heavy metal:** Ions are astringent and antiseptic.
    Adsorbents: Adsorbs noxious, irritant substances and protects the skin or mucosa.
- **Dermal protectives are** magnesium stearate, zinc stearate, calamine, ZnO, starch, boric acid, bentonite.
- **Occlusive protectives:** Collodion, dimethicone.

Irritants and counterirritants

Irritants stimulate sensory nerve ending at the site of application, induce inflammation, produce cooling or warmth, pricking, tingling, hyperesthesia or numbness or vasodilation depending upon nature, or concentration. Irritant with effect of hyperemia and sensory component are **rubefacient.** Stronger irritants increase capillary permeability called **vesicants.** Certain irritants used to relieve pain and inflammation of deeper organs called **counterirritants** used to relieve headache, muscular, joint and pleural pains. Some counterirritants are:

> Volatile oils (turpentine, clove or eucalyptus oil), stearoptenes (camphor, thymol, menthol), mustard seeds, capsicum, canthridin, methylsalicylate, alcohol.

Caustics and escharotics are corrosive and cauterizer respectively used for local tissue destruction like removal of moles, warts, papilloma, condylomata. Some caustics are:

- **Podophyllium resin** (10–25% alcoholic solution or suspension in mineral oil)
- **Silver nitrate**
- **Phenol** 80% w/w solution
- **Trichloroacetic acid** (10–20%)
- **Glacial acetic acid** (undiluted)

Keratolytics

Dissolve intracellular horny layer substance of skin, used for corns, warts, psoriasis, dermatitis, athlete foot, ringworm. Some keratolytics are salicylic acid, resorcinol (used for seborrheic dermatitis, eczema, ringworm), benzoic acid, urea as 5–20%.

Antiseborrheics

Seborrheic dermatitis affects areas rich in sebaceous gland with erythematous scaly lesion. Yeast, *Pityrosporum ovale* has got some roles in its genesis. Drugs used are:
- **Selenium sulfide** (Selsun 2.5% suspension shampoo) helps as antikeratolytic, fungicidal. May produce hypersensitivity.
- **Zinc pyrithione** reduces epidermal turnover and inhibits *P. ovale* often combined to ketoconazole.
- **Corticosteroids** highly effective, but relapse rates are high. Prolong use can produce skin atrophy, purpurae.
- **Antifungals:** Ketoconazole orally or 2% cream gives good results (Nizral 2% ointment or clorimazole 1% solution)
- **Salicylic acid:** Keratolytic with some effects on seborrhea.
- **Sulfur, resorcinol, coaltar; ammoniated mercury** are also effective with minimal antiyeast action. But they are keratolytic and antiseptic.

Antibacterial agents used topically

- **Bacitracin and gramicidin:** These are peptide antibiotics may be combined with neomycin; polymyxin.
- **Mupirocin (pseudomic acid A):** Effective against most gram-positive aerobic bacteria including methicillin-resistant *Staph. aureus.*
- **Polymyxin B:** Prepared in solution or ointment.
- **Neomycin and gentamicin.**

Local antibacterials used for acne

- Clindamycin phosphate
- Erythromycin
- Metronidazole
- Sodium sulfacetamide (10%)

Topical antiviral agents

- Acyclovir
- Penciclovir
- Valacyclovir
- Famiciclovir

Topical antifungal agents

Discussed earlier

Immunomodulators used in skin diseases

- Imiquimod: For genital and perianal warts
- Tacrolimus and pimecrolimus: Macrolide immunosuppressant used for atopic dermatitis.

Sunscreens

The access of solar radiation to the skin may be blocked by 2–5% of an opaque material ointment like titanium oxide, ZnO, or talc magnesium silicate **called physical sunscreen also called sunshades.** Selective absorption of the ultraviolet wavelength is provided by para-aminobenzoic acid (paraminol 10%) which absorbs radiation in the 290–330 mm wavelength. Benzophenones, cinnamates, menthyl anthranilate block UVA. Sunscreens are used as adjunct to vitiligo therapy. Drug induced phototoxicity may prevent skin cancer. Lawsone has significant sunscreen properties. Sun protection factor (SPF) of a given sunscreen measures its effectiveness in absorbing erythrogenic UV light is measured by minimal erythema dose with or without sunscreen in a population which signifies its efficiency. Fair skin individual are advised 15 or above.

Melanizing agents

Increase sensitivity on solar radiation and promote repigmentation of vitiliginous skin. Psoralen (manadenn 10 mg tab, psorline 5 mg tab, 0.25% solution and ointment), methoxsalen (macsoralen 10 mg tab, 1% solution) and trioxsalen (neosoralen 5 mg tabs) are synthetic psoralens. Methoxsalen absorbed better. PUVA (psoralen ultraviolet A) produces significant results in psoriasis, lichen planus, urticaria pigmentosa, atropic dermatitis, cutaneous T cell lymphoma. May cause mottling, erythema, blistering, gastric irritation, nervousness, insomnia, aging of skin. Psoralen is obtained from fruit of *Ammi majus*.

Photochemotheraphy: Electromagnetic radiation classified in different regions based on photon energy. For dermatologists wavelength of 290–320 nm called UVB, wavelength of 320–340 nm called UVA2 and wavelength of 340–400 nm UVA1 and visible wavelength 400–800 nm are important for therapy. These patient should be monitored for concomitant use of other photosensitizing medications such as sulfonamide, thiazide, tetracyclines, NSAID; benzodiazepines.

Mechanism of actions: PUVA acts on 320–400 mm produces two photoreaction. Type I oxygen independent formation of mono- and difunctional adducts of DNA and Type II oxygen dependent, transferring energy to molecule O_2. This phototoxic reaction stimulate melanocyte, antiproliferative, antiinflammatory, immunosuppressive by some unknown mechanism. In psoriasis it decreases DNA dependent proliferation after adduct formation.

Other uses of PUVA are lichen planus, urticaria pigmentosa, atopic dermatitis, cutaneous T cell lymphoma.

PUVA may cause skin cancer, cataract and immunological damage.

Photopheresis: Extracorporeal photopheresis (ECP). After oral administration of methoxsalen, leukocytes are separated from whole blood and exposed to UVA and irradiated cells are returned to patient. Used to treat cutaneous T-cells lymphoma.

Photodynamic therapy: Used for nonmelanoma skin cancer and precancerous active keratosis. Here photosensitizing drugs and visible light, laser and non-laser lights are used for treatment. Agents used for photodynamic therapy are porphyrin and their precursors.

Demelanizing agents

Hydroquinone (melalite), monobenzone (benoquin 20%) or recently developed azelaic acid are used to lighten hyperpigmented patches on skin.

Drugs for acne vulgaris

Under stimulation of androgen, sebaceous

follicles of face and neck produce excessive sebum, and colonise bacteria and yeast (*Propionibacterium acnes, Staph. epidermidis, Pityrosporum ovale*). Bacterial lipase produces fatty acids, irritating follicular ducts causing retention of secretion, hyperkeratosis, comedone may rupture into dermis, causing inflammation and pus formation.

THERAPIES FOR ACNE VULGARIS

A. Systemic Therapy

- Antibiotics (tetracycline/monocycline, erythromycin)
- Estrogen (ethinylestradiol)
- Retinoids (isotretinoin 1 mg/kg daily): Embryopathic, so contraindicated in pregnancy. Etretinate (2nd generation retinoid) used to treat psoriasis; to prevent skin cancer, oral leukoplakia.
- It produces its effect on gene expression by activating two families of receptors, retinoic acid receptor (RAR) and retinoid X receptor (RXR).

B. Topical Therapy

- Benzoyl peroxide (persol 2.5% gel)
- Retinoic acid (transvitamin A 0.05% or retino A 0.025% cream; adapalene; 0.1 %; tazarotene 0.1% gel)
- Topical antibiotics (erythromycin, clindamycin, tetracycline; nadifloxacin)
- Keratolytics (sulfur, salicylic acid, resorcinol)
- Azelaic acid 20% cream
- Anhydrotics: $ZnSO_4$ and $AlCl_3$.

TOPICAL STEROIDS

Has antiinflammatory, immunosuppressive, vasoconstrictor and antiproliferative actions used in: Atopic eczema, contact dermatitis, lichen simplex, seborrheic and irritant dermatitises, psoriasis, varicose eczema. Potent steroid application heals cystic acne, alopecia areata, DLE, hypertrophied scar and keloids, psoriasis of palm, lichen planus (Table 123.1).

Adverse effects of topical steroids: Thinning of epidermis, atrophy, easy bruising, delayed wound healing, superinfection with fungus and bacteria.

Table 123.1: Topical steroids preparations		
Preparation available		
Mild	*Moderate*	*Potent*
Hydrocortisone acetate 0.1–1% (Lycortin)	Fluocinolone acetonide 0.01% (Flucort-H)	Beclomethasone dipropionate (Beclate)
Dexamethasone 0.01% (Eumosone)	Clobetasol butyrate 0.05%, 0.025% (Topicasone)	Betamethasone benzoate
Hydrocortisone butyrate 0.001% (Locoid)	Fluocortolone 0.25% (Colsipan)	Betamethasone valerate 0.12% (Betnovate)
	Hydrocortisone acetate 2.5 % (Wycort)	Halcinonide 0.1% (Cortilate)
		Clobetasol proprionate 0.05% (Lobate)
		Dexamethasone sodium PO_4 0.1%
		Fluocinolone acetonide 0.025% (Flucort)
		Triamcinolone acetonide 0.1% (Ladercort)
		Hydrocortisone butyrate (0.1%)

Table 123.2: Uses of different retinoids

Retinoid name	Uses	Remarks
Tretinoin	Acne; photodamaged skin	0.2, 0.25, 0.1% emollient cream is used
Adapalene	Anti-inflammatory	Stable in sunlight, less irritating
Tazarotene	Psoriasis, acne vulgaris	First FDA approved topical retinoid
Alitretinoin	Kaposi's sarcoma	–
Isotretinion	Nodulocystic, acne vulgaris	Used orally 0.5–2 mg/kg/in acnes

Retinoid (natural and synthetic) exhibits vitamin A activity. 1st generation (Retinel, Tretinoin, Isotretinoin, Alitretinoin), 2nd generation or aromatic retinoids (Acitretin) and 3rd generation or arotenoids (Tazarotene; bexarotene, adapalene). Acute retinoid toxicity is like vitamin A toxicity manifested as dry skin, nose bleeding, conjunctivitis, hair loss, pseudotumor cerebri, moodchanges; teratogenicity.

Other uses of retinoids are inflammatory skin disorders, photoaging, skin malignancies, to normalize skin keratinization, and to enhance penetration of other topical medication, cancer chemoprevention (used systematically and topically) isotretinoin 2 mg/kg/day prevents skin malignancy from xeroderma pigmentosa and nevoid basal cell carcinoma syndrome, cutaneous T cell lymphoma responds to topical and systemic retinoid, *viz.* Bexarotene.

TRICHOGENIC AND ANTITRICHOGENIC AGENTS

(a) **Minoxidil (used topically)**
(b) **Finasteride:** 5α-reductase inhibitor 1 mg/day for 3–6 months promotes hair growth and further loss in androgenic alopecia.

ADR: Erectile dysfunction, loss of libido, ejaculation disorder may occur.

Eflornithine: Irreversible inhibitor of ornithine decarboxylase catalyzing rate limiting step in the biosynthesis of polyamine which is required for cell division and differentiation, affects rate of hair growth, used topically to reduce facial hair growth. Folliculitis stinging, burning sensation may occur. Hair growth restarts after 8 weeks of discontinuation.

Topical Antipruritic Agents

- **Pramoxine hydrochloride** 1% cream. It is a topical anesthetic. Don't apply on eye.
- **Doxepin** 5% cream. H_1 and H_2 antagonists used QD for 8 days. Don't use with MAO-inhibitors.

DRUGS FOR PSORIASIS

- **Acitretin:** Oral dose 25–50 mg/day. Don't use in pregnant woman and patient should not donate blood for 3 years after drug is stopped.
- **Tazarotene:** Used once daily is not more than 20% of body surface.
- **Calcipotriol:** Synthetic vitamin D_3 derivative, used topically for plaque type psoriasis.
- **Biologic agents:** Like T cell modulator alefacept, efalizumab; TNF inhibitors etanercept, infliximab, adalimumab are also used for psoriasis.
- **Miscellaneous:** Folic acid antagonist methotrexate, immunosuppressant cyclosporin, mycophenolate mofatil are effective in psoriasis.

ECTOPARASITICIDES

Lice (Pediculus species); Mites (Sarcoptes)
Drugs used are:
- **Sulphur:** May produce odor so socially unacceptable, repeat application required. Pediculocide and scabicide.
- **Mesulphen (mitigal):** Used for pediculosis and scabies.
- **Benzyl benzoate 25 % (ascabiol):** Used for scabies and pediculosis.

- **Crotamiton (crotorex 10% cream)** is pediculocides, scabicide and antipruritic.
- **Gamma benzene hexachloride (lindane):** Used for pediculosis.
- **Dicophane (DDT):** 1–2% for scabies and pediculosis. It is basically insecticide for mosquitoes. Benzoscab is marked its combination with benzyl benzoate.
- **Tetrethyl thiuram monosulfide** (tetmosol) Scabicide.
- **Permethrin 5%:** Cream applied to pediculosis for 10 minutes and then washed off.
- **Malathoin 0.5%:** Lotion applied on dry hair and after 4–6 hours hairs are combed to remove the nits of lice.
- **Ivermectin:** This anthelminthic drug is effective in scabies and pediculosis. It is the only orally effective drug used for ectoparasite. Dose 0.2 mg/kg.

ANHIDROTICS

Anhidrotics are drugs used to control excess sweating (hyperhidrosis). These may be **systemic anidrotics**, viz. belladonna alkaloids, methantheline or **local anidrotics**, like aluminium chlorhydrate, formalin; glutaraldehyde, esters of hyoscine. Mild hyperhidrosis of feet can be managed by 1:10000 dilution foot bath of $KMnO_4$ or simple talcum powder.

Anhidrotics are deodorants by virtue of their action on sweat glands. Some drugs which retard bacterial decomposition of sweet gland, *viz.* chemical deodorant like sodium carbonate with 20% talc; Aluminum salts, antibacterial drugs like hexachloropane, tetra-chlorosalicylanitide, thiram.

Perfumes by masking odor acts as antidrotics but some of which may produce allergy, dermatitis, photosensitivity.

There is great demand for deodorants nowadays.

124

Antiseptics and Disinfectants

Scmmelweis (1818–1865) demonstrated the value of handwashing with antiseptic solution markedly reduce death rate from puerperal fever. Lister successfully reduced the number of wound infections by prophylactic application of an antiseptic (carbolic acid) to wounds.

Disinfectants or germicides destroy harmful microbes (not usually spores) with the object of preventing transmission of diseases. Disinfectants are suitable for application only to inanimate objects. An antiseptic destroys or inhibits growth of microorganism generally applicable to living tissues. A disinfectant in low concentration or dilution can act as an antiseptic. Detergent cleans surface by lowering surface tension. Sterilization is the process of destroying all life including spores. Disinfection is the killing of infective agents outside the body by direct exposure to chemicals or physical agents. It refers to the action of antiseptics as well as disinfectants.

Antiseptics/disinfectants should be: Stable, cheap, non-staining with agreeable odor, should be cidal, and should destroy spores, active against bacteria, fungi, viruses, protozoa, able to spread through organic films, folds, active in presence of blood, pus, exudates, excreta.

A disinfectant should not corrode or rust instruments and easily washable. Additionally, antiseptic should be:

- Rapid in action and exert prolong protection
- Non-irritants and should not delay healing
- Non-absorbable and produce minimum toxicity, if absorbed.
- Non-sensitizing
- Compatible to soaps and other detergents.

Mechanism of Action of Germicide

It varies and can be grouped into

- Oxidation of bacterial protoplasm
- Denaturing bacterial proteins and enzymes
- Detergent like action

Factors modifying activity of germicide

- Temperature and pH
- Period of contact with microorganism
- Nature of microbe involved
- Size of inoculum
- Presence of blood, pus, etc.

EVALUATION OF ANTISEPTICS AND DISINFECTANTS

Rideal-Walker coefficient: Ratio of minimun concentratrion of test drug required to kill a 24 hours culture of *B. typhosa* in 7.5 minutes at 37.5 °C to that of phenol under similar conditions.

Chick-Martin test: It is an extension of Rideal-Walker test where organic matter, such as suspension of yeast or sterile feces is added to the test medium. The test organism is *B. typhosa,* but a longer contact time is allowed.

Kelsey-Sykes test or capacity test: Four organisms *Ps. aeruginosa, P. vulgaris, E. coli* and *Staph. aureus* and three concentration of different disinfectants diluted with standard and hard water tested simultaneously.

The in-use test: The sample of liquid expressed from mops and other cleaning material in the hospitals are diluted and inoculated in bacterial media. The disinfectants fail the test when more than half of the samples show vigorous growth. The tests given above are of value in the disinfecting objects, but provide no information of possible toxicity or efficacy when in contact with living tissues.

Classification of antiseptics

- **Phenol derivatives:** Phenol, cresol, resorcinol, hexylresorcinol.
- **Oxidizing agents:** Hydrogen peroxide, potassium permanganate, benzoyl peroxide
- **Hallogens:** Iodine, iodophores, chlorine, chlorophores releasing HOCl.

- **Biguanide:** Chlorhexidine.
- **Quarternary ammonium:** Cetrimide, benzalkonium chloride, dequalinium chloride (as gum paint or lozenges)
- Soaps
- **Alcohol:** Ethanol, isopropanol
- **Aldehyde:** Formaldehyde, glutaraldehyde
- **Acid:** Boric and acetic acids
- **Metal salts:** Ammoniated Hg, phenyl, Hg (ic) nitrate, merbromin, silver nitrate, silver sulfadiazine, zinc sulfate, calamme and zinc oxide.
- **Dyes:** Gentian violet, brilliant green, acriflavine, proflavine
- **Furan derivative:** Nitrofurazone.

125

Vaccines and Sera

Host defences against infection may be local or systemic, non-specific or specific, humoral or cellular level.

Active Immunity

May be acquired in three ways:
- Following clinical infection (chickenpox, rubella, measles)
- Following subclinical or inapparent infection (polio, diphtheria)
- Following immunization with an antigen which may be a killed vaccine or a live attenuated vaccine or toxoids.

Advantages of active immunity: Active immunization takes time to develop, but is superior to passive immunity because:
- Duration of protection is long lasting.
- Severe reactions are rare.
- Protective efficacy is superior to passive almost 100%.
- It is cheaper.

Passive immunity can be induced in one body (human or animal) and transferred to another to induce protection against disease. It is readymade antibody induced by:
- Administration of an antibody containing preparation (immunoglobulin or antisera)
- Transfer of antibody across placenta or by human milk.
- Transfer of lymphocyte to induce cellular immunity is still at research level.

Vaccines and sera are biological products which reinforce immunological defence of the body against foreign agencies (mostly infecting organism or their toxins).

Vaccines: Provide active immunity, act as antigen to induce or produce antibodies. On corticosteroid therapy, AIDS and other immune deficiency states they are contraindicated.

Toxoids: They are produced by modified bacterial exotoxins, so that toxicity is lost, but antigenicity is retained. Active immunization may fail with corticosteroids or immunosuppressive therapy.

VACCINES

i. **Killed** (inactivated) contains microorganism killed by heat or chemicals.

ii. **Live attenuated vaccines:** Live bacterias or viruses made avirulent, which grow and multiply in the host body, but they may produce disease in impaired host defences like:
- Leukemia or other malignancies receiving cytotoxic drug.
- SLE
- On corticosteroid therapy, AIDS and other immune deficiency states they are contraindicated.

Difference between attenuated and killed vaccines

	Attenuated vaccine	Killed vaccine
Vaccine dose	Low	High
Antibody	Low	High
Persistence of immunity	Long	Short
Booster	Rearly	Frequently
	Required	Required
Oncogenicity	–	Rare

History of Vaccines

1798	Smallpox
1885	Rabies
1892	Cholera
1913	Diphtheria
1921	BCG
1923	Diphtheria toxoids
1923	Whooping cough
1927	Tetanus toxoids
1937	Influenza and yellow fever
1949	Mumps
1954	Salk polio
1957	Sabin polio
1960	Measles
1962	Rubella
1968	Type C meningococci
1971	Type A meningococci
1976	Hepatitis B

Childhood Immunization at birth

At birth	BCG	OPV	Hepatitis B
6 weeks	OPV	DPT	Hepatitis B
10 weeks	OPV	DPT	
14 weeks	OPV	DPT	
6–9 weeks			Hepatitis B + OPV
9 months			Measles
1–18 months			MMR
5 years			MMR, OPV, DPT (Booster)
10 years	Tetanus	Toxoid	
15–16 years	Tetanus	Toxoid	

Pregnant mother

16–24 weeks, 1st and 2nd doses tetanus toxoid

24–34 weeks, 3rd dose tetanus toxoid

Optional vaccines

Hemophillus	2–6 months 3 doses on 1–2 months booster at 2 years
Influenza	2–4 years
Typhoid	2 years of age

Newer vaccines

Chickenpox	13 years	1 dose at 4–6 weeks
Hepatitis A	2 doses	at 6 months 4–6 weeks interval
Rubella	one dose	for all adolescent girls

Do and Do not Immunization

Do

- Vaccine the children as per immunization
- Maintain vaccine in cold chain
- Keep water bottle in fridge so as to maintain cold chain in power failure.
- Keep different vaccines in different shelves.
- Maintain records of vaccine given.

Do not

- Do not give BCG and measles together.
- Do not postpone vaccination for minor ailments like fever, diarrhea, *etc.*
- Do not mix two vaccines.
- Do not give DPT to child with neurological disorders.

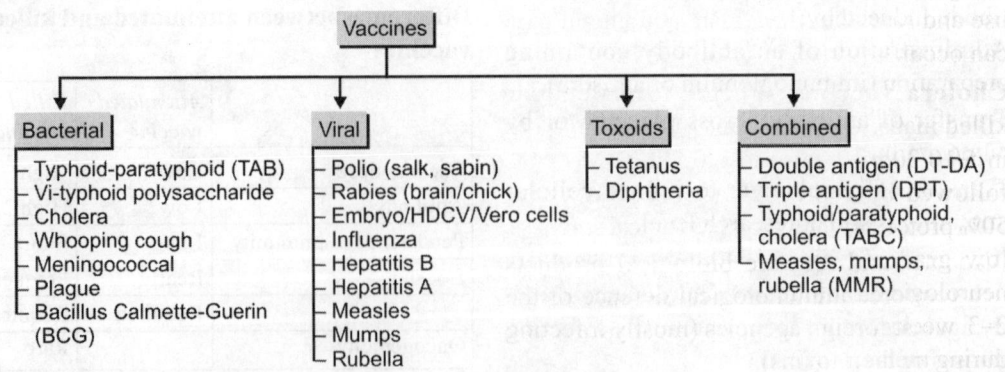

Vaccines

Bacterial
- Typhoid-paratyphoid (TAB)
- Vi-typhoid polysaccharide
- Cholera
- Whooping cough
- Meningococcal
- Plague
- Bacillus Calmette-Guerin (BCG)

Viral
- Polio (salk, sabin)
- Rabies (brain/chick)
- Embryo/HDCV/Vero cells
- Influenza
- Hepatitis B
- Hepatitis A
- Measles
- Mumps
- Rubella

Toxoids
- Tetanus
- Diphtheria

Combined
- Double antigen (DT-DA)
- Triple antigen (DPT)
- Typhoid/paratyphoid, cholera (TABC)
- Measles, mumps, rubella (MMR)

- Do not vaccinate with live vaccines (OPV/ measles/BCG) when patient on immuno-suppressants.
- Do not use reconstituted BCG after 3 hours.
- Do not use reconstituted measle after 6 hours.
- Do not use contaminated, unsterilized needle for vaccination purpose.
- Do not vaccinate with tetanus toxoid frequently, if child is following an immunization schedule.

Bacterial Vaccines

- **Typhoid-paratyphoid A, B (TAB):** 1 mL of suspension contains 1×10^9 S. typhi and 7.5×10^8 each of S. paratyphi A and B in 5 and 10 mL vials, 0.5 mL SC at 2–4 weeks interval is the dose, gives 70% protection in enteric fever. Booster dose every 2–3 years. Fever, tenderness, malaise can occur with first dose for lasting 1–2 days.
- **VI typhoid polysaccharide vaccines (vactyph/typhivax 0.025 mg in 0.5 mL):** Dose 0.5 mL IM or SC). Give 72% protection for 18 months induces longer immunity, with less systemic side effects, but no immunity for paratyphoid A and B. Not recommended for children below 2 years and pregnant women. It contains purified Vi capsular antigen of S. typhi.
- **Typhoid Ty 21a oral vaccines (Typhoral 3 doses):** Prepared from Ty 21a attenuated strain of S.typhi. Produce high cell mediated and humoral antibody. Administered as 3 capsules on alternate days (3 doses) protects for 3 years and gives 70–90% protection. Convenient to use and safe. Diarrhea, rash, abdominal pain can occur.
- **Cholera vaccines:** Phenol/formaldehyde killed inaba; Ogawa strains of Vibrio cholera in 5/10/30 mL vials, dose 0.5 mL IM or SC followed by 1 mL, IM after 4 weeks give 50% protection for 6 months. Topical soreness, low grade fever and aches, occasionally neurological complications may occur. It takes 2–3 weeks to produce immunity so useless during melas.

Oral cholera vaccine (whole cell killed recombinant B-subunits WC/rBS and live CVD 103 HgR are highly immunogenic, safer, protects for 3 years are available in Europe.

- **Typhoid-paratyphoid A, B; cholera (TABC):** Combination of TAB and cholera vaccine available in 5–10 mL vial.
- **Whooping cough (Pertussis):** It is killed vaccine. Dose 0.25–0.5 mL IM or SC thrice at 4 weeks intervals in children below 5 years. Local pain, systemic reaction, high fever, shock, convulsion, focal neurodeficit, altered consciousness, decreased β-adrenergic reactivity can occur. It is a component of triple antigen, so rarely used as such. Adverse reactions are contraindication for next dose. It contains 2×10^{10} B. pertusis organism/mL.
- **Meningococcal A and C vaccines (Meningococcal A and C/Mencevax A and C 0.5 mL amp):** 0.5 mL IM or SC, one dose indicated for prophylaxis of meningitis during epidemic. Contains N. meningitidis A and C 50 μg each per unit in single dose and 10 dose vial.
- **Antiplague vaccine:** Plague bacteria killed in formaldehyde 1 ml IM twice, 2–4 weeks apart. Immunity lasts for 6–8 months, sufficient to cover epidemic. Local and systemic complications are frequent. Contains 2×10^9 Y. pestis organism per ml.
- **Bacillus Calmette-Guerin (BCG):** Developed by Calmette and Guerin (attenuated bovine M. tubercle bacteria). 0.05 mL for neonate and 0.1 mL for older children are injected intracutaneously in left deltoid. A red painless papule appears on 7–10 days above 8 mm diameter with swelling of axillary lymph nodes which dries at 3 months and heals by six months. The protection is unpredictable since it increases body immunity nonspecifically. Used as adjuvant in immunotherapy. Contraindicated with compromised host defence, HIV, pregnancy, Mantoux test positive individual.
- **Typhus vaccines:** Sterile suspension of epidemic and murine, typhus grown in chick embryo in dose of 0.25–1 mL at 7–10 days

interval and booster at yearly may be used as prophylactically to louse-borne, flea-borne typhus.

- **Hemophilus influenzae type B (Hib):** Contains oligosaccharide of *H. influenzae B* (10 μg) conjugated with nontoxic protein 25 μg of CRM_{197} mutant *C. diphtheriae* with alum hydroxide as adjuvant. Dose 0.5 mL IM in 2–6 months of infants for 3 doses; 7–11 months infants, 2 doses or 1 dose for children above 1 year. It protects against *H. influenzae,* meningitis and pneumonia.

Viral Vaccines

Poliomyelitis type 1, 2, 3 viruses are grown in monkey's kidney cells culture for preparation of vaccines.

a. **Oral sabin vaccines** 0.05 mL or 2 drops is directly dropped in mouth. Viruses multiply in intestine to produce active immunity without disease in 0, 6, 10, 14 weeks booster doses at 15–18 months and at school entry. Easy to administer. Simultaneous use below 5 years (pulse polio) has eradicated the wild virus in many countries. This program is going on in India and India is declared as polio-free country.

b. **Inactivated poliomyelitis vaccine** (salk type) preferred for:
   1. Primary immunization in adults because they are prone to vaccine-associated paralysis.
   2. Immunocompromised patient. Three doses of 1 mL in deltoid SC are given at 4–6 weeks interval. Fever, local pain, allergic reaction may occur.
   3. Influenza virus vaccine (inactivated influenza viruses A and B): Two injections of 0.5–1 mL IM, 1–2 months interval are given. Its efficacy is inconsistent because of frequent change of virus antigenicity.

- **Hepatitis B vaccine (Engerix B):** 20 μg/mL virus antigen given IM at 1–6 months, protection offered 99%. Children below 10 years given ½ mL. Especially indicated for blood bank, working surgeon, dentist, health personal, hemodialysis patient, hemophiliac, drug addicts, laboratory technicians should get it. Adverse effects are rare like fever malaise.

- **Mumps virus vaccine:** Cultured in chick embryo, offers protection for 10 years. Post-exposure vaccination may produce clinical disease. This live vaccine is contraindicated in immunodeficient patient. It is live attenuated vaccine. Single dose contains $5000\,TCID_{50}$ (tissue culture infections dose 50%).

- **Measles vaccine live attenuated (rouvax; rimevax):** These are chick embryo cultured. Produces fever, coryza. Immunity lasts for 8 years. Given to children of 9 months of age. Malnourished, chronically ill or tuberculosis patient should be protected to minimize serious complications of measles. It should be given with caution to febrile convulsion and epilepsy patient.

- **Rubella (R-vac):** 0.5 mL deep IM or SC to girls of 1 year to puberty to protect German measles. Contraindicated in pregnancy, febrile illness and untreated TB and female should not conceive for 2 months. Mild fever, rash, cervical and occipital lymph node may enlarge. It is generally given with MMR vaccine. It is live attenuated virus.

- **Smallpox vaccine:** Kept below freezing point, retains its potency for 6 months, and if kept in 0–5 °C, potency is kept for a month. Immunity covers for 5–7 years, but in endemic countries given every 4 years. International certificate is valid for 3 years. Freeze dried vaccine is stable for month at 37–40 °C 0.6 mL inoculated intradermally by scarification. Pregnancy has no contraindication.

- **Measles, mumps, rubella (trimovax):** 0.5 mL given SC. Contraindicated in pregnancy and patient should not conceive within 2 months.

- **Varicella vaccine:** Lyophilized, live attenuated OKa strain of varicella zoster virus grown in human diploid cell culture, which contains $10^{3.3}$ plaque-forming units (PFU) of virus. Dose 0.5 mL SC. Children 1–12 years, 2 doses at 6–10 weeks gap, protects for 10 years.

- **Rabies:** four vaccines are available:
  a. **Antirabic vaccine** carbolized 5% suspension of brain substance containing carbolic acid fixed rabies virus given for post-dogbite patient 2–5 mL in anterior abdominal wall for 14 days. Neuroparalytic complications and encephalitis may occur. Does not give full protection. It is also called neural tissue vaccine (NTV) (simple vaccine).

  b. **Purified chick embryo cell (PCEC) (rabipur):** Virus grown in chick fibroblast inactivated by β-propiolactone. Post-exposure regimen 6 doses of 1 mL given in 0, 3, 14, 30, 90 days. Primary prophylaxis with three doses with booster in one year. Neuroparalytic lesion rare.

  Adverse reactions like local pain, erythema, swelling, and lymph node enlargements may occur.

  c. **Human diploid cell vaccine (HDCV):** Lyophilized inactivated rabies virus grown in human diploid cell culture, prepared with 1 mL of diluent given deep SC in deltoid region. 3 injections given one week apart and booster after 1 year and for veterinary persons every three years. Postexposure course in 0.3, 7, 14, 30, 90 days. Fever joint pain may occur.

  d. **Purified verocell rabies vaccine (PVRV):** Contains inactivated wistar rabies PM/WI 38 1503-3M strain grown in vero continous cell lines, used for pre- and post-exposure immunizaion. Preexposure primary vaccine is done for animal handlers those at risk of animalbite.

TOXOID

- **Tetanus toxoids:** These are formalin treated exotoxin of tetanus bacilli, used routiely, may be fluid or adsorbed. Dose 0.5 mL IM or SC. Fever, local pain and induration may occur. Chloramphenicol administration may interfere with antibody formation, if used simultaneously.

- **Diphtheria toxoids adsorbed:** Modified diphtheria exotoxin adsorbed in aluminum hydroxide, indicated for children below 6 years.

  Mixed antigen

  Double antigen DT-DA

  Diphtheria and tetanus.

  Dose 0.5 mL IM

  Triple antigen (DPT)

  Diphtheria, pertussis; tetanus 0.5 mL IM 4–8 months apart at 3 to 9 months and 18 months of age.

ANTISERA AND IMMUNOGLOBULINS

Normal human γ globulins are concentrated IgG obtained from pooled human plasma used for hepatitis A and B, measles, mumps, poliomyelitis, burn, agammaglobulinemia used IV.

Anti-D globulin (rhiggal) 250–350 μg IM in postpartum or postabortion to Rh-negative mother or inadvertantly administered Rh-positive blood to Rh-negative patients.

Tetanus

a. **Tetanus immunoglobulin (Human) (sii TIG 250 IU):** Prophylactic dose 250–500 IU and therapeutic dose 3000–6000 IU IM.

b. **Tetanus antitoxin (ATS):** Tetanus antitoxin 750 IU, 1500 IU. 50000 IU, 100000 IU IV and rest IM therapeutic. Prophylactic dose 1500–3000 IU; IM or SC. It is inferior to human antitoxin and is prepared from horse.

TYPES OF RABIES ANTISERUM

- **Antirabies serum (ARS):** Obtained from hyperimmunized horse. Dose 40 IU/kg IM and around wound.
- **Human rabies immunoglobulin** (HRIG). Dose 20 IU/kg.

Other Immunoglobulins

- **Hepatitis B immunoglobulin (Hepaglob 100 IU 0.5 mL vial):** 10–18% solution of Human 1 G containing antibodies to hepatitis B given to Hbs Ag positive patient. Dose 1000–2000 IU IM for adult and 32–48 IU/kg for children.

- **Diphtheria antitoxin (ADS):** Dose 20000–40000 IU IM or IV administered to clinical diphtheria patient. It neutralizes exotoxin on the site of infection and circulating in blood, but not which is fixed to the tissues.

- **Gas gangrene antitoxin (AGS):** Prophylactic dose 10000 IU; therapeutic 30000–75000 IU SC/IM/IV prepared from refined equine antitoxin against *Cl. oedematiens, Cl. perfrigens, Cl. septicum.*

- **Anti-snake venum polyvalent:** Dose 20 mL IV and repeated every 1–6 hours till symptoms disappear. Allergy, serum sickness may appear.

Prepared from equine globulin in lyophilized vials with 10 mL. Each 1 mL neutralizes 0–6 mg of cobra; 0.6 mg of russel; 0.45 mg of krait and 0.45 mg of sawscaled viper venum.

Adverse reactions to antisera and immunoglobulin immediate: Urticaria, angioedema, respiratory distress, anaphylaxis (adrenaline should be kept at hand). It is used after skin scratch negative test. Serum sickness, fever, rash, joint pain, lymphadenopathy may occur after 7–12 days or after larger doses or repeated administration.

126

Radioactive Isotopes

The smallest part of an element is called atom, which is made up of a central core called nucleus, surrounded by clouds of electrons, move around nucleus in a defined orbit. The electrons are negatively charged while nucleus is positively charged, which makes an atom electroneutral. The radioactivity is associated with closely packed particles called protons and neutrons. **Atomic number** is the number of protons in the nucleus.

Isotopes are the elements having same atomic numbers (protons) with different mass numbers, *i.e.* varying neutrons. Unstable isotopes are atoms which can give out radiation. They are chemically and metabolically same as stable elements in periodic table, with added power to give radiation can be used to destroy tissues or detected in tissues.

Isobars are atoms having same mass numbers but with different atomic numbers, *e.g.* ^{14}C and ^{14}N. The ratio of neutron to proton in nucleus varies due to variation of number of neutrons. An unstable nucleus has excess of energy and it undergoes spontaneous transformation of the number of protons or neutrons or their arrangements to get stability and excess of energy is liberated in the form of **radioactivity.**

Radioactivity Decay

- **Alpha radiation:** Release of alpha particle (2p + 2n) reduces the atomic number by 2 and mass number by 4.
- **Beta radiation:** Splitting of neutron generates one electron (p particle), one proton and one neutrino neutron.
- **Gamma radiation:** It has no mass or charges. It is in the form of electromagnetic waves.

Half-life of Radioactivity

It is the time taken for radioactive isotope to become half of its original activity.

Five types of transformation take place in nucleus:

1. **α-rays:** Like helium nucleus consists of two protons and neutrons are positively charged.
2. **β-rays:** Negatively charged particles with negligible mass.
3. **γ-rays:** Electromagnetic waves produced by isotopes. Electrically neutral.
4. **Electron capture:** Protons capture an electron from innermost orbit to become neutron and atomic number reduced by one. Emits X-ray.
5. **Isometric transition:** There is emission of γ-ray with reduction in energy level.

Some Units of Radioactivity

Curie (Ci): One curie is 3.7×10^{10} disintegration per second (dps) used for radioactivity of the source. One Becqueral (Bq) = 1 dps.

Rontgen (R): It means exposure dose. 1 R gives rise 2×10^9 ion pairs per cc of air.

Rad is absorbed dose by tissue. 1 Rad = 1.5×10^{12} ion pairs per gram of tissue.

REM is rontgen equivalent in man, *i.e.* biological effect of radiaton is expressed in REM.

Properties of radioisotopes

- Penetrability
- Radioactive decay
- Photographic effect
- Calorigenic effects
- Chemical effect

- Photoelectric effect used for fluoroscopy and γ-ray counting by scintillation counter.

Uses of radioisotopes in medicine

1. **Hematology:** Measurement of blood volume with ^{51}chromium Iron absorption, erythropoiesis and iron kinetics by ^{59}Fe.

Or

Absorption studies of vitamin B_{12} by ^{57}Co folic and ^{3}H in folic acid.

2. **Chemical pathology:**
   - ^{42}KCl and ^{24}NaCl for Na, K and water metabolism.
   - Fat absorption by ^{131}I triolein and oleic acid. ^{47}Ca for calcium kinetics.

3. **CVS:**
   - ^{85}Krypton for pulmonary, and cerebral blood flow.
   - Cardiac output by RIHSA^{131}I human serum albumins.

Thyroid: ^{131}I and $-^{132}$I for uptake and localization of thyroid tissue.

Urinary system: Renal studies using ^{131}I sodium Iodohippurate and kidney localization by ^{203}Hg label chlormerodrin.

Tissue scanning: ^{131}I and ^{99}Tc for thyroid; ^{113}Indium for liver, lung, brain, kidney, bone marrow; ^{99}Tc for liver, brain, spleen; selenomethionine ^{75}Se for parathyroid. Bone scanning by strontium ^{90}Sr.

For assay procedures: Drugs and biologic substances by RIA.

For therapy

- ^{131}I for thyrotoxicosis and thyroid carcinoma
- ^{192}Au and ^{60}Co for treatment of malignancies and secondaries.
- ^{32}P for polycythemia rubra vera.
- ^{90}Yttrium for hypophyseal malignancies.
- ^{182}Tantalum for bladder carcinoma.

It may be used from

Unsealed source: Here radioactive substance is kept in liquid form. Beta ray is the main source of radiation, *viz.* ^{131}I used for thyroid cancer secondaries or ^{32}P used for polycythemia vera.

Sealed source uses gamma radiation, *viz.* radium needle or caesium (^{137}Cs) are preferred as brachytherapy.

Teletherapy (Tele = distant): Here radiation source is away from the patients.

Biological Effects of Radiation

Acute radiation exposure produces nausea, vomiting prostration. On skin (epilation; dermatitis) chronic exposure causes atropy, fibrosis, loss of elasticity, *etc.* On blood: Leukopenia, thrombocytopenia.

Delayed effects are

- Ageing
- Induces neoplasm
- Sterility
- Chromosomal damage

Radioprotectives: *In vivo, viz.* cyanide, catecholamine, para-aminopropiophenon by producing hypoxia.

In vivo and *in vitro*: Cystamine, mercaptoethylamine, cysteine contain in sulfydryl group and very toxic.

Chelating agents like EDTA removes radio elements. Zirconium citrate minimizes tissue deposition.

Beta radiation can be cut out by thick glass or perspex or lead apron, partially used for personal monitoring devices like film bandages containing sensitive plates recording effects of radiations can give some ideas of exposed radiation. Periodic blood count should be done to radiation exposed person to detect abnormal blood picture.

Maximal Permissible Dose

Human beings are always exposed to some amount of background radiation 150 mrem/year from cosmic ray and terrestrial environment. The cosmic rays are higher at higher altitude or in coastal areas. Diagnostic X-ray exposure causes 75 millirem. Maximum permissible dose of radiation for radiation workers (doctors/technician) is 5 mrem/year and for general population 0.5 mrem/year.

127

Immunopharmacology

Immunology deals with self and non self discrimination may be as **Innate** or natural b, **Adaptive** or acquired. Innate is non specific but adaptive is specific against invading pathogens by creation of specific memory cells. The adaptive immunity may be humoral involving B lymphocyte or cellular involving T-lymphocyte. If immune system reacts with self component it becomes auto-immune disease. Therefore it may be compared with double edged showed. All cells exerting immune response either innate or adaptive reside in bone marrow and liver.

The mature lymphocyte and natural killer cells NK cells (A component of innate immunity) are produced from lymphoid stem cells. T and B lymphocyte are produced from mature lymphocyte which exert adaptive immune response. B-lymphocyte on exposure to specific antigen differentiate into plasma cells producing antibody and T cells influenced by thymic hormone migrate to thymus and by stimulus from antigen presenting cells (APC) differentiate into helper T cells (TH cells) and cytotoxic T cells (CTL) which have got specific protein cluster of CD_4^+ and CD_8^+ respectively. Helper T cells outside thymus differentiate in TH_1; TH_2; TH_3 etc. to produce different cytokines viz TH_1 produce interleukin IL-2; interferon and TH_2 produce IL 4;5, etc. Innate immunity cells are neutrophil, basophil, eosinophil, mast cells, macrophages, dendritic cells, natural killer cells.

Adaptive immune response comprises of cell mediated immunity (CM1) and antibody mediated immunity (AMI). CMI is responsible for intracellular pathogens (virus, parasite, fungi), tissue transplant, cancer cells.

Major histocompatibility complex (MHC) also called human leukocyte antigen (HLA) are located in plasma membrane of most body cells helps T cells to recognise foreign cells. MHC-1 are located in nucleated cells. MHC-II are expressed by professional antigen presenting cells like dendritic cells or macrophage.

MHC-1 proteins are presented to surface T cell receptor (TCR). TCD8 cells recognize class-I MHC-1, while TCD4 recognize MHC-II. T-cells activation requires two signals. In absence of second signal it becomes anergic, *i.e.* without response. The first signal to T-Cell receptor is peptide bound MHC molecule and second signal is CD40, CD80, CD86, *i.e.* T-lymphocyte associated antigen-4 is negative feedback. There are two subsets of T-helper cells. TH-1, TH-2. TH-1 produce interferon and IL-2, to produce cell mediated immunity whereas TH-2 produce IL-4, IL-5, IL-6 stimulate B-cells to produce antibody producing plasma cells.

CYTOKINES

These are heterogenous group of proteins with diverse functions like immunomodulation and control of hematopoiesis, *viz.* erythropoietin, thrombopoietin interferons interleukin, etc. which are numbered according to their discovery of cytokines. Interferons are interferon-α, interferon-β and interferon-γ. Interferon-α and β are acid stable whereas interferon-γ is acid labile. Interferon γ enhances immunity.

Some cytokin inhibitors:

- **Anakinra:** Used for rheumatoid arthritis.
- **Rilonacept:** Used for gout. Both are IL-1 inhibitor.

Unwanted immune response:

- **Type-I** Prior sensitisation has resulted this immune response stimulated by CD4 + TH$_2$ cells mediates by IgE. It is also known as anaphylactic reaciton.
- **Type-II** reactions are also called cytotoxic reaction, complement dependent reaction, *viz.* agranulocytosis by drug.
- **Type-III** are also called complex mediated

hypersensitivity when antobody reacts with soluble antigen *viz* Arthus reaction.

- **Type-IV** hypersensitivity or delayed hyper-sensitivity or cell mediated immunity. It is important in skin reactions to drugs and chemicals.

The drugs have been tried to suppress the (cellular or humoral) immunity (immunosuppressants) or stimulate the immunity (immuno-stimulants) which have widespread clinical applications.

The immune manipulation is used to treat autoimmune diseases or organ transplantation, infections and cardiovascular diseases.

Site of action different immuno suppresants   (Cyclosporin; Tacrolimus; sirolimus)

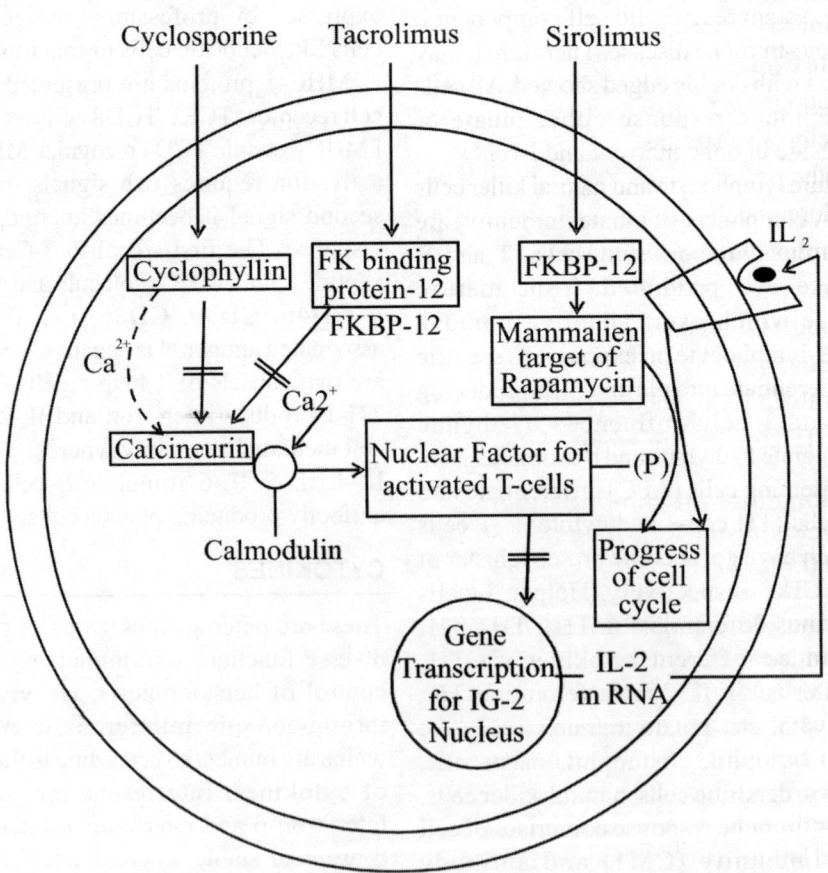

Fig. 127.1: Mechanisms of action of cyclosporine and tacrolimus

Table 127.1: Monoclonal antibodies

Monoclonal antibody	Target subsystem	Used for
Abagovomab	gov	Ovarian cancer
Abciximab	ci (circulation)	Antiplatelet
Adalimumab	lim (musculoskeletal)	Rheumatoid arthritis
Basiliximab	li (lower immunity)	Transplantation
Capromab	Pro (prostate)	Prostate cancer
Infliximab	li	Rheumatoid arthritis
Solanezumab	ne (nervous system)	Alzheimer's disease
Rituximab	tu (miscellaneous tumor)	Non-Hodgkin's lymphoma
Panobaccumab	bac (bacterial)	*Pseudomonas aeruginosa* infection

The drugs are:

1. **Specific T-cell inhibitors**
   Cyclosporine, Tacrolimus.
2. **Proliferation signal inhibitors (PSI)**
   Sirolimus; Everolimus
3. **Cytotoxic drugs**
   - Azathioprine
   - Cyclophosphamide
   - Methotrexate
   - Chlorambucil
4. **Mycophenolate mofetil (MMF)**
5. **Glucocorticoids:** Prednisolone, *etc.*
6. **Antibodies (biologics):**
   - Muromonab CD$_3$
   - Antithymocyte globulin (ATG)
   - Rho (D) immunoglobulin

Site of action different Immunosuppressants (Cyclosporin; Tacrolinus; Sirolimus) (Fig. 127.1)

Cyclosporine (Imusporin 25–50 mg cap: sandimmun neoral 100 mg cap): Cyclic polypeptide with 11 amino acids, obtained from fungus is used for organ transplantation. Selectively inhibits T-lymphocyte proliferation, IL-2, cytokine production and response of inducer T-cells to IL-I. More effective when administered before antigen exposure. Suppresses cell mediated immunity and prevents graft rejection, but host defence mechanism to combat bacterial infection is maintained. Free of toxic effects on bone marrow and RE system. Routinely used for renal, bone marrow, hepatic, cardiac transplantation. In emergency, it is given IV dose 10–15 mg/kg/day gradually reduced to 2–6 mg/kg/day given with milk or fruit juice. Available as imusporin. In autoimmune diseases like rheumatoid arthritis, uveitis, bronchial asthma, inflammatory bowel disease, psoriasis, used with corticosteroid or methotrexate in low doses (2–5 mg/kg/day). It enhances nephrotoxicity of other nephrotoxic drugs like aminoglycosides, vancomycin, amphotericin B. Phenytoin, rifampicin and other enzyme inducer may reject graft because they enhance its metabolism. Whereas erythromycin, ketoconazole inhibit its metabolism to cause toxicity. K$^+$ and potassim sparing drugs should be used judiciously to prevent hyperkalemia.

ADR: Rise in BP, diabetes, anorexia, lethargy, gum hyperplasia, seizure may occur.

Tacrolimus: It is 100 times potent to inhibit helper T cells *via* calcineurin. Used IV or orally. Particularly used for liver transplantation as its absorption is not dependent on bile. Oral absorption variable, metabolized by CYP3A4. Hypertension, hirsutism, gum hyperplasia (less than cyclosporine), diabetes, neurotoxicity, alopecia, diarrhea can occur. Dose 0.05–0.1 mg/kg BD orally, available as tacromus 1 and 5 mg caps. (Fig. 127.1)

Sirolimus: It is macrocyclic lactone produced by *Stractomyces hygroscopicus*. It is like cyclosporine, binds immunophylins and inhibits calcineurin. It blocks response of T-cells to cytokine. Orally used either alone or in combination to other immunosuppressants to prevent rejection of solid organ allograft. Sirolimus containing stents used to prevent restenosis.

Everolimus is a derivative of sirolimus decreases rejection in cardiac transplant patient. It is a new drug of this group with shorter $t\frac{1}{2}$. Sirolimus and everolimus are called proliferation signal inhibitors (PSIs).

Pimecrolimus: It is used topically for atopic eczema as 1% ointment. Its mechanism of action is similar to tactolimus.

Azathioprine: It selectively affects differentiations and functioning of T-cells, inhibits cytolytic lymphocytes and decreases cell mediated immunity. Used to prevent renal and other graft rejection, generally combined with cyclosporine to reduce cyclosporine's toxicity. Also used for autoimmune disorders.

Cyclophosphamide: This alkylating agent spupressing humoral more effective in B-cells compared to T-cells. In bone marrow transplantation, a high dose is given. Low doses are given for pemphigus, SLE and ITP, RA, Crohn's disease; multiple sclerosis.

Methotrexate: Used for rheumatoid arthritis, pemphigus, uveitis, chronic active hepatitis, depresses cytokine production and cellular immunity.

Leflunomide: Is a prodrug, inhibits pyrimidine synthesis, orally active with long $t\frac{1}{2}$. Used to treat RA. Liver damage may occur. **Teriflunomide** is active metabolite of leflunomide.

Hydroxychloroquine: Antimalarial with property to suppress immunity used for RA; SLE.

Chlorambucil: It is used for transplant maintenance and autoimmune diseases. Other cytotoxic drugs like vincristine, cytarabine also have immunosuppressive properties. Dactonomycin D is used with some success in renal transplantation.

Pentostatin may be used for steroid resistant graft *vs* host disease after allogenic stem cell transplantation to prevent rejection.

Glucocorticoids: Sequester lymphocytes and decreases cell mediated immunity. Used in high doses to prevent organ rejection with cyclosporine. Used in all cases of autoimmune diseases. Long-term complications are its limitations.

Mycophenolate mofetil: Obtained from *Penicillium glaucus*. It inhibits lymphocyte proliferation, antibody prodution and cell mediated immunity, better to azathioprine, reduces requirement of cyclosporine. Vomiting and diarrhea may occur. Used as add-on drug to cyclosporine + glucocorticoids in renal transplant. Also used to treat vasculopathy after cardiac implant, stem cell transplant.

Thalidomide: It has anti-inflammatory, immunomodulation and it is an inhibitor of angiogenesis. It inhibits TNFα, and phagocytosis. Used in multiple myeloma; erythema nodosum leprosum. Immunomodulating derivative of thalidomide is called IMIDs like **Linalidomide**.

Pomalidomide is new FDA approved IMiD trialed for relapsed or refractory multiple myeloma.

CC4047 (Actimid) is IMID at investigational level for myelodysplastic syndrome, myeloma, Ca-prostate. Selective cytokines inhibitory drugs SelCIDs are phosphodiesterase-4 inhibitor with anti-TNFα activity are in investigational level.

IMMUNOSUPPRESSANT ANTIBODIES

Monoclonal and Polyclonal Antibodies

Monoclonal antibodies are produced by hydridoma technique by single clone of B cells. Kohlar and Milstein awarded nobel prize for medicine in 1987. They are nonspecific and homogeous used for diagnostic and therapeutic purposes. They specifically block target antigen's function directed against T-lymphocyte, B-lymphocyte, TNF, interleukin. It can be conjugated with chemotherapeutic agent, toxin, radioisotopes. (Radio lebeled anti CD20 *viz* ttrium ibritumomab used for NHL) and can be used as therapeutic agent. They are also used: (i) As immuno-suppressant, (ii) to treat auto-immune diseases, (iii) as antiplatelet, (iv) to treat cancer, (v) to treat viral diseases and (vi) for diagnosis.

The first generations monoclonal antibodies are murine so they produce immune response in majority of recipient with short half-life. These problems are surmounted by chimeric or humanised monoclonal antibody. It contains murine Fab domain and human Fc domain in chimeric or changing both in human.

Nomenclature of monoclonal antibodies: It has got a suffix of mab; prefix varies for different monoclonal antibodies other parts are target subsystem and origin subsystem (*viz.* 'u' for human, 'xi' for chimeric, 'zu' for humanized, *etc.*

Muromonab CD$_3$: Murine monoclonal antibody against CD$_3$ glycoprotein, located near T-cell receptor, postponed nephro- and hepatotoxicities of cycloserine. Aseptic meningitis, intragraft thrombosis, seizure, shock like state, pulmonary edema may occur. High dose corticosteroid reduces reaction. Initial doses release cytokine presented as flu.

Antithymocyte Globulin (ATG): Polyclonal antibody purified from horse and other animals immunized with human thymic lymphocyte. Depletes T-lymphocytes. Used to prevent allograft rejection. May produce serum sickness and anaphylaxis. Cheaper than muromonab CD$_3$. Thymoglobulin (rabbit) 25 mg/vial 1.5 mg/kg/day IV; ATG 100 mg inj. 200 mg/day IV; Lymphoglobulin (equine) 100 mg/vial, dose 10 mg/kg/day IV.

Anti-D immunoglobulin (Rhiggal 250–300 mg IM): It should be used within 72 hours of delivery and abortion. It is IgG having high titer of antibodies against Rh D. Should not be given to infant or Rh +ve patient. Higher dose of 1000–2000 mg given for Rh –ve received inadvertently Rh +ve blood.

TOLERANCE

Immunosuppression has risk of flairing opportunistic infection and secondary tumor, so ultimate goal in organ transplantation or auto-immune disease is to provide antigen-antibody non-responsiveness or tolerance for true care of this conditions.

IMMUNOSTIMULANTS

Enhances immunological response non-specifically, drugs like amantidine, tilorane stimulate humoral immune system. Tetramisole (levamisole) has immunotropic properties. They augment cutaneous delayed hypersensitivity reactions in anergic state. BCG is non-specific stimulant of immunity, used with conventional therapy in treatment of leukemia, melanoma, lung carcinoma. Clofazimine augments phagocytic activity of macrophages.

Antihelmintic levamisole, thalidomide, lenalidomide also modulate immunity.

Immunoglobulin intravenous (IGIV): 2 mg/kg used for immunoglobulin deficiencies like HIV desease, bone marrow transplant, Kawasaki's disease, SLE, refractory ITP. Mechanism: Possibly reduction of T-helper cells, increasing suppressor T-cells and reduction of spontaneous immunoglobulin production and increases antibody catabolism.

Hyperimmune globulin: This is pooled from human and animal donors with high titer of antibody against virus or toxins. Used to treat respiratory syncytials virus or cytomegalovirus, Varicella zoster virus, Herpes virus, hepatitis B, rabies, tetanus digoxin overdose. It is passive transfer of antibodies.

Cytokines like interferon, various interleukins, colony stimulating factor (CSF): Recombinant IL-2 like Aldesleukin used to treat malignant melanoma and renal carcinoma. Filgrastim and sargramostim, recombinant G-CSF and CM-CSF respectively used for chemotherapy-induced myelosuppression. Imiquimod used for genital wart is an immunoresponse modifier.

128

Gene Therapy

Gene therapy is a new approach to treat a disease, but a number of technological, toxicological and ethical problems has to be solved before its widespread use. Only somatic gene therapy by inserting new gene in somatic cell is under trial. Germ cell gene therapy is unethical. Permission for gene therapy is required before it is started. The gene which is transferred is called transgene. Gene may be delevered by *in vivo* or *ex vivo* approach. In *in vivo* it is delivered by either intravenously or directly into tissue of targets. In *ex vivo* the cell is removed from body (*viz.* stem cells from marrows, it is treated out side with vector and genetically altered cell is back into patient). For choosing gene delivery system following things are to be taken into consideration. (i) capacity of how much DNA it can carry, (ii) transinfection capactiy, (iii) life time of transinfected material and (iv) safety issue specialy if virus borne transinfection is taken into consideration. Following are the diseases where gene therapy may be of help.

- Cystic fibrosis: Cystic fibrosis transport regulator gene is inserted in respiratory epithelial cells which regulate expression of an apical chloride channel.

- Growth hormone deficiency cultured myoblast with growth hormone gene is implanted.

- LDL receptor gene is implanted in liver in familial hypercholesterolemia.

- Hypoxanthine phosphoribosyl transferase gene

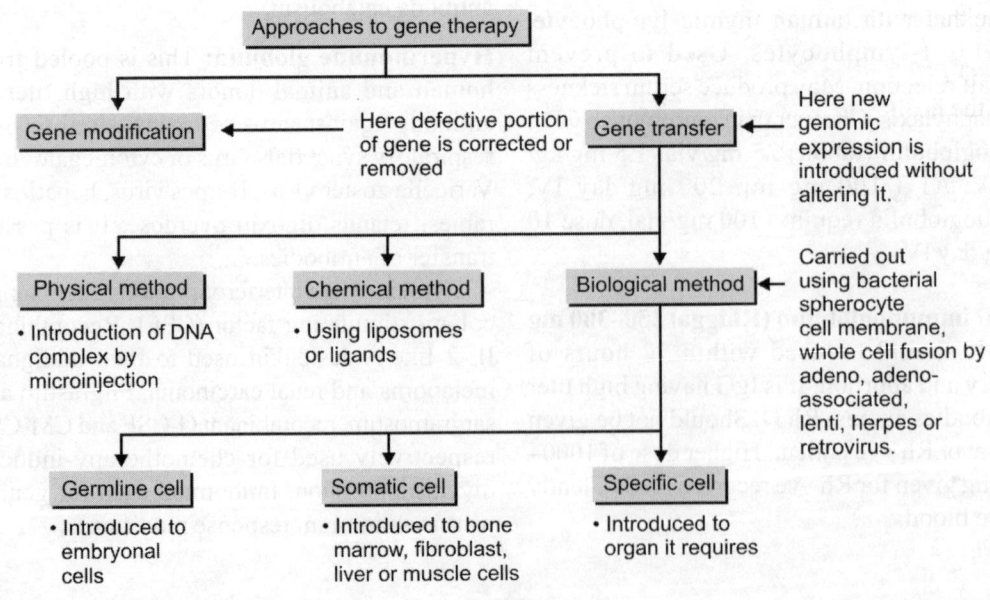

```
                    ┌─────────────────────────────────┐
                    │   Approaches to gene therapy    │
                    └─────────────────────────────────┘

  ┌────────────────────┐   Here defective portion    ┌──────────────┐   Here new
  │ Gene modification  │◄── of gene is corrected or   │ Gene transfer│── genomic
  └────────────────────┘   removed                    └──────────────┘   expression is
                                                                         introduced without
                                                                         altering it.

  ┌─────────────────┐   ┌─────────────────┐   ┌──────────────────┐   Carried out
  │ Physical method │   │ Chemical method │   │ Biological method│◄── using bacterial
  └─────────────────┘   └─────────────────┘   └──────────────────┘   spherocyte
  • Introduction of DNA  • Using liposomes                           cell membrane,
    complex by             or ligands                                whole cell fusion by
    microinjection                                                   adeno, adeno-
                                                                     associated,
                                                                     lenti, herpes or
                                                                     retrovirus.

  ┌─────────────────┐   ┌─────────────────┐   ┌──────────────────┐
  │  Germline cell  │   │  Somatic cell   │   │  Specific cell   │
  └─────────────────┘   └─────────────────┘   └──────────────────┘
  • Introduced to        • Introduced to bone      • Introduced to
    embryonal              marrow, fibroblast,        organ it requires
    cells                  liver or muscle cells
```

is introduced to correct enzyme deficiency in CNS producing neuropsychiatric disorder.

- Gene for tyrosine hydroxylase produces dopamine in basal ganglion in parkinsonism.
- Genes are supplemented to rectify Alzheimer's disease, Huntington's chorea, lateral sclerosis.
- Nerve growth factor gene is implanted in stroke and multiple sclerosis.
- Muscle dystropin gene is administered in Duchenne muscular dystrophy.
- Cancer cells can be selectively killed by genetic therapy and their resistance to chemotherapy can be rectified.
- Human tissue kallikrein genes may by introduced in hypertension.
- In anemia myoblast mediated human erythro-poietin gene can be introduced.
- Genes can be of help to prevent restenosis, introducing genes which inhibit growth of intimal cells.
- Insulin dependent diabetes may be treated by gene producing insulin.
- Hemophilia by introducing factor VIII gene.

Malaria: With vaccine produced by gene alteration.

AIDS by injecting fibroblast expressing HIV envelope glycoprotein gene to augment immunity against HIV.

Gene therapy is only at research level.

Summary procedures

Isolate the healthy gene with its sequence.

Introduce it in carrier vector as cassette for expression and delivery of the vector to the target.

Different types of vector or carrier for gene delivery are viruses (retro, adeno), liposomes, plasmids and physical methods.

New genomic expression as introduced without altering it is carried out by using:

- Bacterial spherocytes
- Erythrocyte cell membrane
- Whole cell fusion by adeno, adeno-associotied Lenti virus, Herpes virus or retrovirus.

Gene therapy may be done *ex vivo, i.e.* tissue cells are isolated and transfected with vector carrying relevant gene which is injected back in patient or *in vivo* where viruses carrying gene injected systematically another promising approach is to block expression of defective gene by antisense oligonucleotides, *viz.* Fomivirsen is antisense oligonucleotide to treat cyto-megalovirus (CMV) and retinitis.

Complications of gene therapy

- Gene silencing, *i.e.* repression of the promoters.
- Genotoxicity, *i.e.* insertional mutagenesis.
- Phenotoxicity, *i.e.* overexpression or ectopic expression of transgene.
- Immunotoxicity to vector or transgene
- Horizontal transmission, *i.e.* infectious vector transferred to the environment.
- Vertical transmission, *i.e.* germline trans-mission of donated DNA.

Drug Schedules

The drugs are sold under Controlled Substance Act (CSA) of the USA are grouped according to potential abuse. According to USP and National formulary, different schedules are given in Table 129.1.

According to Drugs and Cosmetic Act 2001 (10th amendment of India), the different schedules are as follows:

Schedule A	Specimens of prescribed forms
Schedule B	States for drug analysis by Govt. analyzer
Schedule C	Biological products
Schedule D	Exemption from import of drugs
Schedule E	Poisonous substances of Ayurveda
Schedule F	Standard of bacterial vaccines
Schedule FF	Standard of ophthalmic preparation
Schedule F (II)	Standard of surgical dressing
Schedule F (III)	Standard of umbilical tapes
Schedule G	Detailed of drugs leveled with caution
Schedule H	Must be prescribed by registered medical practitioner
Schedule J	List of ailments for which no drug should be claimed for cure
Schedule M	Good manufacturing practices
Schedule M (I)	Factory requirement for manufacturing homeopathic drugs
Schedule M (II)	Factory requirement to produce cosmetics
Schedule M (III)	Factory requirement to produce medical devices
Schedule N	Minimum equipment of pharmacy
Schedule O	Provision applicable to disinfect fluids
Schedule P	Life period of drug
Schedule P (I)	Packing size of drug
Schedule R	Standard of medical contraceptive
Schedule RI	Standard of medical devices
Schedule S	Standard of cosmetics
Schedule T	Requirement of factory for Ayurvedic drugs
Schedules U and U (I)	Manufacturing records
Schedule V	Standard of patent and proprietary drugs
Schedule W	Drugs sold by generic name only
Schedule X	Psychotropic drugs with special license for manufacturing and sold
Schedule Y	Guidelines for clinical trials.

Table 129.1: USP schedules				
Schedule I	*Schedule II*	*Schedule III*	*Schedule IV*	*Schedule V*
With high potential of abuse, *viz.* LSD; heroin	High potential of abuse and physical and psychic dependent potential, *viz.* morphine phenobarbitone	Accepted medical use with restriction, *viz.* chlorphenaramine	Low abuse potential can be refilled for six months, *viz.* benzodiazepines	Minimal abuse and dependence, *viz.* locomotin of OTC drug

Total Parenteral Nutrition

Parenteral nutrition is feeding a person intravenously bypassing usual process of eating and digestion. It is given by a catheter placed in a vein. It supplies all nutritional requirement, may be used in hospital or home. It is used to promote positive nitrogen balance and growth of children.

Indications

i. Complete bowel rest to heal bowel lesion.

ii. Preoperative support

iii. Adjunct to cancer chemo and / or radiation therapy.

Composition

Calorie: As 20–25% dextrose through central vein with water 40ml/kg/day.

Protein: As synthetic amino acid (8–9%) as 200 ml bottle for IV use. The calorie provided by amino acids are not taken into calculation but used as a source of protein. It also prevents fatty infiltrations of liver. Albumin as 10–25 gm/day given to those who loose protein on exudates. Anemia rectified by blood transfusion.

Fats: Safflower oil 10–20% and soya bean oil 10–20% mixed in glycrol with emulsifying agent is given 1V 10%. Supplies caloric 1.1 caloric / ml. Linolenic acid is also added. Weekly 500–1000 ml is required to prevent deficiency syndrome. It is given by peripheral veins. Nothing should be added in fat emulsion.

Technique

Base solution is prepared daily with dextrose and amino acid, to it vitamins and mineral are added.

A 20% solution providing 3.4 Kcal / gram as dextrose (it is not anhydrous). It is hypertonic solution so should be given by central vein in a rate of 5-7 ml/kg/min. Add insulin 10 IU / 250 gm of dextrose to prevent hyperglycemia. Heparin may prevent fibrin plugging.

S.No.	Item	Dose
1.	Zinc	3–4 mg/day
2.	Copper	0.5–1.5 mg/day
3.	Iodine	75–150 mcg/day
4.	Manganese	0.15–0.8 mg/day
5.	Chromium	10–15 mcg/day
6.	Selenium	50–200 mcg/day
7.	Thiamine	3 mg/day
8.	Riboflavin	3 mg/day
9.	Pantothenic acid	15 mg/day
10.	Pyridoxine	4 mg/day
11.	Niacin	40 mg/day
12.	Biotin	60 mg/day
13.	B_{12}	5 mcg/day
14.	Folic acid	400 mcg/day
15.	Vitamin C	100 mg
16.	Vitamine A	3300 IU per week

Start at 1 litre and increase by ½ to 1 litre / day if patient can to tolerate. It is given in 18 hours and in rest 6 hours patient gets 5% dextrose to prevent rebound hypoglycemia. When TPN is withdrawn glucose infusion should be tapered gradually.

Complications of TPN

Azotemia, Hyperglycemia and rebound hypoglycemia on cessation, liver dysfunction, sepsis, allergy, metabolic bone disorders.

A patient on TPN should be strictly monitiored with intake – output chart, weighing, signs of fluid overload, sepsis, blood glucose. Creatinine. Na, K, Ca, Mg, P estimation, liver function test (bilirubin, SGPT), Mg, P estimation, liver function test (bilirubin, SGPT every 3–4 days).

Improvement Sign

- 1.5 kg weight/week weight gain
- Improvement of muscle strength.
- Plasma albumin, transferrin level improvement
- Growth normalization in children.

Index